Concepts of Physical Fitness

Active Lifestyles for Wellness

SEVENTEENTH EDITION

Charles B. Corbin

Arizona State University

Gregory J. Welk

Iowa State University

William R. Corbin

Arizona State University

Karen A. Welk

Mary Greeley Medical Center, Ames, Iowa

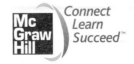
Connect
Learn
Succeed™

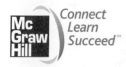

CONCEPTS OF PHYSICAL FITNESS: ACTIVE LIFESTYLES FOR WELLNESS,
SEVENTEENTH EDITION

Published by McGraw-Hill, a business unit of The McGraw-Hill Companies, Inc., 1221 Avenue of the
Americas, New York, NY, 10020. Copyright © 2013 by The McGraw-Hill Companies, Inc. All rights
reserved. Printed in the United States of America. Previous editions © 2011, 2009, 2008, 2006, 2005,
2003, 2000, 1997, 1994, 1991, 1988, 1985, 1981,1978, 1974 and 1970. No part of this publication may be
reproduced or distributed in any form or by any means, or stored in a database or retrieval system, without
the prior written consent of The McGraw-Hill Companies, Inc., including, but not limited to, in any network or other electronic storage or transmission, or broadcast for distance learning.

Some ancillaries, including electronic and print components, may not be available to customers outside
the United States.

This book is printed on acid-free paper.

1 2 3 4 5 6 7 8 9 0 DOW/DOW 1 0 9 8 7 6 5 4 3 2

ISBN 978-0-07-131860-0
MHID 0-07-131860-7

Cover Image: © Brand X Pictures/PunchStock

All credits appearing at the end of the book are considered to be an extension of the copyright page.

The Internet addresses listed in the text were accurate at the time of publication. The inclusion of a
website does not indicate an endorsement by the authors or McGraw-Hill, and McGraw-Hill does not
guarantee the accuracy of the information presented at these sites.

Brief Contents

Contents

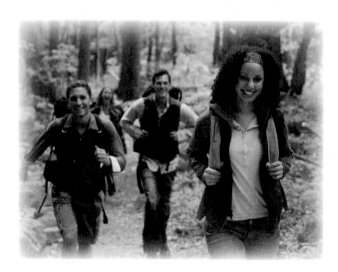

Section IV

Physical Activity: Special Considerations   225

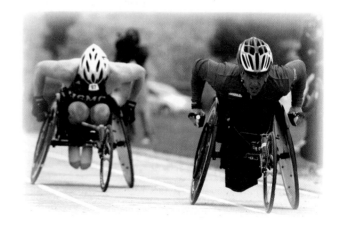

Section V

Nutrition and Body Composition   289

Section VI

Stress Management   367

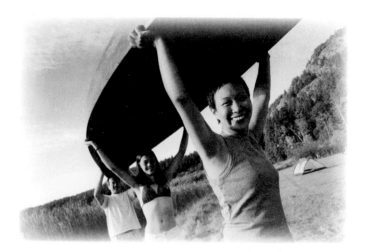

Features

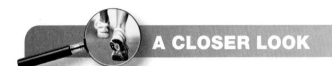
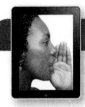

Lab Activities

All end-of-concept Lab Activities are available in *Connect* and can be edited, assigned, completed, submitted, and graded online. Students simply upload completed labs to their instructor.

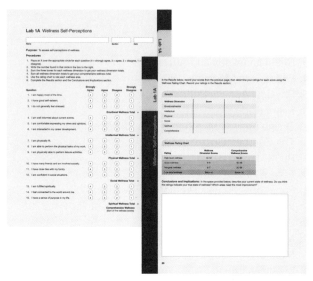

HELP is here!

A proven philosophy for **achieving** health, wellness, and physical fitness

"Health is available to Everyone for a Lifetime, and it's Personal."

A proven approach for **teaching** fitness and wellness

Concise content modules—based on sound learning objectives—highlight key concepts and promote active lifestyles.

With *Connect Fitness and Wellness*

A powerful online, interactive set of tools for learning and behavior change.

A winning combination!

The goal of our program—summarized in the "HELP" philosophy stated above—is to help all people make personal lifestyle changes that promote health, fitness, and wellness over a lifetime. Organized into concise concepts that make it easy for students to learn, *Concepts of Physical Fitness* is integrated with online activities and assessments that enable students to apply the latest research on fitness and wellness to their own lives.

HELP: A proven philosophy for **achieving** lifetime fitness and wellness . . .
"Health is available to Everyone for a Lifetime, and it's Personal"

LEARNING OBJECTIVES

After completing the study of this concept, you will be able to:

▶ Describe the HELP philosophy and discuss its implications in making personal decisions about health, wellness, and fitness.

▶ Define the dimensions of health and wellness, and explain how they interact to influence health and wellness.

▶ Distinguish health-related and skill-related dimensions of physical fitness.

▶ Identify the determinants of health, wellness, and fitness, and explain how they each contribute to health, wellness, and fitness.

▶ Identify related national health goals and show how meeting personal goals can contribute to reaching national goals.

▶ Use health behavior change strategies to carry out self-assessments of personal lifestyles and wellness perceptions.

• Concise modules called "concepts" give instructors flexibility and students a manageable framework for learning and mastering course content. New learning objectives introduce each concept, guiding students on key points and how to assess their progress.

 HELP   **Health is available to Everyone for a Lifetime, and it's Personal**

According to the National Institutes of Health, although genes do not necessarily cause diseases, they do influence our risk of developing diseases, such as cancer, heart disease, and addiction. The interaction between our genes and our environments and experiences is a complex one that is still being studied.

Would knowing you were genetically predisposed to a particular disease change the lifestyle decisions you make?

connect ACTIVITY

• **HELP** activities encourage students to reflect, think critically, and apply the HELP philosophy to their lives.

A CLOSER LOOK

Blue Zones

For his book *Blue Zones*, Dan Buettner researched communities across the world that had higher life expectancies and quality of life than other communities. He identified their common characteristics to try to determine the underlying factors that influence good health. He referred to these communities as "Blue Zones" and came up with nine specific attributes that contributed to the improved health. It is not surprising that physical activity (labeled as "Move Naturally") was at the top of the list. (To see the complete list of principles, visit www.bluezones.com.) Some public health groups and agencies have sought to promote broad application of these principles as the basis for coordinated community health programming. The book, in this case, can be viewed as a guide or recipe for healthy communities. However, it may also be likened to a fad diet that might promise an easy path to health and wellness.

Is it possible for communities to follow these recommendations as part of building a healthy community? Why or why not?

connect ACTIVITY

• The new **A Closer Look** feature focuses on recent and sometimes controversial topics. Additional features include **Technology Update** (advances in technology), **In the News** (late-breaking fitness and wellness information), and **HP 2020** (highlights of the Healthy People 2020 national health goals). New follow-up, critical-thinking questions spur class discussion and personal reflection and are assignable within *Connect*.

Table 10 Exercises for Core Strength   **connect** VIDEO 9

1. Crunch (Curl-Up)

This exercise develops the upper abdominal muscles. Lie on the floor with the knees bent and the arms extended or crossed with hands on shoulders or palms on ears. If desired, legs may rest on bench to increase difficulty. For less resistance, place hands at side of body (do not put hands behind neck). For more resistance, move hands higher. Curl up until shoulder blades leave floor; then roll down to the starting position. Repeat. Note: Twisting the trunk on the curl-up develops the oblique abdominals.

Rectus abdominis
Transversus abdominis
Internal oblique (cut)
External oblique (cut)

3. Crunch with Twist (on Bench)

This exercise strengthens the oblique abdominals and helps prevent or correct lumbar lordosis, abdominal ptosis, and backache. Lie on your back with your feet on a bench, knees bent at 90 degrees. Arms may be extended or on shoulders or hand on ears (the most difficult). Same as crunch except twist the upper trunk so the right shoulder is higher than the left. Reach toward the left knee with the right elbow. Hold. Return and repeat to the opposite side.

Internal oblique
External oblique

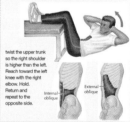

• Detailed, updated illustrations show students exactly how to perform strength training and flexibility exercises, and the core muscles they are improving.

A proven approach for **teaching** behavior change for health, fitness, and wellness

Connect Fitness and Wellness gives students the tools needed to think critically about lifestyle changes and the behavioral skills needed to adopt and maintain healthy lifestyles.

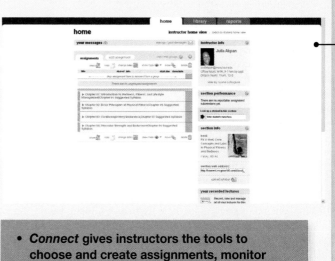

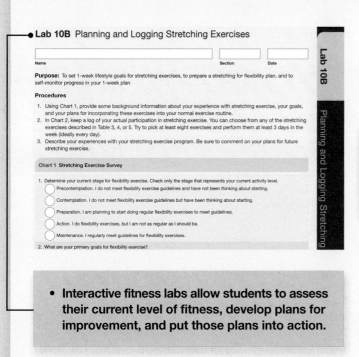

- *Connect* gives instructors the tools to choose and create assignments, monitor student progress, and manage their course more easily and efficiently.

- Interactive fitness labs allow students to assess their current level of fitness, develop plans for improvement, and put those plans into action.

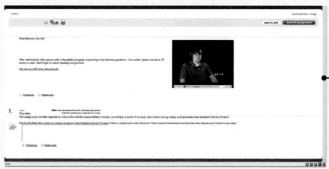

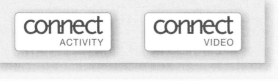

- *Connect* icons link text to additional online assignments and video activities.

- New video clips and video activities engage students, make the concepts relevant, and inspire them to change.

Highlights of the Seventeenth Edition

The seventeenth edition of *Concepts of Physical Fitness* is designed to deliver an integrated print and digital program that continues to be at the cutting edge of physical activity and health promotion, empowering students to take positive steps toward developing a lifelong commitment to healthy and active living. With its hallmark modular approach called "concepts," the new edition has been thoroughly updated and offers several new features designed to enhance student learning.

Extensive revisions to the content in *Connect* add new and exciting materials for easy use by students and instructors. A variety of updated and expanded *Connect* video activities help explain complex issues and provide opportunities for personal reflection and critical thinking. New *Connect* icons 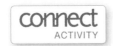 throughout the text guide students to these and additional online assignments that help students apply the material.

Significant revisions have been made in the content to reflect new health guidelines and recommendations. A revised **physical activity pyramid** provides a unique, useful model to help students understand and apply new physical activity guidelines.

Revised concept opener pages now include **learning objectives** that guide student learning and assessment. Each concept also includes an updated **Strategies for Action** section designed to help students use the lab activities to effect personal behavior change.

Each concept also includes a variety of timely features with supplemental content. One new feature, **A Closer Look,** provides information about new and sometimes controversial information related to fitness, health, and wellness. Another, called **HP 2020,** helps students see relationships between their behaviors and broader national health goals. Other updated features in each concept include **Technology Update** (describes advances in health and fitness technology), **In the News** (highlights late-breaking fitness, health, and wellness information), and **HELP** (provides tips to show students how to *help* themselves). Follow-up questions are assignable in *Connect,* helping students develop self-management, critical thinking, and reflection skills and motivating them to apply concepts of fitness, health, and wellness in their own lives.

Key **Web Resources** at the end of each concept provide students with additional online resources that supplement the content just learned. For students who want to know more about a particular topic, a list of **Suggested Readings** is given at the end of each concept.

A detailed summary of new and updated concept-by-concept content follows:

1   Health, Wellness, Fitness, and Healthy Lifestyles: An Introduction
- Reorganized to highlight HELP philosophy
- New information and statistics about Healthy People 2020
- Updated statistics about health and wellness
- Revised model of health, fitness, and wellness

2   Self-Management and Self-Planning Skills for Health Behavior Change
- New content on social-ecological models of health and wellness
- Expanded content on SMART goals
- Specific goal-setting guidelines for people with different levels of experience
- New discussion of "Blue Zones" and characteristics of healthier environments

3   Preparing for Physical Activity
- Updated content on warm-up and stretching guidelines
- Revised CPR guidelines
- Clarification of the distinctions between dynamic and sport-specific warm-ups
- New discussion of "minimalist" running shoes

4   The Health Benefits of Physical Activity
- Revised information about hypokinetic diseases
- Updated information on links between inactivity and metabolic syndrome
- Updates on the *Exercise is Medicine* campaign

5   How Much Physical Activity Is Enough?
- Updated descriptions of exercise training principles
- Revised content on FITT model and applications for exercise prescription
- Updated model of the physical activity pyramid with revised guidelines
- New content on sedentary behavior and independent risks from inactivity

6   Moderate Physical Activity: A Lifestyle Approach
- Clarification on concept of METS and Met-Minutes
- New definitions for vigorous activity and sedentary activity
- New information on health benefits of moderate activity and metabolic fitness
- New content about the built environment and walkability

7   Cardiovascular Fitness
- New content on ACSM fitness guidelines (Frequency–Intensity–Time)
- Revised information on target heart rate calculations and heart rate zones
- Updated content on the benefits of vigorous exercise

8   Vigorous Aerobics, Sports, and Recreational Activities
- Revised presentation of aerobic exercises
- New content on patterns and trends in aerobic exercise, sport, and recreation
- New information on types (and popularity) of group exercises (e.g., Zumba®)
- Expanded content on vigorous recreation and extreme sports

9   Muscle Fitness and Resistance Exercise
- New information about power as a health-related fitness dimension
- New sections on functional fitness and core strength
- New depictions of isometric, isokinetic, and isotonic exercise
- Revised resistance training guidelines
- New graphics and revised content on periodization
- New discussion of the popularity of the P90X fitness program

10   Flexibility
- Expanded content on flexibility fundamentals and importance for health
- Clarification on factors influencing flexibility

- Importance of flexibility for functional fitness
- New content on dynamic stretching (and distinctions from ballistic stretching)
- Revised stretching guidelines

11 Body Mechanics: Posture, Questionable Exercises, and Care of the Back and Neck
- New content on causes of back pain
- Updated information on (and explanations of) microtrauma
- Strategies for correcting postural deviations
- Revised discussion on implications of poor posture
- Enhanced conceptual graphics depicting good posture and good body mechanics

12 Performance Benefits of Physical Activity
- New content on high intensity interval training (HIIT)
- New information on the importance of functional fitness for sports training
- Expanded content and models on periodization

13 Body Composition
- Revised statistics about the prevalence of obesity
- Updated information about links between obesity and health
- Revised content about basal metabolic rate and creeping obesity

14 Nutrition
- New content on MyPlate and applications for diet education
- Updated information on the dietary guidelines and strategies for implementation
- Revised content on trans fat guidelines and fat substitutes
- New content on omega 3 fatty acids, soy, and antioxidants
- New legislation on vending machines and nutritional information requirements

15 Managing Diet and Activity for Healthy Body Fatness
- New conceptual model on energy balance
- Updated information on contributions of light activity to weight control
- New content on "emotional eating" and "mindless eating"

- New model of obesogenic environments and strategies for healthy eating
- New information about public/private partnerships for obesity prevention

16 Stress and Health
- Updated figure depicting stressors and reactions to stress
- New content on discrimination experiences as a source of stress
- Updated information on individualized differences in the stress response

17 Stress Management, Relaxation, and Time Management
- Updated information about mental health benefits of physical activity
- New content and image on time use and implications for stress management
- New content on effective coping strategies
- Clarification between appraisal-focused and emotion-focused coping

18 Evaluating Fitness and Wellness Products: Becoming an Informed Consumer
- New content on nutrition quackery
- Updated information about efforts to combat fraud and quackery
- Discussion of issues with labeling of "herbal" and "natural" supplements
- New content on health literacy
- Recent rulings on exaggerated health claims on fitness shoes
- New discussion of titanium necklaces

19 Toward Optimal Health and Wellness: Planning for Healthy Lifestyle Change
- Reorganized content on factors influencing health and wellness
- Expanded content on inherited risks and using the health-care system
- New content on the impact of environmental factors (including new table)
- Guidelines for adopting healthy lifestyles

Teaching and Learning with *Concepts*

Concepts in Loose-Leaf Format

McGraw-Hill has done a considerable amount of research with college students, not only asking them questions about how they study and use course materials, but also using ethnographic research tools to observe how they study. During the course of this research, students told us they want books and online learning systems that are:

- Light and easy to carry
- Engaging and relevant to their own lives
- Inexpensive
- Supported by digital activities that help them learn and succeed in their course

Based on what we heard from students, we are introducing *Concepts* in a *three-hole punched, loose-leaf* format that is portable, flexible, and cost effective. *Concepts* in loose-leaf format offers these advantages:

- Students will need to carry only the portion of the book that's being covered in class with them.
- In addition to the print version of the book, students will receive an integrated, multimedia eBook, including videos and links to other resources.

Would you still like your students to have a bound book? You will be able to order one through our *Create* system. While you're at it, we can pull out any of the chapters of the book you don't assign. This ensures that students are purchasing only the content that is being assigned to them, making the book 100 percent relevant to your course, more affordable for students, lightweight, and portable.

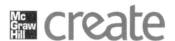

Create, because Customization Matters

Design your ideal course materials with McGraw-Hill's *Create* at **www.mcgrawhillcreate.com**! Rearrange or omit chapters, combine material from other sources, and/or upload your syllabus or any other content you have written to make the perfect resource for your students. Search thousands of leading McGraw-Hill textbooks to find the best content for your students, then arrange it to fit your teaching style. You can even personalize your book's appearance by selecting the cover and adding your name, school, and course information. When you order a *Create* book, you receive a complimentary review copy. Get a printed copy in 3 to 5 business days or an electronic copy (eComp) via email in about an hour.

> Register today at **www.mcgrawhillcreate.com** and craft your course resources to match the way you teach.

CourseSmart

CourseSmart is the world's largest provider of digital course materials. Our catalog includes over 90 percent of the core textbooks in use today in North American higher education as eTextbooks, as well as the largest online catalog of eResources and digital course materials available for instant access. CourseSmart's comprehensive selection gives students, faculty, partners, and institutions a new way to find and access eTextbooks and digital course material in one place. Visit **www.CourseSmart.com** to learn more and to try a sample chapter.

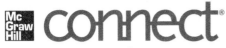 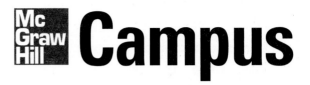

Connect Fitness and Wellness

Connect Fitness and Wellness gives students access to a wealth of interactive online content, including fitness labs and self-assessments, video activities, practice quizzes, and other assignable activities based on the book content. With *Connect*, instructors can easily assign pre-built activities, create and edit assignments, produce video lectures, upload their own articles or videos, cascade assignments, and produce reports for their course sections. All *Connect* content can be accessed directly from within any course management system—all with a single sign-on. *Connect* assignments automatically and instantly feed grades directly to the course management system grade center, and students can access all of their assignments through one homepage. Additionally, the media-rich eBook contains embedded video clips, full-color images, links to discipline specific sites, key terms and definitions, and behavior change tools.

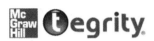

Tegrity Campus

Tegrity Campus is a fully automated, cloud-based lecture-capture solution used in traditional, hybrid, and online courses to record lectures and/or supplementary course content. It's incredibly easy to use, as instructors simply click a button to start the recording, and click another to stop it. From there, the content is uploaded instantly to the Tegrity Cloud, where students are able to access it anytime and anywhere on just about any device. Tegrity's personalized learning features make study time incredibly efficient and more than 7 out of 10 students say the use of Tegrity improved their grades. To learn more about Tegrity, watch a 2-minute Flash demo at **http://tegritycampus.mhhe.com**.

McGraw-Hill Campus™

McGraw-Hill Campus™ is a one-stop teaching and learning experience available to users of any learning management system. This institutional service allows faculty and students to enjoy single sign-on (SSO) access to all McGraw-Hill Higher Education materials, including the award-winning McGraw-Hill *Connect*™ platform, from directly within the institution's website. McGraw-Hill Campus™ provides faculty with instant access to all McGraw-Hill Higher Education teaching materials (e.g., eTextbooks, test banks, PowerPoint slides, animations and learning objects), allowing them to browse, search, and use any instructor ancillary content in our vast library at no additional cost to instructors or students. Students enjoy SSO access to a variety of free products (e.g., quizzes, flash cards, narrated presentations) as well as subscription-based products (e.g., McGraw-Hill *Connect*™). With this program enabled, faculty and students never need to create another account to access McGraw-Hill products and services.

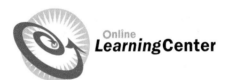

Online Learning Center

The *Concepts of Physical Fitness* Online Learning Center (www.mhhe.com/corbin17e) provides easy access to a variety of resources for instructors:

- PowerPoint presentations
- Instructor's manual
- Test bank
- Image bank

Thank You

Two words that can never be said enough to the many people who have helped the *Concepts* books to be successful, including the thousands of instructors and students who have taught and learned from these books for more than 45 years. We are proud that the *Concepts* books were among the first ever published for use in college fitness and wellness courses; that the *Surgeon General's Report on Physical Activity and Health* adopted definitions from the book; and that instructors have continued to select the *Concepts* books for use in their courses for more than 4 decades.

We listen to those who review our books and to our users, who provide comments by mail, phone, personal conversations, and email. Comments and critiques help us make our books better for both students and instructors. The list of people who have helped us over the years is now nearly two pages long. But we feel that the pages that allow us to acknowledge those who have helped us are well worth it. At the risk of inadvertently failing to mention someone, we want to acknowledge the following people for their role in the development of this book.

First, we would like to acknowledge a few people who have made special contributions over the years. Linus Dowell, Carl Landiss, and Homer Tolson, all of Texas A & M University, were involved in the development of the first *Concepts* book in 1968.

Other pioneers were Jimmy Jones of Henderson State University, who started one of the first *Concepts* classes in 1970 and has led the way in teaching fitness in the years that have followed; Charles Erickson, who started a quality program at Missouri Western; and Al Lesiter, a leader in the East at Mercer Community College in New Jersey. David Laurie and Barbara Gench at Kansas State University, as well as others on that faculty, were instrumental in developing a prototype concepts program, which research has shown to be successful.

A special thanks is extended to Andy Herrick and Jim Whitehead, who have contributed to much of the development of various editions of the book, including excellent suggestions for change. Mark Ahn, Keri Chesney, Chris MacCrate, Guy Mullins, Stephen Hustedde, Greg Nigh, Doreen Mauro, Marc vanHorne, Ken Rudich, and Fred Huff, along with other current or former employees of the

Applied Learning Technologies Institute and the University Technology Office, deserve special recognition.

We would like to thank the following reviewers (in alphabetical order), whose comments and suggestions were helpful in making this edition as complete as possible: Brent Alvar, Chandler-Gilbert Community College; Steve Ball, University of Missouri-Columbia; Michael Bemben, University of Oklahoma-Norman; Cherilyn Cox, Northeast Lakeview College; Jason Crandall, Kentucky Wesleyan College; Carol Lynn Fieser, Tarrant County College; Raymond Gibson, Atlantic Cape Community College; Ken Holliday, Southern State Community College; Katie Hubbard, Lansing Community College; Michelle Ihmels, Iowa State University; Patricia Ochoa, Chattanooga State Community College; Lynn Pantuosco-Hensch, Westfield State University; William Papin, Western Carolina University; Daniel Mark Persson, Southwestern Oklahoma State University; H. Kyle Ryan, Peru State College; Jennifer Spry-Knutson, Des Moines Area Community College-Boone; Sheila Stepp, State University of New York-Orange; Jeffrey Walkuski, State University of New York-Cortland; and Jeffrey Willardson, Eastern Illinois University.

In addition, we want to acknowledge the following: Kelly Adam, Nena Amundson, James Angel, Vincent Angotti, Candi D. Ashley, Jeanne Ashley, Debra Atkinson, Kym Y. Atwood, Mark Bailey, Diane Bartholomew, Carl Beal, Debra A. Beal, Roger Bishop, Eugene B. Blackwell, Ann Bolton, Laura L. Borsdorf, Marika Botha, Amy Bowersock, David S. Brewster, Stanley Brown, Joseph W. Bubenas, Kenneth L. Cameron, Ronnie Carda, Bill Carr, Curt W. Cattau, Robert Clayton, Bridget Cobb, Ruth Cohoon, Sarah Collie, P. Greg Comfort, Cindy Ekstedt Connelly, Karen Cookson, Betsy Danner, J. Jesse DeMello, Linda Gazzillo Diaz, Terry Dibble, John Dippel, Caprice Dodson, Dennis Docheff, Joseph Donnelly, Paul Downing, J. Ellen Eason, Melvin Ezell Jr., Linda Farver, Bridget A. Finley, Pat Floyd, Diane Sanders Flickner, Judy Fox, James A. Gemar, Jeffrey T. Godin, Ragen Gwin, Janet Hamilton, Janelle Handlos, Earlene Hannah, Carole J. Hanson, James Harvey, John Hayes, Lisa Hibbard, Virginia L. Hicks, Robin Hoppenworth, David Horton, Amy Howton, Sister Janice Iverson, Wayne Jacobs, Tony Jadin, Martin W. Johnson, Arthur A. Jones, William B. Karper, Dawn Ketterman-Benner, Todd Kleinfelter, Larry E. Knuth, Jon

Kolb, Craig Koppelman, Richard Krejci, William Kuehl, Mary Jeanne Kuhar, Garry Ladd, Ron Lawman, Jennifer L. H. Lechner, James E. Leone, Keri Lewis, Alexis Hayes Lowe, Paul Luebbers, James Marett, R. Cody McMurtry, Pat McSwegin, Betty McVaigh, John Merriman, Beverly F. Mitchell, Sandra Morgan, Robert J. Mravetz, J. Dirk Nelson, Scott Owen, J. D. Parsley, Charles Pelitera, George Perkins, Judi Phillips, Wiley T. Piazza, Lindy S. Pickard, William Podoll, Karen (Pea) Poole, Robert Pugh, Kelly Quick, Harold L. Rainwater, Robert W. Rausch Jr., Larry Reagan, Matthew Rhea, Laura Richardson, Peter Rehor, Stan Rettew, Mary Rice, Amy P. Richardson, Sharon Rifkin, Rose Schmitz, Garth D. Schoffman, James J. Sheehan, Jan Sholes, Mary Slaughter, Robert L. Slevin, Laurel Smith, Dixie Stanforth, Robert Stokes, Jack Clayton Stovall, Dawn Strout, Frederick C. Surgent, Laura Switzer, Terry R. Tabor, Thomas E. Temples, McKinley Thomas, Paul H. Todd, Susan M. Todd, Don Torok, Maridy Troy, Kenneth R. Turley, Karen Watkins, Kenneth E. Weatherman, John R. Webster, James R. Whitehead, Louise Whitney, Marjorie Avery Willard, Patty Williams, Tillman (Chuck) Williams, Newton Wilkes, Bruce Wilson, Dennis Wilson, Ann Woodard, and Patricia A. Zezula.

We want to acknowledge others who have contributed, including Virginia Atkins, Charles Cicciarella, David Corbin, Ron Hager, Donna Landers, Susan Miller, Robert Pangrazi, Lynda Ransdell, Karen Ward, Darl Waterman, and Weimo Zhu. Among other important contributors are former graduate students who have contributed ideas, made corrections, and contributed in other untold ways to the success of these books. We wish to acknowledge Jeff Boone, Laura Borsdorf, Lisa Chase, Tom Cuddihy, Darren Dale, Bo Fernhall, Ken Fox, Connie Fye, Louie Garcia, Steve Feyrer-Melk, Sarah Keup, Guy LeMasurier, James McClain, Kirk Rose, Jack Rutherford, Cara Sidman, Scott Slava, Dave Thomas, Min Qui Wang, Jim Whitehead, Bridgette Wilde, and Ashley Woodcock. A very special thanks goes to Dave Corbin and Jodi Hickman LeMasurier. Dave and Jodi spent many hours researching photos for this book. We especially appreciate the Spanish translation of vocabulary terms by Julio Morales from Lamar University, as well as the thorough and excellent proofreading by Bob Widen.

Over the years many people have helped with the development of ancillary materials. We wish to thank Jim Whitehead for the suggestion to include the "Take a Stand" feature in the *Connect* materials that accompany the book. Thanks to Ron Hager, Michelle Immels, Lynda Ransdell, Cara Sidman, Marsha Todd, Steve Ball, and Carol Lynn Fieser for their help with *Connect* in preparing and/or piloting some of the labs, quizzes, assignments, and videos.

The authors want to extend thanks to the video production crews at Arizona State University (especially Ken Rudich and Fred Huff), University of Missouri (special thanks to Steve Ball), East Carolina University, and Cara Sidman (University of North Carolina-Wilmington) for their help in developing video resources for *Connect*. A special thanks goes to Mark Ahn from Mark Ahn Creative Services for his excellent work in producing video for *Connect* and for photos used in the book.

We would like to thank all past editors (there have been many), including Michelle Turenne, Carlotta Seely, and Gary O'Brien. Special thanks go to Vicki Malinee, our development editor, who has offered not only editorial help but also excellent suggestions for content, design, and art for the current edition. Finally, we would like to thank the other important people who are responsible for this new edition of the book and the ancillary materials: Scott Harris, Rhona Robbin, Bill Minick, David Patterson, Holly Irish, Debra Kubiak, Nancy Null, Anne Draus, and Patricia Ohlenroth.

Charles B. Corbin
Gregory J. Welk
William R. Corbin
Karen A. Welk

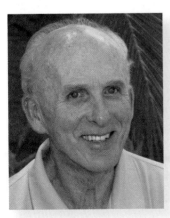
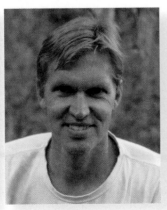
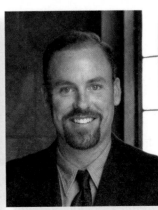
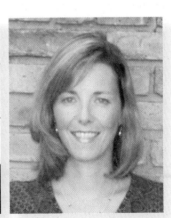

Dedication

The authors wish to dedicate this book in loving memory to Charles Samuel "Charlie" Corbin (April 22, 2004–July 18, 2004), son of Will and Suzi Corbin, grandson of Cathie and Chuck Corbin, and to Alyson Welk (April 30, 1995–June 2, 2003), daughter of Karen and Greg Welk. We also want to dedicate this new edition to our nonauthor wives, non-author children, and grandchildren, whose sacrifices have allowed us to spend the time necessary to create this book. Without their support, this program would not be possible. Thank you, Cathie Corbin, Suzi Corbin, Charles Corbin Jr., Dave Corbin, Katie Corbin, Julia Corbin, Molly Corbin, Lucy Corbin, Colin Welk, Evan Welk, and Grant Welk.

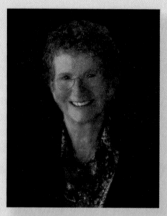

Ruth Lindsey 1926–2005

In Memoriam:
A Tribute to
Our Co-author and
Friend

On May 29, 2005, we lost a great leader and an outstanding advocate for healthy lifestyles, physical activity, and physical education. Our long-time co-author and friend, Ruth Lindsey, will long be remembered for her contributions to the *Concepts* books and to our profession. Ruth was born in 1926 in Kingfisher, Oklahoma, and graduated from high school in Checotah. She earned her BS from Oklahoma State University in 1948, her MS from the University of Wisconsin in 1954, and her doctorate from Indiana University in 1965.

Ruth began her college teaching career at Oklahoma State University (OSU) in 1948, and after brief stints at Monticello College and DePauw University, she returned to OSU in 1956, where she advanced through the ranks to full professor. In 1976, she was a visiting professor at the University of Utah. Ruth then served as professor of physical education at California State University at Long Beach until her retirement in 1988. She continued to contribute as author of the *Concepts* books until 2003.

Ruth was a recognized scholar in physical education with special expertise in biomechanics, kinesiology, questionable exercises, nutrition, and physical activity for senior adults. She actively campaigned against consumer health fraud. She was the author of more than a dozen books, including *Body Mechanics, The Ultimate Fitness Book, Fitness for Life, Concepts of Physical Fitness,* and *Concepts of Fitness and Wellness.* Ruth published numerous papers and served as a leader in many professional organizations. She was an accomplished athlete who won the Oklahoma Women's Fencing Championship and was a low-handicap golfer.

Over the years, hundreds of thousands of students have read Ruth's writings. Her own students and her co-authors will remember her for her command of her subject matter, her attention to detail, the red ink on papers and manuscripts, her concern for her profession, and her personal concern for each individual. Ruth was a woman of principle and character. She will long be remembered for her contributions to our field and for being the kind and caring person that she was. We miss our co-author, our colleague, and our friend.

Health, Wellness, Fitness, and Healthy Lifestyles: An Introduction

LEARNING OBJECTIVES

After completing the study of this concept, you will be able to:

▶ Describe the HELP philosophy and discuss its implications in making personal decisions about health, wellness, and fitness.

▶ Define the dimensions of health and wellness, and explain how they interact to influence health and wellness.

▶ Distinguish health-related and skill-related dimensions of physical fitness.

▶ Identify the determinants of health, wellness, and fitness, and explain how they each contribute to health, wellness, and fitness.

▶ Identify related national health goals and show how meeting personal goals can contribute to reaching national goals.

▶ Use health behavior change strategies to carry out self-assessments of personal lifestyles and wellness perceptions.

Good health, wellness, fitness, and healthy lifestyles are important for all people.

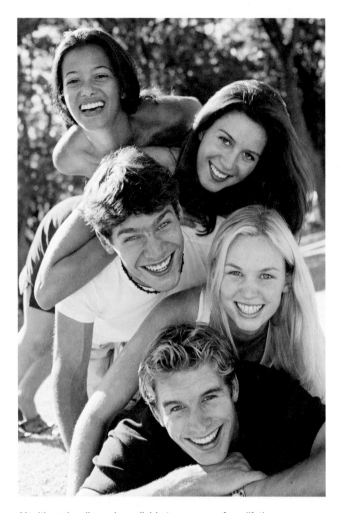

Health and wellness is available to everyone for a lifetime.

Ninety-nine percent of American adults say that "being in good health" is of primary importance. Good health—for them and those they care about—is more important than money and other material things. Having good health, wellness, and fitness can make us feel good, look good, and enjoy life fully. This book is designed to help you achieve good health by providing information to help you make good decisions. You will also learn essential **self-management skills.** With practice, use of these skills promotes healthy lifestyles that lead to good health, wellness, and fitness throughout life. An overview of basic self-management skills is provided in Concept 2.

The HELP Philosophy

The HELP philosophy provides a basis for making healthy lifestyle change possible. The four-letter acronym HELP summarizes the overall philosophy used in this book. Each letter in HELP characterizes an important part of the philosophy: *Health* is available to *Everyone* for a *Lifetime*—and it's *Personal*. The concepts in the book

provide principles and guidelines that help you adopt positive lifestyles. The labs provide experiences for learning behavioral skills needed to maintain these lifestyles.

A personal philosophy that emphasizes health can lead to behaviors that promote it. The *H* in HELP stands for *health*. One theory that has been extensively tested indicates that people who believe in the benefits of healthy lifestyles are more likely to engage in healthy behaviors. The theory also suggests that people who state intentions to put their beliefs into action are likely to adopt behaviors that lead to health, wellness, and fitness.

Everyone can benefit from healthy lifestyles. The *E* in HELP stands for *everyone*. Anyone can change a behavior or lifestyle. Nevertheless, many adults feel ineffective in making lifestyle changes. Physical activity is not just for athletes—it is for all people. Eating well is not just for other people—you can do it, too. All people can learn stress-management techniques and practice healthy lifestyles.

Healthy behaviors are most effective when practiced for a lifetime. The *L* in HELP stands for *lifetime*. Young people sometimes feel immortal because the harmful effects of unhealthy lifestyles are often not immediate. As we grow older, we begin to realize that unhealthy lifestyles have cumulative negative effects. Starting early in life to emphasize healthy behaviors results in long-term health, wellness, and fitness benefits. One study showed that the longer healthy lifestyles are practiced, the greater the beneficial effects. This study also demonstrated that long-term healthy lifestyles can even overcome hereditary predisposition to illness and disease.

Healthy lifestyles should be based on personal needs. The *P* in HELP stands for *personal*. No two people are exactly alike. Just as no single pill cures all illnesses, no single lifestyle prescription exists for good health, wellness, and fitness. Each person must assess personal needs and make lifestyle changes based on those needs.

You can adopt the HELP philosophy. As you progress through this book, consider ways that you can implement the HELP philosophy. In each concept, HELP boxes are provided to stimulate your thinking about key health issues.

National Health Goals

Healthy People 2020 **(HP2020) is a comprehensive set of health promotion and disease prevention objectives with the primary intent of improving the nation's health.** The objectives, developed by experts from hundreds of national health organizations and published in 2010, provide benchmarks to determine progress over the period from 2010 to 2020. The objectives also serve as goals to motivate and guide people in making sound health decisions as well as to provide a focus for public health programs.

The national health goals for the year 2010 were established in 2000. Studies show that significant progress was made in that 10-year period: For example, 23 percent of all goals were met and progress was made on 48 percent. The hope is that similar progress can be made in the 10 years leading to 2020.

In addition to helping change the health of society at large, HP2020 goals also have implications for personal health behavior change. Societal changes can occur only when individuals adjust personal behaviors and work together to make changes that benefit other people. Not all objectives will have personal implications for each individual, but societal awareness of the objectives may lead to future changes in the health of our country.

Specific HP2020 goals are provided at the end of each concept to show the links between the content of this text and the national health goals. Four of the "overarching goals" of HP2020 are described in more detail in the sections that follow. The section at the end of each concept, "Strategies for Action," offers assessment and planning tips for improving health, wellness, and fitness and for working toward meeting HP2020 goals.

A primary goal of HP2020 is to help all people have high-quality, longer lives free of preventable disease, injury, and premature death. Over the past century, the average life expectancy in the United States has increased by 60 percent. Although different reports yield slightly different results, studies have generally shown that Americans now live longer than ever before. Results included in Figure 1 are from the most recent **World Health Organization (WHO)** life expectancy report. These data provide statistics for healthy life expectancy in North American countries. Globally, according to the most current *World Factbook*, Canada ranks 12th, the United States ranks 50th, and Mexico ranks 72nd in life expectancy.

Living a long life is important, but so is having a high-quality life. This means feeling good, looking good, and being happy. It also means being fit enough to enjoy your leisure and to be able do what you want to do without limitation. An index called HALE (Healthy Life Expectancy) is often used to determine the number of years of life a person has a good quality of life as opposed to having illness or impaired function. Figure 1 uses information from HALE to show the number of years of high-quality life (green) and years of life with low quality (orange). Adopting healthy lifestyles when we are young can increase the length of life and can also increase quality of life.

Achieving health equity, eliminating disparities, and improving the health of all groups is another primary goal of HP2020. Health varies greatly with

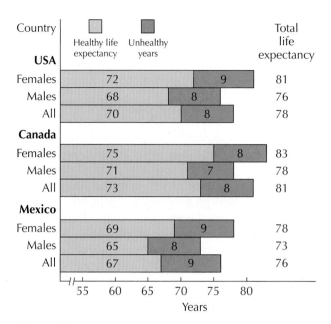

Figure 1 ▶ Healthy life expectancy for North America.
Sources: World Health Organization and National Center for Health Statistics.

ethnicity, income, gender, and age. For example, African Americans, Hispanics, and Native Americans have a shorter life expectancy than White non-Hispanics, and men have a shorter life expectancy than women. Health disparities also exist in quality of life. One method of assessing disparities in quality of life is to compare the number of **healthy days** diverse groups experience each month. Minorities, including African Americans, Hispanics, and Native Americans, experience about 24 healthy days each month compared to 25 for White

Self-management Skills Skills that you learn to help you adopt healthy lifestyles and adhere to them.

Health Optimal well-being that contributes to one's quality of life. It is more than freedom from disease and illness, though freedom from disease is important to good health. Optimal health includes high-level mental, social, emotional, spiritual, and physical wellness within the limits of one's heredity and personal abilities.

World Health Organization (WHO) WHO is the United Nations' agency for health and has 193 member countries. Its principal goal is the attainment of the highest possible level of health for all people. WHO has been instrumental in making health policy and in implementing health programs worldwide since its inception in 1948.

Healthy Days A self-rating of the number of days (per week or month) a person considers himself or herself to be in good or better than good health.

non-Hispanics. People with very low income typically have 22 healthy days per month, compared with 26 days for those with high income. Men have a higher number of healthy days than women.

The reason for such differences in the number of healthy days varies. The relatively higher number of unhealthy days for women is, at least in part, because they live longer and their unhealthy years later in life factor into their average number of healthy days. Disparities in healthy days by level of income may be due to environmental, social, or cultural factors as well as less access to preventive care. Both physical and mental health problems are the most frequent reasons for unhealthy days. Physical illness, pain, depression, anxiety, sleeplessness, and limitations in ability to function or perform enjoyable activities are the problems people most frequently reported.

Another primary goal of HP2020 is to create social and physical environments that promote good health for all. The environment, both social and physical, has much to do with both quality of life and length of life. Environmental factors are discussed in greater detail on page 13 and in several of the later concepts in this book.

The final primary goal of HP2020 is to promote quality of life, healthy development, and healthy behaviors across all stages of life. Healthy days decrease as we age. Young adults experience more healthy days each month than older adults. Over the past two decades, there has been a steady decline in healthy days for the average person, no doubt because of the increase in the number of older adults in our society. The number of healthy days takes its biggest drop after age 75. It is interesting that in recent national surveys older adults (ages 50 to 75) report being happier and more secure than younger people age 20 to 40.

A recent national report (*Blueprint for a Healthier America*) underscores the need to focus future efforts on

prevention and preparedness, including changing both the social and physical environment to increase emphasis on physical activity, nutrition, and prevention of tobacco use. The report indicates that an investment of $10 per person per year in proven community-based programs that focus on healthy lifestyles could save the country $16 per person over a five-year period.

Health and Wellness

Health is more than freedom from illness and disease. Over 60 years ago, the World Health Organization defined health as more than freedom from illness, disease, and debilitating conditions. Prior to that time, you were considered to be "healthy" if you were not sick. HP2020 refers to quality of life in two of its four overarching goals, highlighting the importance of the wellness component of health.

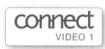

Figure 2 illustrates the modern concept of health. This general state of being is characterized by freedom from disease and debilitating conditions (outer circle), as well as wellness (center circle).

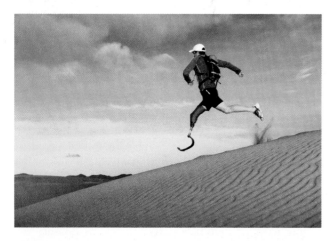

Physical activity is for everyone. An active lifestyle promotes health and wellness.

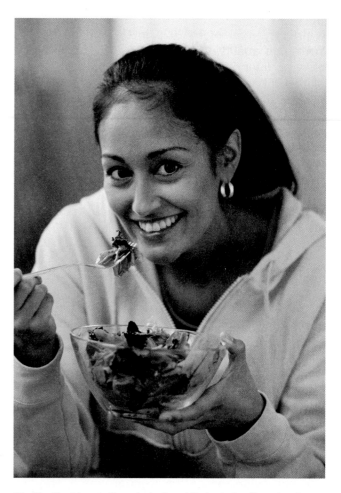

Healthy lifestyles are the principal contributor to health and wellness.

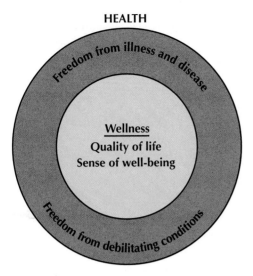

Figure 2 ▶ A model of optimal health, including wellness.

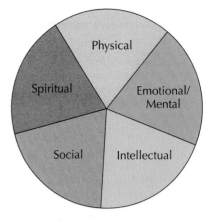

Figure 3 ▶ The dimensions of health and wellness.

Wellness is the positive component of optimal health. Disease, **illness,** and debilitating conditions are negative components that detract from optimal health. Death can be considered the ultimate opposite of optimal health. **Wellness,** in contrast, is the positive component of optimal health. It is characterized by a sense of well-being reflected in optimal functioning, health-related **quality of life,** meaningful work, and a contribution to society. HP2020 objectives use the term *health-related quality of life* to describe a general sense of happiness and satisfaction with life.

Health and wellness are personal. Every individual is unique—and health and wellness are influenced by each person's unique characteristics. Making comparisons to other people on specific characteristics may produce feelings of inadequacy that detract from one's profile of total health and wellness. Each of us has personal limitations and strengths. Focusing on strengths and learning to accommodate weaknesses are essential keys to optimal health and wellness.

Health and wellness are multidimensional. The dimensions of health and wellness include emotional-mental, intellectual, social, spiritual, and physical. Table 1 describes the various dimensions, and Figure 3 illustrates the importance of each one for optimal health and wellness. Some people include environmental and vocational dimensions in addition to the five shown in Figure 3.

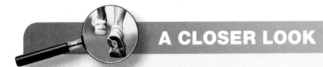

A CLOSER LOOK

Social Determinants of Health

Healthy People 2020 and related documents from the World Health Organization (WHO) emphasize the importance of understanding the determinants of health. The WHO reports outline the importance of *social determinants* in reducing health disparities throughout the world. They note that people's circumstances are shaped by distribution of money, power, and resources at local, national, and global levels, which can result in "unfair but avoidable" differences in health status in different places. For example, the lack of pure water, medical facilities, and medicine result in higher rates of disease (particularly infectious disease) and lower quality of life in third world countries than in more technologically advanced countries.

How do social determinants influence health status within the United States?

ACTIVITY

Illness The ill feeling and/or symptoms associated with a disease or circumstances that upset homeostasis.

Wellness The integration of many different components (social, emotional/mental, spiritual, and physical) that expand one's potential to live (quality of life) and work effectively and to make a significant contribution to society. Wellness reflects how one feels (a sense of well-being) about life, as well as one's ability to function effectively. Wellness, as opposed to illness (a negative), is sometimes described as the positive component of good health.

Quality of Life A term used to describe wellness. An individual with quality of life can enjoyably do the activities of life with little or no limitation and can function independently. Individual quality of life requires a pleasant and supportive community.

Table 1 ▶ Definitions of Health and Wellness Dimensions

Emotional/mental health—Freedom from emotional/mental illnesses, such as clinical depression, and possession of emotional wellness. The goals for the nation's health refer to mental rather than emotional health and wellness. In this book, mental health and wellness are considered to be the same as emotional health and wellness.

Emotional/mental wellness—The ability to cope with daily circumstances and to deal with personal feelings in a positive, optimistic, and constructive manner. A person with emotional wellness is generally characterized as happy instead of depressed.

Intellectual health—Freedom from illnesses that invade the brain and other systems that allow learning. A person with intellectual health also possesses intellectual wellness.

Intellectual wellness—The ability to learn and to use information to enhance the quality of daily living and optimal functioning. A person with intellectual wellness is generally characterized as informed instead of ignorant.

Physical health—Freedom from illnesses that affect the physiological systems of the body, such as the heart and the nervous system. A person with physical health possesses an adequate level of physical fitness and physical wellness.

Physical wellness—The ability to function effectively in meeting the demands of the day's work and to use free time effectively. Physical wellness includes good physical fitness and the possession of useful motor skills. A person with physical wellness is generally characterized as fit instead of unfit.

Social health—Freedom from illnesses or conditions that severely limit functioning in society, including antisocial pathologies.

Social wellness—The ability to interact with others successfully and to establish meaningful relationships that enhance the quality of life for all people involved in the interaction (including self). A person with social wellness is generally characterized as involved instead of lonely.

Spiritual health—The one component of health that is totally composed of the wellness dimension; it is synonymous with spiritual wellness.

Spiritual wellness—The ability to establish a values system and act on the system of beliefs, as well as to establish and carry out meaningful and constructive lifetime goals. Spiritual wellness is often based on a belief in a force greater than the individual that helps her or him contribute to an improved quality of life for all people. A person with spiritual wellness is generally characterized as fulfilled instead of unfulfilled.

In this book, health and wellness are considered to be personal factors, so environmental and vocational wellness are not included in Tables 1 and 2. However, the environment (including your work environment) is very

Table 2 ▶ The Dimensions of Wellness

Wellness Dimension	Negative — — — — — — — Positive	
Emotional/mental	Depressed — — — — — —	Happy
Intellectual	Ignorant — — — — — —	Informed
Physical	Unfit — — — — — — — —	Fit
Social	Lonely — — — — — — —	Involved
Spiritual	Unfulfilled — — — — — —	Fulfilled
Total outlook	Negative — — — — — —	Positive

important to overall personal wellness, and for this reason, environmental factors are prominent in the model of wellness described on page 13 and are featured throughout this book. The final concept in the book links environmental and vocational factors to the personal wellness dimensions described in Table 1.

Wellness reflects how one feels about life, as well as one's ability to function effectively. A positive total outlook on life is essential to each of the wellness dimensions. As illustrated in Table 2, a "well" person is satisfied in work, is spiritually fulfilled, enjoys leisure time, is physically fit, is socially involved, and has a positive emotional/mental outlook. He or she is happy and fulfilled.

The way one perceives each dimension of wellness affects one's total outlook. Researchers use the term *self-perceptions* to describe these feelings. Many researchers believe that self-perceptions about wellness are more important than actual circumstances or a person's actual state of being. For example, a person who has an important job may find less meaning and job satisfaction than another person with a much less important job. Apparently, one of the important factors for a person who has achieved high-level wellness and a positive outlook on life is the ability to reward himself or herself. Some people, however, seem unable to give themselves credit for their successes. The development of a system that allows a person to perceive the self positively is essential, along with the adoption of positive **lifestyles** that encourage improved self-perceptions. The questionnaire in Lab 1A will help you assess your self-perceptions of the various wellness dimensions. For optimal wellness, it is important to find positive feelings about each dimension.

Health and wellness are integrated states of being. The segmented pictures of health and wellness shown in Figure 3 and Tables 1 and 2 are used only to illustrate the multidimensional nature of health and wellness. In reality, health and wellness are integrated states of being that

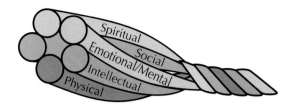

Figure 4 ▶ The integration of wellness dimensions.

can best be depicted as threads woven together to produce a larger, integrated fabric. Each dimension relates to each of the others and overlaps all the others. The overlap is so frequent and so great that the specific contribution of each thread is almost indistinguishable when looking at the total (Figure 4). The total is clearly greater than the sum of the parts.

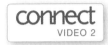

It is possible to possess health and wellness while being ill or possessing a debilitating condition. Many illnesses are curable and may have only a temporary effect on health. Others, such as Type I diabetes, are not curable but can be managed with proper eating, physical activity, and sound medical treatment. Those with manageable conditions may, however, be at risk for other health problems. For example, unmanaged diabetes is associated with a high risk for heart disease and other health problems.

Debilitating conditions, such as the loss of a limb or loss of function in a body part, can contribute to a lower level of functioning or an increased risk for illness and thus to poor health. On the other hand, such conditions need not limit wellness. A person with a debilitating condition who has a positive outlook on life may have better overall health than a person with a poor outlook on life but no debilitating condition.

Just as wellness is possible among those with illness and disability, evidence is accumulating that people with a positive outlook are better able to resist the progress of disease and illness than are those with a negative outlook. Thinking positive thoughts has been associated with enhanced results from various medical treatments and surgical procedures.

Wellness **is a term used by the uninformed as well as experts.** Unfortunately, some individuals and groups have tried to identify wellness with products and services that promise benefits that cannot be documented. Because well-being is a subjective feeling, unscrupulous people can easily make claims of improved wellness for their product or service without facts to back them up.

Holistic health is a term that is similarly abused. Consider that optimal health includes many areas; thus, the term *holistic* (total) is appropriate. In fact, the word *health*

originates from a root word meaning "wholeness." Unfortunately, questionable health practices are sometimes promoted under the guise of holistic health. Care should be used when considering services and products that make claims of wellness and/or holistic health to be sure that they are legitimate.

Physical Fitness

Physical fitness is a multidimensional state of being. **Physical fitness** is the body's ability to function efficiently and effectively. It consists of at least five health-related and six skill-related components, each of which contributes to total quality of life. Physical fitness is associated with a person's ability to work effectively, enjoy leisure time, be healthy, resist **hypokinetic diseases or conditions,** and meet emergency situations. It is related to, but different from, health and wellness.

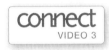

Although the development of physical fitness is the result of many things, optimal physical fitness is not possible without regular physical activity.

The health-related components of physical fitness are directly associated with good health. The five components of health-related physical fitness are body composition, cardiovascular fitness, flexibility, muscular

Lifestyles Patterns of behavior or ways an individual typically lives.

Physical Fitness The body's ability to function efficiently and effectively. It consists of health-related physical fitness and skill-related physical fitness, which have at least 11 components, each of which contributes to total quality of life. Physical fitness also includes metabolic fitness and bone integrity. Physical fitness is associated with a person's ability to work effectively, enjoy leisure time, be healthy, resist hypokinetic diseases, and meet emergency situations. It is related to, but different from, health, wellness, and the psychological, sociological, emotional/mental, and spiritual components. Although the development of physical fitness is the result of many things, optimal physical fitness is not possible without regular exercise.

Hypokinetic Diseases or Conditions *Hypo-* means "under" or "too little," and *-kinetic* means "movement" or "activity." Thus, *hypokinetic* means "too little activity." A hypokinetic disease or condition is one associated with lack of physical activity or too little regular exercise. Examples include heart disease, low back pain, Type II diabetes, and obesity.

Body Composition

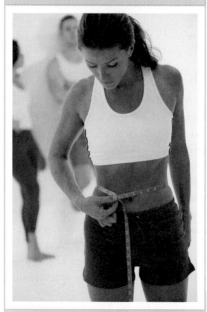

The relative percentage of muscle, fat, bone, and other tissues that make up the body. A fit person has a relatively low, but not too low, percentage of body fat (body fatness).

Muscular Endurance

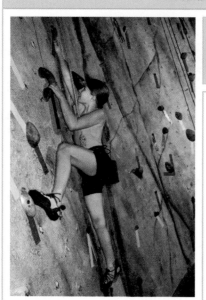

The ability of the muscles to exert themselves repeatedly. A fit person can repeat movements for a long period without undue fatigue.

Cardiovascular Fitness

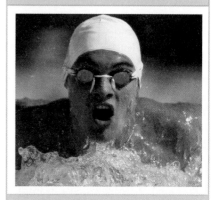

The ability of the heart, blood vessels, blood, and respiratory system to supply nutrients and oxygen to the muscles and the ability of the muscles to utilize fuel to allow sustained exercise. A fit person can persist in physical activity for relatively long periods without undue stress.

Dimensions of Health-Related Physical Fitness

Strength

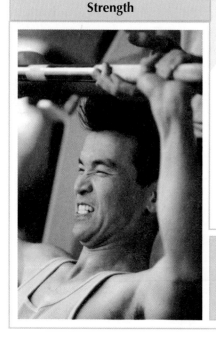

The ability of the muscles to exert an external force or to lift a heavy weight. A fit person can do work or play that involves exerting force, such as lifting or controlling one's own body weight.

Flexibility

The range of motion available in a joint. It is affected by muscle length, joint structure, and other factors. A fit person can move the body joints through a full range of motion in work and in play.

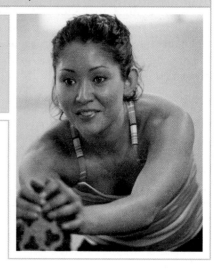

Figure 5 ▶ Components of health-related physical fitness.

endurance, and strength (see Figure 5). Each health–related fitness characteristic has a direct relationship to good health and reduced risk for hypokinetic disease. It is for this reason that the five health-related physical fitness components are emphasized in this book.

Possessing a moderate amount of each component of health-related fitness is essential to disease prevention and health promotion, but it is not essential to have exceptionally high levels of fitness to achieve health benefits. High levels of health-related fitness relate more to performance than to health benefits. For example, moderate amounts of strength are necessary to prevent back and posture problems, whereas high levels of strength contribute most to improved performance in activities such as football and jobs involving heavy lifting.

The skill-related components of physical fitness are associated more with performance than with good health. The components of skill-related physical fitness are agility, balance, coordination, power, reaction time, and speed (see Figure 6). They are called skill-related because people who possess them find it easy to achieve high levels of performance in motor skills, such as those required in sports and in specific types of jobs. Power is sometimes referred to as a combined component of fitness, since it requires both strength (a health-related component) and speed (a skill-related component). Because most experts consider power to be associated more with performance than with good health, 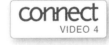 it is classified as a skill-related component of fitness in this book. Skill-related fitness is sometimes called sports fitness or motor fitness.

It is important to recognize that skill-related fitness is multidimensional and highly specific. For example, coordination could be hand-eye coordination, such as batting a ball; foot-eye coordination, such as kicking a ball; or many other possibilities. The six parts of skill-related fitness identified here are those commonly associated with successful sports and work performance. Each could be measured in ways other than those presented in this book. Measurements are provided to help you understand the nature of total physical fitness and to help you make important decisions about lifetime physical activity.

Metabolic fitness is a nonperformance component of total fitness. Physical activity can provide health benefits that are independent of changes in traditional health-related fitness measures. Physical activity promotes good **metabolic fitness,** a state associated with reduced risk for many chronic diseases. People with a cluster of low metabolic fitness characteristics are said to have metabolic syndrome (also known as Syndrome X). Metabolic syndrome is discussed in more detail in Concept 4.

Bone integrity is often considered to be a nonperformance measure of fitness. Traditional definitions do not include **bone integrity** as a part of physical fitness, but some experts feel they should. Like metabolic fitness, bone integrity cannot be assessed with performance measures the way most health-related fitness parts can. Regardless of whether bone integrity is considered a part of fitness or a component of health, strong, healthy bones are important to optimal health and are associated with regular physical activity and sound diet.

The many components of physical fitness are specific but are also interrelated. Physical fitness is a combination of several aspects, rather than a single characteristic. A fit person possesses at least adequate levels of each of the health-related, skill-related, and metabolic fitness components. Some relationships exist among various fitness characteristics, but each component of physical fitness is separate and different from the others. For example, people who possess exceptional strength may not have good cardiovascular fitness, and those who have good coordination do not necessarily possess good flexibility.

Good physical fitness is important, but it is not the same as physical health and wellness. Good physical fitness contributes directly to the physical component of good health and wellness and indirectly to the other four components. Good fitness has been shown to be associated with reduced risk for chronic diseases, such as heart disease, and has been shown to reduce the consequences of many debilitating conditions. In addition, good fitness contributes to wellness by helping us look our best, feel good, and enjoy life. Other physical factors can also influence health and wellness. For example, having good physical skills enhances quality of life by allowing us to participate in enjoyable activities, such as tennis, golf, and bowling. Although fitness can assist us in performing these activities, regular practice is also necessary. Another example is the ability to fight off viral and bacterial infections. Although fitness can promote a strong immune system, other physical factors can influence our susceptibility to these and other conditions.

Metabolic Fitness A positive state of the physiological systems commonly associated with reduced risk for chronic diseases such as diabetes and heart disease. Metabolic fitness is evidenced by healthy blood fat (lipid) profiles, healthy blood pressure, healthy blood sugar and insulin levels, and other nonperformance measures.

Bone Integrity Soundness of the bones is associated with high density and absence of symptoms of deterioration.

Power

The ability to transfer energy into force at a fast rate. Kicking in martial arts and throwing the discus are activities that require considerable power.

Agility

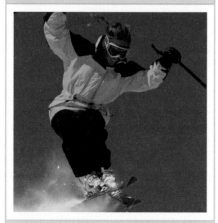

The ability to rapidly and accurately change the direction of the movement of the entire body in space. Skiing and wrestling are examples of activities that require exceptional agility.

Reaction Time

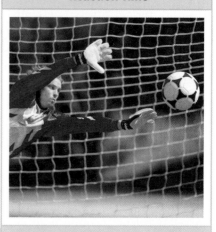

The time elapsed between stimulation and the beginning of reaction to that stimulation. Reacting to a soccer ball and starting a sprint race require good reaction time.

Dimensions of Skill-Related Physical Fitness

Coordination

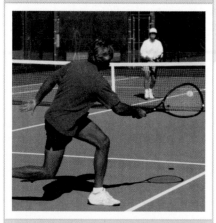

The ability to use the senses with the body parts to perform motor tasks smoothly and accurately. Juggling, hitting a tennis ball, and kicking a ball are examples of activities requiring good coordination.

Speed

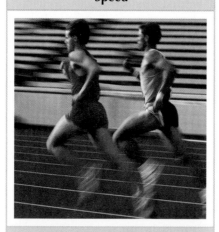

The ability to perform a movement in a short period of time. Sprinters and wide receivers in football need good foot and leg speed.

Balance

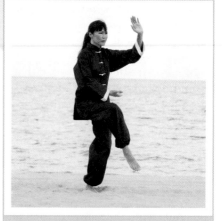

The maintenance of equilibrium while stationary or while moving. Performing tai chi movements and performing stunts on the balance beam are activities that require exceptional balance.

Figure 6 ▶ Components of skill-related physical fitness.

Determinants of Lifelong Health, Wellness, and Fitness

Many factors are important in developing lifetime health, wellness, and fitness, and some are more in your control than others. Figure 7 provides a model for describing many of the factors that contribute to health, wellness, and fitness. Central to the model are health, wellness, and fitness because these are the states of being (shaded in green and gold) that each of us wants to achieve. Around the periphery are the factors that influence these states of being. Those shaded in dark blue are the factors over which you have the least control (heredity, age, and disability). Those shaded in light blue (health care and environmental factors) are factors over which you have some control but less than the factors shaded in red (personal actions/interactions, cognitions, and emotions).

Those shaded in light red are the factors over which you have greatest control (healthy lifestyles).

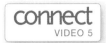

Heredity (human biology) is a factor over which we have little control. Experts estimate that human biology, or heredity, accounts for 16 percent of all health problems, including early death. Heredity influences each part of health-related physical fitness, including our tendencies to build muscle and to deposit body fat. Each of us reaps different benefits from the same healthy lifestyles, based on our hereditary tendencies. Even more important is that predispositions to diseases are inherited. For example, some early deaths are a result of untreatable hereditary conditions (e.g., congenital heart defects). Obviously, some inherited conditions are manageable (e.g., diabetes) with proper medical supervision and appropriate lifestyles.

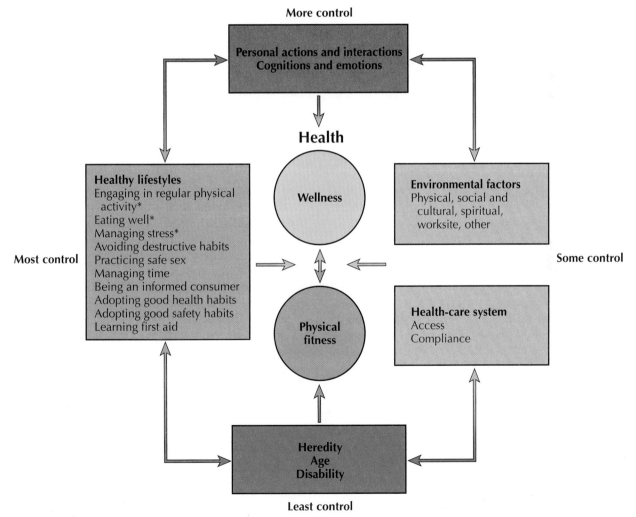

*These lifestyles are viewed as "priority lifestyles."

Figure 7 ► Determinants of health, fitness, and wellness.

HEL P **Health is available to Everyone for a Lifetime, and it's Personal**

According to the National Institutes of Health, although genes do not necessarily cause diseases, they do influence our risk of developing diseases, such as cancer, heart disease, and addiction. The interaction between our genes and our environments and experiences is a complex one that is still being studied.

Would knowing you were genetically predisposed to a particular disease change the lifestyle decisions you make?

TECHNOLOGY UPDATE

Podcasts

Podcasts are compressed digital files containing audio or video that can be downloaded from the Internet to a portable media player or personal computer. The word *Pod* refers to a personal media player, the receiver of the information delivered by a *podcaster.* Originally used to transmit music and news, podcasts of health information are now common.

Do you think you would rely on this type of resource for health-related information? Why or why not?

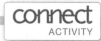

Heredity is a factor over which we have little control and is, therefore, illustrated in dark blue in Figure 7. Each of us can limit the effects of heredity by being aware of our personal family history and by making efforts to best manage those factors over which we do have control.

In the concepts that follow, you will learn more about heredity and how it affects health, wellness, and fitness.

Health, wellness, and fitness are influenced by the aging of our population. In 2030 when post–World War II baby boomers are over the age of 65, adults 65 or older will make up 20 percent of the population. The number of people over 85 will triple by 2050. There are currently more than 100,000 people over the age of 100. The definition of *old* is changing, with most people believing that a person is not old until age 71 or older. Nearly a quarter of the population believes that being old begins at 81.

Whatever the standard for being old, age is a factor over which we have no control. The major health and wellness concerns of older adults include losing health, losing the ability to care for oneself, losing mental abilities, running out of money, being a burden to family, and being alone. Chronic pain is also a major problem among older adults. Nearly 30 percent of adults over 65 experience chronic pain, as opposed to 3 percent of those under 30. Nearly 60 percent of older adults experience frequent pain, as opposed to 17 percent of those under 30. Older adults have 36 percent more unhealthy days than young adults.

Age is shaded in dark blue in Figure 7 because it is a factor that you cannot control. However, healthy lifestyles can reduce the effects of aging on health, wellness, and fitness. As detailed later in this book, healthy lifestyles can extend life and have a positive effect on quality of life.

Disabilities can affect, but they do not necessarily limit, health, wellness, and fitness. Disabilities typically result from factors beyond your control (shaded in dark blue in Figure 7). Many types of disabilities affect health, fitness, and wellness. An objective disability (e.g., loss of a limb, impaired intellectual functioning) can make it difficult to function in certain circumstances but need not limit health, wellness, and fitness. All people have a limitation of one kind or another. Societal efforts to help all people function within their limitations can help everyone, including people with disabilities, have a positive outlook on life and experience a high quality of life. With assistance from an instructor, it is possible for all people to adapt the information in this book for use in promoting heath, wellness, and fitness.

The health-care system affects our ability to overcome illness and improve our quality of life. Approximately 10 percent of unnecessary deaths occur as a result of disparities in the health-care system. The quality of life for those who are sick and those who tend to be sick is influenced greatly by the type of medical care they receive. Health care is not equally available to all. A study by the Institute of Medicine, entitled "Insuring America's Health," indicates that 18,000 people die unnecessarily in the United States each year because they lack health insurance. Those without health insurance are less likely to get high-quality medical care than those with insurance. Many of those without insurance have chronic conditions that go undetected and as a result become untreatable. The passage of the Affordable Health Care Act addresses this issue by enabling all Americans to have health insurance.

Many people fail to seek medical help even though care is accessible. Others seek medical help but fail to comply with medical advice. For example, they do not take prescribed medicine or do not follow up with treatments. Men are less likely to seek medical advice than women. For this reason, treatable conditions sometimes become untreatable. Once men seek medical care, evidence reveals, they get better care than women. Also, more of the medical research has been done on men. This is of concern because treatments for men and women often vary for similar conditions.

Wellness as evidenced by quality of life is also influenced by the health-care system. Traditional medicine, sometimes referred to as the **medical model,** has focused primarily on the treatment of illness with medicine, rather than illness prevention and wellness promotion. Efforts to educate health-care personnel about techniques for promoting wellness have been initiated in recent years. Still, it is often up to the patient to find information about health promotion. For example, a patient with risk factors for heart disease might be advised to eat better or to exercise more, but little specific information may be offered. In Figure 7, the health-care system is in light blue to illustrate the fact that it is a factor over which you may have limited control.

The environment is a major factor affecting our health, wellness, and fitness. Environmental factors account for nearly one-fourth of all early deaths and affect quality of life in many ways. We do have more control over environmental factors than heredity, but they are not totally under our control. For this reason, the environmental factors box is depicted in Figure 7 with a lighter shade of blue than the heredity, age, and disability box.

You can exert personal control by selecting healthy environments rather than by exposing yourself to unhealthy or unsafe environments. This includes your choice of living and work location, as well as the social, spiritual, and intellectual environments. On the other hand, circumstances may make it impossible for you to make the choices you would prefer. Important environmental factors are discussed throughout the text, particularly in Concept 6 and the final concept in the book. Some suggestions for how you can work to alter the environment in a positive way are also discussed in the last concept.

Personal actions, interactions, cognitions, and emotions all have an effect on health, wellness, and fitness. Some people think that good health, wellness, and fitness are totally out of personal control. Others think that they are totally in control. Neither statement is entirely true. While heredity, age, and disability are factors you cannot control, and health care and the environment are factors over which you have limited control, there are things that you can do relating to these factors. You can use your cognitive abilities to learn about your family history and use that information to limit the negative influences of heredity. You can learn how to adapt to disabilities and personal limitations, as well as to the aging process. You can research the health-care system and the environment to minimize the problems associated with them.

Your personal interactions also influence your health, wellness, and fitness. You are not alone in this world. Your various environments, and how you interact with them, influence you greatly. You have a choice about the environments in which you place yourself and the people with whom you interact in these environments.

Humans have the ability to think (cognitions) and to use critical thinking to make choices and to determine the actions they take and the interactions they engage in. Emotions also affect personal actions and interactions. A major goal of this book is to help you learn self-management skills designed to help you use your cognitive abilities to solve problems and make good decisions about good health, wellness, and fitness, as well as to help you to be in control of your emotions when taking action and making decisions that affect your health.

None of us makes perfect decisions all of the time. Sometimes we take actions and make choices based on inadequate information, faulty thinking, pressure from others, or negative influences from our emotions. While the focus of this book is on healthy lifestyles, all of the factors that influence health, wellness, and fitness will be discussed in greater detail in the concepts that follow. The goal is to help you consider all factors and to make informed decisions that will lead to healthful behaviors. Some strategies for action for each of the factors are presented in the final concept of this book.

Lifestyle change, more than any other factor, is the best way to prevent illness and early death in our society. Statistics show that more than half of early deaths are the result of chronic diseases caused by unhealthy lifestyles. Many of these chronic diseases are targeted in the HP2020 report, and many of the new health objectives focus on them. As shown in Figure 7, these lifestyles affect health, wellness, and physical fitness. The double-headed arrow between health/wellness and physical fitness illustrates the interaction between these factors. Physical fitness is important to health and wellness development and vice versa.

The major causes of early death have shifted from infectious diseases to chronic lifestyle-related conditions. Scientific advances and improvements in medicine and health care have dramatically reduced the incidence of infectious diseases over the past 100 years (see Table 3). Diphtheria and polio, both major causes of death in the 20th century, have been virtually eliminated in Western culture. Smallpox was globally eradicated in 1977.

Medical Model The focus of the health-care system on treating illness with medicine, with little emphasis on prevention or wellness promotion.

In the News

Health, Wellness, and Fitness: The Good News

The Gallup-Healthways Well-Being Index® provides an indicator of how U.S. residents rate their health and well-being over time. More than 1,000 adults are surveyed every day and results are summarized each month. In addition to the overall Well-Being Index, separate indices monitor life adjustment, emotional health, physical health, healthy behaviors, work environment, and health access. The indices track trends at the national level as well as by state, major cities, and congressional districts. Visit the Well-Being Index at www.well-beingindex.com to see how Americans feel about their health and well-being.

What do you think is needed to promote health and well-being at the local, state, and national level?

Table 3 ▶ Major Causes of Death in the United States			
Current Rank	**Cause**	**1900 Rank**	**Cause**
1	Heart disease	1	Pneumonia*
2	Cancer	2	Tuberculosis*
3	Lower respiratory disease	3	Diarrhea/enteritis*
4	Stroke	4	Heart disease
5	Injuries/accidents	5	Stroke
6	Alzheimer's disease	6	Liver disease
7	Diabetes	7	Injuries
8	Influenza/pneumonia*	8	Cancer
9	Kidney disease	9	Senility
10	Suicide	10	Diphtheria*

*Infectious diseases: The only diseases among the top ten that are primarily infectious in nature today are influenza/pneumonia.

Infectious diseases have been replaced with chronic lifestyle-related conditions as the major causes of death. Four of the top seven current causes of death (heart disease, cancer, stroke, and diabetes) fall into this category. While heart disease remains the leading killer among all adults, National Cancer Institute statistics indicate that cancer is the leading cause of death for adults under the age of 85. Death rates have recently decreased for 8 of the top 10 causes of death. The incidence of kidney disease was unchanged, and suicide increased 1 percent.

HIV/AIDS, formerly in the top 10 causes of death, is now 15th. The drop is primarily because of the development of treatments to increase the life expectancy of those infected. Many among the top 10 are referred to as chronic lifestyle-related conditions because alteration of lifestyles can result in reduced risk for these conditions.

Healthy lifestyles are critical to wellness. Just as unhealthy lifestyles are the principal causes of modern-day illnesses, such as heart disease, cancer, and diabetes, healthy lifestyles can result in the improved feeling of wellness that is critical to optimal health. In recognizing the importance of "years of healthy life," the Public Health Service also recognizes what it calls "measures of well-being." This well-being, or wellness, is associated with social, emotional/mental, spiritual, and physical functioning. Being physically active and eating well are two healthy lifestyles that can improve well-being and add years of quality living. Many of the healthy lifestyles associated with good physical fitness and optimal wellness will be discussed in detail later in this book. The Healthy Lifestyle Questionnaire at the end of this concept gives you the opportunity to assess your current lifestyles.

Regular physical activity, sound nutrition, and stress management are priority healthy lifestyles. Three of the lifestyles listed in Figure 7 are considered to be priority healthy lifestyles: engaging in regular **physical activity** or **exercise,** eating well, and managing

Physical Activity Generally considered to be a broad term used to describe all forms of large muscle movements, including sports, dance, games, work, lifestyle activities, and exercise for fitness. In this book, *exercise* and *physical activity* will often be used interchangeably to make reading less repetitive and more interesting.

Exercise Physical activity done for the purpose of getting physically fit.

stress. There are several reasons for placing priority on these lifestyles. First, they affect the lives of all people. Second, they are lifestyles in which large numbers of people can make improvement. Finally, modest changes in these behaviors can make dramatic improvements in individual and public health. For example, statistics suggest that modest changes in physical activity patterns and nutrition can prevent more than 400,000 deaths annually. Stress also has a major impact on drug, alcohol, and smoking behavior, so managing stress can help individuals minimize or avoid those behaviors.

The other healthy lifestyles listed in Figure 7 are also very important for good health. The reason that they are not emphasized as priority lifestyles is that they do not affect everyone as much as the first three do. Many healthy lifestyles will be discussed in this book, but the focus is on the priority healthy lifestyles because virtually all people can achieve positive wellness benefits if they adopt them.

The "actual causes" of most deaths are due to unhealthy lifestyles. As illustrated in Table 3, chronic diseases (e.g., heart diseases, cancer) are the direct causes of most deaths in our society. Public health experts have used epidemiological statistics to show that unhealthy lifestyles such as tobacco use, inactivity, and poor eating actually cause the chronic diseases and for this reason are referred to as the "actual causes of death." Tobacco is the leading actual cause of death, but inactivity and poor diet account for the next largest percentage of deaths (see Table 4). The percentage

Table 4 ▶ Actual Causes of Death in the United States		
Rank	Actual Cause	Percentage of Deaths
1	Tobacco use	18.1
2	Inactivity/poor diet	16.6
3	Alcohol consumption	3.5
4	Microbial agents (flu, pneumonia)	3.1
5	Toxic agents	2.3
6	Motor vehicles	1.8
7	Firearms	1.2
8	Sexual behavior	0.8
9	Illicit drug use	0.7
10	Other	<.05

Source: Mokdad et al.

of deaths attributed to inactivity and poor diet has recently been questioned, but their overall influence on health is indisputable. The information presented throughout this book is designed to help you change behaviors to reduce your risk for early death from the actual causes listed in Table 4.

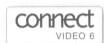
VIDEO 6

Strategies for Action

Self-assessments of lifestyles will help you determine areas in which you may need changes to promote optimal health, wellness, and fitness. The Healthy Lifestyle Questionnaire in the lab resource materials will help you assess your current lifestyle behaviors to determine if they are contributing positively to your health, wellness, and fitness. Because this questionnaire contains some very personal information, answering all the questions honestly will help you get an accurate assessment. As you continue your study, refer back to this questionnaire to see if your lifestyles have changed.

Initial self-assessments of wellness and fitness will provide information for self-comparison. It is important to assess your wellness and fitness at an early stage. These early assessments will only be estimates. As you continue your study, you will have the opportunity to do more comprehensive self-assessments that will allow you to see how accurate your early estimates were.

In Lab 1A, you will estimate your wellness using a Wellness Self-Perceptions questionnaire, which assesses five wellness dimensions. Remember, wellness is a state of being that is influenced by healthy lifestyles. Because other factors, such as heredity, environment, and health care, affect wellness, it is possible to have good wellness scores even if you do not do well on the lifestyle questionnaire. However, over a lifetime, unhealthy lifestyles will catch up with you and have an influence on your wellness and fitness. As each individual makes progress toward improving wellness, we move closer to meeting the HP2020 goal of living long, high-quality lives.

ACTIVITY

Web Resources

American Medical Association (AMA) **www.ama-assn.org**

Centers for Disease Control and Prevention (CDC) **www.cdc.gov**

Health Canada **http://www.hc-sc.gc.ca**

Healthier United States **www.healthfinder.gov**

Healthy People 2020 **www.healthypeople.gov/HP2020**

Institute of Medicine **www.iom.edu**

Kaiser Permanente, HealthAlliance Hospital, CDC, and the Institute for Healthcare Improvement. 2011. **http://xnet.kp.org/newscenter/pointofview/2010/032410healthylife.html**

National Center for Chronic Disease Prevention and Health Promotion Publications **http://www.cdc.gov/chronicdisease/index.htm**

President's Council on Fitness, Sports, and Nutrition **www.fitness.gov**

Robert Wood Johnson Foundation **www.rwjf.org**

Trust for America's Health **http://healthyamericans.org/**

U. S. Government Healthcare **www.HealthCare.gov**

Well-Being Index—Gallup Poll **www.gallup.com/poll/wellbeing.aspx**

World Health Organization **www.who.int**

Web Podcasts (Selected Websites)

Arizona State University on iTunes U—Introduction to Exercise and Wellness **http://itunes.asu.edu**

CDC **www2a.cdc.gov/podcasts**

Johns Hopkins Medicine Podcasts **www.hopkinsmedicine.org/news/audio/podcasts/Podcasts.html**

Journal of the American Medical Association Podcasts **http://jama.ama-assn.org/misc/audiocommentary.dtl**

University of Maryland—Medical Podcasts (Medically Speaking) **www.umm.edu/podcasts/?source-google&gclid=CNS2g7_8oo0CFRfOggodmDi_5g**

U.S. Food and Drug Administration **www.fda.gov/AboutFDA/ContactFDA/StayInformed/RSSFeeds/ucm144574.htm**

U.S. Government Podcasts—Health Podcasts from the U.S. Government **www.usa.gov/Topics/Reference-Shelf/Libraries/Podcasts/Health.shtml**

Suggested Readings

Central Intelligence Agency. 2011. *The World Factbook.* Washington, DC: CIA. Available at **https://www.cia.gov/library/publications/the-world-factbook/**

Owen, N., et al. 2010. Too much sitting: The population health science of sedentary behavior. *Exercise and Sport Sciences Reviews.* 38(3):105–1113.

Sebastiani, P., et al. 2010. Genetic signatures of exceptional longevity in humans. *Science.* Published online July 1, 2010, **www.sciencemag.org**

Trust for America's Health. 2008. *Blueprint for a Healthier America.* Washington, DC: Trust for America's Health. Available at **http://healthyamericans.org/report/55/blueprint-for-healthier-america**

United Nations Report on Non-Communicable Diseases. 2011. Available at **www.un.org/en/ga/president/65/issues/**

World Health Organization. 2011. *World Report on Disability.* Geneva: WHO. Available at **www.who.int/publications/en**

World Health Statistics 2012. Available at **www.who.int/gho/publications/world_health_statistics/2012/en/index.html**

Healthy People 2020

The *Healthy People 2020* goals provide health targets for the nation to achieve by the year 2020. The following goals relate specifically to the content of this concept:

- Create a society in which all people live long, healthy lives.
- Promote quality of life, healthy development, and healthy behaviors (including being active, eating well, and avoiding destructive habits) across all stages of life.
- Attain high-quality, longer lives free of preventable disease, injury, and premature death.
- Achieve health equity, eliminate disparities, and improve the health of all groups.
- Create social and physical environments that promote good health for all.
- Increase public awareness and understanding of the determinants of health, disease, and disability.

The national health goals emphasize "high-quality" living and "quality of life." How do these national goals relate to health, wellness, and fitness as defined in this concept?

Lab Resource Materials: The Healthy Lifestyle Questionnaire

The purpose of this questionnaire is to help you analyze your lifestyle behaviors and to help you make decisions concerning good health and wellness for the future. Information on this Healthy Lifestyle Questionnaire is of a personal nature. For this reason, this questionnaire is not designed to be submitted to your instructor. **It is for your information only.** Answer each question as honestly as possible, and use the scoring information to help assess your lifestyle.

Directions: Place an X over the "yes" circle to answer yes. If you answer "no," make no mark. Score the questionnaire using the procedures that follow.

(yes) **1.** I accumulate 30 minutes of moderate physical activity most days of the week (brisk walking, stair climbing, yard work, or home chores).

(yes) **2.** I do vigorous activity that elevates my heart rate for 20 minutes at least 3 days a week.

(yes) **3.** I do exercises for flexibility at least 3 days a week.

(yes) **4.** I do exercises for muscle fitness at least 2 days a week.

(yes) **5.** I eat three regular meals each day.

(yes) **6.** I select appropriate servings from the major food groups each day.

(yes) **7.** I restrict the amount of fat in my diet.

(yes) **8.** I consume only as many calories as I expend each day.

(yes) **9.** I am able to identify situations in daily life that cause stress.

(yes) **10.** I take time out during the day to relax and recover from daily stress.

(yes) **11.** I find time for family, friends, and things I especially enjoy doing.

(yes) **12.** I regularly perform exercises designed to relieve tension.

(yes) **13.** I do not smoke or use other tobacco products.

(yes) **14.** I do not abuse alcohol.

(yes) **15.** I do not abuse drugs (prescription or illegal).

(yes) **16.** I take over-the-counter drugs sparingly and use them only according to directions.

(yes) **17.** I abstain from sex or limit sexual activity to a safe partner.

(yes) **18.** I practice safe procedures for avoiding sexually transmitted infections (STIs).

(yes) **19.** I use seat belts and adhere to the speed limit when I drive.

(yes) **20.** I have a smoke detector in my house and check it regularly to see that it is working.

(yes) **21.** I have had training to perform CPR if called on in an emergency.

(yes) **22.** I can perform the Heimlich maneuver effectively if called on in an emergency.

(yes) **23.** I brush my teeth at least twice a day and floss at least once a day.

(yes) **24.** I get an adequate amount of sleep each night.

(yes) **25.** I do regular self-exams, have regular medical checkups, and seek medical advice when symptoms are present.

(yes) **26.** When I receive advice and/or medication from a physician, I follow the advice and take the medication as prescribed.

(yes) **27.** I read product labels and investigate their effectiveness before I buy them.

(yes) **28.** I avoid using products that have not been shown by research to be effective.

(yes) **29.** I recycle paper, glass, and aluminum.

(yes) **30.** I practice environmental protection, such as carpooling and energy conservation.

Overall Score—Total "Yes" Answers

Scoring: Give yourself 1 point for each "yes" answer. Add your scores for each of the lifestyle behaviors. To calculate your overall score, sum the totals for all lifestyles.

Physical Activity

1. ☐
2. ☐
3. ☐
4. ☐
☐ Total +

Nutrition

5. ☐
6. ☐
7. ☐
8. ☐
☐ Total +

Managing Stress

9. ☐
10. ☐
11. ☐
12. ☐
☐ Total +

Avoiding Destructive Habits

13. ☐
14. ☐
15. ☐
16. ☐
☐ Total +

Practicing Safe Sex

17. ☐
18. ☐
☐ Total +

Adopting Safety Habits

19. ☐
20. ☐
☐

Knowing First Aid

21. ☐
22. ☐
☐ Total +

Personal Health Habits

23. ☐
24. ☐
☐ Total +

Using Medical Advice

25. ☐
26. ☐
☐ Total +

Being an Informed Consumer

27. ☐
28. ☐
☐ Total +

Protecting the Environment

29. ☐
30. ☐
☐ Total =

Sum All Totals for Overall Score

☐

Interpreting Scores: Scores of 3 or 4 on the four-item scales indicate generally positive lifestyles. For the two-item scales, a score of 2 indicates the presence of positive lifestyles. An overall score of 26 or more is a good indicator of healthy lifestyle behaviors. It is important to consider the following special note when interpreting scores.

Special Note: Your scores on the Healthy Lifestyle Questionnaire should be interpreted with caution. There are several reasons for this. First, all lifestyle behaviors do not pose the same risks. For example, using tobacco or abusing drugs has immediate negative effects on health and wellness, whereas others, such as knowing first aid, may have only occasional use. Second, you may score well on one item in a scale but not on another. If one item indicates an unhealthy lifestyle in an area that poses a serious health risk, your lifestyle may appear to be healthier than it really is. For example, you could get a score of 3 on the destructive habits scale and be a regular smoker. For this reason, the overall score can be particularly deceiving.

Strategies for Change: In the space to the right, make some notes concerning the healthy lifestyle areas in which you could make some changes. You can refer to these notes later to see if you have made progress.

Healthy Lifestyle Ratings

Rating	Two-Item Scores	Four-Item Scores	Overall Scores
Positive lifestyles	2	3 or 4	26 to 30*
Consider changes	Less than 2	Less than 3	Less than 26

*See Special Note.

Lab 1A Wellness Self-Perceptions

Name	**Section** **Date**

Purpose: To assess self-perceptions of wellness

Procedures

1. Place an X over the appropriate circle for each question (4 = strongly agree, 3 = agree, 2 = disagree, 1 = strongly disagree).
2. Write the number found in that circle in the box to the right.
3. Sum the three boxes for each wellness dimension to get your wellness dimension totals.
4. Sum all wellness dimension totals to get your comprehensive wellness total.
5. Use the rating chart to rate each wellness area.
6. Complete the Results section and the Conclusions and Implications section.

Question	Strongly Agree	Agree	Disagree	Strongly Disagree	Score
1. I am happy most of the time.	4	3	2	1	
2. I have good self-esteem.	4	3	2	1	
3. I do not generally feel stressed.	4	3	2	1	
			Emotional Wellness Total	=	
4. I am well informed about current events.	4	3	2	1	
5. I am comfortable expressing my views and opinions.	4	3	2	1	
6. I am interested in my career development.	4	3	2	1	
			Intellectual Wellness Total	=	
7. I am physically fit.	4	3	2	1	
8. I am able to perform the physical tasks of my work.	4	3	2	1	
9. I am physically able to perform leisure activities.	4	3	2	1	
			Physical Wellness Total	=	
10. I have many friends and am involved socially.	4	3	2	1	
11. I have close ties with my family.	4	3	2	1	
12. I am confident in social situations.	4	3	2	1	
			Social Wellness Total	=	
13. I am fulfilled spiritually.	4	3	2	1	
14. I feel connected to the world around me.	4	3	2	1	
15. I have a sense of purpose in my life.	4	3	2	1	
			Spiritual Wellness Total	=	
			Comprehensive Wellness (Sum of five wellness scores)		

In the Results below, record your scores from the previous page; then determine your ratings for each score using the Wellness Rating Chart. Record your ratings in the Results section.

Results

Wellness Dimension	Score	Rating
Emotional/mental		
Intellectual		
Physical		
Social		
Spiritual		
Comprehensive		

Wellness Rating Chart

Rating	Wellness Dimension Scores	Comprehensive Wellness Scores
High-level wellness	10–12	50–60
Good wellness	8–9	40–49
Marginal wellness	6–7	30–39
Low-level wellness	Below 6	Below 30

Conclusions and Implications: In the space provided below, describe your current state of wellness. Do you think the ratings indicate your true state of wellness? Which areas need the most improvement?

Self-Management and Self-Planning Skills for Health Behavior Change

LEARNING OBJECTIVES

After completing the study of this concept, you will be able to:

▶ Identify and define the five stages of change and explain how the stages relate to making lifestyle changes.

▶ Describe the four key factors that influence health behaviors, describe components in each category, and explain how the factors relate to stages of change.

▶ Identify and describe the self-management skills that predispose and enable you to change and reinforce changes once you have made them.

▶ Identify and describe the six steps in self-planning and explain how they can be used to make personal plans for behavior change.

▶ Conduct self-assessments of your current stages for health behaviors and your self-management skills for making health behavior change.

▶ Identify related national health goals and show how meeting personal goals can contribute to reaching national goals.

Learning and regularly using self-management skills can help you adopt and maintain healthy lifestyles throughout life.

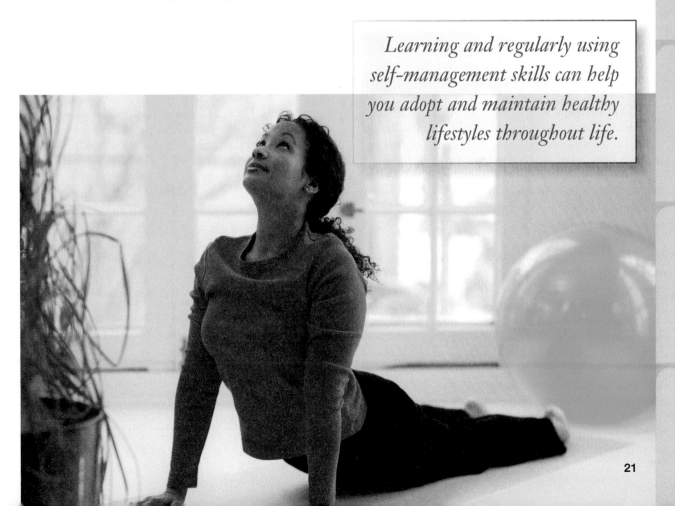

Reducing illness and debilitating conditions and promoting wellness and fitness are important public health goals. As noted in Concept 1, adopting healthy lifestyles is a key factor in health, wellness, and fitness promotion, but evidence suggests that many people are not able to make changes, even when they want to do so. Experts have determined that people who practice healthy lifestyles possess certain characteristics. These characteristics, including personal responsibility, can be modified to improve the health behaviors of all people. Researchers have also identified several special skills, referred to as self-management skills, that can be useful in altering factors related to adherence and ultimately in making lifestyle changes. Like any skill, self-management skills must be practiced if they are to be useful. The factors relating to adherence and the self-management skills described in this concept can be applied to a wide variety of healthy lifestyles. The early sections of this book focus on using self-management skills to become and stay active throughout life. Later sections focus on using these skills to adopt other healthy lifestyles that promote good health and wellness. In the final section, you get an opportunity to use the skills to make informed choices and plan for healthy living.

Making Lifestyle Changes

Many adults want to make lifestyle changes but find changes hard to make. Results of several national public opinion polls show that adults often have difficulty making desired lifestyle changes. Examples include those who believe that physical activity is important but do not get enough exercise to promote good health, those who have tried numerous times to lose weight but have failed, those who know good nutrition is good for health but do not eat well, and those who feel stress on a regular basis but have not found a way to become less stressed. Changes in other lifestyles are frequently desired but often not accomplished. More information about public opinion polls related to health is presented in the "In the News" feature.

Practicing one healthy lifestyle does not mean you will practice another, though adopting one healthy behavior often leads to the adoption of another. College students are more likely to participate in regular physical activity than are older adults. However, they are also much more likely to eat poorly and abuse alcohol. Many young women adopt low-fat diets to avoid weight gain and smoke because they mistakenly believe that smoking will contribute to long-term weight maintenance. These examples illustrate the fact that practicing one healthy lifestyle does not ensure **adherence** to another. However, there is evidence that making one lifestyle change often makes it easier to make other changes. For example, smokers who

have started regular physical activity programs often see improvements in fitness and general well-being and decide to stop smoking.

People do not make lifestyle changes overnight. People progress forward and backward through several stages of change. When asked about a specific healthy lifestyle, people commonly respond with yes or no answers. If asked, "Do you exercise regularly?" the answer is yes or no. When asked, "Do you eat well?" the answer is yes or no. We know that there are many different stages of lifestyle behavior.

James Prochaska (a well-known health psychologist) and his colleagues developed the Transtheoretical Model to explain the importance of **stages of change** for understanding behavior. They suggest that lifestyle changes occur in at least five different stages, as illustrated in Figure 1. The stages were originally developed to help clarify negative lifestyles, such as smoking. Smokers who are not considering stopping are at the stage of precontemplation. Those who are thinking about stopping are classified in the contemplation stage. Those who have bought a nicotine patch or a book about smoking cessation are in the preparation stage. They have moved beyond contemplation and are preparing to take action. The action stage occurs when the smoker makes a change in behavior, even a small one, such as cutting back on the number of cigarettes smoked. The fifth stage, maintenance, is reached when a person finally stops smoking for a relatively long time (e.g., 6 months).

The stages of change model (as illustrated in Figure 1) has been applied to positive lifestyles as well as negative ones. Those who are totally sedentary are considered to be in the precontemplation stage. Contemplators are thinking about becoming active. A person at the preparation stage may have bought a pair of walking shoes and appropriate clothing for activity. Those who have started activity, even if infrequent, are at the stage of action. Those who have been exercising regularly for at least 6 months are at the stage of maintenance.

Whether the lifestyle is positive or negative, people move from one stage to another in an upward or a downward

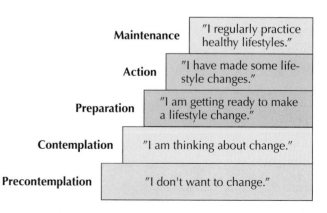

Figure 1 ▶ Stages of lifestyle change.

In the News

Public Opinion Polls about Health, Wellness, and Fitness

Many organizations, both profit and nonprofit, regularly poll Americans concerning their health, wellness, and fitness, as well as their attitudes about these subjects. Among the most well known polls are those by CBS/New York Times, USA Today/CNN/Gallup, NBC/Washington Post, and Trust for America's Health/Robert Wood Johnson Foundation. Some results of surveys by the various polls include the following:

- 76 percent of Americans favor increasing funding for prevention programs.

- 77 percent believe that prevention programs will save money over the long run.

- 72 percent want more investment in prevention—even if it does not save money—because it will prevent disease and save lives.

- 57 percent want to invest in prevention—even if money is not saved—if it improves quality of life (wellness).

- 50 percent believe that more money should be spent on medical and health research.

These results are from different sources and from different types of polls but they collectively show an interest in health, prevention, and wellness. While Americans overwhelmingly support these ideas, there is relatively little money invested in prevention and health promotion research. Funding is often in jeopardy for existing work-site wellness programs and school health/physical education programs.

Why is it hard for organizations to invest more fully in prevention?

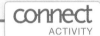

direction. Individuals in the action stage may move on to maintenance or revert to contemplation. Smokers who succeed in quitting permanently report having stopped and started dozens of times before reaching lifetime maintenance. Similarly, those attempting to adopt positive lifestyles, such as eating well, often move back and forth from one stage to another, depending on their life circumstances.

Once maintenance is attained, relapse is less likely to occur. Although complete relapse is possible, it is generally less likely after the maintenance stage is reached. At the maintenance stage, the behavior has been integrated into a personal lifestyle, and it becomes easier to sustain. For example, a person who has been active for years does not have to undergo the same thought processes as a beginning exerciser—the behavior becomes automatic and habitual. Similarly, a nonsmoker is not tempted to smoke in the same way as a person who is trying to quit.

Factors That Promote Lifestyle Change

Various factors have been found to influence the adoption and maintenance of healthy lifestyles. A variety of theories have been proposed to understand health behavior (e.g., Social Cognitive Theory, Self-Determination Theory, Theory of Planned Behavior, Theory of Reasoned Action). Each theory offers some unique attributes or concepts, but they share many of the same components. The previously mentioned Transtheoretical Model integrates elements from multiple theories and can be viewed as a "meta-theory." The distinction between a "theory" and a "model" is

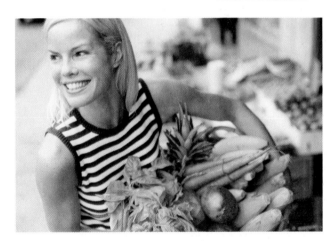

Access to healthy foods is an important predisposing factor for good nutrition.

important in this case. The Transtheoretical Model does not provide a new explanation of behavior (a theory) but rather a guide or map that makes using and applying the theories easier (a model). The unique advantage of the Transtheoretical Model is that it demonstrates that behavior is influenced in different ways depending on the stage of change a person has reached.

Another meta-theory that has been used to explain the challenges of changing health behaviors is the

Adherence Adopting and sticking with healthy behaviors, such as regular physical activity or sound nutrition, as part of your lifestyle.

Stage of Change The level of motivational readiness to adopt a specific health behavior.

Social-Ecological Model. This model also integrates multiple theories, but a key point in this model is that a person's behavior is strongly influenced by the nature of the environment in which she or he lives. If you are in a supportive social environment and have access to healthy foods and activity resources, adopting healthier lifestyles is easier.

You do not need a thorough understanding of the theories and models, but you should be aware of the basic principles. Concepts from both the Transtheoretical and Social-Ecological models have been combined to provide a simpler way to understand the various factors that influence behavior. For ease of understanding, the various factors are classified as **personal, predisposing, enabling, and reinforcing factors** (see Figure 2). Predisposing factors help precontemplators get going—moving them toward contemplation or even preparation. Enabling factors help those in contemplation or preparation take a step toward action. Reinforcing factors move people from action to maintenance and help those in maintenance stay there.

Personal factors affect health behaviors but are often out of your personal control. Age, gender, heredity, social status, and current health and fitness levels are all personal factors that affect your health behaviors. For example, there are significant differences in health behaviors among people of various ages. According to one survey, young adults between the ages of 18 and 34 are more likely to smoke (30 percent) than those 65 and older (13 percent). On the other hand, young adults are much more likely than older adults to be physically active.

Gender differences are illustrated by the fact that women use health services more often than men. Women are more likely than men to have identified a primary care doctor and are more likely to participate in regular health screenings. As you will discover in more detail later in this book, heredity plays a role in health behaviors. For example, some people have a hereditary predisposition to gain weight, and this may affect their eating behaviors.

Age, gender, and heredity are factors you cannot control. Other personal factors that relate to health behaviors include social status and current health and

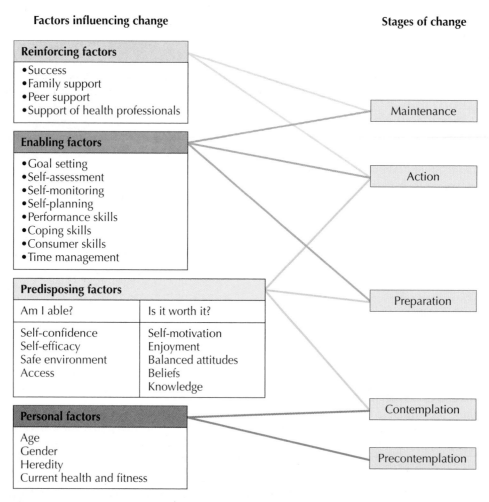

Figure 2 ▶ Factors that influence health behaviors at various stages of change.

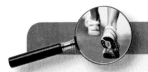

A CLOSER LOOK

Blue Zones

For his book *Blue Zones,* Dan Buettner researched communities across the world that had higher life expectancies and quality of life than other communities. He identified their common characteristics to try to determine the underlying factors that influence good health. He referred to these communities as "Blue Zones" and came up with nine specific attributes that contributed to the improved health. It is not surprising that physical activity (labeled as "Move Naturally") was at the top of the list. (To see the complete list of principles, visit www.bluezones.com.) Some public health groups and agencies have sought to promote broad application of these principles as the basis for coordinated community health programming. The book, in this case, can be viewed as a guide or recipe for healthy communities. However, it may also be likened to a fad diet that might promise an easy path to health and wellness.

Is it possible for communities to follow these recommendations as part of building a healthy community? Why or why not?

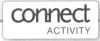

fitness status. Evidence indicates that people of lower socioeconomic status and those with poor health and fitness are less likely to contemplate or participate in activity and other healthy behaviors. No matter what personal characteristics you have, you can change your health behaviors. If you have several personal factors that do not favor healthy lifestyles, it is important to do something to change your behaviors. Making an effort to modify the factors that predispose, enable, and reinforce healthy lifestyles is essential. As shown in Figure 2, the factors influence behavior at different stages of change.

Predisposing factors are important in getting you started with the process of change. Several predisposing factors can help you move from contemplation to preparation and then to taking action with regard to healthy behavior. A person who possesses many of the predisposing factors is said to have self-motivation (also called intrinsic motivation). If you are self-motivated, you will answer positively to two basic questions: "Am I able?" and "Is it worth it?"

"Am I able to do regular activity?" "Am I able to change my diet or to stop smoking?" Figure 2 includes a list of four factors that help you say, "Yes, I am able." Two of these factors are **self-confidence** and **self-efficacy.** Both have to do with having positive perceptions about your own ability. People with positive self-perceptions are more self-motivated and feel they are capable of making behavior changes for health improvement. Other factors that help you feel you are able to do a healthy behavior include easy access and a safe environment. For example, people who have easy access to exercise equipment at home or the workplace or who have a place to exercise within 10 minutes of home are more likely to be active than those who do not. Similarly, access to healthy food options is critical for adopting a healthy diet. A supportive physical and social environment can also make it easier to adopt healthy habits.

"Is it worth it?" People who say yes to this question are willing to make an effort to change their behaviors. Predisposing factors that make it worth it to change behaviors include enjoying the activity, balancing positive and negative attitudes, believing 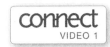 in the benefits of a behavior, and having knowledge of the health benefits of a behavior (see Figure 2). If you enjoy something and feel good about it (have positive attitudes and beliefs), you will be self-motivated to do it. It will be

Personal Factors Factors, such as age or gender, related to healthy lifestyle adherence but not typically under personal control.

Predisposing Factors Factors that make you more likely to adopt a healthy lifestyle, such as participation in regular physical activity, as part of your normal routine.

Enabling Factors Factors that help you carry out your healthy lifestyle plan.

Reinforcing Factors Factors that provide encouragement to maintain healthy lifestyles, such as physical activity, for a lifetime.

Self-Confidence The belief that you can be successful at something (for example, the belief that you can be successful in sports and physical activities and can improve your physical fitness).

Self-Efficacy Confidence that you can perform a specific task (a type of specific self-confidence).

Table 1 ▶ Self-Management Skills for Changing Predisposing Factors

Self-Management Skill	How Is It Useful?
Overcoming Barriers	**Lifestyle Example**
Develop skills that make it possible to overcome problems or challenges in adopting or maintaining healthy behaviors. By conquering challenges, you learn skills that help you overcome other barriers to healthy lifestyles.	A person is tempted by snack foods and candy provided by co-workers. Learning to resist these foods takes discipline, but overcoming barriers builds confidence that helps the person stay focused on long-term goals.
Building Self-Confidence and Motivation	**Lifestyle Example**
Take small steps that allow success. With each small step, confidence and motivation increase and you develop the feeling "I can do that."	A person says, "I would like to be more active, but I have never been good at physical activities." Starting with a 10-minute walk, the person sees that "I can do it." Over time, the person becomes confident and motivated to do more physical activity.
Balancing Attitudes	**Lifestyle Example**
Learn to balance positive and negative attitudes. Developing positive attitudes and reducing negative attitudes helps you adhere to a healthy lifestyle.	A person does not do activity because he or she lacks support from friends, has no equipment, and does not like to get sweaty. These are negatives. Shifting the balance to positive things, such as fun, good health, and good appearance, can help promote activity.
Building Knowledge and Changing Beliefs	**Lifestyle Example**
Build your beliefs on sound information. Knowledge does not always change beliefs, but awareness of the facts can play a role in achieving good health.	A person says, "I don't think what I eat has much to do with my health and wellness." Acquiring knowledge is fundamental to being an educated person. Studying the facts about nutrition can provide the basis for changes in beliefs and lifestyles.

worth it. The lifestyle examples provided in Table 1 will help you understand how to apply these predisposing factors to your own lifestyle.

Enabling factors move you from the beginning stages of change to action and maintenance. A variety of skills help you follow through with decisions to make changes in behaviors. Figure 2 lists eight self-management skills that contribute to behavior change. The labs in each concept provide opportunities to learn and apply these self-management skills to your lifestyle. Table 2 explains the importance of each skill and how each one can contribute to behavior change.

Reinforcing factors help you adhere to lifestyle changes. Once you have reached the action or maintenance stage, it is important to stay at this high level. Reinforcing factors help you stick with a behavior change (see Figure 2).

One of the most important reinforcing factors is success. If you change a behavior and experience success, this makes you want to keep doing the behavior. If attempts to change a behavior result in failure, you may conclude that the behavior does not work and give up on it. Planning for success is essential for adhering to healthy lifestyle changes. Using the self-management

skills described in this concept and throughout this book can help you plan effectively and achieve success.

Social support from family, peers, and health professionals can also be reinforcing. There are, however, different kinds of support and some are more helpful than others. Support for well-informed personal choices is referred to as support of autonomy. One example is

HELP   Health is available to Everyone for a Lifetime, and it's Personal

Friends may have a bigger impact on us than we realize. A recent study followed people over 32 years to examine the impact of social connections on health and health outcomes. According to the study, people are more likely to become obese if a friend becomes obese. Similar relationships were found for adult siblings and spouses, though the connection between friends appears stronger. This relationship was not found for neighbors. The authors suggested that there is a clustering of health behaviors in social groups that explain the shared outcomes.

Do your friends hurt or help you maintain a healthy lifestyle?

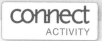

Table 2 ► Self-Management Skills for Changing Enabling Factors	
Self-Management Skill	**How Is It Useful?**
Goal-Setting Skills	**Lifestyle Example**
Establish what you want to achieve in the future. Goals should be realistic and achievable. Learning to set goals for behavior change is especially important for beginners.	A person wants to lose body fat. Setting a goal of losing 50 pounds makes success unlikely. Setting a process goal of restricting 200 calories a day or expending 200 more a day for several weeks makes success more likely.
Self-Assessment Skills	**Lifestyle Example**
Assess your own fitness, health, and wellness and learn to interpret your own self-assessment results. It takes practice to become good at doing self-assessments.	A person wants to know his or her health strengths and weaknesses. The best procedure is to select good tests and self-administer them. Practicing the assessments in this book will help you become good at self-assessment.
Self-Monitoring Skills	**Lifestyle Example**
Monitor your behavior by keeping records. Many people think they adhere to healthy lifestyles, but they do not. They have a distorted view of what they actually do. Self-monitoring gives you a true picture of your own behavior and progress.	In spite of restricting calories, a person can't understand why he or she is not losing weight. Keeping records may show that the person is not counting all the calories. Learning to keep records of progress contributes to adherence.
Self-Planning Skills	**Lifestyle Example**
Plan for yourself rather than having others do all the planning for you.	A person wants to be more active, to eat better, and to manage stress. Self-planning skills will help him or her plan a personal activity, nutrition, or stress-management program.
Performance Skills	**Lifestyle Example**
Learn the skills necessary for performing specific tasks, such as sports or relaxation. These skills can help you feel confident and enjoy activities.	A person avoids physical activity because he or she does not have the physical skills equal to those of peers. Learning sports or other motor skills allows this person to choose to be active.
Coping Skills	**Lifestyle Example**
Develop a new way of thinking about things. Using this skill, you can see situations in more than one way and learn to think more positively.	A person is stressed and frequently anxious. Learning stress–management skills, such as relaxation, can help a person cope. Like all skills, stress-management skills must be practiced to be effective.
Consumer Skills	**Lifestyle Example**
Gain knowledge about products and services. You may also need to rethink untrue beliefs that lead to poor consumer decisions.	A person avoids seeking medical help when sick. Instead, the person takes an unproven remedy. Learning consumer skills provides knowledge for making sound medical decisions.
Time-Management Skills	**Lifestyle Example**
Keep records similar to self-monitoring, focusing on total time use rather than specific behaviors. Skillful monitoring of time can help you plan and adhere to healthy lifestyles.	A person wants more quality time with family and friends. Monitoring time can help him or her reallocate time to spend it in ways that are more consistent with personal priorities.

encouragement from family, friends, or a doctor for starting and sticking to a nutritious diet. The supporting person might ask, "How can I help you meet your goals?" One goal of this book is to help you take control of your own behaviors concerning your personal health, fitness, and wellness.

Not all feedback is perceived as reinforcing and supportive. Although the people providing the feedback may feel they are being helpful and supportive, some feedback may be perceived as applying pressure or as an attempt to control behavior. Scolding a person for not sticking to a diet, for example, or offering the suggestion that "you are not going to get anywhere if you don't stick to your diet," will often be perceived as applying pressure. If you want to help friends and family make behavior changes, avoid applying pressure and attempt to provide positive forms of support. Research also suggests it is desirable to promote autonomy and freedom of choice so that change is

Table 3 ► Self-Management Skills for Changing Reinforcing Factors	
Self-Management Skill	**How Is It Useful?**
Social Support	**Lifestyle Example**
Obtain the support of others for healthy lifestyles. You learn how to get support from family and friends for your autonomous decisions. Support of a doctor can help.	A person has gradually developed a plan to be active. Friends and loved ones encourage activity and help the person develop a schedule that will allow and encourage regular activity.
Relapse Prevention	**Lifestyle Example**
Stick with a healthy behavior once you have adopted it. It can be easy to relapse to an unhealthy lifestyle. Skills such as avoiding high-risk situations and learning how to say no help you avoid relapse.	A person stops smoking. To stay at maintenance, the person can learn to avoid situations where there is pressure to smoke. He or she can learn methods of saying no to those who offer tobacco.

self-directed. Table 3 provides life-style examples of the key reinforcing factors of social support and relapse prevention.

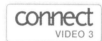

Self-Management Skills

Learning self-management skills can help you alter factors that lead to healthy lifestyle change. Personal, predisposing, enabling, and reinforcing factors influence the way you live. These factors are of little practical significance, however, unless they can be altered to promote healthy lifestyles. Learning self-management skills (sometimes called self-regulation skills) can help you change the predisposing, enabling, and reinforcing factors described in Tables 1 (page 26), 2 (page 27), and 3. In fact, some of the enabling factors are self-management skills. Learning these skills takes practice, but with effort anyone can learn them. This book offers many opportunities to learn and practice self-management skills.

It takes time to change unhealthy lifestyles. People in Western cultures are used to seeing things happen quickly. We flip a switch, and the lights come on. We want food quickly, and thousands of fast-food restaurants provide it. The expectation that we should have what we want when we want it has led us to expect instantaneous changes in health, wellness, and fitness. Unfortunately, there is no quick way to health. There is no pill that can reverse the effects of a lifetime of sedentary living, poor eating, or tobacco use. Changing your lifestyle is the key. But lifestyles that have been practiced for years are not easy to change. As you progress through this book, you will have the opportunity to learn how to implement self-management skills. Learning these skills is the surest way to make permanent lifestyle changes.

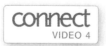

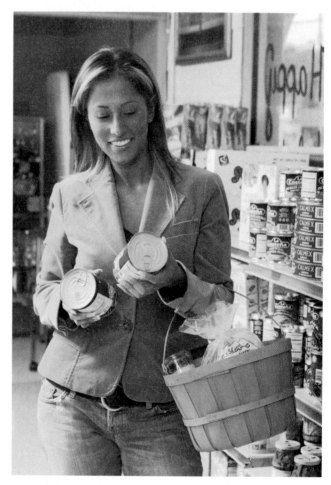

Adopting healthy lifestyle habits requires extra discipline and effort.

Self-Planning for Healthy Lifestyles

Self-planning is a particularly important self-management skill. In the final concept in this book, after you have studied a variety of concepts and self-management skills, you will have the opportunity to develop a personal plan for several healthy lifestyles. Several self-management skills, including self-assessment, self-monitoring, and goal-setting, are used in the six-step self-planning process (see Table 4).

Step 1: Clarifying Reasons

Clarifying your reasons for behavior change is the first step in program planning. People at precontemplation stage are not considering a change in behavior; they see no need. It's when they reach the contemplation stage that they consider changes in behavior. One of the most common and most powerful reasons for contemplating a change in a lifestyle is the recommendation of a doctor, often after a visit associated with an illness. Other common reasons are to improve personal appearance, lose weight, increase energy levels, improve the ability to perform daily tasks, and improve quality of life (wellness). Identifying your reasons for wanting to change helps you determine which behaviors to change first and

helps you establish specific goals. Reflect on your reasons for wanting to make lifestyle changes before moving on to step 2.

Step 2: Identifying Needs

Self-assessments are useful in establishing personal needs, planning your program, and evaluating your progress. You have already done some self-assessments of wellness, current activity levels, and current lifestyles. In the labs for this concept and others that follow, you will make additional assessments. The results of these assessments help you build personal profiles for a variety of health behaviors that can be used as the basis for program planning. With practice, self-assessments become more accurate. For this reason, it is important to repeat self-assessments and to pay careful attention to the procedures for performing them. If questions arise, get a professional opinion rather than making an error.

Table 4 ► Self-Planning Skills

Self-Planning	Description	Self-Management Skill
1. Clarifying reasons	Knowing the general reasons for changing a behavior helps you determine the type of behavior change that is most important for you at a specific point in time. If losing weight is the reason for wanting to change behavior, altering eating and activity patterns will be emphasized.	Results of the Self-Management Skills Questionnaire (Lab 2B) will help you determine which self-management skills you use regularly and the ones you might need to develop.
2. Identifying needs	If you know your strengths and weaknesses, you can plan to build on your strengths and overcome weaknesses.	Self-assessment: In the concepts that follow, you will learn how to assess different health, wellness, and fitness characteristics. Learning these self-assessments will help you identify needs.
3. Setting personal goals	Goals are more specific than reasons (see step 1). Establishing specific things that you want to accomplish can provide a basis for feedback that your program is working.	Goal setting: Guidelines in this concept will help you set goals. In subsequent concepts, you will establish goals for different lifestyles.
4. Selecting program components	A personal plan should include the specific program components that will meet your needs and goals based on steps 1–3. Examples include meal plans for nutrition and specific activities for your physical activity plan.	Many self-management skills, including time management, consumer, and performance skills, are useful in developing plans for a variety of healthy behaviors.
5. Writing your plan	Once program components, such as meal plans for nutrition and specific activities for physical activity, have been determined, you should put your plan in writing. This establishes your intentions and increases your chances of adherence.	Self-planning: This includes writing down the time of day, day of the week, and other details you will include in your plan.
6. Evaluating progress	Once you have used your plan, you will know what works and what does not. Periodic self-assessments can help you modify the plan to make it better.	Self-monitoring: This skill is used in keeping records (logs) and determining if goals are met. Self-assessment: This skill is used to help you determine if goals are met.

Periodic self-assessments can help determine if you are meeting health, wellness, and fitness standards and making progress toward personal health goals. When performed properly, self-assessments help you determine if you have met your goals and if you are meeting health standards (e.g., meeting health fitness standards, eating appropriate amounts of nutrients). Self-assessments also offer a measure of independence and can help you avoid unnecessary and expensive tests. They serve as a screening procedure to determine if you need professional assistance. However, because self-assessments may not be as accurate as tests by health and medical professionals, it is wise to have periodic tests by an expert to see if your self-assessments are accurate.

Self-assessments also have the advantage of consistent error rather than variable error. The best type of assessments are done by highly qualified experts using precise instruments. Following directions and practicing assessment techniques will reduce error significantly. Still, errors will occur. One advantage of a self-assessment is that the person doing the assessment is always the same—you. Even if you make an error in a self-assessment, it is likely to be consistent over time, especially if you use the same equipment each time you make the assessment. For example, scales have limitations for monitoring changes in weight (and fat). But if you measure your own weight using a home scale and your measurement always shows your weight to be 2 pounds higher than it really is, you have made a consistent error. You can determine if you are improving because you know the error exists. Variable errors are likely when different instruments are used, when different people make the assessments, and when procedures vary from test to test. Differences in scores are harder to explain with variable forms of error because they are not consistent.

Step 3: Setting Personal Goals

There are differences between short-term and long-term goals. **Short-term goals** are goals that you can accomplish in days or weeks. **Long-term goals** take longer to accomplish—sometimes months or even years.

There are differences between general goals and SMART goals. **General goals** are broad statements of your reasons for wanting to accomplish something. Examples include changing a behavior such as eating better or being more active, or changing a physical characteristic such as losing weight or getting fit. **SMART goals** are less general and have several important characteristics. SMART goals are specific (*S*). A specific goal provides details, such as limiting calories to a specific number each day. SMART goals are measurable (*M*).

They allow you to perform assessments before you establish your goals and again later to see if you have met your goals. SMART goals are attainable (*A*). They are neither too hard, nor too easy. If the goal is too hard, failure is likely, which is discouraging. If the goal is too easy, it is not challenging. SMART goals are also relevant (*R*). They are your personal goals and should have meaning to you personally. Personally relevant goals provide motivation. Finally, SMART goals are timely (*T*). Timely goals are especially meaningful when you begin a program for making personal changes. Choosing goals that are timely helps you focus on the most salient changes that you want to make.

There are differences between behavioral and outcome goals. A **behavioral goal** is associated with something you do. An example of a specific short-term behavioral goal is *to perform 30 minutes of brisk walking 6 days a week for the next 2 weeks.* It is a behavioral goal because it refers to a behavior (something you do). An **outcome goal** is associated with a physical characteristic (e.g., lowering your body weight, lowering your blood pressure, building strength). Typically, it takes weeks or months to reach outcome goals. This is because outcome goals depend on many things other than your behavior. For example, your heredity affects your body fat and muscle development.

Different factors influence your success in meeting goals. Consider these factors when setting your goals:

- *Outcome goals are not recommended as short-term goals because they take time to achieve.* Typically, it takes weeks or months to reach outcome goals so they make better long-term goals than short-term goals.

- *Outcome goals depend on many things other than your lifestyle behavior.* For example, your heredity affects your ability to achieve an outcome goal such as achieving a certain body weight and or achieving a fitness standard. The same lifestyle change program may produce different results for different people. For this reason, goals must vary from person to person, especially outcome goals. For example, two people may establish an outcome goal of losing 5 pounds over a 6-week period. Because we inherit predispositions to body composition, one person may meet the goal, while another may not, even if both strictly adhere to the same diet. A similar example can be used for fitness and physical activity. People not only inherit a predisposition to fitness but also inherit a predisposition to benefit from training. In other words, if 10 people do the same physical activities, there will be 10 different results. One person may improve performance by 60 percent, while another might improve only 10 percent. This

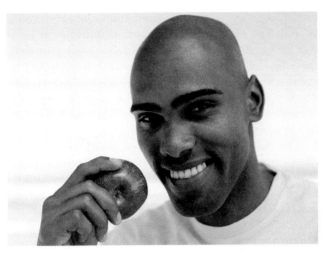

A goal to consume more fruits and vegetables is an example of a behavioral goal.

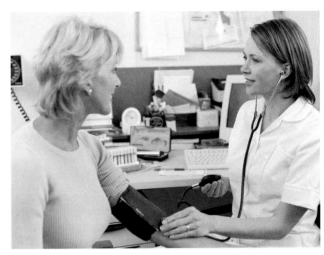

Reducing blood pressure is an example of an outcome goal.

makes it hard for beginners to set realistic outcome goals. Too often, people set a goal based on a comparative standard rather than on a standard that is possible for the individual to achieve in a short time.

Guidelines for beginners differ from guidelines for people who are more experienced when setting goals. Beginners should consider these guidelines:

- *Start with general long-term goals in mind.* It is good to have your goals in mind when you begin a program. But beginners may want to use general rather than specific long-term goals. You may choose either behavioral or outcome goals, but keep them general. For example, choose a goal of losing weight or getting fit. Getting too specific can be discouraging for reasons discussed above.

- *Focus on SMART short-term behavioral objectives.* As noted previously, an example of a specific short-term behavioral goal is *to perform 30 minutes of brisk walking 6 days a week for the next 2 weeks.* It is a behavioral goal because it refers to a behavior (something you do). It is a SMART goal because it is specific, measurable, attainable, realistic, and timely. When using behavioral goals the principal factor associated with success

is your willingness to give effort. No matter who you are, you can accomplish a behavioral goal if you give regular effort. This type of goal will help you keep your motivation level high and prevent you from being discouraged.

- *Avoid frequent outcome self-assessments, focus on self-monitoring of behavior.* A self-assessment before setting goals helps you to set SMART goals. Self-assessments can also help you see if you have met your goals. For beginners, however, frequent self-assessment—especially of

---

Short-Term Goals Statements of intent to change a behavior or achieve an outcome in a period of days or weeks.

Long-Term Goals Statements of intent to change behavior or achieve a specific outcome in a period of months or years.

General Goals Broad statements of your reasons for wanting to accomplish something. Examples include changing a behavior such as eating better or being more active, or changing a physical characteristic such as losing weight or getting fit.

SMART Goals Goals that are Specific (*S*), Measurable (*M*), Attainable (*A*), Relevant (*R*) and Timely (*T*).

Behavioral Goal A statement of intent to perform a specific behavior (changing a lifestyle) for a specific period of time. An example is "I will walk for 15 minutes each morning before work."

Outcome Goal A statement of intent to achieve a specific test score (attainment of a specific standard) associated with good health, wellness, or fitness. An example is "I will lower my body fat by 3 percent."

Make your personal goals **SMART**.

S = Specific
M = Measurable
A = Attainable
R = Relevant
T = Timely

outcomes—is discouraged. For example, if the long-term goal is to lose weight, weighing frequently can be discouraging and even deceiving. Self-monitoring of behavior is encouraged however. For the walking goal discussed above, keeping an activity log of your daily participation will help you comply.

- *Use a series of short-term goals to make progress toward long-term goals.* Once short-term behavioral goals are reached, establish new ones. After meeting a series of short-term goals, consider goal-setting guidelines for more experienced people.

Experienced people should consider these guidelines:

- *Start with SMART long-term goals.* Experience helps people realize that it takes time to meet long-term goals, especially outcome goals. Both SMART behavioral and outcome goals can be considered.

- *Use a series of short-term SMART goals (both behavioral and outcome) as a means of accomplishing long-term goals.* Even experienced people are more likely to achieve success if they realize that setting and meeting a series of SMART short-term goals is important. For example, a person who has high blood pressure (160 systolic) may set a long-term outcome goal of lowering systolic blood pressure to 120 over a period of 6 months. Several behavioral goals can be established for the 6-month period, including taking blood pressure medication (daily), performing 30 minutes of moderate physical activity each day, and limiting salt in the diet to less than 100 percent of the recommended dietary allowance. If the long-term outcome goal is realistic, adhering to SMART short-term behavioral goals will result in achieving the outcome goal.

- *Use self-assessments and self-monitoring to determine if you are making progress.* Self-assessments can be more frequent for the experienced. Still, avoid expecting too much, especially for outcome goals. Self-monitoring of behavioral goals is good, even for the experienced. If you commit to the behavior and stick to your plan, the outcomes will follow.

Maintenance goals are also appropriate once goals have been achieved or when improvements aren't necessary. For example, the person who lowers systolic blood pressure from 160 to 120 need not continue to lower the new healthy blood pressure. Once a healthy outcome goal has been achieved, a new outcome goal of maintaining a systolic blood pressure of 120 is appropriate. Behavioral goals will also have to be modified. For the person who has reduced blood pressure to a healthy level, medication levels might be reduced for maintenance.

Maintenance goals are appropriate in other areas as well. For example, dietary restriction and extra exercise for weight maintenance will likely be different from those for losing weight. When a person reaches a healthy level of fitness, maintenance may be the goal rather than continued improvement. You cannot improve forever; at some point, attempting to do so may be counterproductive to health.

The self-management skills of social support and relapse prevention described in Table 3 are useful in maintenance. Several applications (apps) are now available to help you get social support and prevent relapse (see *Technology Update*).

Making improvement can motivate you to reach long-term goals. As noted earlier, setting short-term goals that are both attainable and realistic will help you reach your long-term goals. Meeting short-term goals encourages and motivates you to continue with your healthy lifestyle plan. Don't expect to set perfect goals all the time. No matter how much self-assessing and self-monitoring you do, you may sometimes set goals too low or too high. If the goal is set too low, it is easily achieved, and a new, higher goal can be established. If the goal is set too high, you may fail to reach it, even though you have made considerable progress toward the goal.

Rather than becoming discouraged when a goal is not met, consider the improvement you have made. Improvement, no matter how small, means that you are moving toward your goal. Also, you can measure your improvement and use it to help set future goals. Of course, periodic self-assessments and good record keeping (self-monitoring) are necessary to keep track of improvements accurately.

Putting your goals in writing helps formalize them. If you don't write them down, your goals will be easy to forget. Writing them helps establish a commitment to yourself and clearly establishes your goals. You can revise them if necessary. Written goals are not cast in concrete.

Step 4: Selecting Program Components

You can choose from many different program components to meet your goals. Concept 1 described 10 types of lifestyle change, ranging from priority lifestyles (physical activity, nutrition, and stress management) to avoiding destructive habits and adopting positive safety and personal health habits. The components depend on the goals of your program. For example, if the goal is to become more fit and physically

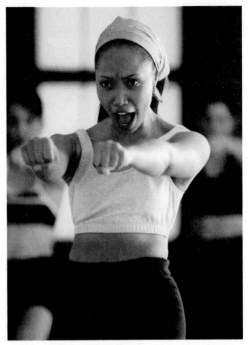

Self-planning can help you implement a variety of changes to enhance health, wellness, and fitness.

active, the program components will be the activities you choose. You will want to identify activities that match your abilities and that you enjoy. You will want to select activities that build the type of fitness you want to improve.

Other examples of program components are preparing menus for healthy eating, participating in stress-management activities, planning to attend meetings to help avoid destructive habits, and attending a series of classes to learn CPR and first aid. Preparing a list of program components that will help you meet your specific goals will prepare you for step 5, writing your plan.

Step 5: Writing Your Plan

Preparing a written plan can improve your adherence to the plan. A written plan is a pledge, or a promise, to be active. Research shows that intentions to be active are more likely to be acted on when put in writing. In the concepts that follow, you will be given the opportunity to prepare written plans for all of the activities in the physical activity pyramid, as well as for other healthy lifestyles. A good written plan includes daily plans with scheduled times and other program details. For example, the daily written plan for stress management could include the time of day when specific program activities are conducted (e.g., 15-minute quiet time at noon, yoga class from 5:30 to 6:30). An activity plan would include a schedule of the activities for each day of the week, including starting and finishing time and specific details concerning the activities to be performed. A dietary plan would include specific menus for each meal and between-meal snacks.

In the labs that accompany the final concept of this book, you will write plans for several different lifestyles. By then you will have learned a variety of self-management skills that will assist you.

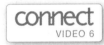
VIDEO 6

Step 6: Evaluating Progress

Self-assessment and self-monitoring can help you evaluate progress. Once you have written a plan, you will want to determine your effectiveness in sticking with your plan. Keeping written records is one type of self-monitoring.

Self-monitoring is a good way to assess success in meeting behavioral goals. Keeping a dietary log or using a pedometer to keep track of steps are examples of self-monitoring. Self-assessments are a good way to see if you have met outcome goals.

Throughout this book, you will learn to self-assess a variety of outcomes (e.g., fitness, body fatness) and self-monitor behaviors (e.g., diet, physical activities, stress-management activities). In step 2 in program planning, you used self-assessments to determine your needs and to help you plan your goals (step 3). Once you have tried your program, you can use the same self-assessments and self-monitoring strategies to evaluate the effectiveness of your program. You can see if you have met the goals you established for yourself.

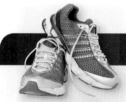

Strategies for Action

To be effective, self-management and self-planning skills require a commitment to make changes in lifestyle. As indicated in Figure 1 on page 22, change occurs stage by stage, and an individual is likely to be at different stages for different health behaviors. For example, a person may be at the maintenance stage for physical activity but at the contemplation stage for adopting sound nutrition practices. In this book, many self-management skills are described for use in progressing from one stage to another. Different skills are important, depending on your current stage and the lifestyle behavior you are attempting to change.

The lab worksheets that accompany each concept will help you learn the self-assessment, self-management, and self-planning skills necessary for behavior change. Self-assessments of current health, wellness, and fitness status, as well as self-monitoring of your current lifestyle, can help you determine your reasons for making change and help you establish SMART goals for change. Like all skills, practice is necessary to improve self-management skills. Table 5 refers you to labs in the text designed to enhance specific self-management skills.

Assessing self-management skills that influence healthy lifestyles provides a basis for changing your health, wellness, or fitness. Self-assessments of your current health, wellness, and fitness status, as well as self-monitoring of your current lifestyles, can help you determine your reasons and establish reasonable goals for healthy lifestyle change. The Healthy Lifestyle Questionnaire and the Wellness Self-Perceptions Questionnaire you took in Concept 1 got you started. In this concept you can use the Stage of Change Questionnaire (Lab 2A) to help you decide which lifestyles you might need to modify. You can use the Self-Management Skills Questionnaire (Lab 2B) to determine which self-management skills you may need to improve to help you make effective changes in your lifestyles. In later concepts, you will have the opportunity to make self-assessments for a variety of lifestyles.

Table 5 ▶ Opportunities for Learning Self-Management Skills

Self-Management Skill	Lab Number
Overcoming barriers	6B, 15A, 17A, 24B
Building self-confidence and motivation	2A, 2B
Balancing attitudes	1A, 2A, 2B, 3C, 8A, 19B
Building knowledge and beliefs	1A, 4A, 7A, 12B, 14A, 15A, 15B, 18A, 18B, 19A, 19B, 20A, 21A, 22A, 22B, 23A, 23B
Goal setting	6A, 8B, 9B, 10C, 10D, 11C, 14B, 24B, 24C
Self-assessment	1A, 2A, 3A, 3C, 4A, 5A, 5B, 6B, 7B, 8A, 9A, 10A, 10B, 10D, 11A, 11B, 12A, 12B, 13A, 13B, 13C, 14A, 15B, 16A, 16B, 22A, 22B, 23B, 24A, 24B, 24C
Self-monitoring	2A, 5A, 6A, 7A, 8A, 8B, 9B, 10C, 11C, 17A, 17D, 19A, 22B, 24B, 24C
Self-planning	6A, 8B, 9B, 10C, 10D, 11C, 14B, 24B, 24C
Performance skills	3B, 12A, 17C
Adopting coping skills	16A, 16B, 17A, 17B, 17C, 17D
Learning consumer skills	14B, 15A, 18A, 20A, 23A, 23B, 24B, 24C
Managing time	17A
Finding social support	17D
Preventing relapse	15A, 19B, 24B, 24C

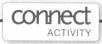

connect
ACTIVITY

Web Resources

ACSM's Fit Society Page **www.acsm.org/access-public-information/newsletters/fit-society-page**

ACSM's *Health and Fitness Journal* **www.acsm.org/access-public-information/acsm-journals/acsm's-health-fitness-journal**

American Heart Association Health and Fitness Center **www.heart.org/HEARTORG/**

American Red Cross **www.redcross.org**

Centers for Disease Control and Prevention (overcoming barriers) **www.cdc.gov/physicalactivity/everyone/getactive/barriers.html**

Healthy People 2020 **www.healthypeople.gov/HP2020**

National Heart Lung and Blood Institute—Health Behavior Change **www.nhlbi.nih.gov/health/public/heart/obesity/lose_wt/index.htm**

Robert Wood Johnson Foundation **www.rwjf.org**

SMART goals **www.projectsmart.co.uk/smart-goals.html**

Trust for America's Health—BluePrint for Healthier America **http://healthyamericans.org/report/55/blueprint-for-healthier-america**

Well-Being Index—Gallup Poll **www.gallup.com/poll/wellbeing.aspx**

Suggested Readings

Benson, G. A., et al. 2011. Telephone-based support for weight loss surgery. *ACSM's Health and Fitness Journal* 15(1):13–19.

Buettner, D. 2008. *The Blue Zones: Lessons for Living Longer from People Who've Lived the Longest.* Washington: DC: The National Geographic Society.

Glantz, K., B. K. Rimer, and K. Viswanath (Eds.). 2008. *Health Behavior and Health Education.* 4th ed. San Francisco: John Wiley and Sons.

Manson, P., and C. C. Butler. 2010. *Health Behavior Change: A Guide for Practitioners.* New York: Churchill Livingstone/ Elsevier.

Marcus, B. E., and L. Forsyth. 2009. *Motivating People to Be Physically Active.* 2nd ed. Champaign, IL: Human Kinetics.

Martin, L. R., et al. 2010. *Health Behavior Change and Treatment Adherence: Evidence-Based Guidelines for Improving Health Care.* New York: Oxford University Press.

Pate, R. R., et al. 2011. Overcoming barriers to physical activity. *ACSM's Health and Fitness Journal* 15(1):7–12.

Pekmezi, D., et al. 2010. Using the transtheoretical model to promote physical activity. *ACSM's Health and Fitness Journal* 14(4):8–13.

Simons-Morton, B., McLeroy, K. R., and M. L. Wendel. 2012. *Behavior Theory in Health Promotion Practice and Research.* Burlington, MA: Jones and Bartlett Learning.

Sullivan, G. S., and J. P. Strode. 2010. Motivation through goal setting: A self-determined perspective. *Strategies* 23(6):19–23.

Taylor, S. E. 2008. *Health Psychology.* 7th ed. New York: McGraw-Hill Higher Education.

White, S. M., E. L. Mailey, and E. McAuley. 2010. Leading a physically active lifestyle: Effective individual behavior change strategy. *ACSM's Health and Fitness Journal* 14(1):8–15.

Whiteley, J. A., and L. A. Milliken. 2011. Making weight loss a family affair. *ACSM's Health and Fitness Journal* 15(2):8–12.

Healthy People 2020

The objectives listed below are societal goals designed to help all Americans improve their health between now and the year 2020. They were selected because they relate to the content of this concept.

- Promote quality of life, healthy development, and healthy behaviors (including being active, eating well, and avoiding destructive habits) across all stages of life.

- Create a society in which all people live long, healthy lives.

- Attain high-quality, longer lives free of preventable disease, injury, and premature death.

- Increase public awareness and understanding of the determinants of health, disease, and disability.

- Increase health literacy of the population.

A national goal is to promote health behaviors across all stages of life. Explain how using self-management skills can help individuals change health behaviors and how individual change can contribute to achieving national goals.

connect
ACTIVITY

Lab Resource Materials

Use the diagram below in answering the questions in Lab 2A. It is a reproduction of Figure 2 and includes factors that influence change in healthy behaviors.

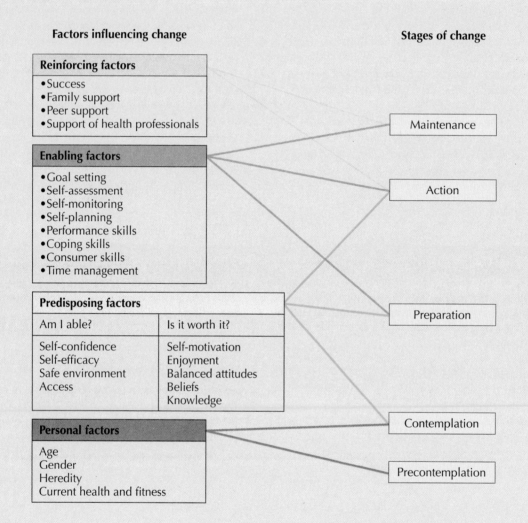

Lab 2A The Stage of Change Questionnaire

Name	**Section**	**Date**

Purpose: To help assess your current level in the stage of change hierarchy for a variety of health behaviors

Procedures

1. Determine your "readiness for change" different health behaviors using the Stage of Change Questionnaire.
2. Evaluate predisposing, enabling, and reinforcing factors for several selected behaviors.
3. Answer the questions in the Conclusions and Implications section.

Results: Complete the Stage of Change Questionnaire on the next page. List two behaviors (below) that you are interested in improving. Beside the behaviors, write your current stage for that behavior.

Behavior 1: _____   **Current Stage?**_____

Behavior 2: _____   **Current Stage?** _____

Conclusions and Implications: For each behavior, discuss the enabling, predisposing, and reinforcing factors that you think are particularly important for you as you work to change this behavior (refer to the stages of change model and Tables 1, 2, and 3 in the text).

Behavior 1:

Behavior 2:

Stage of Change Questionnaire (make one choice for each question)

1. Physical Activity

☐ Precontemplation—I am not active, and I do not plan to start.
☐ Contemplation—I am not active, but I am thinking about starting.
☐ Preparation—I am getting ready to become active.
☐ Action—I do some activity but need to do more.
☐ Maintenance—I have been active regularly for several months.

2. Eating Well (Nutrition)

☐ Precontemplation—I do not eat well and don't plan to change.
☐ Contemplation—I do not eat well but am thinking about change.
☐ Preparation—I am planning to change my diet.
☐ Action—I sometimes eat well but need to do more.
☐ Maintenance—I have eaten well regularly for several months.

3. Managing Stress

☐ Precontemplation—I do not manage stress well and plan no changes.
☐ Contemplation—I am thinking about making changes to manage stress.
☐ Preparation—I am planning to change to manage stress better.
☐ Action—I sometimes take steps to manage stress better but need to do more.
☐ Maintenance—I have used good stress-management techniques for several months.

4. Adopting Good Safety Habits (e.g., seat belt use, safe storage of medicine)

☐ Precontemplation—I have at least one unsafe habit but plan no changes.
☐ Contemplation—I am thinking about making changes regarding a safety habit.
☐ Preparation—I am planning to make a change regarding a safety habit.
☐ Action—I have taken action concerning a habit but need to do more.
☐ Maintenance—I have no safety habits that need to change (I practice good safety).

5. Adopting Good Personal Health Habits (e.g., brushing and flossing, adequate sleep)

☐ Precontemplation—I have at least one health habit that needs change but plan no changes.
☐ Contemplation—I am thinking about making changes related to a health habit.
☐ Preparation—I am planning to make a change regarding a health habit.
☐ Action—I have taken action concerning a habit but need to do more.
☐ Maintenance—I have no health habits that need to change.

6. Learning First Aid (e.g., CPR/First Aid)

☐ Precontemplation—I do not know CPR/first aid and do not plan to learn.
☐ Contemplation—I am thinking about learning CPR/first aid.
☐ Preparation—I have made plans to learn CPR/first aid.
☐ Action—I once knew CPR/first aid but need an update.
☐ Maintenance—I am up-to-date on my CPR/first aid and will keep updated.

Questions 7 and 8 are highly personal. Answer for your own use, but do not record answers on this sheet.

7. Avoiding Destructive Habits (e.g., tobacco, drugs, alcohol)

☐ Precontemplation—I have at least one destructive habit but plan no change.
☐ Contemplation—I am thinking about making changes related to a destructive habit.
☐ Preparation—I am planning to make a change regarding a destructive habit.
☐ Action—I have taken action concerning a habit but need to do more.
☐ Maintenance—I have no destructive habits or have stopped the habit for months.

8. Practicing Safe Sex

☐ Precontemplation—I have practiced unsafe sex and plan no change.
☐ Contemplation—I am thinking about making changes to an unsafe habit.
☐ Preparation—I am planning to make a change regarding an unsafe habit.
☐ Action—I have taken action concerning a habit but need to do more.
☐ Maintenance—I do not practice unsafe sex or have stopped the habit for months.

Lab 2B The Self-Management Skills Questionnaire

Name   **Section**   **Date**

Purpose: To help you assess your self-management skills that are important for three priority lifestyles (physical activity, healthy nutrition, stress management)

Procedures

1. Each question in the questionnaire on pages 41 and 42 reflects one of the self-management strategies described in this text. Each of the 12 questions requires an answer about three different healthy behaviors. Answer each question using a 3 for very true, 2 for somewhat true, or 1 for not true. Record the number of your answer in the appropriate box for each of the three healthy lifestyles.
2. After you have answered all 12 questions for each of the three lifestyles, total the three columns to get a total score for physical activity, nutrition, and stress management.
3. Determine your rating for each lifestyle using the Self-Management Skills Rating Chart. Record your rating in the Results section.
4. Answer the questions in the Conclusions and Implications section.

Results: Record your rating for each of three healthy lifestyles in the chart below.

Self-Management Skills Rating Chart

Rating	Score
Good	30–36
Marginal	24–29
Needs improvement	<24

Self-Management Skills Results	Rating
Physical activity	
Nutrition	
Stress management	

Conclusions and Implications: In several sentences, discuss your ratings regarding self-management skills related to physical activity. You may have a good total score but still have several self-management skills on which you need improvement. Comment on your overall scores and those individual self-management skills on which you had scores of 1 (not true).

In several sentences, discuss your ratings regarding self-management skills related to nutrition. You may have a good total score but still have several self-management skills on which you need improvement. Comment on your overall scores and those individual self-management skills on which you had scores of 1 (not true).

In several sentences, discuss your ratings regarding self-management skills related to stress management. You may have a good total score but still have several self-management skills on which you need improvement. Comment on your overall scores and those individual self-management skills on which you had scores of 1 (not true).

The Self-Management Skills Questionnaire	Very true	Somewhat true	Not true	Activity Score	Nutrition Score	Stress Score
1. I regularly self-assess: (self-assessment)						
personal physical fitness and physical activity levels	3	2	1			
the contents of my diet	3	2	1			
personal stress levels	3	2	1			
2. I self-monitor and keep records concerning: (self-monitoring)						
physical activity	3	2	1			
diet	3	2	1			
stress in my life	3	2	1			
3. I set realistic and attainable goals for: (goal setting)						
physical activity	3	2	1			
eating behaviors	3	2	1			
reducing stress in my life	3	2	1			
4. I have a personal written or formal plan for: (self-planning)						
regular physical activity	3	2	1			
what I eat	3	2	1			
managing stress in my life	3	2	1			
5. I possess the skills to: (performance skills)						
perform a variety of physical activities	3	2	1			
analyze my diet	3	2	1			
manage stress (e.g., progressive relaxation)	3	2	1			
6. I have positive attitudes about: (balancing attitudes)						
my ability to stick with an activity plan	3	2	1			
my ability to stick to a nutrition plan	3	2	1			
my ability to manage stress in my life	3	2	1			
7. I can overcome barriers that I encounter: (overcoming barriers)						
in my attempts to be physically active	3	2	1			
in my attempts to stick to a nutrition plan	3	2	1			
in my attempts to manage stress in my life	3	2	1			

The Self-Management Skills Questionnaire	Very true	Somewhat true	Not true	Activity Score	Nutrition Score	Stress Score
8. I know how to identify misinformation: (consumer skills)						
relating to fitness and physical activity	3	2	1			
relating to nutrition	3	2	1			
relating to stress management	3	2	1			
9. I am able to get social support for my efforts to: (social support)						
be active	3	2	1			
stick to a healthy nutrition plan	3	2	1			
manage stress in my life	3	2	1			
10. When I have problems, I can get back to: (relapse prevention)						
my regular physical activity	3	2	1			
my nutrition plan	3	2	1			
my plan for managing stress	3	2	1			
11. I am able to adapt my thinking to: (coping strategies)						
stick with my activity plan	3	2	1			
stick with my nutrition plan	3	2	1			
stick with my stress-management plan	3	2	1			
12. I am able to manage my time to: (time management)						
stick with my physical activity plan	3	2	1			
shop for and prepare nutritious food	3	2	1			
perform stress-management activities	3	2	1			

Total Activity Score

Total Nutrition Score

Total Stress Score

Preparing for Physical Activity

LEARNING OBJECTIVES

After completing the study of this concept, you will be able to:

▶ Identify and describe key factors for safely participating in a moderate to vigorous physical activity program.

▶ Describe the warm-up, the workout, and the cool-down and explain why each is important.

▶ Explain the potential risks associated with exposure to heat, cold, and altitude and describe precautions that can be taken to prevent problems.

▶ Identify the factors that contribute to soreness and injury from physical activity and describe steps that can be taken to recover from them.

▶ Identify and describe the common positive and negative attitudes about physical activity and explain how they relate to regular participation.

▶ Identify related national health goals and show how meeting personal goals can contribute to reaching national goals.

▶ Assess your readiness for physical activity and demonstrate appropriate warm-up activities.

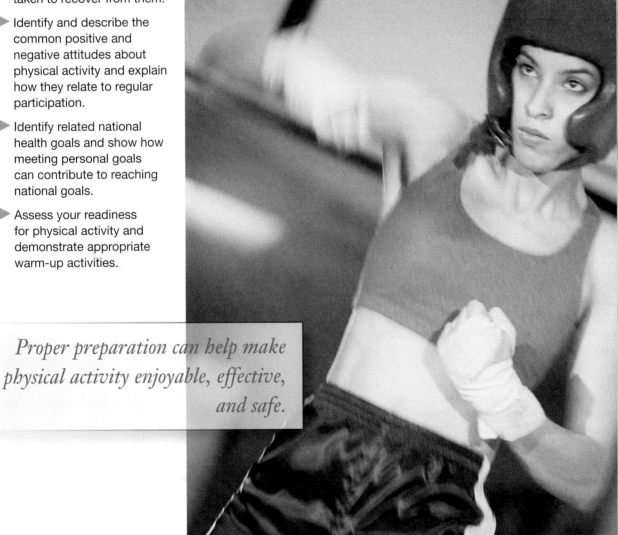

Proper preparation can help make physical activity enjoyable, effective, and safe.

For people just beginning a physical activity program, adequate preparation may be the key to persistence. For those who have been regularly active for some time, sound preparation can help reduce risk of injury and make activity more enjoyable. For long-term maintenance, physical activity must be something that is a part of a person's normal lifestyle. Some factors that will help you prepare for and make physical activity a part of your normal routine are presented in this concept.

Factors to Consider Prior to Physical Activity

Screening before beginning regular physical activity is important to establish medical readiness. The most recent guidelines for exercise testing and prescription of the American College of Sports Medicine (ACSM) suggest that there are two types of pre-participation screening: self-guided screening and professionally guided screening. For self-guided screening, the ACSM endorses the basic recommendation of the *Surgeon General's Report on Physical Activity and Health*, that "previously inactive men over age of 40 and women over age 50, and people at high risk of cardiovascular disease (CVD) should first consult a physician before embarking on a program to which they are unaccustomed."

An alternative method of self-screening involves the use of the Physical Activity Readiness Questionnaire (**PAR-Q**). This seven-item questionnaire was designed by the British Columbia (Canada) Ministry of Health to help people know when it is advisable to seek medical consultation prior to beginning or altering an exercise program. The goal is to prevent unnecessary medical examinations while helping people to be reasonably assured that regular moderate physical activity is appropriate. Other self-administered surveys recommended by the ACSM include those given at a physician's office or those administered by certified health and fitness professionals (e.g., AHA/ACSM Pre-participation Screening Questionnaire). If a pre-participation questionnaire indicates the need, medical clearance is recommended. A **clinical exercise test** may also be appropriate. Those who do not identify health concerns using a self-screening questionnaire (e.g., all "no" answers on the PAR-Q) typically are cleared for moderate self-planned activity programs. For more vigorous exercise and sports, additional screening may be appropriate.

ACSM has developed additional guidelines to standardize professionally guided screening (e.g., assessments conducted by a medical doctor or certified health/fitness professional). As noted in Table 1, the ACSM divides people into three general risk categories: low, moderate, and high risk. Some of the risk factors used

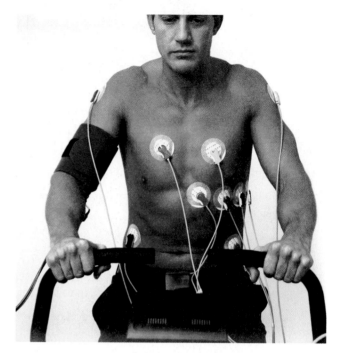

A clinical exercise test—an example of professionally guided screening—is recommended for some individuals to ensure they can exercise safely.

Table 1 ▶ American College of Sports Medicine Risk Stratification Categories and Criteria

Stratification Category	Criteria
Low risk	People who have no heart disease symptoms and have no more than one of the risk factors listed below
Moderate risk	People without heart disease symptoms who have two or more of the risk factors listed below
High risk	People with known pulmonary or metabolic disease, OR one or more signs or symptoms in the list below

Risk Factors

Family history of heart disease; smoker; high blood pressure (hypertension); high cholesterol; abnormal blood glucose levels; obesity (high BMI, excess waist girth); sedentary lifestyle; low HDL cholesterol level; men age 45 or older; women age 55 or older

Signs and Symptoms

Chest, neck, or jaw pain from lack of oxygen to the heart; shortness of breath at rest or in mild exercise; dizziness or fainting; difficult or labored breathing when lying, sitting, or standing; ankle swelling; fast heartbeat or heart palpitations; pain in the legs from poor circulation; heart murmur; unusual fatigue or shortness of breath with usual activities

Source: American College of Sports Medicine.

to identify risk categories are identifiable without professional consultation (e.g., age, family history, smoking, sedentary lifestyle), while others may require professional screening (e.g., blood cholesterol, blood glucose). Many health clubs now offer professional screening for these variables. Individuals found to be at risk are then referred to medical follow-up. Low-risk people who are apparently healthy are typically cleared for moderate and many forms of vigorous activity without a medical exam or an exercise test. Those with moderate risk can participate in low to moderate activity without a medical exam or exercise test; however, both are recommended before initiating vigorous programs. For those in the high-risk category, a comprehensive medical exam is necessary before starting either a moderate or high-intensity program and before taking an exercise test. For those just beginning a program or those resuming physical activity after an injury or illness, consultation with a physician is always wise, no matter what your age or medical condition.

Consideration should also be given to altering exercise patterns if you have an illness or a temporary sickness, such as a cold or the flu. The immune system and other body systems may be weaker at this time, and medicines (even over-the-counter ones) may alter responses to exercise. It is best to work back gradually to your normal routine after illness.

There is no way to be absolutely sure that you are medically sound to begin a physical activity program. Even a thorough exam by a physician cannot guarantee that a person does not have some limitations that may cause a problem during exercise. Use of the PAR-Q (see Lab 3A) and adherence to the ACSM guidelines are advised to help minimize the 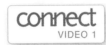 risk while preventing unnecessary medical cost. However, if you are unsure about your readiness for activity, a medical exam and a clinical exercise test are the surest ways to make certain that you are ready to participate.

It is important to dress properly for physical activity. Clothing should be appropriate for the type of activity being performed and the conditions in which you are participating. Comfort is a much more important consideration than looks. Table 2 provides guidelines for dressing for activity.

Shoes are an important consideration for safe and effective exercise. Decisions about shoes should be based on intended use (e.g., running, tennis), shoe and foot characteristics, and comfort. Shoes are designed for specific activities, and performance will typically be best if you select and use them for their intended purpose and fit, rather than how they look. Hybrid shoes, known

---

Table 2 ▶ Selecting Appropriate Clothing for Activity

General Guidelines

- Avoid clothing that is too tight or that restricts movement.
- Material in contact with skin should be porous.
- Clothing should protect against wind and rain but allow for heat loss and evaporation—e.g., Gortex, Coolmax.
- Wear layers so that a layer can be removed if not needed.
- Wear socks for most activities to prevent blisters, abrasions, odor, and excessive shoe wear.
- Socks should be absorbent and fit properly.
- Do not use nonporous clothing that traps sweat to lose weight; these garments prevent evaporation and cooling.

Special Considerations

- Consider eye protection for racquetball and other sports.
- Women should wear an exercise bra for support.
- Men should consider an athletic supporter for support.
- Wear helmets and padding for activities with risk of falling, such as biking or inline skating.
- Wear reflective clothing for night activities.
- Wear water shoes for some aquatic activities.
- Consider lace-up ankle braces to prevent injury.
- Consider a mouthpiece for basketball and other contact sports.

---

as "cross-trainers," can be a versatile option, but they typically don't provide the needed features for specific activities. For example, they may lack the cushioning and support needed for running and the ankle support for activities such as basketball. Features of common activity shoes are highlighted in Figure 1.

Most shoes have very thin sockliners, but supplemental inserts can be purchased to provide more cushioning and support. Custom orthotics can also be used to correct alignment problems or minimize foot injuries (e.g., plantar fasciitis). A very important, and frequently neglected, consideration is to replace shoes after extended use. Runners typically replace shoes every 4 to 6 months (or 400 to 600 miles), even if the outer appearance of the shoe is still good. The main functions of athletic shoes are to reduce shock from impact and protect the foot—one of the best prevention strategies for avoiding injuries is to replace your shoes on a regular basis.

PAR-Q An acronym for Physical Activity Readiness Questionnaire; designed to help determine if you are medically suited to begin an exercise program.

Clinical Exercise Test A test, typically administered on a treadmill, in which exercise is gradually increased in intensity while the heart is monitored by an EKG. Symptoms not present at rest, such as an abnormal EKG, may be present in an exercise test.

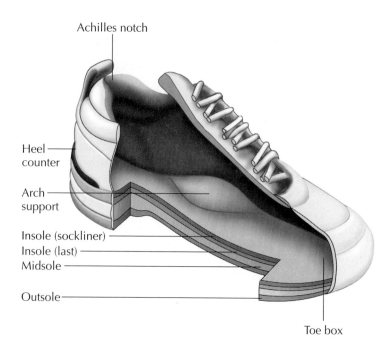

Achilles notch: Protects tendon

Heel counter: Cradles heel to provide movement control; reduces slippage and blistering; a stiff counter reduces pronation

Arch support: Supports arch; height and shape of arch should vary with foot characteristics

Insole (sockliner): Removable layer for additional shock and sweat absorption; can be replaced periodically and/or customized

Insole (last): Refers to shape of shoe bed; curved (allows more mobility; better for those with high, rigid arches); straight (controls excessive motion, better for those with abnormal pronation); or semicurved (moderate flexibility and stability)

Midsole: Provides cushion, stability, and motion control; important for shock absorption

Outsole: Provides traction; determines shoe flexibility; type depends on intended purpose of shoe

Toe box: Should have adequate height to wiggle toes and prevent rubbing on top of toes and adequate length so toes do not contact front of shoe

Figure 1 ▶ Anatomy of an activity shoe.

Factors to Consider during Daily Physical Activity

There are three components of the daily activity program: the warm-up, the workout, and the cool-down. The key component of a fitness program is the daily workout. Experts agree, however, that the workout should be preceded by a warm-up and followed by a cool-down. The warm-up prepares the body for physical activity, and the **cool-down** returns the body to rest and promotes effective recovery by aiding the return of blood from the working muscles to the heart (see Figure 2).

A general warm-up is recommended prior to vigorous exercise. ACSM recommends a general aerobic and muscular endurance **warm-up** consisting of a minimum of 5 to 10 minutes of low-to-moderate aerobic and muscular endurance activity prior to a vigorous workout. Some examples of warm-up activities include walking, slow jogging, slow swimming, slow biking, or low-intensity sport specific movements (e.g., a layup drill in basketball). The general warm-up is intended to prepare the heart, blood vessels, muscles, and other bodily systems for more vigorous activity to follow. The ACSM indicates that the general warm-up increases body temperature and reduces the potential for after-exercise muscle soreness and stiffness, as well as allowing the body to adapt to the demand of the workout that follows. This general warm-up also decreases the risk of irregular heartbeats associated with poor coronary circulation. For those performing moderate activities for their workout (e.g., walk, bike ride, swim), no special general warm-up is necessary since the activity itself is light to moderate in nature. Starting at a slower pace and gradually increasing intensity is recommended.

Consider a muscle-stretching warm-up. Until recently, a muscle-stretching warm-up (stretch warm-up) was recommended after the general warm-up and prior to the workout. A stretch warm-up was thought to help reduce risk of injury, reduce soreness after exercise, and improve performance in sports activities. Recent studies have questioned the value of the stretch warm-up in preventing injury. A recent review also indicates that while stretching may reduce soreness in some, reductions in soreness are only modest. Several studies have indicated that stretching before sports and other types of activities that require strength and power can result in reduced performance. A recent review, however, indicates that performance is only affected if the stretches last 60 seconds or longer. As noted in Concept 10, the recommended length of stretching exercises is 15 to 30 seconds.

The recent evidence, however, does not mean that you should not do a stretch warm-up. Those planning to participate in sports such as gymnastics and diving typically perform a stretch warm-up as do those who perform recreational activities such as dance. For those who have been doing a stretch warm-up prior to other activities, and enjoy it, there is no reason not to continue. A sample of a stretch warm-up is included in Lab 3B. For best results, the stretch warm-up should be done after the general warm-up because stretch is most effective when the muscles are warm. If you plan to do activities in your

TECHNOLOGY UPDATE

Minimalist Running

Running shoes have historically emphasized high-tech shock absorption and cushioning technology, but "minimalist" running and even barefoot running have become increasingly popular. One company best known for making shoe soles has captured runners' imagination with a line of shoes known as the Vibram FiveFingers®. The shoes (which look more like slippers or gloves for your feet) are designed to simulate the feeling of barefoot running while providing protection. They allow you to more easily adopt a forefoot running style rather than striking first on your heel. This change in stride is thought to improve balance, reduce impacts, and improve propulsion. Some studies show that the shoes may reduce chronic knee problems, but it is too early to determine the long-term effects on health or performance. While there is some evidence to support this new approach, experts note that it takes time to retrain your gait. Runners that switch too abruptly can expect to experience considerable soreness, particularly in the calf muscle. Almost all shoe companies now make minimalist shoes or forefoot running shoes and there are varieties for different sports or activities. Advocates of forefoot running include Alberto Salazar, a former U.S. marathon runner and current running coach. Search "minimalist running" or "forefoot running" on the Internet to learn more.

How open would you be to minimalist shoes or forefoot running?

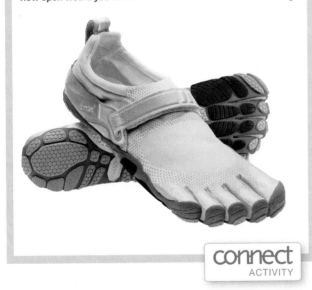

connect
ACTIVITY

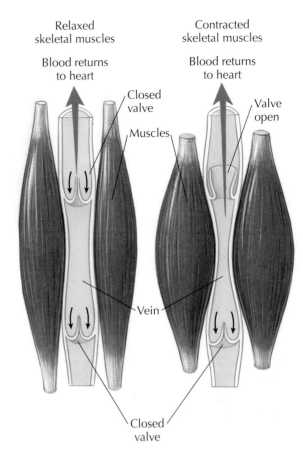

Figure 2 ▶ Muscle contractions help the veins return blood to the heart.

You may choose to do flexibility exercises as part of your workout or after your workout (as part of the cool-down).

Consider other warm-up options. People who plan to perform resistance training or play a vigorous sport should consider a **dynamic warm-up** or a **sport-specific warm-up**. A dynamic warm-up includes the performance

Cool-Down Light to moderate activity done after a workout to help the body recover; often consisting of the same exercises used in the warm-up.

Warm-Up Light to moderate physical activity performed before a more vigorous workout, including a general aerobic/muscular endurance warm-up and often a stretch warm-up.

Dynamic Warm-Up The performance of calisthenics of gradually increasing intensity (e.g., jumping jacks, jumping, skipping).

Sport-Specific Warm-Up The performance of sports-related movements of gradual intensity (e.g., layup drill in basketball, swinging a club in golf or racket in tennis).

workout that involve strength and power, you should not do stretches that last longer than 60 seconds.

The stretch warm-up is not intended to substitute for a regular program of stretching to build flexibility. In other words, if you have not trained regularly to build flexibility, a warm-up is not the best way to get flexible.

of calisthenics of gradually increasing intensity. Those interested in high-level performance (e.g., movements requiring great force, and fast movements) should choose a dynamic warm-up of calisthenics that simulates the types of movements to be used in the vigorous phase of the workout or event. The sport-specific warm-up includes sports-related movements of gradual intensity. Examples include performing layup, shooting, and other drills before a basketball game or swinging a golf club or tennis racket before playing. A general warm-up may be performed before the dynamic and sports-related warm-up or may be used as a general warm-up; however, the initial activities should be of moderate intensity and gradually increase in intensity. As noted previously, if the workout is of moderate intensity, no warm-up is necessary (e.g., 30-minute brisk walk). Some people who plan to perform a more vigorous workout may prefer only a general warm-up.

The workout is the principal component of an activity program and occurs after the warm-up and before the cool-down. The **workout,** also referred to as the conditioning phase of a training session, is the component of the physical activity program that is designed to provide health and other benefits, depending on the type of activity performed (see Concept 4). Workout information, including appropriate frequency, intensity, and length of time for many types of physical activities in the physical activity pyramid (Concept 5), is included in subsequent concepts.

A cool-down after the workout promotes an effective recovery from physical activity. The ACSM recommends a 5- to 10-minute cool-down similar to the general warm-up (e.g., light to moderate activity) after a vigorous workout. In addition to helping reduce metabolic by-products, the general cool-down helps the cardiovascular system (heart rate and blood pressure) return to a normal state.

During physical activity, the heart pumps a large amount of blood to supply the working muscles with the oxygen necessary to keep moving. The muscles squeeze the veins (see Figure 2), which forces the blood back to the heart. Valves in the veins prevent the blood from flowing backward. As long as exercise continues, muscles move the blood back to the heart, where it is once again pumped to the body. If exercise is stopped abruptly, the blood is left in the area of the working muscles and has no way to get back to the heart. In the case of a runner, the blood pools in the legs. Because the heart has less blood to pump, blood pressure may drop. This can result in dizziness and can even cause a person to pass out. The best way to prevent this problem is to slow down gradually after exercise and keep moving until blood pressure and heart rate have returned to

HELP   **Health is available to Everyone for a Lifetime, and it's Personal**

Exercising can lead to serious heat-related problems if the body becomes dehydrated. The body's thirst mechanism usually lags behind the true need for fluids. Experts recommend drinking 1 to 2 cups of water or another hydrating liquid before exercise and then an additional cup every 20 minutes thereafter.

Do you follow these guidelines or could you be dehydrated during or after your typical exercise sessions? What strategies can you use to drink more water?

connect ACTIVITY

near resting values. This phase is especially important for those with cardiovascular risk factors or disease.

The cool-down can also include a stretching phase. Stretching the muscles at the end of the workout, or after the workout, can help relieve muscle spasms in fatigued muscles, and stretching is more effective in building flexibility when the muscles are warm. The ACSM recommends 10-plus minutes for stretching to build flexibility. To be effective, as a complete flexibility program, stretching performed in a cool-down would need to be personalized and include exercises for all muscle groups (see Concept 10).

Physical Activity in the Heat and Cold

Physical activity in hot and humid environments challenges the body's heat loss mechanisms. During vigorous activity, the body produces heat, which must be dissipated to regulate body temperature. The body has several ways to dissipate heat. *Conduction* is the transfer of heat from a hot body to a cold body. *Convection* is the transfer of heat through the air or any other medium. Fans and wind can facilitate heat loss by convection and help regulate temperature. The primary method of cooling is through *evaporation* of sweat. The chemical process involved in evaporation transfers heat from the body and reduces the body temperature. When conditions are humid, the effectiveness of evaporation is reduced, since the air is already saturated with moisture. This is why it is difficult to regulate body temperature when conditions are hot and humid.

Heat-related illness can occur if proper hydration is not maintained. Maximum sweat rates during physical activity in the heat can approach 1–2 liters per hour. If this fluid is not replaced, **dehydration** can occur. If

connect VIDEO 2

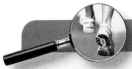

A CLOSER LOOK

CPR Guidelines and AEDs

To be prepared for physical activity, you also need to be prepared for emergencies. For example, it is important to know basic first aid and cardiopulmonary resuscitation (CPR) if needed. Guidelines from the American Heart Association (AHA) have been revised, shifting the order used for performing CPR. The previous method used the A-B-C method to denote *airway, breathing,* and *compressions.* The new guidelines emphasize doing compressions first (C-A-B). Proper certification is recommended, but the guidelines were revised to get more people to help even when not certified (some CPR is better than no CPR). If a person is unresponsive, call for help and begin chest compressions immediately, then open the airway and give mouth-to-mouth rescue breaths along with alternating compressions. Also, automated external defibrillators (AED) are available in many public places, including fitness centers and schools. The AHA offers free online training for CPR and AED devices (visit www.heart.org and search for "Heartsaver® First Aid CPR AED"). The AHA also has a 3-minute video on YouTube titled *AHA Guidelines for CPR* that shows the basic steps.

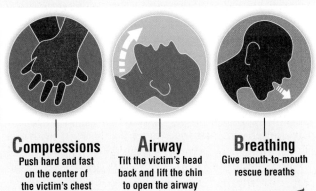

Compressions
Push hard and fast on the center of the victim's chest

Airway
Tilt the victim's head back and lift the chin to open the airway

Breathing
Give mouth-to-mouth rescue breaths

American Heart Association
Learn and Live

©2010 American Heart Association 10/10DS3849

How might the revised guidelines encourage more bystanders to help in a crisis situation? Would you be more inclined to provide aid?

connect ACTIVITY

---

dehydration is not corrected with water or other fluid-replacement drinks, it becomes increasingly difficult for the body to maintain normal body temperatures. At some point, the rate of sweating decreases as the body begins to conserve its remaining water. It shunts blood to the skin to transfer excess heat directly to the environment, but this is less effective than evaporation. **Hyperthermia** and associated heat-related problems can result (see Table 3).

One way to monitor the amount of fluid loss is to monitor the color of your urine. The American College of Sports Medicine indicates that clear (almost colorless) urine produced in large volumes indicates that you are hydrated. As water in the body is reduced, the urine

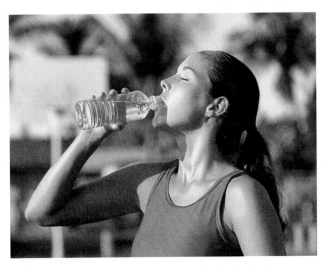

Adequate hydration is critical for safe exercise in the heat.

Table 3 ▶ Types of Heat-Related Problems

Problem	Symptoms	Severity
Heat cramps	Muscle cramps, especially in muscles most used in exercise	Least severe
Heat exhaustion	Muscle cramps, weakness, dizziness, headache, nausea, clammy skin, paleness	Moderately severe
Heatstroke	Hot, flushed skin; dry skin (lack of sweating); dizziness; fast pulse; unconsciousness; high temperature	Extremely severe

Workout The component of a total physical activity program designed to produce health, wellness, fitness, and other benefits using appropriate amounts of different types of physical activity.

Dehydration Excessive loss of water from the body, usually through perspiration, urination, or evaporation.

Hyperthermia Excessively high body temperature caused by excessive heat production or impaired heat loss capacity. Heatstroke is a hyperthermic condition.

Find air temperature on the top; then find the humidity on the left. Find the heat index where the columns meet.

Relative Humidity (%)	Air Temperature (Degrees F)										
	70	75	80	85	90	95	100	105	110	115	120
100	72	80	91	108	132						
95	71	79	89	105	128						
90	71	79	88	102	122						
85	71	78	87	99	117	141					
80	71	78	86	97	113	136					
75	70	77	86	95	109	130					
70	70	77	85	93	106	124	144				
65	70	76	83	91	102	119	138				
60	70	76	82	90	100	114	132	149			
55	69	75	81	89	98	110	126	142			
50	69	75	81	88	96	107	120	135	150		
45	68	74	80	87	95	104	115	129	143		
40	68	74	79	86	93	101	110	123	137	151	
35	67	73	79	85	91	98	107	118	130	143	
30	67	73	78	84	90	96	104	113	123	135	148
25	66	72	77	83	88	94	101	109	117	127	139
20	66	72	77	82	87	93	99	105	112	120	130
15	65	71	76	81	86	91	97	102	108	115	123
10	65	70	75	80	85	90	95	100	105	111	116
5	64	69	74	79	84	88	93	97	102	107	111
0	64	69	73	78	83	87	91	95	99	103	107

"Apparent Temperatures"
(Heat Index)

■ = Extreme danger zone
■ = Danger zone
□ = Extreme caution zone
□ = Caution zone
□ = Safe

Figure 3 ▶ Heat index values (apparent temperatures).

Source: Data from National Oceanic and Atmospheric Administration.

becomes more concentrated and is a darker yellow color. This indicates dehydration and a need for fluid replacement. Dietary supplements that contain amphetamine derivatives and/or creatine may contribute to undetected dehydration among some individuals.

Acclimatization improves the body's tolerance in the heat. Individuals with good fitness will respond better to activity in the heat than individuals with poor fitness. With regular exposure, the body adapts to the heat. The majority of the adaptation to hot environments occurs in 7 to 14 days, but complete acclimatization can take up to 30 days. As you adapt to the heat, your body becomes conditioned to sweat earlier, to sweat more profusely, and to distribute the sweat more effectively around the body, and the composition of sweat is altered. This process makes it easier for your body to maintain a safe body temperature.

Precautions should be taken when doing physical activity in hot and humid environments. The **heat index** (also referred to as apparent temperature) combines temperature and humidity to help you determine when an environment is safe for activity. The combination of high temperature and humidity presents the greatest risk of heat-related problems in exercise. Physical activity is safe when the apparent temperature is below 80°F (26.7°C). Figure 3 shows the risk of exercise at progressively higher apparent temperatures.

Consider the following guidelines for exercising in the heat and humidity.

- Limit or cancel activity if the apparent temperature reaches the danger zone (see Figure 3).

- Drink fluids before, during, and after vigorous activity. Guidelines suggest about 2 cups before activity and about 1 cup for each 15–20 minutes during activity. After activity, drink about 2 cups for each pound of weight lost. The thirst mechanism lags behind the body's actual need for fluid, so drink even if you don't feel thirsty. Fluid-replacement beverages (e.g., Gatorade, Powerade) are designed to provide added energy (from carbohydrates) without impeding hydration. If you choose to use one of these beverages, select one that contains electrolytes and no more than 4 to 8 percent carbohydrates.

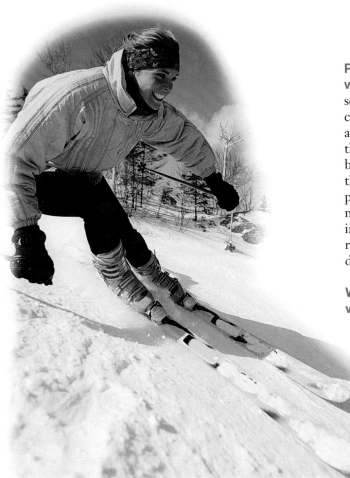

Wind, cold, and altitude present some additional challenges for winter exercise.

- Avoid extreme fluid intake. Drinking too much water can cause a condition called **hyponatremia,** sometimes referred to as "water intoxication." It occurs when you drink too much water, resulting in the dilution of the electrolytes in the blood; interestingly, it has symptoms similar to those of dehydration. If left untreated, it can result in loss of consciousness and even death.

- Gradually expose yourself to physical activity in hot and humid environments to facilitate acclimatization.

- Dress properly for exercise in the heat and humidity. Wear white or light colors that reflect rather than absorb heat. Select wickable clothes instead of cotton to aid evaporative cooling. Rubber, plastic, or other nonporous clothing is especially dangerous. A porous hat or cap can help when exercising in direct sunlight.

- Watch for signs of heat stress (see Table 3). If signs are present, stop immediately, get out of the heat, remove excess clothing, and drink cool water. Seek medical attention if symptoms progress. Consider cold water immersion for heat stroke.

Physical activity in exceptionally cold and windy weather can be dangerous. Activity in the cold presents the opposite problems as exercise in the heat. In the cold, the primary goal is to retain the body's heat and avoid **hypothermia** and frostbite. Early signs of hypothermia include shivering and cold extremities caused by blood shunted to the body core to conserve heat. As the core temperature continues to drop, heart rate, respiration, and reflexes are depressed. Subsequently, cognitive functions decrease, speech and movement become impaired, and bizarre behavior may occur. Frostbite results from water crystallizing in the tissues, causing cell destruction.

When doing activity in cold, wet, and windy weather, precautions should be taken. A combination of cold and wind (windchill) poses the greatest danger for cold-related problems during exercise. Research conducted in Canada, in cooperation with the U.S. National Weather Service, produced tables for determining **windchill factor** and the time of exposure necessary to get frostbite (see Figure 4). Consider the following guidelines for performing physical activity in cold and wind:

- Limit or cancel activity if the windchill factor reaches the danger zone (see Figure 4).

- Dress properly. Wear light clothing in several layers rather than one heavy garment. The layer of clothing closest to the body should transfer (wick) moisture away from the skin to a second, more absorbent layer.

Heat Index An index based on a combination of temperature and humidity that is used to determine if it is dangerous to perform physical activity in hot, humid weather (also called apparent temperature).

Hyponatremia A condition caused by excess water intake, called "water intoxication," that results in a dilution of electrolytes, leading to serious medical complications.

Hypothermia Excessively low body temperature (less than 95°F), characterized by uncontrollable shivering, loss of coordination, and mental confusion.

Windchill Factor An index that uses air temperature and wind speed to determine the chilling effect of the environment on humans.

Actual Temperature Reading (Degrees F)	Estimated Wind Speed (mph)									Minutes to Frostbite
	Calm	5	10	15	20	25	30	35	40	
40	40	36	34	32	30	29	28	27	27	
30	30	25	21	19	17	16	15	14	13	
20	20	13	9	6	4	3	1	0	-1	
10	10	1	-4	-7	-9	-11	-12	-14	-15	
0	0	-11	-16	-19	-22	-24	-26	-27	-29	30
-10	-10	-22	-28	-32	-35	-37	-39	-41	-43	10
-20	-20	-34	-41	-45	-48	-51	-53	-55	-57	5
-30	-30	-46	-53	-58	-61	-64	-67	-69	-71	
-40	-40	-57	-66	-71	-74	-78	-80	-82	-84	

☐ = Caution Zone   ☐ = Risk Zone   ☐ = High Risk Zone   ☐ = Extreme Danger Zone

Figure 4 ▶ Windchill factor chart.

Source: National Weather Service.

Polypropylene and capilene are examples of wickable fabrics. A porous windbreaker keeps wind from cooling the body and allows the release of body heat. The hands, feet, nose, and ears are most susceptible to frostbite, so they should be covered. Wear a hat or cap, mask, and mittens. Mittens are warmer than gloves. A light coating of petroleum jelly on exposed body parts can be helpful.

- Keep from getting wet in cold weather. If you get wet because of unavoidable circumstances, seek a warm place to dry off.

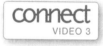

Physical Activity in Other Environments

High altitude may limit performance and require adaptation of normal physical activity. The ability to do vigorous physical tasks is diminished as altitude increases. Breathing rate and heart rates are more elevated at high altitude. With proper acclimation (gradual exposure), the body adjusts to the lower oxygen pressure found at high altitude, and performance improves. Nevertheless, performance ability at high altitudes, especially for activities requiring cardiovascular fitness, is usually less than would be expected at sea level. At extremely high altitudes, the ability to perform vigorous physical activity may be impossible without an extra oxygen supply. When moving from sea level to a high altitude, vigorous exercise should be done with caution. Acclimation to high altitudes requires a minimum of 2 weeks and may

not be complete for several months. Care should be taken to drink adequate water at high altitude.

Exposure to air pollution should be limited. Various pollutants can cause poor performance and, in some cases, health problems. Ozone, a pollutant produced primarily by the sun's reaction to car exhaust, can cause symptoms, including headache, coughing, and eye irritation. Similar symptoms result from exposure to carbon monoxide, a tasteless and odorless gas, caused by combustion of oil, gasoline, and/or cigarette smoke. Most news media in metropolitan areas now provide updates on ozone and carbon monoxide levels in their weather reports. When levels of these pollutants reach moderate levels, some people may need to modify their exercise. When levels are high, some may need to postpone exercise. Exercisers wishing to avoid ozone and carbon monoxide may want to exercise indoors early in the morning or later in the evening and avoid areas with a high concentration of traffic.

Plant pollens, dust, and other pollutants in the air may cause allergic reactions for certain people. Weather reports of pollens and particulates may help exercisers determine the best times for their activities and when to avoid vigorous activities.

Soreness and Injury

Understanding soreness can help you persist in physical activity and avoid problems. A common experience for many exercisers is a certain degree of muscle soreness that occurs 24–48 hours after intense exercise. This soreness, termed delayed-onset muscle soreness **(DOMS)**, typically occurs when muscles are exercised at levels beyond their normal use. Some people mistakenly believe that lactic acid is the cause of muscle soreness. Lactic acid (a by-product of anaerobic metabolism) is produced during vigorous exercise, but levels return to normal within 30 minutes after exercise, while DOMS occurs 24 hours after exercise. DOMS is caused by microscopic muscle tears that result from the excessive loads on the muscles. Soreness is not a normal part of the body's response to exercise but occurs if an individual violates the principle of progression and does more exercise than the body is prepared for. While it may be uncomfortable to some, it has no long-term consequences and does not predispose one to muscle injury. To reduce the likelihood of DOMS, it is important to progress your program gradually.

The most common injuries incurred in physical activity are sprains and strains. A strain occurs when the fibers in a muscle are injured. Common activity-related injuries are hamstring strains that occur after a vigorous sprint. Other commonly strained muscles include the muscles in the front of the thigh, the low back, and the calf.

A sprain is an injury to a ligament—the connective tissue that connects bones to bones. The most common sprain is to the ankle; frequently, the ankle is rolled to the outside (inversion) when jumping or running. Other common sprains are to the knee, the shoulder, and the wrist.

Tendonitis is an inflammation of the tendon; it is most often a result of overuse rather than trauma. Tendonitis can be painful but often does not swell to the extent that sprains do. For this reason, elevation and compression are not as effective as ice and rest. A physician should be consulted for an appropriate diagnosis.

Being able to treat minor injuries will help reduce their negative effects. Minor injuries, such as muscle strains and sprains, are common to those who are persistent in their exercise. If a serious injury should occur or if symptoms persist, it is important to get immediate medical attention. However, for minor injuries, following the **RICE** formula will help you reduce the pain and speed recovery. In this acronym, *R* stands for *rest*. Muscle sprains and strains heal best if the injured area is rested. Rest helps you avoid further damage to the muscle. *I* stands for *ice*. The quick application of cold (ice or ice water) to a minor injury minimizes swelling and speeds recovery. Cold should be applied to as large a surface area as possible (soaking is best). If ice is used, it should be wrapped to avoid direct contact with the skin. Apply cold for 20 minutes, three times a day, allowing 1 hour between applications. *C* stands for *compression*.

Wrapping or compressing the injured area also helps minimize swelling and speeds recovery. Elastic bandages or elastic socks are good for applying compression. Care should be taken to avoid wrapping an injury too tightly because this can result in loss of circulation to the area. *E* stands for *elevation*. Keeping the injured area elevated (above the level of the heart) is effective in minimizing swelling. If pain or swelling does not diminish after 24 to 48 hours, or if there is any doubt about the seriousness of an injury, seek medical help. Some experts recommend adding a *P* to RICE (PRICE) to indicate that *prevention* (P) is as important as treatment of injuries. Building strength and flexibility, warming up, beginning gradually when starting a new activity, and wearing protective equipment, such as lace-up ankle braces, are simple methods of prevention.

Taking over-the-counter pain remedies can help reduce the pain of muscle strains and sprains. Aspirin and ibuprofen (e.g., Excedrin, Motrin) have anti-inflammatory properties. However, acetaminophen (e.g., Tylenol) does not. It may reduce the pain but will not reduce inflammation.

Muscle cramps can be relieved by statically stretching a muscle. Muscle cramps are pains in the large muscles that result when the muscles contract vigorously for a continued period of time. Muscle cramps are usually not considered to be an injury, but they are painful and may seem like an injury. They are usually short in duration and can often be relieved with proper treatment. Cramps can result from lack of fluid replacement (dehydration), from fatigue, and from a blow directly to a muscle. Static stretching can help relieve some cramps. For example, the calf muscle, which often cramps among runners and other sports participants, can be relieved using the calf stretcher exercise, which is part of the warm-up in this concept.

Attitudes about Physical Activity

Knowing the most common reasons for inactivity can help you avoid sedentary living. Most people want to be active but find many barriers get in the way.

DOMS An acronym for delayed-onset muscle soreness, a common malady that follows relatively vigorous activity, especially among beginners.

RICE An acronym for rest, ice, compression, and elevation; a method of treating minor injuries.

Table 4 ▶ Common Reasons People Give for Not Being Active

Reason	Description	Strategy for Change
I don't have the time.	This is the number one reason people give for not exercising. Invariably, those who feel they don't have time know they should do more exercise. They say they plan to do more in the future when "things are less hectic." Young people say they will have more time to exercise in the future. Older people say they wish they had taken the time to be active when they were younger.	Planning a daily schedule can help you find the time for activity and avoid wasting time on things that are less important. Learning the facts in the concepts that follow will help you see the importance of activity and how you can include it in your schedule with a minimum of effort and with time efficiency.
It's too inconvenient.	Many who avoid physical activity do so because it is inconvenient. They say, "It takes too long to get to the gym" and "It makes me sweaty and messes up my hair."	If you have to travel more than 10 minutes to do activity or if you do not have easy access to equipment, you will avoid activity. Locating facilities and finding a time when you can shower is important.
I just don't enjoy it.	Many do not find activity to be enjoyable or invigorating. These people may assume that all forms of activity have to be strenuous and fatiguing.	There are many activities to choose from. If you don't enjoy vigorous activity, try more moderate forms of activity, such as walking.
I'm no good at physical activity.	"People might laugh at me," "Sports make me nervous," and "I am not good at physical activities" are reasons some people give for not being active. Some people lack confidence in their own abilities. This may be because of past experiences in physical education or sports.	With properly selected activities, even those who have never enjoyed exercise can get hooked. Building skills can help, as can changing your way of thinking. Avoiding comparisons with others can help you feel successful.
I am not fit, so I avoid activity.	Some people avoid exercise because of health reasons. Some who are unfit lack energy. Starting slowly can build fitness gradually and help you realize that you can do it.	There are good medical reasons for not doing activity, but many people with problems can benefit from exercise if it is properly designed. If necessary, get help adapting activity to meet your needs.
I have no place to be active, especially in bad weather.	Regular activity is more convenient if facilities are easy to reach and the weather is good. Opportunities have increased considerably in recent years. Some of the most popular activities require little equipment, can be done in or near home, and are inexpensive.	If you cannot find a place, if it is not safe, or if it is too expensive, consider using low-cost equipment at home, such as rubber bands or calisthenics. Lifestyle activity can be done by anyone at almost any time.
I am too old.	As people grow older, many begin to feel that activity is something they cannot do. For most people, this is simply not true! Properly planned exercise for older adults is not only safe but also has many health benefits—e.g., longer life, fewer illnesses, an improved sense of well-being, and optimal functioning.	Older people who are just beginning activity should start slowly. Lifestyle activities are a good choice. Setting realistic goals can help, as can learning to do resistance training and flexibility exercises.

The most common reasons given by people who do not do regular physical activity are listed in Table 4. Experts consider many of these attitudes to be barriers that can be overcome. In fact, as mentioned in Concept 2, a key self-management skill that predicts long-term behavior change is the ability to overcome barriers. The strategies in Table 4 can help inactive people become more active.

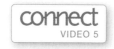

Knowing the reasons people give for being active can help you adopt positive attitudes toward activity. To enhance the promotion of physical activity in society, many researchers have sought to determine why some people choose to be active and others do not. The most common reasons for physical activity are highlighted in Table 5. The table also offers strategies for changing behaviors.

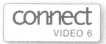

Table 5 ▶ Common Reasons for Doing Regular Physical Activity

Reason	Description	Strategy for Change
I do activity for my health, wellness, and fitness.	Surveys show this is the number one reason for doing regular physical activity. Unfortunately, many adults say that a "doctor's order to exercise" would be the most likely reason to get them to begin a program. For some, however, waiting for a doctor's order may be too late.	Gaining information contained in this book will help you see the value of regular physical activity. Performing the self-assessments in the various concepts will help you determine the areas in which you need personal improvement.
I do activity to improve my appearance.	In our society, looking good is highly valued; thus, physical attractiveness is a major reason people participate in regular exercise. Regular activity can contribute to looking your best.	Setting realistic goals and avoiding comparisons with others can help you be more successful.
I do activity because I enjoy it.	A majority of adults say that enjoyment is of paramount importance in deciding to be active. Statements include the "peak experience," the "runner's high," or "spinning free." The sense of fun, well-being, and general enjoyment associated with physical activity is well documented.	People who do not enjoy activity often lack performance skills or feel that they are not competent in activity. Improving skills with practice, setting realistic goals, and adopting a new way of thinking can help you be successful and enjoy activities.
I do activity because it relaxes me.	Relaxation and release from tension rank high as reasons people do regular activity. It is known that activity in the form of sports and games provides a catharsis, or outlet, for the frustrations of daily activities. Regular exercise can help reduce depression and anxiety.	Activities such as walking, jogging, or cycling are ways of getting some quiet time away from the job or the stresses of daily living. In a later concept, you will learn about exercises that you can do to reduce stress.
I like the challenge and sense of personal accomplishment I get from physical activity.	A sense of personal accomplishment is frequently a reason for people doing activity. In some cases, it is learning a new skill, such as racquetball or tennis; in other cases, it is running a mile or doing a certain number of crunches. The challenge of doing something you have never done before is apparently a powerful experience.	Taking lessons to learn skills or attempting activities new to you can provide the challenge that makes activity interesting. Also, adopting a new way of thinking allows you to focus on the task rather than on competition with others.
I like the social involvement I get from physical activities.	Physical activity can have social benefits. People say, "It is a good way to spend time with members of my family." "It is a good way to spend time with close friends." "Being part of the team is satisfying." Activity settings can also provide an opportunity for making new friends.	If you find activity to be socially unrewarding, you may have to find activities that you, your family, or your friends enjoy. Taking lessons together can help. Also, finding a friend with similar skills can help. Focus on the activity rather than the outcome.
Competition is the main reason I enjoy physical activity.	"The thrill of victory" and "sports competition" are two reasons given for being active. For many, the competitive experience is very satisfying.	Some people simply do not enjoy competing. If this is the case for you, select noncompetitive individual activities.
Physical activity helps me feel good about myself.	For many people, participation in physical activity is an important part of their identity. They feel better about themselves when they are regularly participating.	Physical activity is something that is self-determined and within your control. Participation can help you feel good about yourself, build your confidence, and increase your self-esteem.
Physical activity provides opportunities to get fresh air.	Being outside and experiencing nature are reasons that some people give for being physically active.	Many activities provide opportunities to be outside. If this is an important reason for you, seek out parks and outdoor settings for your activities.

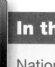

In the News

National Physical Activity Plan

Public health experts realize that comprehensive efforts are needed to increase participation in physical activity in society. The Centers for Disease Control and Prevention (CDC) led efforts to create a National Physical Activity Plan to provide a framework for coordinated action (www.physicalactivityplan.org). The plan includes specific strategies for how activity can be promoted through different settings (business, education, health care, mass media, parks/recreation, public health, transportation, and nonprofits). Each sector presents strategies aimed at promoting physical activity. Each strategy also outlines specific tactics that communities, organizations and agencies, and individuals can use to address the strategy. Separate strategies for promoting physical activity are provided for each sector. Recommendations are also provided to help communities, organizations, agencies, and individuals apply these strategies.

Does this type of coordinated effort help increase participation in physical activity? Why or why not?

Strategies for Action

Screening for risks can help make activity safer. Athletes in competitive sports often undergo pre-participation physical examinations to screen for potential cardiac arrhythmias or conditions known to increase risks during exercise. Recreational athletes may not take the same precautions. The best advice is to get a physical prior to beginning serious training. This is especially critical if you have a family history of heart problems. Lab 3A will help you determine if you should consult a physician.

A proper warm-up can prepare your body for activity and a gradual cool-down can improve recovery. Lab 3B provides a sample flexibility-based warm-up and cool-down routine that may be helpful. Determine what works best for your needs.

Assess your attitudes concerning physical activity. Active people generally have more positive attitudes than negative ones. This is referred to as a "positive balance of attitudes." The questionnaire in Lab 3C gives you the opportunity to assess your balance of attitudes. If you have a "negative balance" score, you can analyze your attitudes and determine how you can change them to view activity more favorably.

Web Resources

American College of Sports Medicine (ACSM) Position Statements **www.acsm.org/access-public-information/position-stands**

- Exercise and Acute Cardiovascular Events
- Exertional Heat Illness during Training and Competition
- Exercise and Fluid Replacement
- Prevention of Cold Injuries during Exercise

ACSM's Fit Society Page **www.acsm.org/access-public-information/newsletters/fit-society-page**

ACSM's Health and Fitness Journal **www.acsm.org/access-public-information/acsm-journals/acsm's-health-fitness-journal**

American Red Cross (AED information) **www.redcross.org**

Med Watch **www.fda.gov/medwatch**
National Athletic Trainers Association **www.nata.org**
WebMD **www.webmd.com**

Suggested Readings

ACSM. 2010. *ACSM's Guidelines for Exercise Testing and Prescription.* 8th ed. Philadelphia: Lippincott, Williams & Wilkins.

ACSM. 2010. *ACSM's Resource Manual for Guidelines for Exercise Testing and Prescription.* 6th ed. Philadelphia: Lippincott, Williams & Wilkins.

Barwood, M. J., Thelwell, R. C., and M. J. Tipton. 2008. Psychological skills training improves exercise performance in the heat. *Medicine and Science in Sports and Exercise* 40(2):387–396.

Bernardot, D. 2007. Timing of energy and fluid intake. *ACSM's Health and Fitness Journal* 11(4):13–19.

Carlson, M. 2012. Exercising in the cold. *ACSM's Health and Fitness Journal.* 16(1):8–12.

Fradkin, A., et al. 2009. Warm-up and physical performance: What is the relationship? A systematic review with meta analysis (abstract). *Medicine and Science in Sports and Exercise* 41(5 Supplement):151–152.

Henschke, N., and C. C. Lin. 2011. Stretching before or after exercise does not reduce delayed-onset muscle soreness. *British Journal of Sports Medicine* 45:1249–1250.

Herbert, R. D., de Noronha, M., and S. J. Kamper. 2011. Stretching to prevent or reduce muscle soreness after exercise. *Cochrane Database Systematic Reviews* 7:CD0045771.

Kay, A. D., and A. J. Blazevich. 2011. Effect of acute static stretch on maximal muscle performance: A systematic review. *Medicine and Science in Sports and Exercise* 44(1):154–164.

Lowry, R., et al. 2007. Physical activity–related injury and body mass index among U.S. high school students. *Journal of Physical Activity and Health* 4(3):225–342.

Perberdy, M. A., and J. P. Ornato. 2008. Progress in resuscitation: An evolution, not a revolution. *Journal of the American Medical Asssociation* 299(10):1188–1190.

Rea, T. D., et al. 2010. CPR with chest compression alone or with rescue breathing. *New England Journal of Medicine* 363(5):423–433.

Stover, B., and B. Murray. 2007. Drink up: Science of hydration. *ACSM's Health and Fitness Journal* 11(3):7–12.

Walter, T., et al. 2011. Active movement warm-up routines. *Journal of Physical Education Recreation and Dance* 82(3):23–31.

Young, S. 2010. From static stretching to dynamic exercise: Changing the warm-up paradigm. *Strategies* 24(1):13–17.

Healthy People 2020

The objectives listed below are societal goals designed to help all Americans improve their health between now and the year 2020. They were selected because they relate to the content of this concept.

- Reduce sports and recreation injuries.
- Reduce injuries from overexertion.
- Reduce emergency department visits for nonfatal injuries.

- Increase the proportion of public and private schools that require students to wear appropriate protective gear when engaged in school-sponsored physical activities.
- Increase health literacy of the population.

A national goal is to reduce sports and recreational injuries, as well as injuries from overexertion. Explain how using the information related to preparing for exercise can help you and others contribute to meeting this national goal.

connect
ACTIVITY

Lab 3A Readiness for Physical Activity

Name	**Section**	**Date**

Purpose: To help you determine your physical readiness for participation in a program of regular exercise

Procedures

1. Read the directions on the "PAR-Q & You" on page 60.
2. Answer each of the seven questions on the form.
3. If you answered "yes" to one or more of the questions, follow the directions just below the PAR-Q questions regarding medical consultation.
4. If you answered "no" to all seven questions, follow the directions at the lower left-hand corner of the PAR-Q.
5. Answer the five questions about physical readiness for sports or vigorous training in Chart 1 below.
6. Record your scores below and answer the question in the Conclusions and Implications section.

Results

Chart 1 Physical Readiness for Sports or Vigorous Training

Answer the PAR-Q before using this chart. If your answer to any of these questions is "yes," you should consult with your personal physician by telephone or in person to determine if you have a potential problem with sports or vigorous training.

Yes	No	
☐	☐	**1.** Do you plan to participate on an organized team that will play intense competitive sports (e.g., varsity team, professional team)?
☐	☐	**2.** If you plan to participate in a collision sport (even on a less organized basis), such as football, boxing, rugby, or ice hockey, have you been knocked unconscious more than one time?
☐	☐	**3.** Do you currently have symptoms from a previous muscle injury?
☐	☐	**4.** Do you currently have symptoms from a previous back injury, or do you experience back pain as a result of involvement in physical activity?
☐	☐	**5.** Do you have any other symptoms during physical activity that give you reason to be concerned about your health?

Determine your PAR-Q score. Place an X over the circle that includes the number of "yes" answers that you had for the PAR-Q (see page 60).

(0) (1) (2) (3) (4) (5) (6) (7)

Determine your readiness for sports or rigorous training (see Chart 1 above). Place an X over the number of "yes" answers that you had for the Physical Readiness for Sports or Vigorous Training chart.

(0) (1) (2) (3) (4) (5)

Conclusions and Implications: In several sentences, discuss your readiness for physical activity. Base your comments on your questionnaire results and the types of physical activities you plan to perform in the future.

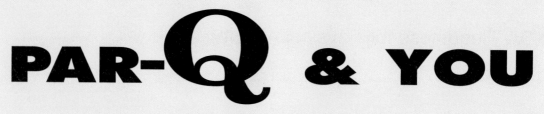

Regular physical activity is fun and healthy, and increasingly more people are starting to become more active every day. Being more active is very safe for most people. However, some people should check with their doctor before they start becoming much more physically active.

If you are planning to become much more physically active than you are now, start by answering the seven questions in the box below. If you are between the ages of fifteen and sixty-nine, the PAR-Q will tell you if you should check with your doctor before you start. If you are over sixty-nine years of age, and you are not used to being very active, check with your doctor.

Common sense is your best guide when you answer these questions. Please read the questions carefully and answer each one honestly: check YES or NO.

YES	NO	
☐	☐	1. Has your doctor ever said that you have a heart condition <u>and</u> that you should only do physical activity recommended by a doctor?
☐	☐	2. Do you feel pain in your chest when you do physical activity?
☐	☐	3. In the past month, have you had chest pain when you were not doing physical activity?
☐	☐	4. Do you lose your balance because of dizziness or do you ever lose consciousness?
☐	☐	5. Do you have a bone or joint problem that could be made worse by a change in your physical activity?
☐	☐	6. Is your doctor currently prescribing drugs (for example, water pills) for your blood pressure or heart condition?
☐	☐	7. Do you know of <u>any other reason</u> you should not do physical activity?

If
you
answered

Yes

YES to one or more questions

Talk with your doctor by phone or in person BEFORE you start becoming much more physically active or BEFORE you have a fitness appraisal. Tell your doctor about the PAR-Q and which questions you answered YES.

- You may be able to do any activity you want—as long as you start slowly and build up gradually. Or you may need to restrict your activities to those that are safe for you. Talk with your doctor about the kinds of activities you wish to participate in and follow his or her advice.
- Find out which community programs are safe and helpful for you.

No

NO to all questions

If you answered NO honestly to <u>all</u> PAR-Q questions, you can be reasonably sure that you can

- Start becoming much more physically active—begin slowly and build up gradually. This is the safest and easiest way to go.
- Take part in a fitness appraisal—this is an excellent way to determine your basic fitness so that you can plan the best way for you to live actively.

DELAY BECOMING MUCH MORE ACTIVE:

- If you are not feeling well because of a temporary illness, such as a cold or a fever—wait until you feel better or
- If you are or may be pregnant—talk to your doctor before you start becoming more active.

Please note: If your health changes so that you then answer YES to any of the above questions, tell your fitness or health professional. Ask whether you should change your physical activity plan.

<u>Informed Use of the PAR-Q:</u> The Canadian Society for Exercise Physiology, Health Canada, and their agents assume no liability for persons who undertake physical activity, and if in doubt after completing this questionnaire, consult your doctor prior to physical activity.

You are encouraged to copy the PAR-Q but only if you use the entire form

*Developed by the British Columbia Ministry of Health.
Produced by the British Columbia Ministry of Health and the Department of National Health & Welfare

Physical Activity Readiness
Questionnaire • PAR-Q
(revised 2002)

Note: It is important that you answer all questions honestly. The PAR-Q is a scientifically and medically researched pre-exercise selection device. It complements exercise programs, exercise testing procedures, and the liability considerations attendant with such programs and testing procedures. PAR-Q, like any other pre-exercise screening device, will misclassify a small percentage of prospective participants, but no pre-exercise screening method can entirely avoid this problem.

Lab 3B The Stretch Warm-Up and Cool-Down

Name	**Section** **Date**

Purpose: To familiarize you with a sample group of stretch warm-up and cool-down exercises

Procedures

1. Perform a 2- to 5-minute cardiovascular warm-up (walk, jog, slow jump rope, swim).
2. Perform the exercises in Chart 1 on page 62, including the alternative exercises, three times each. Hold the stretch for 15 to 30 seconds.
3. Complete the Results section below and answer the questions in the Conclusions and Implications section.

Results: In the following, put an X over the circle that represents the amount of tightness you felt when performing each of the stretching warm-up and cool-down exercises. Tightness indicates that you may have shortness of a specific muscle group and that stretching exercises at times other than the warm-up or cool-down are needed.

Amount of Tightness

	None	Moderate	Severe
Calf stretch	◯	◯	◯
Hamstring stretch	◯	◯	◯
Leg hug	◯	◯	◯
Seated side stretch	◯	◯	◯
Zipper	◯	◯	◯

Alternative Exercises

Side stretch	◯	◯	◯
Hip and thigh stretch	◯	◯	◯
One-leg stretch	◯	◯	◯

Conclusions and Implications: The general cardiovascular warm-up is recommended for all people. In addition, you may want to consider a stretch warm-up and stretch cool-down (as shown in this lab), or a dynamic or sport-specific warm-up option. In several sentences, discuss your experiences with the warm-up/cool-down and what you would plan to use in the future.

Chart 1 Sample warm-up and cool-down exercises

The exercises shown here can be used before a workout as a warm-up or after a workout as a cool-down. Perform these exercises slowly, preferably after completing a cardiovascular warm-up. Do not bounce. Hold each stretch for at least 15–30 seconds. Perform each exercise at least once and up to three times. Other stretching exercises are presented in the concept on flexibility, and they can be used in a warm-up or cool-down.

Cardiovascular Warm-Up

Before you perform a vigorous workout, walk or jog slowly for 2 minutes or more. After exercise, do the same. Do this portion of the warm-up prior to muscle stretching.

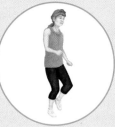

Calf Stretch

This exercise stretches the calf muscles (gastrocnemius and soleus). Face a wall with your feet 2 or 3 feet away. Step forward on your left foot to allow both hands to touch the wall. Keep the heel of your right foot on the ground, toe turned in slightly, knee straight, and buttocks tucked in. Lean forward by bending your front knee and arms and allowing your head to move nearer the wall. Hold. Repeat with the other leg.

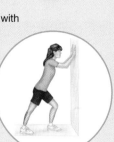

Hamstring Stretch

This exercise stretches the muscles of the back of the upper leg (hamstrings) as well as those of the hip, knee, and ankle. Lie on your back. Bring the right knee to your chest and grasp the toes with the right hand. Place the left hand on the back of the right thigh. Pull the knee toward the chest, push the heel toward the ceiling, and pull the toes toward the shin. Attempt to straighten the knee. Stretch and hold. Repeat with the other leg.

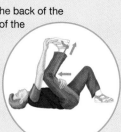

Leg Hug

This exercise stretches the hip and back extensor muscles. Lie on your back. Bend one leg and grasp your thigh under the knee. Hug it to your chest. Keep the other leg straight and on the floor. Hold. Repeat with the opposite leg.

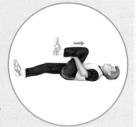

Seated Side Stretch

This exercise stretches the muscles of the trunk. Begin in a seated position with the legs crossed. Stretch the left arm over the head to the right. Bend at the waist (to right), reaching as far as possible to the left with the right arm. Hold. Do not let the trunk rotate. Repeat to the opposite side. For less stretch, the overhead arm may be bent. This exercise can be done in the standing position but is less effective.

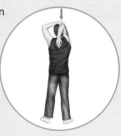

Zipper

This exercise stretches the muscle on the back of the arm (triceps) and the lower chest muscles (pecs). Lift the right arm and reach behind the head and down the spine (as if pulling up a zipper). With the left hand, push down on the right elbow and hold. Reverse arm position and repeat.

ALTERNATE EXERCISES

Because of location (wet or hard surface), you may choose to substitute exercises that do not require you to lie down. The side stretch (standing) can be substituted for the seated side stretch, the hip and thigh stretch for the leg hug (does not stretch the same muscles), and the one-leg stretch (standing) for the hamstring stretch.

Side Stretch

This exercise stretches the trunk lateral flexors. Stand with feet shoulder-width apart. Stretch left arm overhead to right. Bend to right at waist reaching as far as possible with left arm; reach as far as possible with right arm. Hold. Do not let trunk rotate or lower back arch. Repeat on opposite side. Note: This exercise is made more effective if a weight is held down at the side in the hand opposite the side being stretched. More stretch will occur if the hip on the stretched side is dropped and most of the weight is borne by the opposite foot.

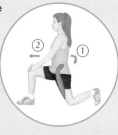

Hip and Thigh Stretch

This exercise stretches the hip (iliopsoas) and thigh muscles (quadriceps) and is useful for people with lordosis and back problems. Place right knee directly above right ankle and stretch left leg backward so knee touches floor. If necessary, place hands on floor for balance.
1. Tilt the pelvis backward by tucking in the abdomen and flattening the back.
2. Then shift the weight forward until a stretch is felt on the front of the thigh: hold. Repeat on opposite side. Caution: Do not bend front knee more than 90 degrees.

One-Leg Stretch

This exercise stretches the lower back muscles. Stand with one foot on a bench, keeping both legs straight. Contract the hamstrings and gluteals by pressing down on bench with the heel for three seconds; then relax and bend the trunk forward, toward the knee. Hold for 10–15 seconds. Return to starting position and repeat with opposite leg. As flexibility improves, the arms can be used to pull the chest toward the legs. Do not allow either knee to lock. This exercise is useful in relief of backache and correction of swayback.

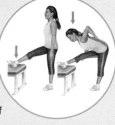

Lab 3C Physical Activity Attitude Questionnaire

Name	Section	Date

Purpose: To evaluate your feelings about physical activity and to determine the specific reasons you do or do not participate in regular physical activity

Directions: The term *physical activity* in the following statements refers to all kinds of activities, including sports, formal exercises, and informal activities, such as jogging and cycling. Make an X over the circle that best represents your answer to each question.

	Strongly Disagree	Disagree	Undecided	Agree	Strongly Agree	Item Score	Attitude Score
1. I should do physical activity regularly for my health.	1	2	3	4	5		Health and Fitness Score
2. Doing regular physical activity is good for my fitness and wellness.	1	2	3	4	5	+ =	
3. Regular exercise helps me look my best.	1	2	3	4	5		Appearance Score
4. I feel more physically attractive when I do regular physical activity.	1	2	3	4	5	+ =	
5. One of the main reasons I do regular physical activity is that it is fun.	1	2	3	4	5		Enjoyment Score
6. The most enjoyable part of my day is when I am exercising or doing a sport.	1	2	3	4	5	+ =	
7. Taking part in physical activity helps me relax.	1	2	3	4	5		Relaxation Score
8. Physical activity helps me get away from the pressures of daily living.	1	2	3	4	5	+ =	
9. The challenge of physical training is one reason I do physical activity.	1	2	3	4	5		Challenge Score
10. I like to see if I can master sports and activities that are new to me.	1	2	3	4	5	+ =	
11. I like to do physical activity that involves other people.	1	2	3	4	5		Social Score
12. Exercise offers me the opportunity to meet other people.	1	2	3	4	5	+ =	
13. Competition is a good way to make physical activity fun.	1	2	3	4	5		Competition Score
14. I like to see how my physical abilities compare with those of others.	1	2	3	4	5	+ =	
15. When I do regular exercise, I feel better than when I don't.	1	2	3	4	5		Feeling Good Score
16. My ability to do physical activity is something that makes me proud.	1	2	3	4	5	+ =	
17. I like to do outdoor activities.	1	2	3	4	5		Outdoor Score
18. Experiencing nature is something I look forward to when exercising.	1	2	3	4	5	+ =	

Procedures

1. Read and answer each question in the questionnaire.
2. Write the number in the circle of your answer in the box labeled "Item Score."
3. Add scores for each pair of scores and record in the "Attitude Score" box.
4. Record each attitude score and a rating for each score (use Rating Chart) in the chart below.
5. Record the number of good and excellent scores in the box provided. Use the score in the box to determine your rating using the Balance of Feelings Rating Chart.

Results: Record your results as indicated in the Procedures section.

Physical Activity Attitude Questionnaire Results

Attitude	Score	Rating
Health and fitness		
Appearance		
Enjoyment		
Relaxation		
Challenge		
Social		
Competition		
Feeling good		
Outdoor		

How many good or excellent scores do you have?

Balance of Feeling Score

Having 5 or more in the box above indicates that you have a positive balance of feelings (more positive than negative attitudes).

Attitude Rating Chart

Rating Category	Attitude Score
Excellent	9–10
Good	7–8
Fair	5–6
Poor	3–4
Very poor	2

Balance of Feelings Rating Chart

Excellent	6–9
Good	5
Fair	4
Poor	2–3
Very poor	0–1

In a few sentences, discuss your "balance of feelings" rating. Having more positive than negative scores (positive balance of feelings) increases the probability of being active. Include comments on whether you think your ratings suggest that you will be active or inactive and whether your ratings are really indicative of your feelings. Do you think that the scores on which you were rated poor or very poor might be reasons you would avoid physical activity? Explain.

The Health Benefits of Physical Activity

LEARNING OBJECTIVES

After completing the study of this concept, you will be able to:

▶ Define the term *hypokinetic* and explain how physical activity can reduce risk of hypokinetic diseases and conditions.

▶ Identify several cardiovascular diseases/conditions associated with physical inactivity and explain how physical activity can help to reduce risk.

▶ Describe metabolic syndrome and explain how physical activity can help to reduce risk of this hypokinetic condition.

▶ Describe additional hypokinetic conditions and explain how physical activity can help reduce risk of them.

▶ Explain the role of physical activity in preventing conditions associated with aging.

▶ Explain the role of physical activity in promoting optimal wellness.

▶ Present an overview of the health and wellness benefits of physical activity and fitness.

▶ Identify related national health goals and show how meeting personal goals can contribute to reaching national goals.

▶ Assess your heart disease risk factors.

> *Physical activity and good physical fitness can reduce the risk of illness and contribute to optimal health and wellness.*

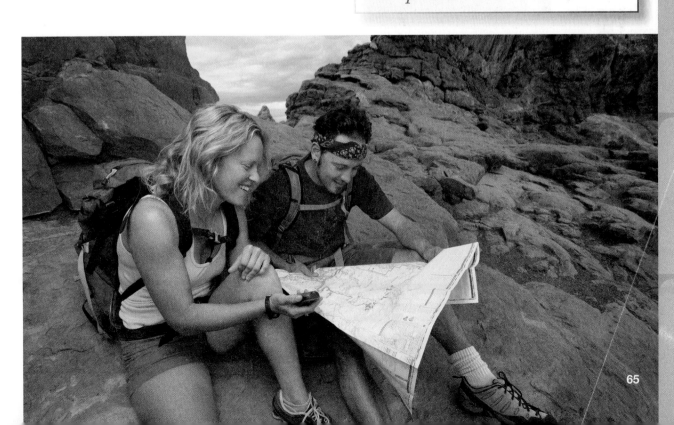

The landmark *Surgeon General's Report on Physical Activity and Health* informed the general public of the risks of sedentary living and the health benefits of physical activity. Since that document was published, even more evidence has accumulated supporting the benefits of an active lifestyle. The first chapter of ACSM's *Guidelines for Exercise Testing and Prescription* and Chapter 2 of the 2008 *Physical Activity Guidelines for Americans* are devoted to the benefits and risks associated with physical activity. Both *Healthy People 2020 and Achieving Health for All* (Canada) highlight the importance of regular physical activity for improving population health in the 21st century. This concept summarizes the health benefits of regular physical activity and good fitness.

Physical Activity and Hypokinetic Diseases

Regular physical activity and good fitness can promote good health, help prevent disease, and be a part of disease treatment. There are three major ways in which regular physical activity and good fitness can contribute to optimal health and wellness. First, they can aid in disease/illness prevention. There is considerable evidence that the risk of **hypokinetic diseases or conditions** can be greatly reduced among people who do regular physical activity and achieve good physical fitness. Virtually all **chronic diseases** that plague society are considered to be hypokinetic, though some relate more to inactivity than others. Nearly three-quarters of all deaths among those 18 and older are a result of chronic diseases. Leading public health officials have suggested that physical activity may offer the most promising public health solution to control chronic diseases, much as immunization controls infectious diseases.

Second, physical activity and fitness can be significant contributors to disease/illness treatment. Even with the best disease prevention practices, some people will become ill. Regular exercise and good fitness have been shown to be effective in alleviating symptoms and aiding rehabilitation after illness for such hypokinetic conditions as diabetes, heart disease, and back pain.

Finally, physical activity and fitness contribute to quality of life and wellness, the positive component of good health. In the process, they aid in meeting many other national health goals.

Too many adults suffer from hypokinetic disease, and the economic cost is high. In 1961, Kraus and Raab coined the term *hypokinetic disease* to describe health problems associated with lack of physical activity. They showed how sedentary living, or as they called it, "take it easy" living, contributes to the leading killer diseases in our society.

A public advocacy group coined the term **sedentary death syndrome (SeDS)** to describe inactive living and associated hypokinetic disease risk factors. They indicate that SeDS is responsible for the epidemic of chronic disease in our society and resulting increases in health costs. In the next few years, expenditures for health care are expected to account for one-fifth of all spending in the United States.

Regular physical activity over a lifetime may overcome the effects of inherited risk. People with a family history of disease may believe they can do nothing because their heredity works against them. There is no doubt that heredity significantly affects risk for early death from hypokinetic diseases. New studies of twins, however, suggest that active people are less likely to die early than inactive people with similar genes. This suggests that long-term adherence to physical activity can overcome other risk factors, such as heredity.

In the News

The Surgeon General's Vision for a Healthy and Fit Nation

A government report by the Surgeon General's Office (*The Surgeon General's Vision for a Healthy and Fit Nation*) emphasizes the importance of healthy lifestyles for improving our nation's health. The report specifically focuses on "helping Americans lead healthier lives through better nutrition and regular physical activity." Combating overweight and obesity through healthy choices is the major goal. The report emphasizes that the current epidemic of overweight and obesity threatens the historic progress we have made in increasing the quality and years of healthy life in Americans. Projections suggest that if trends continue, the current generation will have a shorter lifespan (on average) than their parents.

Does this projected outcome surprise you? What needs to happen to reverse this trend?

connect
ACTIVITY

Physical Activity and Cardiovascular Diseases

The various types of cardiovascular disease are the leading killers in automated societies. There are many forms of **cardiovascular disease (CVD).** Some are classified as **coronary heart disease (CHD)** because they affect the heart muscle and the blood vessels that supply the heart. **Coronary occlusion** (heart attack) is a type of CHD. **Atherosclerosis** and **arteriosclerosis** are two conditions that increase risk for heart attack and are considered to be types of CHD. **Angina pectoris** (chest or arm pain), which occurs when the oxygen supply to the heart muscle is diminished, is sometimes considered to be a type of CHD, though it is really a symptom of poor circulation.

Hypertension (high blood pressure), **stroke** (brain attack), **peripheral vascular disease,** and **congestive heart failure** are other forms of CVD. Inactivity relates in some way to each of these types of disease.

In the United States, CVD accounts for more than 34 percent of all deaths. More than 81 million people currently have one or more forms of CVD. Men are more likely to suffer from heart disease than women, although the differences have narrowed in recent years. African American, Hispanic, and Native American populations are at higher than normal risk. Heart disease and stroke death rates are similar in the United States, Canada, Great Britain, Australia, and other automated societies.

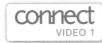

There is a wealth of statistical evidence that physical inactivity is a primary risk factor for CHD. Much of the research relating inactivity to heart disease has come from occupational studies that show a high incidence of heart disease in people involved only in sedentary work. There are limitations in some of these studies but they collectively present convincing evidence that the inactive individual has an increased risk for coronary heart disease. A study summarizing all of the important occupational studies shows a 90 percent reduced risk for coronary heart disease for those in active versus inactive occupations.

The American Heart Association, after carefully examining the research literature, elevated sedentary living from a secondary to a primary risk factor, comparable to high blood pressure, high blood cholesterol, obesity, and cigarette smoke. The reason for this change is that inactivity increases risk in multiple ways and large numbers of adults are sedentary and vulnerable to these risks. The *Surgeon General's Report*

on Physical Activity and Health concluded that "physical inactivity is causally linked to atherosclerosis and coronary heart disease."

Hypokinetic Diseases or Conditions *Hypo-* means "under" or "too little" and *kinetic* means "movement" or "activity." Thus, *hypokinetic* means "too little activity." A hypokinetic disease or condition is associated with lack of physical activity or too little regular exercise. Examples include heart disease, low back pain, and Type II diabetes.

Chronic Diseases Diseases or illnesses associated with lifestyle or environmental factors, as opposed to infectious diseases; hypokinetic diseases are considered to be chronic diseases.

Sedentary Death Syndrome (SeDS) A group of symptoms associated with sedentary living, including low health-related fitness (low cardiovascular fitness and weak muscles), low bone density, and the presence of metabolic syndrome (poor metabolic fitness).

Cardiovascular Disease (CVD) A broad classification of diseases of the heart and blood vessels that includes CHD, high blood pressure, stroke, and peripheral vascular disease.

Coronary Heart Disease (CHD) Diseases of the heart muscle and the blood vessels that supply it with oxygen, including heart attack.

Coronary Occlusion The blocking of the coronary blood vessels; sometimes called heart attack.

Atherosclerosis The deposition of materials along the arterial walls; a type of arteriosclerosis.

Arteriosclerosis Hardening of the arteries due to conditions that cause the arterial walls to become thick, hard, and nonelastic.

Angina Pectoris Chest or arm pain resulting from reduced oxygen supply to the heart muscle.

Hypertension High blood pressure; excessive pressure against the walls of the arteries that can damage the heart, kidneys, and other organs of the body.

Stroke A condition in which the brain, or part of the brain, receives insufficient oxygen as a result of diminished blood supply; sometimes called apoplexy or cerebrovascular accident (CVA).

Peripheral Vascular Disease A lack of oxygen supply to the working muscles and tissues of the arms and legs, resulting from decreased blood flow.

Congestive Heart Failure The inability of the heart muscle to pump the blood at a life-sustaining rate.

Physical Activity and the Healthy Heart

Regular exercise increases the heart muscle's ability to pump oxygen-rich blood. A fit heart muscle can handle extra demands placed on it. Through regular exercise, the heart muscle gets stronger, contracts more forcefully, and therefore pumps more blood with each beat. The heart is just like any other muscle—it must be exercised regularly to stay fit. The fit heart also has open, clear arteries free of atherosclerosis (see Figure 1).

The "normal" resting heart rate is said to be 72 beats per minute (bpm). However, resting rates of 50 to 85 bpm are common. People who regularly do physical activity typically have lower resting heart rates than people who do no regular activity. Some endurance athletes have heart rates in the 30 and 40 bpm range, which is considered healthy or normal. Although resting heart rate is *not* considered to be a good measure of health or fitness, decreases in individual heart rate following training reflect positive adaptations. Low heart rates in response to a standard amount of physical activity *are* a good indicator of fitness. The bicycle and step tests presented later in this book use your heart rate response to a standard amount of exercise to estimate your cardiovascular fitness.

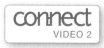

Physical Activity and Atherosclerosis

Atherosclerosis, which begins early in life, is implicated in many cardiovascular diseases. Atherosclerosis is a condition that contributes to heart attack, stroke, hypertension, angina pectoris, and peripheral vascular disease. Deposits on the walls of arteries restrict blood flow and oxygen supply to the tissues. Atherosclerosis of the coronary arteries, the vessels that supply the heart muscle with oxygen, is particularly harmful. If these arteries become narrowed, the blood supply to the heart muscle is diminished, and angina pectoris may occur. Atherosclerosis increases the risk of heart attack because a fibrous clot is more likely to obstruct a narrowed artery than a healthy, open one.

Current theory suggests that atherosclerosis begins when damage occurs to the cells of the inner wall, or endothelium, of the artery (see Figure 2). Substances associated with blood clotting are attracted to the damaged area. These substances seem to cause the migration of smooth muscle cells, commonly found only in the middle wall of the artery (media), to the endothelium. In the later stages, fats (including cholesterol) and other substances are thought to be deposited, forming plaques, or protrusions, that diminish the internal diameter of the artery. This process was once thought to occur later in life but research indicates that the first signs of atherosclerosis begin in early childhood.

Regular physical activity can help prevent atherosclerosis by lowering blood lipid levels. There are several kinds of **lipids** (fats) in the bloodstream, including **lipoproteins,** phospholipids, triglycerides, and cholesterol. Cholesterol is the most well known, but it is not the only culprit. Many blood fats are manufactured by the body itself, whereas others are ingested in high-fat foods, particularly saturated fats (fats that are solid at room temperature).

As noted earlier, blood lipids are thought to contribute to the development of atherosclerotic deposits on the inner walls of the artery. One substance, called

Figure 1 ► The fit heart muscle.

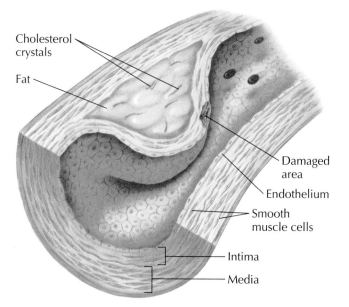

Figure 2 ► Atherosclerosis.

low-density lipoprotein (LDL), is a major contributor to the development of atherosclerosis. LDL is basically a core of cholesterol surrounded by protein and another substance that makes it water soluble. The benefit of regular exercise is that it can reduce blood lipid levels, including LDL-C (the cholesterol core of LDL). People with high total cholesterol and LDL levels have a higher than normal risk for heart disease (see Table 1). New evidence indicates that there are subtypes of LDL cholesterol (characterized by their small size and high density) that pose even greater risks. These subtypes are hard to measure and not included in most current blood tests, but future research will no doubt help us better understand and measure them.

Triglycerides are another type of blood lipid. Elevated levels of triglycerides are related to heart disease. Triglycerides lose some of their ability to predict heart disease with the presence of other risk factors, so high levels are more difficult to interpret than other blood lipids. Normal levels are considered to be 150 mg/dL or less. Values of 151 to 199 are borderline, 200 to 499 are high, and above 500 are very high. It would be wise to include triglycerides in a blood lipid profile. Physical activity is often prescribed as part of a treatment for high triglyceride levels.

Regular physical activity can help prevent atherosclerosis by increasing HDL in the blood. Whereas LDLs carry a core of cholesterol that is involved in the development of atherosclerosis, **high-density lipoprotein (HDL)** picks up cholesterol and carries it to the liver, where it is eliminated from the body. HDL is often called the "good cholesterol" and is desirable. When having a blood test, ask for information about HDL as well as the other measures included in Table 1. Individuals who have regular physical activity usually have lower total cholesterol, lower LDL, and higher HDL levels than inactive people.

Regular physical activity can help prevent atherosclerosis by reducing blood coagulants. **Fibrin** and platelets (types of cells involved in blood coagulation) deposit at the site of an injury on the wall of the artery, contributing to the process of plaque buildup, or atherosclerosis. Regular physical activity has been shown to reduce fibrin levels in the blood. The breakdown of fibrin seems to reduce platelet adhesiveness and the concentration of platelets in the blood.

Other indicators of inflammation of the arteries are predictive of atherosclerosis. Recently, a number of other constituents in the blood have been shown to be associated with risk for cardiovascular disease. Among these are indicators of inflammation inside the arteries, such as C-reactive protein (CRP), interleukin-6 (IL-6), Chlamydia pneumonia heat shock protein (Cp-HSP60), and tumor necrosis factor-a (TNF-a). These compounds are not necessarily causes of atherosclerosis, but they are indicators of inflammatory processes that lead to plaque formation. Inflammatory processes also soften existing plaque and increase the likelihood of plaque rupture or the formation of clots, which can directly precipitate heart attacks.

The inner wall of the artery (endothelium) was once thought to be a relatively passive layer of tissue that merely lines the artery. However, recent evidence suggests that it is an active layer of tissue that functions in several ways in addition to providing a protective barrier. For example, sensing units in the endothelium stimulate production of agents that regulate blood flow by dilating and constricting the artery. The released substances can help prevent the buildup of deposits on the arterial wall. However, when the inner wall of the artery ceases to function effectively, it increases the risk of plaque buildup.

CRP is one of the most studied indicators of a dysfunctional endothelium. Screening for elevated levels of CRP is now commonly done to identify patients that may be at risk

Table 1 ▶ Cholesterol Classifications (mg/dL)*				
	Total (TC)	LDL-C	HDL-C	TC/HDL-C
Optimal	– – –	<100	– – –	
Near optimal	– – –	100–129	– – –	– – –
Desirable	<200	– – –	60+	– – –
Borderline	200–239	130–159	40–59	3.6–5.0
High risk	240+	160–189	<40	5.0+
Very high risk	– – –	>190	– – –	– – –

Source: Third Report of the National Cholesterol Education Program.
*Different classification systems are used for each of the four measures (two to five categories). Blank (---) spaces are included for categories not used for each measure.

Lipids All fats and fatty substances.

Lipoproteins Fat-carrying proteins in the blood.

Low-Density Lipoprotein (LDL) A core of cholesterol surrounded by protein; the core is often called "bad cholesterol."

Triglycerides A type of blood fat associated with increased risk for heart disease.

High-Density Lipoprotein (HDL) A blood substance that picks up cholesterol and helps remove it from the body; often called "good cholesterol."

Fibrin A sticky, threadlike substance that, in combination with blood cells, forms a blood clot.

for heart disease. Preliminary standards from the American Heart Association suggest that levels below 1 mg/L indicate low risk, levels between 1 mg/L and 3 mg/L indicate moderate risk, and above 3 mg/L indicate high risk.

High levels of the amino acid homocysteine have also been associated with increased risk for heart disease, though the American Heart Association says it is too early to begin screening for it. Tentative fasting values have been established at 5 to 15 millimoles per liter of blood for the normal range, 16 to 30 as moderate, 31 to 100 as intermediate, and above 100 as high. Recent research suggests that healthy lifestyles can help reduce the risk of arterial inflammation. For example, studies show that regular physical activity can promote endothelial health, and nutrition can help reduce markers of inflammation. Adequate levels of folic acid, vitamins B-6 and B-12 help prevent high blood homocysteine levels, so eating foods that ensure adequate daily intake of these vitamins is recommended.

Physical Activity and Heart Attack

Regular physical activity reduces the risk for heart attack, the most prevalent and serious of all cardiovascular diseases. A heart attack (coronary occlusion) occurs when a coronary artery is blocked (see Figure 3). A clot, or thrombus, is the most common cause, reducing or cutting off blood flow and oxygen to the heart muscle. If the blocked coronary artery supplies a major portion of the heart muscle, death will occur within minutes. Occlusions of lesser arteries may result in angina pectoris or a nonfatal heart attack.

People who perform regular physical activity have half the risk for a first heart attack, compared with those who are sedentary. Possible reasons are less atherosclerosis, greater diameter of arteries, and less chance of a clot forming.

Regular exercise can improve coronary circulation and, thus, reduce the chances of a heart attack or dying from one. Within the heart, many tiny branches extend from the major coronary arteries. All of these vessels supply blood to the heart muscle. Active people are likely to have greater blood-carrying capacity in these vessels, probably because the vessels are larger and more elastic. Also, the active person may have a more profuse distribution of arteries within the heart muscle (see Figure 4), which results in greater blood flow. A few studies show that physical activity may promote the growth of "extra" blood vessels, which are thought to open up to provide the heart muscle with the necessary blood and oxygen when the oxygen supply is diminished, as in a heart attack. Blood flow from extra blood vessels is referred to as **coronary collateral circulation.**

Improved coronary circulation may provide protection against a heart attack because a larger artery would require more atherosclerosis to occlude it. In addition, the development of collateral blood vessels supplying the heart may diminish the effects of a heart attack, as these extra (or collateral) blood vessels may take over the function of regular blood vessels.

The heart of an inactive person is less able to resist stress and is more susceptible to an emotional storm that may precipitate a heart attack. The heart is rendered inefficient by one or more of the following circumstances: high heart rate, high blood pressure, and excessive stimulation. All of these conditions require the

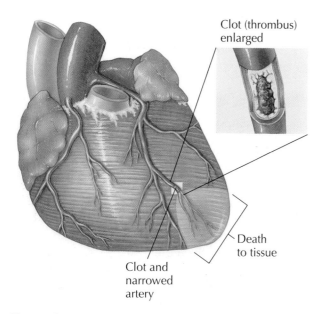

Clot (thrombus) enlarged

Death to tissue

Clot and narrowed artery

Figure 3 ▶ Heart attack.

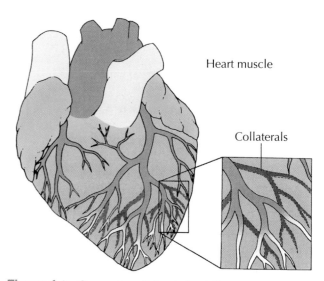

Heart muscle

Collaterals

Figure 4 ▶ Coronary collateral circulation.

heart to use more oxygen than is normal and decrease its ability to adapt to stressful situations.

The inefficient heart beats rapidly because it is dominated by the **sympathetic nervous system,** which speeds up the heart rate. Thus, the heart continuously beats rapidly, even at rest, and never has a true rest period. High blood pressure also makes the heart work harder and contributes to its inefficiency.

Research indicates that regular physical activity can:

- lead to dominance of the **parasympathetic nervous system,** which slows heart rate and helps the heart work efficiently;
- help the heart rate return to normal faster after emotional stress;
- strengthen the heart muscle, making it better able to weather an **emotional storm;**
- reduce hormonal effects on the heart, thus lessening the chances of circulatory problems;
- reduce the risk of sudden death from ventricular fibrillation (arrhythmic heartbeat).

Regular physical activity is one effective means of rehabilitation for a person who has coronary heart disease or who has had a heart attack. Not only does regular physical activity seem to reduce the risk of developing coronary heart disease, but those who already have the condition may reduce the symptoms of the disease through regular exercise. For people who have had heart attacks, regular and progressive exercise can be an effective prescription when carried out under the supervision of a physician. Remember, however, that exercise is not the treatment of preference for all heart attack victims. In some cases, it is harmful.

Physical Activity and Other Cardiovascular Diseases

Regular physical activity is associated with a reduced risk for high blood pressure (hypertension). "Normal" **systolic blood pressure** is 120 mm Hg or less and normal **diastolic blood pressure** is 80 mm Hg or less. Prehypertension is a condition that exists when your blood pressure is higher than normal but not high enough to be considered hypertension (see Table 2). Prehypertension has been linked to higher than normal risk of heart attack and, though not as serious as hypertension, should be taken seriously. Nearly one-third of American adults have high blood pressure. High blood pressure is associated with heart disease, stroke, diabetes, and many other diseases. African Americans, Hispanics, and Native Americans have higher incidence than White non-Hispanics. Older people have higher incidence than younger people.

Table 2 ▶ Blood Pressure Classifications for Adults*

Category	Systolic Blood Pressure (mm Hg)	Diastolic Blood Pressure (mm Hg)
Normal	<120	<80
Prehypertensive	121–139	81–89
Stage 1 hypertension	140–159	90–99
Stage 2 hypertension	>160	>100

Source: National Heart, Lung, and Blood Institute.
*Not taking antihypertensive drugs and not acutely ill. When the systolic and diastolic blood pressure categories vary, the higher reading determines the blood pressure classification.

High blood pressure is sometimes referred to as the "silent killer" because nearly one-third of people with elevated blood pressure do not know they have it. It is important to monitor your blood pressure on a regular basis. With practice and good equipment, you can accurately measure your own blood pressure. Because blood pressure can be elevated by emotions and circumstances, a single measurement may not be accurate, so at least two separate measurements are recommended. While self-assessments can be helpful, they are not a substitute for periodic assessments by a qualified medical person.

Exceptionally low blood pressures (below 100 systolic and 60 diastolic) do not pose the same risks to health as

Coronary Collateral Circulation Circulation of blood to the heart muscle associated with the blood-carrying capacity of a specific vessel or development of collateral vessels (extra blood vessels).

Sympathetic Nervous System The branch of the autonomic nervous system that prepares the body for activity by speeding up the heart rate.

Parasympathetic Nervous System The branch of the autonomic nervous system that slows the heart rate.

Emotional Storm A traumatic emotional experience that is likely to affect the human organism physiologically.

Systolic Blood Pressure The upper blood pressure number, often called working blood pressure. It represents the pressure in the arteries at its highest level just after the heart beats.

Diastolic Blood Pressure The lower blood pressure number, often called "resting pressure." It is the pressure in the arteries at its lowest level occurring just before the next beat of the heart.

TECHNOLOGY UPDATE

Heart360

Physical inactivity is one of the primary risks for cardiovascular disease. The American Heart Association has released a free, Web-based tracking tool (www.Heart360 .org) that allows individuals to record and monitor changes in key risk factors over time, including blood pressure, cholesterol, blood glucose, inactivity, and body mass index (BMI). With this tool, you create a secure "health vault" account to save confidential health data. The site evaluates your risk profiles and provides links to educational resources. If your physician has a provider account, you can share results with your physician.

Would this type of tool help you adopt heart-healthy lifestyles? Would the connection with your physician make you more accountable?

connect
ACTIVITY

Many factors in addition to healthy lifestyle have led to a significant reduction in cardiovascular disease deaths in recent years. While lifestyle changes such as being active, eating well, managing stress, and abstaining from tobacco use are important in the prevention and treatment of cardiovascular diseases, a variety of other factors have contributed to the recent decrease in deaths associated with the diseases. Heart disease is still the leading killer of both men and women. In the late 1990s deaths exceeded one million per year, but death rates from heart disease have decreased by more than 29 percent. Some of the reasons for that decline, other than healthy lifestyle change, include earlier and better detection (e.g., exercise tests, angiograms,

high blood pressure but can cause dizziness, fainting, and lack of tolerance to change in body positions.

A recent research summary indicates that the effects of physical activity on blood pressure are more dramatic than previously thought and are independent of age, body fatness, and other factors. Inactive, less fit individuals have a 30 to 50 percent greater chance of being hypertensive than active, fit people. Regular physical activity can also be one effective method of reducing blood pressure for those with prehypertension or hypertension. Physical inactivity in middle age is associated with risk for high blood pressure later in life. The most plausible reason is a reduction in resistance to blood flow in the blood vessels, probably resulting from dilation of the vessels.

Regular physical activity can help reduce the risk for stroke. Stroke is a major killer of adults. People with high blood pressure and atherosclerosis are susceptible to stroke. Since regular exercise and good fitness are important to the prevention of high blood pressure and atherosclerosis, exercise and fitness are considered helpful in the prevention of stroke.

Regular physical activity is helpful in preventing peripheral vascular disease. People who exercise regularly have better blood flow to the working muscles and other tissues than inactive, unfit people. Since peripheral vascular disease is associated with poor circulation to the extremities, regular exercise can be considered one method of preventing this condition.

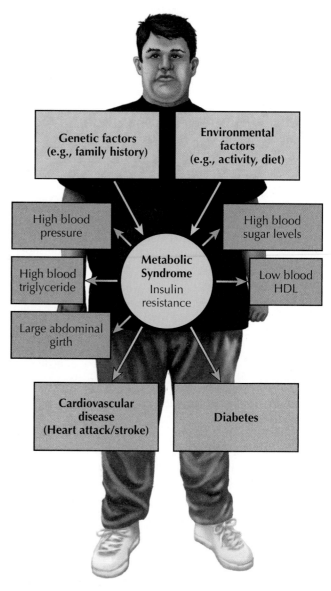

Figure 5 ▶ Mechanism and effects of metabolic syndrome.

CT scans) and better emergency care. Improved medications for lowering blood fat levels (e.g., blood thinners, including aspirin) and lowering blood pressure levels have also played a role and less invasive surgical methods (e.g., angioplasty, stents) and improvements in postcoronary care.

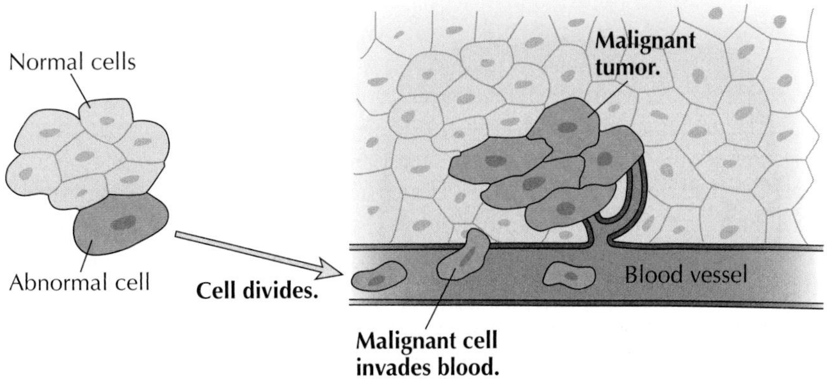

Physical Activity and Metabolic Syndrome

Physical inactivity is associated with metabolic syndrome. Metabolic syndrome is the opposite of good metabolic fitness, as discussed in Concept 1. Several groups, including the American Heart Association and the American Medical Association, have defined the characteristics of metabolic syndrome (see Figure 5). People with at least three of the following characteristics have metabolic syndrome: blood pressure above 130/85, a fasting blood sugar level of 100 or higher, blood triglycerides of 150 or above, a low blood HDL level (less than 40 for men and less than 50 for women), and/or a high abdominal circumference (equal to or above 40 inches for men or 35 inches for women).

People with metabolic syndrome have a higher than normal risk of chronic diseases, such as diabetes, heart disease, and stroke. A questionnaire developed by researchers who conducted the Framingham Heart Study uses metabolic measures and several other measures to predict heart disease. This questionnaire is better at predicting heart disease than metabolic syndrome alone, but metabolic syndrome is a better predictor of diabetes. Lab 4A at the end of the concept can be used by those who do not have the necessary metabolic syndrome measures, though having a metabolic fitness assessment is advised periodically, especially as you grow older.

Physical Activity and Other Hypokinetic Conditions

Physical activity reduces the risk of some forms of cancer. According to the American Cancer Society (ACS), cancer is a group of many different conditions characterized by abnormal, uncontrolled cell growth. As illustrated in Figure 6, the abnormal cells divide, forming **malignant tumors (carcinomas).** If the abnormal cells reach the blood, they can spread, causing tumors elsewhere in the body. **Benign tumors** are generally

Figure 6 ▶ The spread of cancer (metastasis).

not considered to be cancerous because their growth is restricted to a specific area of the body by a protective membrane. The first editions of this book did not include any form of cancer as a hypokinetic disease. We now know, however, that overall death rates from some types of cancer are lower among active people than those who are sedentary. These cancers are described in Table 3 with possible reasons for the cancer/inactivity link. The

Table 3 ▶ Physical Activity and Cancer

Cancer Type	Effect of Physical Activity
Colon	Exercise speeds movement of food and cancer-causing substances through the digestive system, and reduces prostaglandins (substances linked to cancer in the colon).
Breast	Exercise decreases the amount of exposure of breast tissue to circulating estrogen. Lower body fat is also associated with lower estrogen levels. Early life activity is deemed important for both reasons. Fatigue from therapy is reduced by exercise.
Rectal	Similar to colon cancer, exercise leads to more regular bowel movements and reduces "transit time."
Prostate	Fatigue from therapy is reduced by exercise. Regular exercise, especially vigorous exercise, may reduce death rate.

Malignant Tumors (carcinomas) An uncontrolled and dangerous growth capable of spreading to other areas; a cancerous tumor.

Benign Tumors An abnormal growth of tissue confined to a particular area; not considered to be cancer.

entries in Table 3 are listed in order based on the strength of evidence supporting the cancer/inactivity link.

As indicated in Concept 1, cancer is a leading cause of death. In the United States cancer causes more than 560,000 deaths annually. However, the five-year survival rate for people diagnosed with cancer is up 50 percent over the past three decades. Many factors are responsible, including early diagnosis and improved medical treatments. Healthy lifestyles can also play a role. The American Cancer Society (ACS) guidelines highlight the importance of regular physical activity and a healthy diet in preventing cancer and early death. Physical activity is also considered to be important to 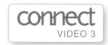 the wellness of the cancer patient in many ways, including improved quality of life, physical functioning, and self-esteem, as well as less dependence on others, reduced risk for other diseases, and reduced fatigue from disease or disease therapy. The ACS and the Lance Armstrong Foundation (www.Livestrong.org) are two good sources of information about cancer and cancer treatments.

Physical activity plays a role in the management and treatment of Type II diabetes. Diabetes mellitus (diabetes) is a group of disorders that results when there is too much sugar in the blood. It occurs when the body does not make enough **insulin** or when the body is not able to use insulin effectively.

Type I diabetes, or insulin-dependent diabetes, accounts for a relatively small number of the diabetes cases and is not considered to be a hypokinetic condition. Type II diabetes (often not insulin-dependent) was formerly called "adult-onset diabetes." Reports indicate more cases of Type II diabetes among children than in the past, in part because of better record keeping but also because of increases in obesity among children in recent years.

Diabetes is the seventh leading cause of death among people over 40. It accounts for at least 10 percent of all short-term hospital stays and has a major impact on health-care costs in Western society. According to the American Diabetes Association (ADA), there are nearly 24 million people in the United States with diabetes (7.8 percent of the population). Unfortunately, 5.7 million of those don't know it. An estimated additional 57 million are prediabetic; they have metabolic profiles characteristic of those with diabetes (see Web Resources, ADA, or Canadian Diabetes Association, for more statistics).

People who perform regular physical activity are less likely to suffer from Type II diabetes than sedentary people. For people with Type II diabetes, regular physical activity can help reduce body fatness, decrease **insulin resistance,** improve **insulin sensitivity,** and improve the body's ability to clear sugar from the blood

in a reasonable time. With sound nutritional habits and proper medication, physical activity can be useful in the management of both types of diabetes.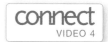

Regular physical activity is important to maintaining bone density and decreasing risk for osteoporosis. As noted in Concept 1, some experts consider bone integrity to be a health-related component of physical fitness. Bone density cannot be self-assessed. It is measured using a dual X-ray absorptiometry (DXA) machine, an expensive and sophisticated form of X-ray machine that can also be used to measure body fatness. Healthy bones are dense and strong. When bones lose calcium and become less dense, they become porous and are at risk for fracture. The bones of young children are not especially dense, but during adolescence and early adulthood (see Figure 7), bones increase in density to a level higher than any other time in life (peak bone density). Though bone density often begins to decrease in young adulthood, it is not until older adulthood that bone loss becomes dramatic. Over time, if bone loss continues, older adults become susceptible to a condition called **osteoporosis** (bone density drops below the osteoporosis threshold). Some will have crossed the fracture threshold, putting them at risk for fractures, especially to the hip, vertebrae, and other "soft" or "spongy" bones of the skeletal system. Active people have a higher peak bone mass and are more resistant to osteoporosis (see blue line in Figure 7) than sedentary people (see red line in Figure 7).

Women, especially postmenopausal women, have a higher risk of osteoporosis than men, but it is a disease of both sexes. Although Figure 7 reflects the combined bone density status for men and women, males typically have a higher peak bone mass than females, and for this reason, males can lose more bone density over time without reaching the osteoporosis or fracture threshold. More women reach the osteoporosis and fracture thresholds at

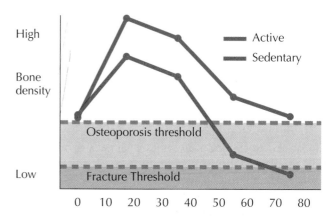

Figure 7 ▶ Changes in bone density with age.

earlier ages than men. Other risk factors for osteoporosis are age, family history/heredity, frame size, smoking, caffeine use, alcohol use, current or previous eating disorders, early menstruation, low dietary calcium intake, low body fat, amenorrhea, and extended bed rest.

The National Osteoporosis Foundation (NOF) recommends five steps to bone health and osteoporosis prevention:

- Get daily recommended amounts of calcium and vitamin D. Eat a diet rich in both nutrients. Exposure to the sun provides a source of vitamin D. The NOF recommends 1,000 mg of calcium daily for people under 50, and 1,200 mg for those over 50. Adults under age 50 need 400–800 IU of vitamin D, and adults over 50 need 800–1,000 units. If you have difficulty getting enough of these nutrients from food or sunlight, your health-care provider may recommend a supplement.

- Engage in regular weight-bearing exercise. Weight-bearing exercise (e.g., walking, dancing, jogging) and resistance training are good choices. The load bearing and pull of muscles build bone density.

- Avoid smoking and excessive alcohol.

- Talk to your health-care provider about bone health.

- When appropriate, have a bone density test and take medication. There is no cure for osteoporosis, but the FDA has approved a variety of treatments for osteoporosis to help reduce bone loss over time. When appropriate, a physician may prescribe FDA-approved medications such as raloxifene (sold as Evista), alendronate (sold as Fosamax), or other approved drugs. Hormone treatments such as thyroid-based Calcitonin treatments and estrogen are approved. Estrogen replacement therapy (ERT), also known as hormone replacement treatment (HRT), can reduce risk of osteoporosis among postmenopausal women, but may increase risk for cancer and other diseases. Medical consultation based on individual factors is recommended.

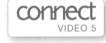

Active people who possess good muscle fitness are less likely to have back and musculoskeletal problems than are inactive, unfit people. Because few people die from it, back pain does not receive the attention given to such medical problems as heart disease and cancer. But back pain is the second leading medical complaint in the United States, second only to headaches. Only the common cold and the flu cause more days lost from work. At some point in our lives, approximately 80 percent of all adults experience back pain that limits the ability to function normally. In National Safety Council data, the back was the most frequently injured of all body parts, and the injury rate was double that of any other part of the body.

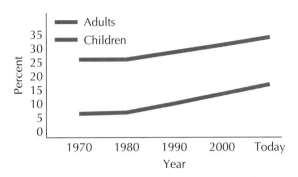

Figure 8 ▶ Incidence of obesity.
Source: National Center for Health Statistics.

The great majority of back ailments are the result of poor muscle strength, low levels of endurance, and poor flexibility. Tests on patients with back problems show weakness and lack of flexibility in key muscle groups.

Lack of fitness is probably the leading reason for back pain in Western society. Other factors also increase the risk of back ailments, including poor posture, improper lifting and work habits, heredity, and disease states such as scoliosis and arthritis.

Physical activity is important in maintaining a healthy body weight and avoiding the numerous health conditions associated with obesity. National studies indicate that more than two-thirds of adults are overweight and more than one-third are obese (32.2 percent of men and 35.5 percent of women). Nearly a third of children are either overweight or obese. From 1950 through 1980, obesity (15 percent) and overweight were fairly stable but increased dramatically from 1980 to the present. In the past few years the rate of increase in overweight and obesity has not been as dramatic as during the previous decade (see Figure 8). Obesity is not a disease state in itself but is a hypokinetic condition associated with a multitude of far-reaching complications. Research has shown that fat people who are fit

Insulin   A hormone secreted by the pancreas that regulates levels of sugar in the blood.

Insulin Resistance   A condition that occurs when insulin becomes ineffective or less effective than necessary to regulate sugar levels in the blood.

Insulin Sensitivity   A person with insulin resistance (see previous definition) is said to have decreased insulin sensitivity. The body's cells are not sensitive to insulin, so they resist it and sugar levels are not regulated effectively.

Osteoporosis   A condition associated with low bone density and subsequent bone fragility, leading to high risk for fracture.

are not at especially high risk for early death. However, when high body fatness is accompanied by low cardio-vascular and low metabolic fitness, risk for early death increases substantially. For more information on obesity, see Concept 13.

Physical activity reduces the risk and severity of a variety of common emotional/mental health disorders. Nearly half of adult Americans will report having a mental health disorder at some point in life. A recent summary of studies revealed that there are several emotional/mental disorders associated with inactive lifestyles.

Depression is a stress-related condition experienced by many adults. Thirty-three percent of inactive adults report that they often feel depressed. For some, depression is a serious disorder that physical activity alone will not cure; however, research indicates that activity, combined with other forms of therapy, can be effective.

Anxiety is an emotional condition characterized by worry, self-doubt, and apprehension. More than a few studies have shown that symptoms of anxiety can be reduced by regular activity. Low-fit people who do regular aerobic activity seem to benefit the most. In one study, one-third of active people felt that regular activity helped them cope better with life's pressures.

Physical activity is also associated with better and more restful sleep. People with insomnia (the inability to sleep) seem to benefit from regular activity if it is not done too vigorously right before going to bed. A recent study indicates that 52 percent of the population feel that physical activity helps them sleep better. Regular aerobic activity is associated with reduced brain activation, which can result in greater ability to relax or fall asleep.

A final benefit of regular exercise is increased self-esteem. Improvements in fitness, appearance, and the ability to perform new tasks can improve self-confidence.

Physical activity can help the immune system fight illness. Until recently, infectious disease and other diseases of the immune system were not considered to be hypokinetic. Recent evidence indicates that regular moderate to vigorous activity can actually aid the immune system in fighting disease. Each of us is born with an "innate immune system," which includes anatomical and physiological barriers, such as skin, mucous membranes, body temperature, and chemical mediators that help prevent and resist disease. We also develop an "acquired immune system" in the form of special disease-fighting cells that help us resist disease. Figure 9 shows a J-shaped curve that illustrates the benefits of exercise to acquired immune function. Sedentary people have more risk than those who do moderate activity, but with very high and sustained vigorous activity, such as extended high performance training, immune system function actually decreases.

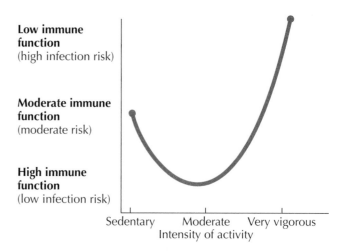

Figure 9 ▶ Physical activity and immune function.

Regular moderate and reasonable amounts of vigorous activity have been shown to reduce incidence of colds and days of sickness from infection. The immune system benefit may extend to other immune system disorders as well. There is evidence that regular physical activity can enhance treatment effectiveness and improve quality of life for those with HIV/AIDS. However, as Figure 9 indicates, too much exercise may cause problems rather than solve them.

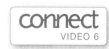

Physical activity during pregnancy can benefit both the mother and the child. In the not too distant past, exercise during pregnancy was discouraged. Over the years, evidence has shown that appropriate exercise (including resistance training and moderate to vigorous aerobic exercise) by pregnant women can help prevent excess weight gain, help retain pre-pregnancy fitness levels, and result in shorter, less complicated labor. Physical activity does not cause damage to the baby or miscarriage and may help the baby developmentally.

Pregnant women are nearly twice as likely to be sedentary (fail to meet current activity guidelines) than other women in spite of the fact that guidelines from the American College of Obstetricians and Gynecologists indicate that most women should meet national guidelines as described in this book. More intense exercise is appropriate in many cases but should be done with "close medical supervision."

Regular physical activity can have positive effects on some nonhypokinetic conditions. The following nonhypokinetic conditions can benefit from physical activity:

• *Arthritis.* Many, if not most, arthritics are in a deconditioned state resulting from a lack of activity. The traditional advice that arthritics should avoid physical activity is now being modified in view of the findings that carefully prescribed exercise has a variety of benefits. Common problems for both those with rheumatoid arthritis (RA) and osteoarthritis (OA) are decreased strength, loss of range of motion, and poor cardiovascular endurance. Well-planned exercise, designed to meet the needs of the specific type of arthritis of the individual, can be beneficial in preventing and treating impairments, and enhancing function, general fitness, and well-being.

- *Asthma*. Asthmatics often have physical activity limitations, but with proper management activity can be part of their daily life. In fact, when done properly, activity can reduce airway reactivity and medication use. Because exercise can trigger bronchial constriction, it is important to choose appropriate types of activity and to use inhaled medications to prevent bronchial constriction caused by exercise or other triggers, such as cold weather. Asthmatics should avoid cold weather exercise.

- *Premenstrual syndrome (PMS)*. PMS, a mixture of physical and emotional symptoms that occurs prior to menstruation, has many causes. However, changes in lifestyle, including regular exercise, may be effective in relieving PMS symptoms.

- *Cystic fibrosis*. A recent review indicates that exercise helps cystic fibrosis patients by facilitating systemic improvements and, more importantly, enhancing quality of life.

- *Other conditions*. Low- to moderate-intensity aerobic activity and resistance training are prescribed for some people who have chronic pain (persistent pain without relief) and/or fibromyalgia (chronic muscle pain). Evidence also suggests that active people have a reduced chance of having gallstones than inactive people. Activity may also decrease risk of impotence.

Physical Activity and Aging

Regular physical activity can improve fitness and functioning among older adults. Approximately 30 percent of adults age 70 and over have difficulty with one or more activities of daily living. Women have more limitations than men, and low-income groups have more limitations than higher-income groups. Nearly one-half of these adults also get no assistance in coping with their limitations.

The inability to function effectively as you grow older is associated with lack of fitness and inactive lifestyles. This loss of function is sometimes referred to as "acquired aging," as opposed to "time-dependent" aging. Because so many people experience limitations in daily activities and find it difficult to get assistance, it is especially important for older people to stay active and fit.

In general, older adults are much less active than younger adults. Losses in muscle fitness are associated with loss of balance, greater risk of falling, and less

ability to function independently. Studies also show that exercise can enhance cognitive functioning and perhaps reduce risk for dementia. Though the amount of activity performed must be adapted as people grow older, fitness benefits discussed in the next section and throughout this book apply to people of all ages.

Regular physical activity can compress illness into a shorter period of our life. An important national health goal is to increase the years of healthy life. Living longer is important, but being able to function effectively during all years of life is equally—if not more—important. *Compression of illness*, also called compression of morbidity, refers to shortening the total number of years that illnesses and disabilities occur. Healthy lifestyles, including regular physical activity, have been shown to compress illness and increase years of effective functioning. Inactive people not only have a shorter lifespan, but also have more years of illness and disability than active people.

Recent evidence indicates that Alzheimer's disease and dementia are hypokinetic conditions. More than a few studies indicate that factors relating to heart health also contribute to brain health. The studies indicate that physical and challenging mental activities are especially important for preventing decline in cognitive function and reducing the risk of developing Alzheimer's and dementia. Although additional research is needed, this is important news for physicians and public health officials looking for ways to reduce the prevalence of Alzheimer's disease.

Physical Activity, Health, and Wellness

Good health-related physical fitness and regular physical activity contribute to optimal wellness. Regular physical activity and good fitness not only help prevent illness (see Figure 10) and disease but also promote quality of life and wellness. Good health-related physical fitness can help you look good, feel good, and enjoy life. Specific benefits of wellness associated with good fitness are the following:

- *Good physical fitness can help an individual work effectively and efficiently*. A person who can resist fatigue, muscle soreness, back problems, and other symptoms associated with poor health-related fitness is capable of working productively and having energy left over at the end of the day.

- *Good physical fitness can help an individual enjoy leisure time*. A fit person is more likely to get and stay involved in leisure-time activities than an unfit person. Enjoying your leisure time may not add years to your life but can add life to your years.

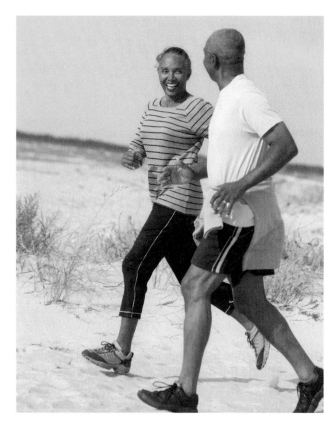

Regular physical activity promotes healthy aging and high quality of life.

- *Good physical fitness is essential to effective living.* Although the need for each component of physical fitness is specific to each individual, every person requires enough fitness to perform normal daily activities without undue fatigue. Whether it be walking, performing household chores, or merely enjoying the simple things in life without pain or fear of injury, good fitness is important to all people.

- *Physical fitness is the basis for dynamic and creative activity.* Though the following quotation by former President John F. Kennedy is more than 50 years old, it clearly points out the importance of physical fitness:

"The relationship between the soundness of the body and the activity of the mind is subtle and complex. Much is not yet understood, but we know what the Greeks knew: that intelligence and skill can only function at the peak of their capacity when the body is healthy and strong, and that hardy spirits and tough minds usually inhabit sound bodies. Physical fitness is the basis of all activities in our society; if our bodies grow soft and inactive, if we fail to encourage physical development and prowess, we will undermine our capacity for thought, for work, and for the use of those skills vital to an expanding and complex America."

President Kennedy's belief that activity and fitness are associated with intellectual functioning has now been backed up with research. A recent research summary suggests that, though modest, the effect of activity and fitness on intellectual functioning is positive. One study shows activity to foster new brain cell growth. Time taken to be active during the day has been shown to help children learn more, even though less time is spent in intellectual pursuits.

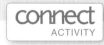 **connect**
VIDEO 7

- *Good physical fitness may help you function safely and handle unexpected emergencies.* Emergencies are never expected, but, when they do arise, they often demand performance that requires good fitness. For example, flood victims may need to fill sandbags for hours without rest, and accident victims may be required to walk or run long distances for help.

Physical activity is a major part of most employee health promotion programs. Companies have come to understand the importance of promoting healthy lifestyles among their employees. Work-site health promotion programs typically use a broad focus on promoting a variety of healthy lifestyles, but physical activity is considered the mainstay of most programs. To facilitate active lifestyles, many companies build their own fitness centers inside the workplace or provide free or reduced-cost memberships for employees. Work-site programs that promote activity can reduce risk factors in employees and help companies control the high cost of health care. Companies that offer comprehensive programs frequently save more than $4 for each dollar invested. The expansion of work-site health programs is viewed as a critical public health priority and one of the most promising approaches for controlling health-care costs.

Too much activity can lead to hyperkinetic conditions. The information presented in this concept points out the health benefits of physical activity performed in appropriate amounts. When done in excess or incorrectly, physical activity can result in

Health and Wellness Benefits of Physical Activity and Fitness

Improved Cardiovascular Health
- Stronger heart muscle fitness and health
- Lower heart rate
- Better electric stability of heart
- Decreased sympathetic control of heart
- Increased O_2 to brain
- Reduced blood fat, including low-density lipoproteins (LDLs)
- Increased protective high-density lipoproteins (HDLs)
- Delayed development of atherosclerosis
- Increased work capacity
- Improved peripheral circulation
- Improved coronary circulation
- Resistance to "emotional storm"
- Reduced risk for heart attack
- Reduced risk for stroke
- Reduced risk for hypertension
- Greater chance of surviving a heart attack
- Increased oxygen-carrying capacity of the blood

Improved Strength and Muscular Endurance
- Greater work efficiency
- Less chance for muscle injury
- Reduced risk for low back problems
- Improved performance in sports
- Quicker recovery after hard work
- Improved ability to meet emergencies

Resistance to Fatigue
- Ability to enjoy leisure
- Improved quality of life
- Improved ability to meet some stressors

Other Health Benefits
- Decreased diabetes risk
- Quality of life for diabetics
- Improved metabolic fitness
- Extended life
- Decrease in dysfunctional years
- Aids for some people who have arthritis, PMS, asthma, chronic pain, fibromyalgia, or impotence
- Improved immune system

Enhanced Mental Health and Function
- Relief of depression
- Improved sleep habits
- Fewer stress symptoms
- Ability to enjoy leisure and work
- Improved brain function

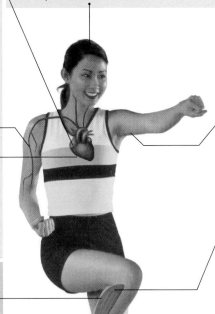

Improved Wellness
- Improved quality of life
- Leisure-time enjoyment
- Improved work capacity
- Ability to meet emergencies
- Improved creative capacity

Opportunity for Successful Experience and Social Interactions
- Improved self-concept
- Opportunity to recognize and accept personal limitations
- Improved sense of well-being
- Enjoyment of life and fun
- Improved quality of life

Improved Appearance
- Better figure/physique
- Better posture
- Fat control

Greater Lean Body Mass and Less Body Fat
- Greater work efficiency
- Less susceptibility to disease
- Improved appearance
- Less incidence of self-concept problems related to obesity

Improved Flexibility
- Greater work efficiency
- Less chance of muscle injury
- Less chance of joint injury
- Decreased chance of developing low back problems
- Improved sports performance

Bone Development
- Greater peak bone density
- Less chance of developing osteoporosis

Reduced Cancer Risk
- Reduced risk for colon and breast cancer
- Possible reduced risk for rectal and prostate cancers

Reduced Effect of Acquired Aging
- Improved ability to function in daily life
- Better short-term memory
- Fewer illnesses
- Greater mobility
- Greater independence
- Greater ability to operate an automobile
- Lower risk for dementia

Figure 10 ▶ Health and wellness benefits of physical activity and fitness.

hyperkinetic conditions. The most common hyperkinetic condition is overuse injury to muscles, connective tissue, and bones. Recently, anorexia nervosa and body neurosis have been identified as conditions associated with inappropriate amounts of physical activity. These conditions will be discussed in the concept on performance.

Hyperkinetic Conditions Diseases/illnesses or health conditions caused, or contributed to, by too much physical activity.

Physical activity is now recognized as effective "medicine" for prevention of chronic disease. Since physical activity is still not widely prescribed or promoted by medical professionals, the American College of Sports Medicine (ACSM) initiated a program called "Exercise Is Medicine (EIM)" designed to "encourage primary care physicians, and other health care providers, to assess and review every patient's physical activity program at every visit." The initiative has taken off both in the United States and internationally. The website (www.exerciseismedicine.org) provides information to the general public, healthcare providers, health and fitness professionals, and the media.

There are many positive lifestyles that can reduce the risk for disease and promote health and wellness. Inactivity, poor nutrition, smoking, and inability to cope with stress are all risk factors associated with various diseases (see Table 4). Changing these behaviors can dramatically reduce the risk for chronic diseases. Recognize, however, that three risk factors (age, heredity, and gender) are not within your control.

By adopting healthy lifestyles, you can take control over the preventable disease risks. For example, controlling body fatness reduces the risk for diabetes, hypertension, and back problems. Altering your diet can reduce the chances of developing high levels of blood lipids and reduce the risk for atherosclerosis. Being active and adopting healthy lifestyles is a proactive approach to health and wellness. While reducing risk can alter the probability of disease, it does not assure disease immunity.

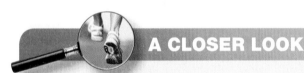

A CLOSER LOOK

Exercise Is Medicine

Although the health benefits of physical activity are readily accepted by scientists, it is not always integrated into medical practice. The "Exercise Is Medicine" initiative from the American College of Sports Medicine offers considerable promise for advancing the promotion of physical activity. Specific programming is also targeted for college campuses. Visit the website (www.exerciseismedicine.org) to review the overall goals of this bold international health initiative.

Think of the title "Exercise Is Medicine" and explain why you believe it was chosen. Would you take exercise more seriously if it was recommended by your physician?

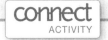
connect
ACTIVITY

Table 4 ▶ Hypokinetic Disease Risk Factors

Factors That Cannot Be Altered

1. *Age.* As you grow older, your risk of contracting hypokinetic diseases increases. For example, the risk for heart disease is approximately three times as great after 60 as before. The risk of back pain is considerably greater after 40.
2. *Heredity.* People who have a family history of hypokinetic disease are more likely to develop a hypokinetic condition, such as heart disease, hypertension, back problems, obesity, high blood lipid levels, and other problems. African Americans are 45 percent more likely to have high blood pressure than Caucasians; therefore, they suffer strokes at an earlier age with more severe consequences.
3. *Gender.* Men have a higher incidence of many hypokinetic conditions than women. However, differences between men and women have decreased recently. This is especially true for heart disease, the leading cause of death for both men and women. Postmenopausal women have a higher heart disease risk than premenopausal women.

Factors That Can Be Altered

4. *Regular physical activity.* Regular exercise can help reduce the risk for hypokinetic disease.
5. *Diet.* A clear association exists between hypokinetic disease and certain types of diets. The excessive intake of saturated fats, such as animal fats, is linked to atherosclerosis and other forms of heart disease. Excessive salt in the diet is associated with high blood pressure.
6. *Stress.* People who are subject to excessive stress are predisposed to various hypokinetic diseases, including heart disease and back pain. Statistics indicate that hypokinetic conditions are common among those in certain high-stress jobs and those having Type A personality profiles.
7. *Tobacco use.* Smokers have five times the risk of heart attack as nonsmokers. Most striking is the difference in risk between older women smokers and nonsmokers. Tobacco use is also associated with the increased risk for high blood pressure, cancer, and several other medical conditions. Apparently, the more you use, the greater the risk. Stopping tobacco use even after many years can significantly reduce the hypokinetic disease risk.
8. *Body (fatness).* Having too much body fat is a primary risk factor for heart disease and is a risk factor for other hypokinetic conditions as well. For example, loss of fat can result in relief from symptoms of Type II diabetes, can reduce problems associated with certain types of back pain, and can reduce the risks of surgery.
9. *Blood lipids, blood glucose, and blood pressure levels.* High scores on these factors are associated with health problems, such as heart disease and diabetes. Risk increases considerably when several of these measures are high.
10. *Diseases.* People who have one hypokinetic disease are more likely to develop a second or even a third condition. For example, if you have diabetes,* your risk of having a heart attack or stroke increases dramatically. Although you may not be entirely able to alter the extent to which you develop certain diseases and conditions, reducing your risk and following your doctor's advice can improve your odds significantly.

*Some types of diabetes cannot be altered.

Strategies for Action

A self-assessment of risk factors can help you modify your lifestyle to reduce risk for heart disease. The Heart Disease Risk Factor Questionnaire in Lab 4A will help you assess your personal risk factors for heart disease. It is not a substitute, however, for a regular medical exam that includes an assessment of other cardiovascular disease risk factors, such as cholesterol and blood glucose. This will allow you to use more sophisticated and accurate risk factor assessments (see the Heart360.org tool highlighted in the *Technology Update* feature).

It is never too early to start being active to improve health. Many of the studies presented in this concept indicate that being "active for a lifetime" prevents health problems. Young adults often think "I'll worry about these problems when I get older." But what you do early in life has much to do with your current health, as well as your health later in life.

Subsequent concepts in this book cover the different components of health-related fitness and the type and amount of activity needed to improve these components. The lab activities in each of these concepts and the culminating lab activity at the end of this book are designed to help you begin planning *now* for lifelong physical activity.

Web Resources

Alzheimer's Association **www.alz.org**

American Cancer Society **www.cancer.org**

American Congress of Obstetricians and Gynecologists **www.acog.org**

American Diabetes Association **www.diabetes.org**

American Heart Association **www.americanheart.org**

American Lung Association **www.lungusa.org**

Arthritis Foundation **www.arthritis.org**

Canadian Diabetes Association **www.diabetes.ca**

Centers for Disease Control and Prevention **www.cdc.gov**

Exercise Is Medicine **www.exerciseismedicine.org**

Framingham Heart Study Risk Questionnaires and Surveys **www.framinghamheartstudy.org**

Healthy People 2020 **www.healthypeople/2020/**

Lance Armstrong Foundation **www.livestrong.org**

National Osteoporosis Foundation **www.nof.org**

National Stroke Association **www.stroke.org**

Physical Activity 360 **www.physicalactivity360.org**

Surgeon General **www.surgeongeneral.gov**

Women's Health Initiative **www.nhlbi.nih.gov/whi/**

U.S. Physical Activity Guidelines **http://www.health.gov/paguidelines/**

YouTube video ("23 and 1/2 Hours") by Mike Evans http://www.youtube.com/watch?v=aUaInS6HIGo

Suggested Readings

ACSM. 2010. *ACSM's Guidelines for Exercise Testing and Prescription.* 8th ed. Philadelphia: Lippincott, Williams & Wilkins, Chapter 1.

Baker, L. D., et al. 2010 Effects of aerobic exercise on middle cognitive impairment. *Archives of Neurology* 67(1):71–79.

Blanchard, C. M. 2012. Heart disease and physical activity: Looking beyond patient characteristics. *Exercise and Sports Sciences Reviews* 40(1):30–36.

Chodzko-Zajko, W. J., et al., 2009. Exercise and physical activity for older adults. *Medicine & Science in Sports & Exercise* 41(7):1510–1530.

Egan, B. M., et al. 2010. US trends in prevalence, awareness, treatment, and control of hypertension, 1988–2008. *Journal of the American Medical Association* 303(20):2043–2050.

Flegal, K. M. 2010. Prevalence and trends in obesity among US adults. *Journal of the American Medical Association* 303(3):235–241.

Geda, Y. E., et al. 2010. Physical exercise, aging, and mild cognitive impairment. *Archives of Neurology* 67(1): 80–86.

Gunter, K. B., et al. 2012. Physical activity in childhood may be key to optimizing lifespan skeletal health. *Exercise and Sports Sciences Reviews* 40(1):13–21.

Ogden, C. L., et al. 2010. Prevalence of high body mass index in U.S. children and adolescents. *Journal of the American Medical Association* 303(3):242–249.

Regensteiner, J. G., et al. (Eds.). 2009. *Diabetes and Exercise.* Totowa, NJ: Humana Press.

Sorace, P., et al. 2010. Peripheral arterial disease. *ACSM's Health and Fitness Journal* 14(1):16–22.

Tangka, F. K., et al. 2010. Cancer treatment costs in the United States. *Cancer.* Published online May 10, 2010, **www.canceronlinejournal.com**

Umpierre, D., et al. 2011. Physical activity advice only or structured exercise training and association with HbA$_{1c}$

levels in Type 2 Diabetes: A systematic review and meta-analysis. *Journal of the American Medical Association* 305(17):1790–1799.

U.S. Department of Health and Human Services. 2008. *2008 Physical Activity Guidelines for Americans.* Washington, DC: USDHHS. Available at **www.health.gov/paguidelines**

Wheatley, C. M., Wilkins, B. W., and Snyder, E. M. 2011. Exercise is medicine in cystic fibrosis. *Exercise & Sport Sciences Reviews.* 39(3):155–160.

Willey, J. Z., et al. 2011. Lower prevalence of silent brain infarcts in the physically active: The Northern Manhattan Study. *Neurology* 76(24):2112–2118.

Healthy People 2020

The objectives listed below are societal goals designed to help all Americans improve their health between now and the year 2020. They were selected because they relate to the content of this concept.

- Attain high-quality, longer lives free of preventable disease, injury, and premature death.

- Increase overall cardiovascular health; reduce heart disease, stroke, high blood pressure, and high blood cholesterol; increase screening; increase awareness; and increase emergency treatment by professionals or bystanders.

- Reduce cancer incidence and death rates, increase cancer patient longevity, increase survivor's quality of life, and increase cancer screening.

- Reduce diabetes incidence and death rates; increase diabetes screening, education, and care.

- Reduce depression and increase screening for depression and mental health.

- Reduce osteoporosis (related hip fractures), pain of arthritis, and limitations from chronic back pain.

- Increase percentage of college students receiving risk factor information.

- Decrease activity limitations, especially in older adults and disabled.

- Increase percentage of physicians who counsel or educate patients about exercise.

A national goal is to increase the percentage of college students receiving risk factor information. How can your campus or community health center have a bigger impact on student health and wellness? Provide suggestions along with examples of current efforts.

connect
ACTIVITY

Lab 4A Assessing Heart Disease Risk Factors

Name _____   Section _____   Date _____

Purpose: To assess your risk of developing coronary heart disease. See page 84 for directions.

Heart Disease Risk Factor Questionnaire

Risk Points

	1	2	3	4	Score
Unalterable Factors					
1. How old are you?	30 or less	31–40	41–54	55+	
2. Do you have a history of heart disease in your family?	None	Grandparent with heart disease	Parent with heart disease	More than one with heart disease	
3. What is your gender?	Female		Male		
			Total Unalterable Risk Score		
Alterable Factors					
4. Do you get regular physical activity?	4–5 days a week	3 days a week	Fewer than 3 days a week	No	
5. Do you have a high-fat diet?	No	Slightly high in fat	Above normal in fat	Eat a lot of meat and fried and fatty foods	
6. Are you under much stress?	Less than normal	Normal	Slightly above normal	Quite high	
7. Do you use tobacco?	No	Cigar or pipe	Less than 1/2 pack a day or use smokeless tobacco	More than 1/2 pack a day	
8. What is your percentage of body fat?*	F = 17–28% M = 10–20%	29–31% 21–23%	32–35% 24–30%	35+% 30+%	
9. What is the systolic number in your blood pressure?	120	121–140	141–160	160+	
10. Do you have other diseases?	No	Ulcer	Diabetes**	Both	

Extra Points: Add points for as many of the following test results as you have available: 1 point for CRP above 3, 1 point for homocysteine above 100, 3 points for LDL above 130, 3 points for TC/HDL-C above 4. If only total cholesterol is available, add 1 point for a score of 200–240 or 3 points for scores above 240.

Total Alterable Risk Score _____

Extra Points _____

Grand Total Risk Score _____

Adapted from *CAD Risk Assessor*, William J. Stone. Reprinted by permission.

*If unknown, estimate your body fat percentage or see Lab 13A.

**Diabetes is a risk factor that is often not alterable.

Procedures

1. Complete the 10 questions and the extra points, if available, on the Heart Disease Risk Factor Questionnaire by circling the answer that is most appropriate for *you* (see front of this lab).
2. Look at the top of the column for each of your answers. In the box provided at the right of each question, write down the number of risk points for that answer.
3. Determine your unalterable risk score by adding the risk points for questions 1, 2, and 3.
4. Determine your alterable risk score by adding the risk points for questions 4 through 10.
5. Determine your total heart disease risk score by adding the scores obtained in steps 3 and 4.
6. Look up your risk ratings on the Heart Disease Risk Rating Scale and record them in the Results section. Answer the questions in the Conclusions and Implications section.

Results: Write your risk scores and risk ratings in the appropriate boxes below.

Heart Disease Risk Scores and Ratings

	Score	Rating
Unalterable risk		
Alterable risk		
Total heart disease risk		

Heart Disease Risk Rating Chart

Rating	Unalterable Score	Alterable Score	Total Score
Very high	9 or more	21 or more	31 or more
High	7–8	15–20	26–30
Average	5–6	11–14	16–25
Low	4 or less	10 or less	15 or less

Conclusions and Implications: The higher your score on the Heart Disease Risk Factor Questionnaire, the greater your heart disease risk. In several sentences, discuss your risk for heart disease. Which of the risk factors do you need to control to reduce your risk for heart disease? Why?

How Much Physical Activity Is Enough?

LEARNING OBJECTIVES

After completing the study of this concept, you will be able to:

▶ Describe each of the key principles of physical activity and explain how the principles relate to each other in helping you achieve health, wellness, and fitness.

▶ Name the four elements of the FITT formula and explain how the formula relates to the concepts of *threshold of training* and *target zones* for different types of physical activity.

▶ List the five steps in the physical activity pyramid and identify the FIT formula for each.

▶ Describe the physical activity patterns of adults, differentiating among groups based on age, gender, and ethnicity.

▶ Describe the four fitness zones used for self-assessments of physical fitness and explain how each level relates to health and performance.

▶ Identify related national health goals and show how meeting personal goals can contribute to reaching national goals.

▶ Self-assess your current activity level for each step of the physical activity pyramid and estimate your current health and skill-related physical fitness.

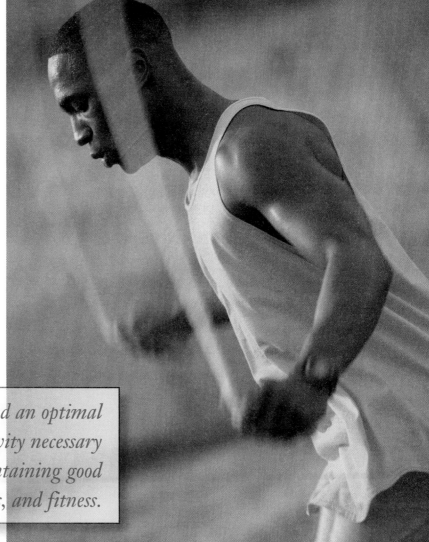

There is a minimal and an optimal amount of physical activity necessary for developing and maintaining good health, wellness, and fitness.

Physical activity is a behavior that leads to fitness, health, and wellness. However, for physical activity to have an optimal effect, the appropriate amount of activity must be performed. This concept describes the basic principles of physical activity, including the FITT formula, and key concepts such as *threshold of training* and *target zones*. Use the physical activity pyramid to help understand and remember physical activity guidelines for different types of activities.

The Principles of Physical Activity

Overload is necessary to achieve the health, wellness, and fitness benefits of physical activity. The **overload principle,** the most basic of all physical activity principles, indicates that doing "more than normal" is necessary if benefits are to occur. In order for a muscle (including the heart muscle) to get stronger, it must be overloaded, or worked against a load greater than normal. To increase flexibility, a muscle must be stretched longer than is normal. To increase muscular endurance, muscles must be 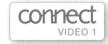 exposed to sustained exercise for a longer than normal period. The health benefits associated with metabolic fitness seem to require less overload than for health-related fitness improvement, but overload is required, just the same.

Increase physical activity progressively for safe and effective results. The **principle of progression** indicates that overload should occur in a gradual progression rather than in major bursts. Failure to adhere to this principle can result in excess soreness or injury. Although some tightness or fatigue is common after exercise, it is not necessary to feel sore in order to improve. Training is most effective when the sessions become progressively more challenging over time.

The benefits of physical activity are specific to the form of activity performed. The **principle of specificity** states that to benefit from physical activity you must overload specifically for that benefit. For example, strength-building exercises may do little for developing cardiovascular fitness, and stretching exercises may do little for altering body composition or metabolic fitness.

Overload is also specific to each body part. If you exercise the legs, you build fitness of the legs. If you exercise the arms, you build fitness of the arms. Some gymnasts, for example, have good upper body development but poor leg development, whereas some soccer players have well-developed legs but lack upper body development.

Specificity is important in designing your warm-up, workout, and cool-down programs for specific activities. Training is most effective when it closely resembles the activity for which you are preparing. For example, if your goal is to improve performance in putting the shot, it is not enough to strengthen the arm muscles. You should train using exercises that require overload of all muscles used and that require motions similar to those used in putting the shot.

The benefits achieved from overload last only as long as overload continues. The **principle of reversibility** is the overload principle in reverse. To put it simply, if you don't use it, you lose it. Some people have the mistaken impression that if they achieve a health or fitness benefit it will last forever. Although there is evidence that you can maintain health benefits with less physical activity than it took to achieve them, if you do not engage in regular physical activity, any benefits attained will gradually erode.

In general, the more physical activity you do, the more benefits you receive. Just as there is a correct dosage of medicine for treatment of illness, there is a correct dosage of physical activity for promoting health benefits and the development of physical fitness. Though there are some exceptions, a considerable amount of research indicates that benefits from physical activity follow a **dose-response relationship**—the more physical activity you perform, the more benefits you gain.

Figure 1 illustrates the overall pattern of the dose-response relationship. The red bar indicates the high risk for hypokinetic disease and early death for those who are inactive. A modest increase in physical activity, such as the

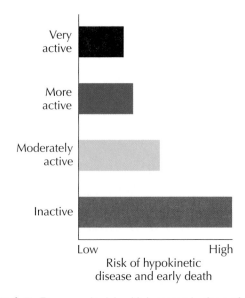

Figure 1 ▶ Decrease in risk with increase in dose of activity.

In the News

Quantity and Quality of Exercise

The American College of Sports Medicine (ACSM) released a new position statement that provides specific guidelines about the amount of physical activity necessary for developing fitness and achieving health benefits. The report ("Quantity and quality of exercise for developing and maintaining cardiorespiratory, musculoskeletal, and neuromotor fitness in apparently healthy adults: Guidance for prescribing exercise") notes that *"the scientific evidence demonstrating the beneficial effects of exercise is indisputable, and the benefits of exercise far outweigh the risks in most adults."* The report emphasizes the importance of developing an "individualized" program based on personal needs.

Why is it important to focus on individual needs? What specific needs do you have and how does this impact your exercise program?

connect
ACTIVITY

30 minutes of moderate activity recommended in the new activity guidelines, results in a substantial decrease in risk and early death (green bar). Additional activity (blue bar) has extra benefits, but the benefits are not as great as those that come from making the change from being inactive to doing some activity. As the black bar indicates, very high levels of activity produce little additional health benefit.

As you learned in Concept 4, the "dose" of activity necessary to get one benefit is not the same as the "dose" for another. For example, changes in cholesterol levels resulting from physical activity may change at a different rate than changes in blood pressure. Many benefits in health, wellness, and fitness are obtained with moderate amounts of activity, so the key is to be at least active enough to obtain these benefits.

The rate of improvement levels off as you become more fit, and at some point maintenance is an appropriate goal. In physical fitness, more is not always better. The **principle of diminished returns** indicates that as you get fitter, you may not get as big a benefit for each additional amount of activity you perform. As shown in Figure 1, the risk of hypokinetic disease and early death is nearly cut in half by moving from being sedentary (red bar) to becoming moderately active (green). More activity (blue) and much activity (black) provide further reduction in risk, but the reduction in risk is diminished for each additional amount of activity.

Clearly, the more activity you perform, the more benefits you get. Beginners benefit the most from becoming active and should strive first to become moderately active. More active people get additional benefits if they do more, but (based on the principle of diminishing returns) they should not expect to continue to improve at the same rate.

Rest is needed to allow the body to adapt to exercise. The **principle of rest and recovery** indicates that you should allow time for recuperation after overload. Proper rest is needed within intense periods of activity, and appropriate rest is needed between training sessions. Rest provides time for the body to adapt to the stimulus provided during the workout. Failure to take sufficient rest can lead to overuse injuries, fatigue, and reduced performance. For recreational exercisers, rest generally implies taking a day off between bouts of exercise or alternating hard and easy days of exercise.

Overload Principle You must perform physical activity in greater than normal amounts (overload) to get an improvement in physical fitness or health benefits.

Principle of Progression You need to gradually increase overload to achieve optimal benefits.

Principle of Specificity Specific types of exercise are needed to improve each fitness component or the fitness of a specific part of the body.

Principle of Reversibility Disuse or inactivity results in loss of benefits achieved as a result of overload.

Dose-Response Relationship A term adopted from medicine. With medicine, it is important to know what response (benefit) will occur from taking a specific dose. When studying physical activity, it is important to know what dose provides the best response (most benefits). The contents of this book are designed to help you choose the best doses of activity for the responses (benefits) you desire.

Principle of Diminished Returns The more benefits you gain as a result of activity, the harder additional benefits are to achieve.

Principle of Rest and Recovery You need adequate rest to allow the body to adapt to and recover from exercise.

All people benefit from physical activity, but the benefits are unique for each person. Heredity, age, gender, ethnicity, lifestyles, current fitness and health status, and a variety of other factors make each person unique at any point in time. The **principle of individuality** indicates that the benefits of physical activity vary from individual to individual based on each person's unique characteristics.

The FITT Formula

The acronyms FITT and FIT help you remember important variables for applying the overload principle. For physical activity to be effective, each type of activity must be done with enough frequency, with enough intensity, and for a long enough time. The first letters from four words spell **FITT** and can be considered as the formula for achieving health, wellness, and fitness benefits.

Frequency (how often)—Physical activity must be performed regularly to be effective. Most benefits require at least 3 days and up to 6 days of activity per week, but frequency ultimately depends on the specific activity and the benefit desired.

Intensity (how hard)—Physical activity must be intense enough to require more exertion (overload) than normal to produce benefits. The appropriate intensity varies with the desired benefit. Health benefits from metabolic fitness require only moderate activity, but performance benefits require more vigorous activity.

Time (how long)—Physical activity must be done for an adequate length of time to be effective. The length of the activity session depends on the type of activity and the expected benefit.

Type (kind of activity)—The benefits derived depend on the type of activity performed. For example, moderate activity must be done at least 5 days a week, while muscle fitness activity may be done as few as 2 days a week.

When determining the formula for each type of activity, the shorter acronym (FIT) can be used because you have already determined the activity type. In the following section, you will learn 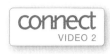 more about the **FIT** formula for each activity in the physical activity pyramid. In subsequent concepts, each formula is described in greater detail.

The pattern and volume of physical activity are important considerations. Two factors, pattern and volume of physical activity, need to be considered when applying the FITT formula. Pattern refers to the way in which you accumulate your exercise. Volume refers to the total amount of exercise that you perform each day. It is a combination of the intensity of your exercise sessions and the total amount of time spent in exercise. Some experts refer to FITT-PV when discussing pattern (*P*) and volume (*V*) of exercise. The ACSM suggests that the recommended volume of exercise for achieving health benefits can be accumulated in several short bouts (10 minutes or longer) or performed in one longer bout to reach a daily total of 30 minutes. Other patterns of exercise include intermittent versus continuous exercise, and different patterns of exercise for muscle fitness (e.g., periodization). The ACSM discourages the "weekend warrior" pattern that includes no regular exercise but "a large total volume" of exercise on one day of the week, typically on a weekend day. Concepts that follow discuss various patterns of exercise and show how they can be used to accumulate the desired volume of exercise for each day.

Threshold of training and *target zone* help you use the FIT formula. The **threshold of training** is the minimum amount of activity (frequency, intensity, and time) necessary to produce benefits. Depending on the benefit expected, slightly more than normal activity may not be enough to promote health, wellness, or fitness benefits. The **target zone** begins at the threshold of training and stops at the point where the activity becomes counterproductive. Figure 2 illustrates the threshold of training and target zone concepts.

Some people incorrectly associate threshold of training and target zones with only cardiovascular fitness. As the principle of specificity suggests, each component of fitness, including metabolic fitness, has its own FIT formula and its own threshold and target zone. The target and threshold levels for **health benefits** are different from those for achieving **performance benefits** associated with high levels of physical fitness.

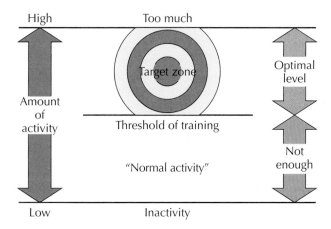

Figure 2 ▶ Physical activity target zone.

It takes time for activity to produce health, wellness, and fitness benefits, even when the FIT formula is properly applied. Sometimes people beginning a physical activity program expect to see immediate results. They expect to see large losses in body fat or great increases in muscle strength in a few days. Evidence shows, however, that improvements in health-related physical fitness and the associated health benefits take several weeks to become apparent. Though some people report psychological benefits, such as "feeling better" and a "sense of personal accomplishment" almost immediately after beginning regular exercise, the physiological changes take considerably longer to be realized. Proper preparation for physical activity includes learning not to expect too much too soon and not to do too much too soon. Attempts to get fit fast will probably be counterproductive, resulting in soreness and even injury. The key is to start slowly, stay with it, and enjoy yourself. Benefits will come to those who persist.

Many organizations have developed physical activity guidelines based on sound principles. To help the general public determine the appropriate FIT formula for each type of physical activity, various organizations have developed guidelines. The earliest guidelines were developed by ACSM. Over the years, guidelines have also been developed by the American Heart Association (AHA), the Office of the Surgeon General (OSG), the Institute of Medicine (IOM), the U.S. Department of Health and Human Services (DHHS), and the Centers for Disease Control and Prevention (CDC). The FITT formula used in this book is based on information from several of these sources, most prominently the DHHS *Physical Activity Guidelines for Americans*, the ACSM's guidelines for exercise prescription, and the ACSM's new position on quality and quantity of exercise (see In the News, page 87).

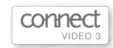

The Physical Activity Pyramid

The physical activity pyramid classifies activities by type and associated benefits. The **physical activity pyramid** (see Figure 3) was created to help readers better understand the five basic *types* of physical activity (e.g., the last *T* in FITT). Over the years, it has proven to be a useful model for illustrating how each type of activity contributes to the development of health, wellness, and physical fitness. The pyramid depicts five different steps. Each step represents a step toward achieving health, wellness, and fitness. Inactivity is shown below the pyramid because it does not represent a step toward active living. Placement in the pyramid is not

meant to suggest that higher steps are more important than lower steps. Activities from all steps are important for optimal health, wellness, and fitness. Key concepts illustrated by the physical activity pyramid include the following:

- Each type of activity has its own FIT formula and unique health, wellness, and physical fitness benefits.
- The different types of physical activity can be combined to meet activity guidelines.
- Extended periods of inactivity can be harmful to your health.
- Eating well (sound nutrition) is an important companion behavior to physical activity (see energy balance scale at the top of Figure 3).

Each of the five steps of the physical activity pyramid are discussed in greater detail in the paragraphs that follow as well as in Concepts 6, 8, 9, and 10.

Inactivity can be hazardous to your health. The five steps in the physical activity pyramid illustrate the different types of physical activity (Figure 3). Recent evidence suggests that minimizing inactivity may be just as important as being active. For children, the physical activity guidelines published by the National Association for Sport

Principle of Individuality Overload provides unique benefits to each individual based on the unique characteristics of that person.

FITT, FIT A formula used to describe the frequency, intensity, time, and type of physical activity necessary to produce benefits. When the type of activity has been determined, the second *T* is dropped and the shorter acronym FIT is used.

Threshold of Training The minimum amount of physical activity that will produce health and fitness benefits.

Target Zone The amounts of physical activity that produce optimal health and fitness benefits.

Health Benefits The results of physical activity that provide protection from hypokinetic disease or early death.

Performance Benefits The results of physical activity that improve physical fitness and physical performance capabilities.

Physical Activity Pyramid Different types of activities contribute to the development of health and physical fitness. Activities lower in the pyramid require more frequent participation, whereas activities higher in the pyramid require less frequency.

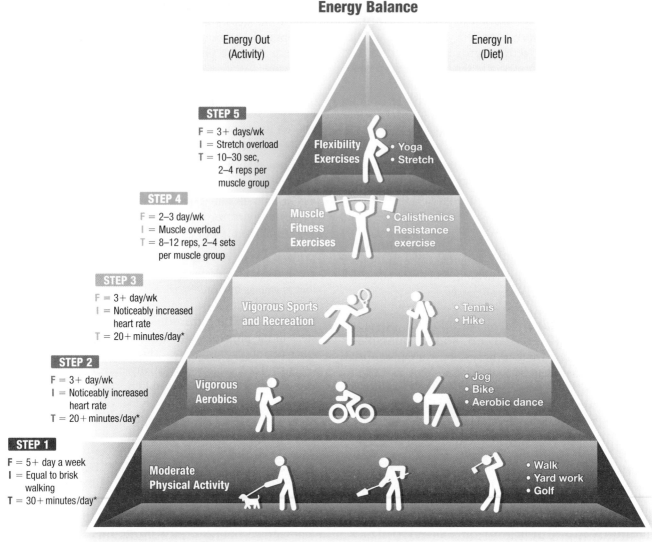

Figure 3 ▶ The physical activity pyramid.

Source: C. B. Corbin

and Physical Education (NASPE) recommend periods of inactivity should not exceed 2 hours at a time. One goal of Healthy People 2020 is to reduce the proportion of youth who are inactive for long periods of time (defined as viewing television and videos or playing computer games more than 2 hours a day).

It is interesting that *Healthy People 2020* does not have a goal for reducing inactivity for adults, inasmuch as many adults sit for many hours each day. An editorial in the *British Journal of Sports Medicine* suggests that sitting for hours provides "harmful signals" to the body's systems. Another study of 17,000 Canadians showed that those who sit more have higher rates of chronic disease and death than those who sit less, independent of the amount of activity they performed. Yet another study showed that among adults the death rates from all causes

are significantly related to the amount of television a person watches. Surveys indicate that people in Western cultures spend more than half of their time sitting, often in front of a television or a computer.

Although regular physical activity from the five steps of the physical activity pyramid is recommended, evidence suggests that even "sub-threshold" amounts of activity can have health benefits (e.g., standing while working and walking while talking on the phone). Sub-threshold exercise is described in more detail in Concepts 6, 13, and 15.

Moderate activities provide many benefits for modest amounts of effort. Moderate aerobic activities equal in intensity to brisk walking provide significant health benefits. For a variety of reasons, they are depicted as step 1 of the physical activity pyramid (see Figure 3).

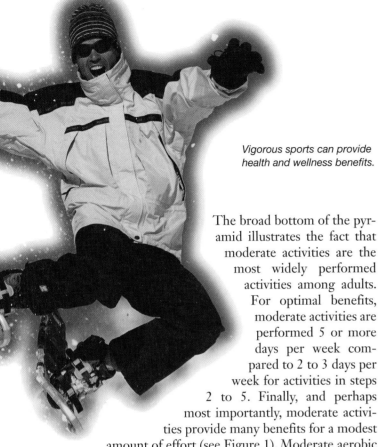

Vigorous sports can provide health and wellness benefits.

The broad bottom of the pyramid illustrates the fact that moderate activities are the most widely performed activities among adults. For optimal benefits, moderate activities are performed 5 or more days per week compared to 2 to 3 days per week for activities in steps 2 to 5. Finally, and perhaps most importantly, moderate activities provide many benefits for a modest amount of effort (see Figure 1). Moderate aerobic activities, such as walking to and from work, climbing the stairs rather than taking an elevator, or doing brisk housework when done as part of the normal daily routine are often referred to as lifestyle physical activities. Moderate activities that are not part of the normal daily routine, such as taking a walk or a bike ride, can also be planned specifically to increase activity levels.

Studies indicate that individuals with active jobs have reduced risks for many chronic conditions. Those who actively commute (bike or walk) to work or to run errands have also been found to have better health profiles. The regular accumulation of activity as a part of one's lifestyle is sufficient to promote positive improvements in metabolic fitness, and these improvements can positively impact health. Additional activity from the other layers of the pyramid are strongly recommended. Moderate activity can be viewed as the baseline, or minimal, activity that should be performed. A summary of the FIT formula for moderate activity is illustrated in step 1 of Figure 3.

Vigorous aerobic activity provides additional health benefits. **Vigorous aerobic activities** (step 2) are of greater intensity than moderate activities (step 1). The greater intensity results in significantly higher heart rates and higher oxygen consumption. Because of its greater intensity, vigorous aerobics can be performed as few as 3 days a week and are especially good for building

cardiovascular fitness and helping to control body fatness. Examples of vigorous aerobic activities, sometimes referred to as active aerobics, are jogging, biking, and aerobic dance. Vigorous aerobic activities can provide metabolic fitness and health benefits similar to moderate activities and can be performed instead of, or in combination with, moderate activities to meet national activity guidelines.

Vigorous sports and recreation activities can provide similar benefits as vigorous aerobic activity. **Vigorous sports and recreation** are activities of similar intensity to vigorous aerobics. Some sports, such as golf and bowling, can be classified as moderate aerobic activities because they are of a lower intensity. Vigorous sports and recreation activities (see Figure 3, step 3) can be performed instead of, or in combination with, vigorous aerobic activities or moderate activities, to meet national activity guidelines.

Muscle fitness exercises are important for optimal fitness and health. There are muscle fitness benefits from many different activities, including vocational activities that require lifting, active sports such as gymnastics and wrestling, and recreational activities such as rock climbing. The muscle fitness activities included at step 4 of the pyramid are those that are planned specifically to build strength and muscular endurance, such as resistance training and calisthenics. The many health and performance benefits of muscle fitness exercises are described in Concept 9. A general description of the FIT formula for muscle fitness exercises is included in Figure 3 (step 4).

Flexibility exercises are important for building and maintaining flexibility. There are flexibility benefits from many different activities, including sports such as gymnastics and diving. The flexibility exercises included at step 5 of the pyramid are those that are planned specifically to build flexibility, such as stretching exercises and yoga. The many benefits of flexibility exercises are described in Concept 10. A general

Moderate Aerobic Activities Aerobic activities equal in intensity to a brisk walk are referred to as moderate activities (see step 1 of the activity pyramid).

Vigorous Aerobic Activities Vigorous aerobic activities that elevate the heart rate and are greater in intensity than a brisk walk (see step 2 of the activity pyramid).

Vigorous Sports and Recreation Sports such as soccer and volleyball, or recreational activities such as hiking, that elevate the heart rate and are of greater intensity than a brisk walk. (See step 3 of the physical activity pyramid.)

TECHNOLOGY UPDATE

Active Workstations

To avoid the health dangers of sitting, one possible solution is to work while standing or moving. A company called Trek Desk sells desks that mount over standard treadmills, offering considerable potential for promoting activity in worksite settings.

Would you use this type of technology to get additional activity if it was available on campus or at your work setting?

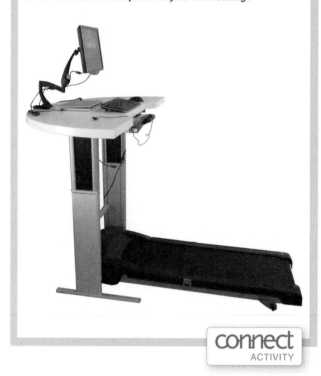

connect
ACTIVITY

description of the FIT formula for flexibility exercises is included in Figure 3 (step 5).

Energy balance is important for maintaining a healthy body composition. Weight management requires that energy intake be matched by energy expenditure. The FIT formula messages in the physical activity pyramid provide general information about the amounts of activity (energy expenditure) necessary for general health and fitness benefits. But these amounts may not be enough for weight management (or weight loss). Current physical activity guidelines suggest that 45 to 60 minutes of daily moderate activity may be necessary (as opposed to 30 minutes).

The balance scale at the top of the pyramid in Figure 3 illustrates the importance of balancing energy intake with energy expenditure. More information about maintaining energy balance for body composition is included in Concepts 14 and 15.

Some important factors should be considered when using the physical activity pyramid. The physical activity pyramid is a useful model for describing different types of activity, their benefits, and the FIT formula for each level. However, as the American College of Sports Medicine points out, physical activity guidelines "cannot be implemented in an overly rigid fashion and recommendations presented should be used with careful attention to the goals of the individual." The following guidelines for using the pyramid should also be considered:

- *No single activity provides all of the benefits.* Many people wonder "What is the perfect form of physical activity?" There is no single activity that can provide all of the health, wellness, and fitness benefits. It is best to perform activities from all steps of the pyramid because each type of activity has different benefits.

- *Something is better than nothing.* Some people may say, "I just don't have time to do all of the activities in the pyramid." This could lead some to throw up their hands in despair, concluding, "I just won't do anything at all." Evidence indicates that something is better than nothing, so try to do a little activity and add more as time allows.

- *Activities from steps 2 and 3 can be used instead of, or in combination with, those from step 1 to achieve health and fitness benefits.* While more people typically perform moderate activities (step 1), many prefer more vigorous activities from steps 2 and 3 of the pyramid. Both provide health benefits and the two can be combined to meet activity guidelines (see Concept 8).

- *Activities from steps 4 and 5 are useful even if you are limited in performing activities at other levels.* It is best to include some activities from steps 1, 2, and 3, but muscular exercise and flexibility exercise do provide benefits on their own.

- *Good planning will allow you to schedule activities from all steps in a reasonable amount of time.* In subsequent concepts, you will learn more about each step of the pyramid, as well as how to plan a total physical activity program.

- *Specific activity recommendations exist for youth. Children are different from adults, and they have different needs for activity.* According to guidelines, children should accumulate at least 60 minutes, and up to several hours, of age-appropriate physical activity on most, if not all, days of the week. The guidelines also recommend minimizing periods of inactivity (periods of 2 or more hours). Adults play a major role in shaping children's current and future activity patterns.

- *Specific guidelines exist for older adults.* Specific activity guidelines are available for adults 65 and older. The guidelines are similar to those for younger adults but differ in some important ways. The guidelines for intensity of aerobic activity take into account the older adult's activity level (see Concept 7). Also, older adults typically do more repetitions and use less resistance when doing muscle fitness exercise (see Concept 9), flexibility exercises become more important, and exercise for balance is recommended.

Physical Activity Patterns

National health goals have been established for each type of activity illustrated in the physical activity pyramid. The percentages of adults 18 and over meeting the national goals for moderate and vigorous activity are presented in Table 1. Adults who did either moderate activity 5 days a week for at least 30 minutes a day OR vigorous activity for 3 days a week for at least 20 minutes a day met the guideline. The survey was conducted before the announcement of the most recent guidelines and did not include people who combined moderate and vigorous activity. The percentages of adults meeting muscle fitness exercise and flexibility exercise goals are presented in Table 2. The good news is that the numbers in Table 1 show higher percentages of adults meeting activity goals than in the past. Currently 35 percent of adults meet the national goal for aerobic activity, up from 30 percent 10 years earlier. The not-so-good news is that more than 50 percent of adults do the minimum amount of activity necessary for gaining the health and fitness benefits of aerobic exercise. Fewer adults meet guidelines for muscle fitness and flexibility exercise than for moderate or vigorous activity.

Table 1 ▶ Percentages of Adults Who Meet National Activity Goals for Moderate or Vigorous Aerobic Physical Activity

Classification Group		Percent
Gender	Male	37
	Female	33
	General Population	35
Age	18–24	43
	25–64	36
	65–74	35
Ethnicity	White[a]	38
	Hispanic[b]	28
	Black[c]	29

Source: Center for Disease Control and Prevention.
[a]Non-Hispanic. [b]Hispanic/Latino. [c]African American

Table 2 ▶ Percentage of Adults Who Meet National Activity Goals by Gender, Age, Income, Ethnicity, and Disability

	Gender		
	Male	Female	All
Moderate	16	13	14
Vigorous	25	22	23
Muscle fitness	27	23	19
Flexibility	29	31	30
	Age		
	18–24	25–44	45–65
Moderate	14	16	13
Vigorous	28[a]	28[a]	22
Muscle fitness	19	27	23
Flexibility	30	29	31
	Income		
	Low	Medium	High
Moderate	11	14	17
Vigorous	16	20	25
Muscle fitness	18	22	36
Flexibility	— — —	— — —	— — —

	Ethnicity			
	White[b]	Hispanic[c]	Black[d]	Asian[e]
Moderate	16	10	10	23
Vigorous	24	17	19	20
Muscle fitness	28	21	30	28
Flexibility	31	22	26	34

	Disability	
	With	Without
Moderate	12	16
Vigorous	13	25
Muscle fitness	14	20
Flexibility	29	31

Source: National Health Interview Survey.
Values represent percentages of adults who reach national goals for each of four types of activity and percentages of adults who get no leisure activity.
[a]Data available for 18–44, same statistic used for both.
[b]Non-Hispanic. [c]Hispanic/Latino. [d]African American. [e]Or Pacific Islander.

The proportion of people meeting national health goals varies based on age. Children are the most active group in Western society. During adolescence, activity starts to decrease, but teens still do more activity than young adults. Activity levels of all types decrease from young adulthood to ages 65 and over (see Tables 1 and 2).

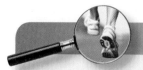

A CLOSER LOOK

Physical Activity Patterns

Patterns of physical activity vary considerably by gender, age, ethnicity, socio-economic status, and other demographic variables. Researchers at the Centers for Disease Control and Prevention (CDC) conduct regular surveillance of physical activity and other health behaviors to understand patterns and trends in the population. One of the more frequently cited survey instruments is the Behavioral Risk Factor Surveillance System (BRFSS). Based on the data, approximately 50 percent of Americans report getting regular physical activity (defined in this survey as 30+ minutes of moderate physical activity 5 or more days per week, or vigorous physical activity for 20+ minutes 3 or more days per week). The website for the BRFSS (www.cdc.gov/brfss/) allows users to examine patterns and trends in health behaviors by a variety of demographic variables and to see the activity levels within specific states.

How do patterns or trends look in your state?

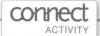
connect
ACTIVITY

HELP **Health is available to Everyone for a Lifetime, and it's Personal**

The U.S. *Physical Activity Guidelines* from the Centers for Disease Control (CDC) indicate that adults should get a minimum of 150 minutes of moderate activity each week (e.g., 30 minutes five days a week). However, performing 75 minutes of vigorous activity per week also meets the guidelines.

Do you think 150 minutes of moderate activity or 75 minutes of vigorous activity per week is a realistic goal for most people?

connect
ACTIVITY

The proportion of adults meeting national health goals varies based on income, education, and disability status. People at or near poverty levels are more than twice as likely to be totally inactive during leisure time, compared with those with high income. Low-income people are also much less likely to meet national health goals for activity than middle- to high-income people. High school dropouts are three times more likely to be totally inactive than college graduates and meet national activity goals less frequently. Adults with one or more physical disabilities have a high probability of being inactive. Minority groups have high rates of inactivity, and as illustrated in Tables 1 and 2, White non-Hispanic people are more likely to meet national activity goals than Hispanic and Black Americans. While no information was provided in the most recent survey for Asian Americans, previous surveys indicate that they are similar in activity levels to White non-Hispanics.

Physical Fitness Standards

Health-based criterion-referenced standards are recommended for rating your fitness. This concept has focused on the amount of physical activity necessary to get health and fitness benefits. Another question to be answered is "How much physical fitness is enough?" Most experts recommend **health-based criterion-referenced standards** to rate your current fitness. These standards

are based on how much fitness is needed for good health. Other standards use norms or percentiles that compare a person's fitness against a reference population. Knowing how you compare with other people is not that important. In fact, such comparisons have been shown to be discouraging to many people. Determining if your fitness is adequate to enhance your health and wellness is more relevant.

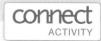
connect
VIDEO 5

Table 3 ▶ The Four Fitness Zones

High-Performance Zone

Reaching this zone provides additional health benefits and is important to high-level performance. However, high performance scores are hard for some people to achieve, and for many people high-level performance is not important. So reaching this zone may be more important to some than others.

Good Fitness Zone

If you reach the good fitness zone, you have enough of a specific fitness component to help reduce health risk. However, staying active (in addition to reaching this fitness zone) is important.

Marginal Zone

Marginal scores indicate that some improvement is in order, but you are nearing minimal health standards set by experts.

Low-Fit Zone

If you score low in fitness, you are probably less fit than you should be for your own good health and wellness.

Health-Based Criterion-Referenced Standards

The amount of a specific type of fitness necessary to gain a health or wellness benefit.

In this book, four different rating zones are used (see Table 3). In the concepts that follow, you will perform many different self-assessments to determine your fitness zone for each part of fitness. The long-term goal is to achieve the "good fitness zone," a standard associated with good health. People in the low fitness zone have a higher risk than those in the other three zones and a goal should be to first strive to move out of the low zone into the marginal zone. Those in the marginal zone are at lower risk than those in the low fitness zone, but should strive to move into the good fitness zone.

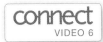

With reasonable amounts of physical activity over time, most people should be able to improve their fitness enough to make it into this range. For personal reasons, some may wish to aim for the high performance zone. Attaining this level may provide some additional health benefits but the effort required is great. Reaching the high performance zone will be important for those interested in high-level performance, but should not be a goal of those in the low fitness or marginal zones until the good fitness zone is reached.

Strategies for Action

A self-assessment of your current activity at each level of the pyramid can help you determine future activity goals.   Lab 5A provides you with the opportunity to assess your physical activity at each level of the pyramid. Lab 5B offers a general assessment of fitness. Later you will develop a program of activity, and these assessments will provide a basis for program planning.

Self-assessments of physical fitness can help you prepare a fitness profile that can be used in program planning.   In the concepts that follow, you will learn to perform a variety of self-assessments of fitness and will learn the scores that are necessary on these assessments to reach the good fitness zone as described in Table 3. In the meantime, you can complete Lab 5B. This lab will help you understand the nature of each part of fitness and estimate your current fitness level for each type of fitness. When you complete the more detailed self-assessments later in the book, you will be able to determine the accuracy of your estimates.

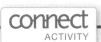

Web Resources

Centers for Disease Control and Prevention (CDC)
www.cdc.gov
Health Canada **http://www.hc-sc.gc.ca**
Healthy People 2020 **www.healthypeople.gov/HP2020**
Let's Move **www.letsmove.gov**
Morbidity and Mortality Weekly Reports **www.cdc.gov/mmwr**
Physical Activity Guidelines for Americans **www.health.gov/paguidelines**

Suggested Readings

ACSM. 2010. *ACSM's Guidelines for Exercise Testing and Prescription.* 8th ed. Philadelphia: Lippincott, Williams & Wilkins.
Barnes, P. M., et al. 2009. Early release of selected estimates based on data from the January–June 2009 *National Health Interview Survey.* National Center for Health Statistics. Available at **www.cdc.gov/nchs/nhis/released200912.htm**
Bassett, D. R., P. Freedson, and S. Kozey. 2010. Medical hazards of prolonged sitting. *Exercise and Sport Sciences Reviews* 38(3):101–102.
Blair, S. N. 2009. Physical inactivity: The biggest public health problem of the 21st century. *British Journal of Sports Medicine* 43(1):1–2.
Centers for Disease Control and Prevention. 2007. Prevalence of regular physical activity among adults—United States. *Morbidity and Mortality Weekly Reports* 56(46):1209–1212.
Dunstan, D. W., et al. 2010. Television viewing time and mortality. *Circulation* 121(3):384–391.
Ekblom-Bak, E., et al. 2010. Are we facing a new paradigm of inactivity physiology? *British Journal of Sports Medicine* 10:1136.
Fulton, J. E., Wargo, J., and F. Loustalot. 2011. Healthy People 2020: Physical activity objectives for the future. *President's Council on Fitness, Sports, and Nutrition Research Digest* 12(2):1–16. Available at **http://fitness.gov/resources-and-grants/council-research/**

Garber, C. E. et al. 2011. Quantity and quality of exercise for developing and maintaining cardiorespiratory, musculoskeletal, and neuromotor fitness in apparently healthy adults: Guidance for prescribing exercise. *Medicine and Science in Sports and Exercise* 43(7):1334–1359.

Kohl, H. W., and T. Murray. 2012. *Foundations of Physical Activity and Public Health*. Champaign, IL: Human Kinetics.

Owen, N., et al. 2010. Too much sitting: The population health science of sedentary behavior. *Exercise and Sport Sciences Reviews* 38(3):105–113.

Pescatello, L. S., et al. 2009. A preview of ACSM's guidelines for exercise testing and prescription: Eighth edition. *ACSM's Health and Fitness Journal* 13(4):23–26.

Pleis, J. R., and B. W. Ward. 2009. Summary health statistics for U. S. Adults: National Health Interview Survey. *Vital Health Statistics* 10(242):74–75.

White, S. M., et al. 2010. Leading a physically active lifestyle: Effective individual behavior change strategies. *ACSM's Health and Fitness Journal* 14(1):8–15.

United States Department of Health and Human Services. 2008. *2008 Physical Activity Guidelines for Americans.* Washington: USDHHS. Available at **www.health.gov/paguidelines**

Healthy People 2020

The objectives listed below are societal goals designed to help all Americans improve their health between now and the year 2020. They were selected because they relate to the content of this concept.

- Reduce proportion of adults who do no leisure-time activity.

- Increase proportion of adults who meet guidelines for aerobic activity.

- Increase proportion of adults who meet guidelines for muscle fitness activity.

- Increase access to employee-based exercise facilities and programs.

- Increase proportion of trips made by walking.

- Increase proportion of youth who meet guidelines for TV viewing and computer use and overuse (overuse is 2 hours a day or more).

- Increase schools with activity spaces that can be used in non-school hours.

It is important to not only develop active lifestyles but also to minimize time spent being inactive (or sedentary). A specific Healthy People 2020 goal focuses on reducing the percentage of people who watch more than 2 hours of TV per day. What can you do to reduce the amount of time you spend being sedentary?

Lab 5A Self-Assessment of Physical Activity

Name	Section	Date

Purpose: To estimate your current levels of physical activity from each category of the physical activity pyramid

Procedures

1. Place an X over the circle that characterizes your participation in each category in the pyramid. Place an X over one circle below the yellow box at the bottom of the pyramid to indicate days of inactivity.
2. Determine if you met the national goal for each type of activity. In the Results section of the chart on the next page, place an X over the "yes" circle if you meet the goal in each area or an X over the "no" circle if you do not meet the goal.

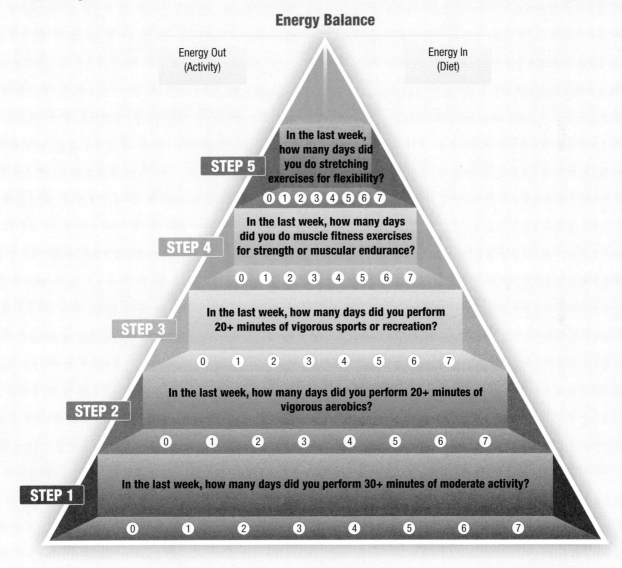

Energy Balance

Energy Out
(Activity)

Energy In
(Diet)

STEP 5 In the last week, how many days did you do stretching exercises for flexibility?
0 1 2 3 4 5 6 7

STEP 4 In the last week, how many days did you do muscle fitness exercises for strength or muscular endurance?
0 1 2 3 4 5 6 7

STEP 3 In the last week, how many days did you perform 20+ minutes of vigorous sports or recreation?
0 1 2 3 4 5 6 7

STEP 2 In the last week, how many days did you perform 20+ minutes of vigorous aerobics?
0 1 2 3 4 5 6 7

STEP 1 In the last week, how many days did you perform 30+ minutes of moderate activity?
0 1 2 3 4 5 6 7

Inactivity

In the last week, how many days did you fail to do any activities from the 5 steps above?

0 1 2 3 4 5 6 7

Results

Activity Type	Step	National Goal	Did You Meet the National Health Goal?	
Moderate activity	1	5 days or more	Yes	No
Vigorous activity	2 and 3	3 days or more	Yes	No
Muscle fitness	4	2 days or more	Yes	No
Flexibility exercises	5	3 days or more	Yes	No
Inactivity	—	Avoid total inactivity	Yes	No

Conclusions and Implications: In the space below, write a brief paper describing your current physical activity patterns. Do you meet the national health goals in all areas? If not, in what types of activity from the pyramid do you need to improve? Are the answers you gave for the past week typical of your regular activity patterns? If you meet all national health goals, explain why you think this is so. Do you think that meeting the goals in the pyramid on the previous page indicates good activity patterns for you?

Write your physical activity assessment paper in the space below.

Lab 5B Estimating Your Fitness

Name	Section	Date

Purpose: To help you better understand each of the 11 components of health-related and skill-related physical fitness and to help you estimate your current levels of physical fitness

Special Note: The activities performed in the lab are *not intended as valid tests of physical fitness.* Completing the activities will help you better understand each component of fitness and help you estimate your current fitness levels. You should not rely primarily on the results of the activities to make your estimates. Rather, you should rely on previous fitness tests you have taken and your own best judgment of your current fitness. Later in this book, you will learn how to perform accurate assessments of each fitness component and determine the accuracy of your estimates.

Procedures

1. Consider a warm-up before and cool-down after. Perform each of the activities described in Chart 1 on page 100.
2. Use past fitness test performances and your own judgment to estimate your current levels for each of the health-related and skill-related physical fitness parts. Low fitness = improvement definitely needed, marginal fitness = some improvement necessary, good fitness = adequate for healthy daily living.
3. Place an X in the appropriate circle for your fitness estimate in the Results section.

Results

Fitness Component	Low Fitness	Marginal Fitness	Good Fitness
Balance	○	○	○
Power	○	○	○
Agility	○	○	○
Reaction time	○	○	○
Speed	○	○	○
Coordination	○	○	○
Cardiovascular fitness	○	○	○
Flexibility	○	○	○
Body composition	○	○	○
Strength	○	○	○
Muscular endurance	○	○	○

Conclusions and Implications: In several sentences, discuss the information you used to make your estimates of physical fitness. How confident are you that these estimates are accurate?

Directions: Attempt each of the activities in Chart 1. Place an X in the circle next to each component of physical fitness to indicate that you have attempted the activity.

Chart 1 Physical Fitness Activities

Balance ◯

1. *One-foot balance.* Stand on one foot; press up so that the weight is on the ball of the foot with the heel off the floor. Hold the hands and the other leg straight out in front for 10 seconds.

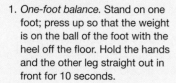

Power ◯

2. *Standing long jump.* Stand with the toes behind a line. Using no run or hop step, jump as far as possible. Men must jump their height plus 6 inches. Women must jump their height only.

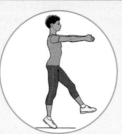

Agility ◯

3. *Paper ball pickup.* Place two wadded paper balls on the floor 5 feet away. Run until both feet cross the line, pick up the first ball, and return both feet behind the starting line. Repeat with the second ball. Finish in 5 seconds.

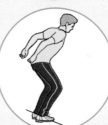

5'

Reaction Time ◯

4. *Paper drop.* Have a partner hold a sheet of notebook paper so that the side edge is between your thumb and index finger, about the width of your hand from the top of the page. When your partner drops the paper, catch it before it slips through the thumb and finger. Do not lower your hand to catch the paper.

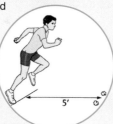

Speed ◯

5. *Double-heel click.* With the feet apart, jump up and tap the heels together twice before you hit the ground. You must land with your feet at least 3 inches apart.

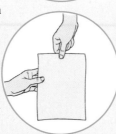

Coordination ◯

6. *Paper ball bounce.* Wad up a sheet of notebook paper into a ball. Bounce the ball back and forth between the right and left hands. Keep the hands open and palms up. Bounce the ball three times with each hand (six times total), alternating hands for each bounce.

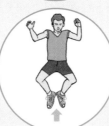

Cardiovascular Fitness ◯

7. *Run in place.* Run in place for 1½ minutes (120 steps per minute). Rest for 1 minute and count the heart rate for 30 seconds. A heart rate of 60 (for 30 sec.) or lower passes. A step is counted each time the right foot hits the floor.

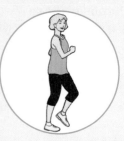

Flexibility ◯

8. *Backsaver toe touch.* Sit on the floor with one foot against a wall. Bend the other knee. Bend forward at the hips. After three warm-up trials, reach forward and touch your closed fists to the wall. Bend forward slowly; do not bounce. Repeat with the other leg straight. Pass if fists touch the wall with each leg straight.

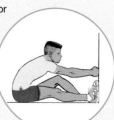

Body Composition ◯

9. *The pinch.* Have a partner pinch a fold of fat on the back of your upper arm (body fatness), halfway between the tip of the elbow and the tip of the shoulder.

Men: no greater than 3/4 inch

Women: no greater than 1 inch

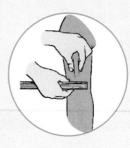

Strength ◯

10. *Push-up.* Lie face down on the floor. Place the hands under the shoulders. Keeping the legs and body straight, press off the floor until the arms are fully extended. Women repeat once; men, three times.

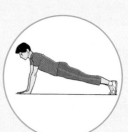

Muscular Endurance ◯

11. *Side leg raise.* Lie on the floor on your side. Lift your leg up and to the side of the body until your feet are 24 to 36 inches apart. Keep the knee and pelvis facing forward. Do not rotate so that the knees face the ceiling. Perform 10 with each leg.

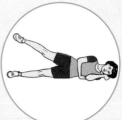

Moderate Physical Activity: A Lifestyle Approach

LEARNING OBJECTIVES

After completing the study of this concept, you will be able to:

▶ Define moderate physical activity and differentiate it from light and vigorous physical activity.

▶ Describe the health benefits of moderate physical activity, and explain why moderate physical activity is the most popular form of physical activity.

▶ Describe and explain the FIT formula for moderate physical activity.

▶ Plan a personal moderate physical activity program based on SMART goals, and self-monitor your plan.

▶ Evaluate your current environment and determine ways to modify it to encourage moderate physical activity.

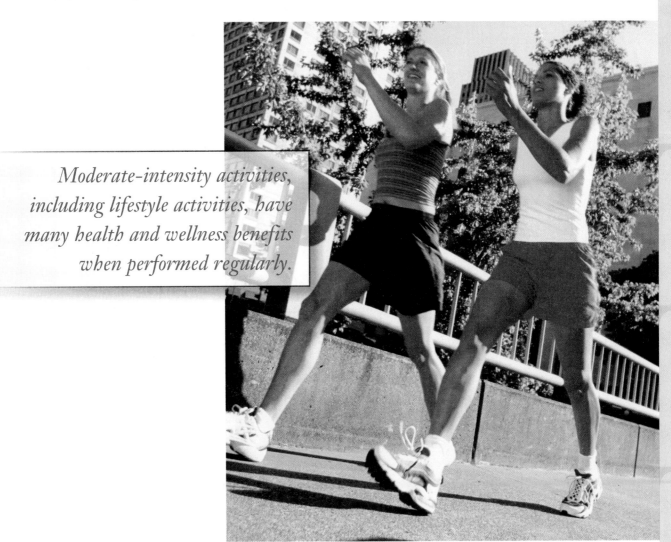

Moderate-intensity activities, including lifestyle activities, have many health and wellness benefits when performed regularly.

Humans are clearly meant to move, but the nature of our society has made it difficult for many people to lead active lifestyles. Cars, motorized golf carts, snowblowers, elevators, remote control devices, and email are just some of the modern conveniences that have reduced the amount of activity in our daily lives. Only a small percentage of adults get enough regular physical activity to promote health and wellness benefits. Moderate-intensity physical activity (which includes many lifestyle tasks done as part of normal daily living), provides most of the benefits associated with active living. In Concept 5, you were provided with an overview of each type of physical activity. In this concept, you will learn in more detail about **moderate physical activity,** the FIT formula for achieving it, and how to plan a personal program to incorporate moderate physical activity into your daily routine.

Adopting an Active Lifestyle

Moderate physical activity is the foundation of an active lifestyle. Moderate physical activity is included at the base of the physical activity pyramid (see Figure 1) because it can be performed by virtually all people,

regardless of fitness level or age. Moderate activities include some activities of daily living as well as less intense sports and recreational activities. Taking a brisk walk is the most obvious example of incorporating moderate activity into daily living. However, activities of daily living, such as walking the dog, gardening, mowing the lawn, carpentry, or housework can count as moderate activities. Moderate sports and recreational activities not considered to be vigorous enough to be placed at step 3 of the physical activity pyramid can also be used to meet the moderate physical activity guideline (e.g., playing catch, shooting baskets, recreational bike riding, and casual rollerblading).

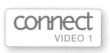

Moderate physical activity can be distinguished from "light" activity and "vigorous" activity. Scientists have devised a method to classify levels of activity by intensity. With this system, all activities are compared against the amount of energy expended at rest.

Resting energy expenditure is defined as 1 "metabolic equivalent" or 1 **MET.** Other activities are then assigned values in multiples of METS. For generally healthy adults, moderate-intensity activities require an energy expenditure of 3.0 to 6.0 METS. This means that they require between three and six times the energy expended while at rest. Moderate-intensity activities are often referred to as **aerobic physical activities** because the aerobic metabolism can typically meet the energy demand of the activity. This allows moderate-intensity (aerobic) activities to be performed comfortably for extended periods of time by most people.

Activities above 6 METS are considered to be **vigorous physical activities** and these cannot usually be maintained as easily unless a person has a good level of fitness. Examples include more structured aerobic activities (e.g., jogging, biking, swimming) or vigorous sports (e.g., soccer). Activities below 3.0 METS can be classified as "light intensity" but researchers now distinguish **light activity** (1.5 to 3.0 METS) from **sedentary activity** (1.0 to 1.5 METS) which primarily captures sitting and lying time. Examples of light

Energy Balance

Energy Out (Activity)

Energy In (Diet)

- **STEP 5** Flexibility Exercises
  - Yoga
  - Stretch
- **STEP 4** Muscle Fitness Exercises
  - Calisthenics
  - Resistance exercise
- **STEP 3** Vigorous Sports and Recreation
  - Tennis
  - Hike
- **STEP 2** Vigorous Aerobics
  - Jog
  - Bike
  - Aerobic dance
- **STEP 1** Moderate Physical Activity
  - Walk
  - Yard work
  - Golf

Avoid Inactivity

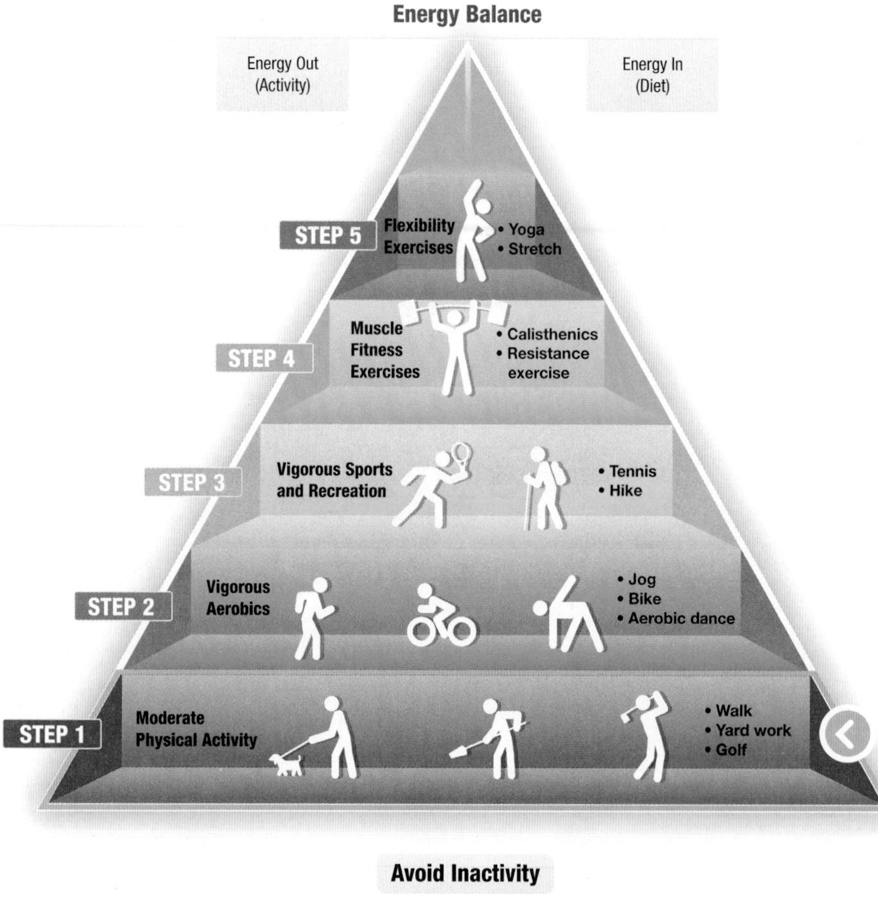

Figure 1 ► The physical activity pyramid, step 1: moderate physical activity.
Source: C. B. Corbin

In the News

Sedentary Time Can Be Harmful

Along with finding ways to get daily moderate activity, recent evidence suggests that it is also important to minimize time spent being sedentary. Recent studies have consistently shown that excess time spent sitting can have negative health consequences, even if you are a physically active person. One study showed that time spent watching TV was associated with risk of being overweight regardless of physical activity level. Another study showed that sedentary behavior (sitting time) was associated with mortality after adjusting for smoking status, diet, and level of physical activity. Avoiding sustained periods of sitting seems to be important for reducing these risks.

What can you do to avoid extended periods of sitting during the day?

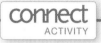

activities include lower-intensity activities of daily living such as showering, grocery shopping, washing dishes, and casual walking. While public health goals focus on moderate activity, minimizing time spent in sedentary activity is also important (see In the News). Distinctions among the types of activities are summarized in Table 1.

Because moderate activities are relatively easy to perform, they are popular among adults. Walking is the most popular of all leisure-time activities among adults. According to the National Sporting Goods Association, 96 million Americans say they walk for exercise, nearly twice the number that participate in the second and third most popular activities, exercising with equipment and swimming. Women walk more than men, and young adults (18–29) walk less than older adults, probably because of more involvement in sports and other vigorous activities. Walking behavior ranges from occasional walks to walking regularly to meet national physical activity guidelines. As many as 40 to 50 percent of adults say they walk, but less than half that number report walking 30 minutes or more at least 5 days a week.

Walking is popular in all age groups, but participation in other moderate activities varies with age. Interestingly, while overall activity levels tend to decline with age, involvement in lifestyle activity actually tends to increase. This is because many older adults move away from vigorous sports and recreation and spend more time in lifestyle activities, such as gardening and golf. Older adults tend to have more time and money for these types of recreational activities, and the lower intensity may be appealing.

The advantage of moderate activity is that there are many opportunities to be active. Finding enjoyable activities that fit into your daily routine is the key to adopting a more active lifestyle.

Moderate Physical Activities Activities equal in intensity to brisk walking; activities three to six times as intense as lying or sitting at rest (3–6 METs).

MET One MET equals the amount of energy a person expends at rest. METs are multiples of resting activity (2 METs equal twice the resting energy expenditure).

Aerobic Physical Activities *Aerobic* means "in the presence of oxygen." Aerobic activities are activities or exercise for which the body is able to supply adequate oxygen to sustain performance for long periods of time.

Vigorous Physical Activities Activities that are more vigorous than moderate activities with intensities at least six times as intense as lying or sitting at rest (>6 METS).

Light Activities Activities that involve standing and/or slow movements with intensities 1.5 to 3 times as intense as lying or sitting at rest (1.5–3.0 METS).

Sedentary Activities Activities that involve lying or sitting with intensities similar to (or just slightly higher) than rest (1.0–1.5 METS).

Table 1 ▶ Classifications of Physical Activity Intensities for Generally Healthy Adults

Classification	Intensity Range	Examples
Sedentary	1.0–1.5 METS	Sitting, lying
Light	1.5–3.0 METS	Showering, grocery shopping, playing musical instrument, washing dishes
Moderate	3.0–6.0 METS	Walking briskly, mowing lawn, playing table tennis, doing carpentry
Vigorous	>6.0 METS	Hiking, jogging, digging ditches, playing soccer

Table 2 ▶ Classification of Moderate Physical Activities for People of Different Fitness Levels

	Activity Classification by Fitness Level			
Sample Lifestyle Activities	Low Fitness	Marginal Fitness	Good Fitness	High Performance
Washing your face, dressing, typing, driving a car	Light	Very light/light	Very light	Very light
Normal walking, walking downstairs, bowling, mopping	Moderate	Moderate	Light	Light
Brisk walking, lawn mowing, shoveling, social dancing	Vigorous	Moderate/Vigorous	Moderate	Moderate

Activity classifications vary, depending on one's level of fitness. Normal walking is considered light activity for a person with good fitness (see Table 1), but for a person with low to marginal fitness the same activity is considered moderate. Similarly, brisk walking may be a vigorous activity (rather than moderate) for individuals with low fitness. Table 2 helps you determine the type of lifestyle activity considered moderate for you. Beginners with low fitness should start with normal rather than brisk walking, for example. In Concept 7, you will learn to assess your current fitness level. You may want to refer back to Table 2 after you have made self-assessments of your fitness.

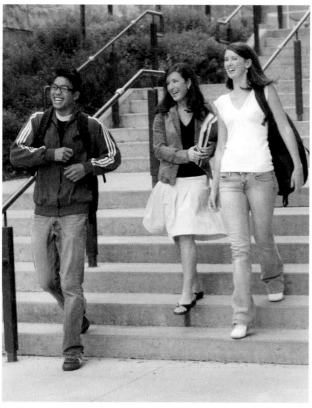

Brief walks throughout the day can help you meet recommended levels of moderate activity.

The Health and Wellness Benefits of Moderate Physical Activity

Moderate activity provides significant health benefits. Research has clearly shown that even modest amounts of moderate activity have significant health benefits. Two early studies paved the way for this line of research. One study reported that postal workers who delivered mail had fewer health problems than workers who sorted mail. Another study reported that drivers of double-decker buses in England had more health problems than conductors who climbed the stairs during the day to collect the tickets. The studies controlled for other lifestyle factors, so the improved health was attributed to the extra activity accumulated throughout the day. Since then, hundreds of studies have further confirmed the importance of moderate activity for good health. However, as described in Concept 5, additional health benefits are possible if vigorous physical activity is also performed.

Moderate activity promotes metabolic fitness. Metabolic fitness is fitness of the systems that provide the energy for effective daily living. Indicators of good metabolic fitness include normal blood lipid levels, normal blood pressure, normal blood sugar levels, and healthy body fat levels. Moderate physical activity promotes metabolic fitness by keeping the metabolic system active. Building and maintaining cardiovascular fitness requires a regular challenge to the cardiovascular system and building metabolic fitness requires a similar regular challenge to the metabolic system. Individuals with good levels of fitness will receive primarily **metabolic fitness benefits** from moderate activity, but those with low fitness will likely receive metabolic and **cardiovascular fitness benefits.** Moderate activity is particularly important for the large segments of the population that do not participate in other forms of regular exercise. As previously described, some activity is clearly better than none.

Moderate physical activity has wellness benefits. The health benefits from physical activity are impressive, but the **wellness benefits** may have a bigger impact on our daily lives. Numerous studies have shown that physical activity is associated with improved quality of life (QOL), but it has proven difficult to determine the contributing factors or underlying mechanisms. The influence may be due to reduced stress, improved cognition, better sleep, improved self-esteem, reduced fatigue or (more likely) a combination of many different effects. A recent study in college students sought to isolate some of the underlying effects. The study reported that students who were more physically active had more positive feeling states ("*pleasant-activated feelings*") than students who were less physically active even after controlling for sleep and previous days' activity and feeling states. They also noted that feeling states improved on days when people reported performing more activity than normal. The wellness benefits can impact young people every day whereas health benefits may not be noticed until a person gets older.

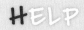

Regular activity is important to achieving health, fitness, and wellness benefits. For the benefits of activity to be optimal, it is important to exercise regularly. The specific benefits from moderate activity tend to be more dependent on frequency than on intensity. This is sometimes referred to as the **last bout effect,** because the effects are short term (i.e., attributable to the last bout of activity performed). For example, regular exercise promotes metabolic fitness by creating the stimulus that helps maintain insulin sensitivity and improve glucose regulation. Another example is the beneficial effect of exercise on stress management. In this case, the periodic stimulus from exercise helps directly counter the negative physical and physiological responses to stress. To maximize the benefits of physical activity, it is important to try to get some activity every day.

Sustained light-intensity activity may provide health benefits and promote weight control. The new physical activity guidelines have recommended that activities be at least moderate in intensity. However, evidence suggests that the accumulation of light-intensity activity can have benefits, especially in those who are sedentary. Some researchers have referred to this type of activity as *Non-Exercise Activity Thermogenesis (NEAT)* to emphasize the substantial number of calories that can be burned by performing light-intensity activity. Meeting the recommendation for moderate activity is best, but beginning some activity, even light activity, is better than doing nothing at all.

How Much Moderate Physical Activity Is Enough?

There is a FIT formula for moderate physical activity. The concept of a threshold of training is used in this book to describe the minimum activity needed for

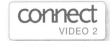

HELP **Health is available to Everyone for a Lifetime, and it's Personal**

Walking is by far the most commonly reported moderate activity, but people often go out of their way to avoid walking (such as driving around the lot to find the closest parking spot; waiting for an elevator rather than climbing a few flights of stairs).

Do you view walking as a "means to an end" (i.e., simply as a way to get around) or as an "end in itself" (i.e., as a way to get more physical activity)? How might this perception influence your activity patterns?

benefits. As described in Concept 5, public health guidelines endorsed by the ACSM, the AHA, and the CDC have recommended that adults accumulate 150 minutes of moderate-intensity activity each week, an amount equal to 30 minutes 5 days a week. The recommendation highlighted in the original *Surgeon General's Report on Physical Activity* called for adults to accumulate about 1,000 kcal/week (or about 150 kcal/day) from moderate activity. Table 3 summarizes the threshold levels for frequency, intensity, and time (duration). Note that these are considered minimal, or threshold, levels. The target zone calls for the accumulation of 30 or more minutes a day. Physical activity above the recommended minimum provides additional health benefits.

Activity bouts of 10 minutes are recommended, but shorter durations of moderate activity have benefits. National physical activity guidelines suggest that moderate activity bouts should be 10 minutes in length or longer for optimal health and fitness benefits. Nevertheless, short-duration moderate activity, sometimes referred to as "incidental physical activity," accumulated throughout the day is also beneficial. The specification of 10-minute sessions in the guidelines is somewhat arbitrary as there is no absolute threshold defining how

Metabolic Fitness Benefits Improvements in metabolic function that reduce risks of diabetes and metabolic syndrome.

Cardiovascular Fitness Benefits Improvements in cardiovascular function that contribute to cardiovascular fitness.

Wellness Benefits Increases in quality of life and well-being.

Last Bout Effect A short-term effect associated with the last bout of activity. Typically related to improvements in metabolic fitness.

Table 3 ▶ The FIT Formula for Moderate Physical Activity

	Threshold of Training (minimum)[a]	Target Zone (optimal)
Frequency	At least 5 days a week	5–7 days a week
Intensity[b]	• Equal to brisk walking[b] • Approximately 150 calories accumulated per day • 3 to 5 METs[b]	• Equal to brisk to fast walking[b] • Approximately 150–300 calories accumulated per day • 3 to 6 METs[b]
Time (duration)[c]	30 minutes or three 10-minute sessions per day	30–60 minutes or more accumulated in sessions of at least 10 minutes

[a]150 minutes per week is recommended by DHHS.

[b]Heart rate and relative perceived exertion can also be used to determine intensity (see Concept 7).

[c]Depends on fitness level (see Table 2).

long activity sessions must be. In general, the main focus should be on the total volume of moderate activity performed.

Vigorous activity can substitute for moderate activity. The U.S. Physical Activity Guidelines released by the Department of Health and Human Services (DHHS) provide some flexibility for meeting activity guidelines. Rather than requiring activity on 5 different days, the DHHS guidelines specify that 150 minutes of moderate physical activity can be accumulated during the week. If you fail to meet the 30-minute guideline on 1 day, you can make it up on another and still meet the guideline. Vigorous-intensity activity can also be substituted to meet the weekly targets. According to the DHHS guidelines, each minute of vigorous activity counts as 2 minutes of moderate. Therefore, the guideline can also be met by performing 75 minutes of vigorous activity instead of 150 minutes of moderate activity.

The guidelines can also be expressed in total "MET-minutes." To compute MET-minutes, you simply multiply the MET level of the activity you performed by the number of minutes. For example, a 60-minute brisk walk (approximately 3 METS) would yield 180 MET-minutes (3 METS × 60 minutes). However, note that this same volume can also be achieved with a 30-minute run that requires approximately 6 METS (6 METS × 30 minutes). A total of 500 MET-minutes per week is recommended to meet the minimum guidelines.

Special moderate activity guidelines have been developed for children, older adults, and adults with chronic health conditions. Guidelines for physical activity depend on the unique needs of the target population. Children need more physical activity than adults (at least 60 minutes and up to several hours of activity each day).

Guidelines are also different for older adults and adults with chronic conditions. As previously described (see Table 2), activity that is moderate for young adults may be too intense for some older individuals or those with health problems. Because of this, the guidelines recommend that these individuals should focus on tracking minutes of activity. This allows the intensity to be a self-determined level that corresponds to a person's relative level of fitness.

Monitoring and Promoting Physical Activity Behavior

Many people use pedometers to monitor daily activity levels. Digital pedometers are a popular self-monitoring tool used to track physical activity patterns. They provide information about the number of steps a person takes. Stride length and weight can be entered into most pedometers to provide estimates of distance traveled and/or calories burned. Some newer pedometers include timers, which track the total amount of time spent moving; some allow step information to be stored over a series of days.

Pedometers provide a helpful reminder about the importance of being active during the day. They also are useful for tracking activity patterns over a series of days. The interest in and popularity of pedometers has resulted in media stories promoting the standard of 10,000 steps as the level of activity needed for good health. This standard was originally developed in Japan, where pedometers were popular before elsewhere in the world. Experts have warned against using an absolute step count standard for all people as it would be too hard for some and not hard enough for others based on personal activity patterns.

Studies on large numbers of people provide data to help classify people into activity categories based on step counts (see Table 4), but actual step goals should vary from person to person. Wear the pedometer for 1 week to establish a baseline step count (average steps per day). Then, set a goal of increasing steps per day by 1,000 to

Table 4 ▶ Activity Classification for Pedometer Step Counts in Healthy Adults

Category		Steps/Day
Sedentary		< 5,000
Low active		5,000–6,999
Somewhat active	Threshold	7,000–9,999
Active	Target Zone	10,000–12,500
Very active		> 12,500

Source: Based on values from Tudor-Locke.

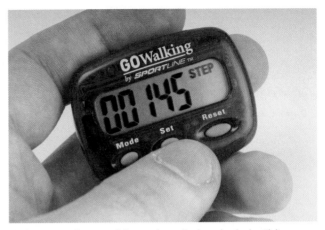

Pedometers offer a useful way of monitoring physical activity.

3,000 steps. Keep records of daily step counts to help you determine if you are meeting your goal. Setting a goal that you are likely to meet will help you find success. As you meet your goal, increase your step counts gradually.

Pedometers do have some limitations as indicators of total physical activity. A person with longer legs will accumulate fewer steps over the same distance than someone with shorter strides (due to a longer stride length). A person running will also accumulate fewer steps over the same distance than a person who walks. There is considerable variability in the quality (and accuracy) of commercial pedometers, so it is important to consider this when purchasing one.

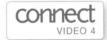

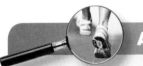 **A CLOSER LOOK**

Every Body Walk

Every Body Walk is a national movement committed to "get Americans up and moving." The organization has developed a variety of social media applications that help to connect organizations, people, and communities across the country. Customized (free) apps for smartphones are available to help track and personalize your walking plan, connect with walking communities, and share stories. Associated Facebook links and Twitter feeds (follow @everybodywalk) provide inspirational messages and opportunities to network and share stories. The website (www.everybodywalk.org) features a hub for walking-related blogs and video clips showing how groups across America are finding a new sense of community through walking.

What are other ways social media can be used to spur community involvement in physical activity?

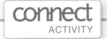

Energy expenditure can be used to monitor physical activity. As shown in Table 3, an energy expenditure of between 150 and 300 kcal/day from physical activity is sufficient for meeting physical activity guidelines. While not as simple as tracking time, calories expended from physical activity can be estimated if the approximate MET value of the activity is known. The energy cost of resting energy expenditure (1 MET) is approximately 1 calorie per kilogram of body weight per hour (1 kcal/kg/hour). An activity such as brisk walking (4 mph) requires an energy expenditure of about 4 METs, or 4 kcal/kg/hour. A 150 lb. person (~ 70 kg) walking for an hour would expend about 280 kcal (4 kcal/kg/hour × 70 kg × 1 hr.). Note that a 30-minute walk would burn approximately 150 calories and satisfy the guideline.

Commercial fitness equipment can provide energy expenditure estimates. The devices use an estimated MET level based on the selected intensity or a measured heart rate (if a heart rate sensor is used). The timer on the machine then tracks the time of the workout, and this allows calories to be estimated during the workout. The estimate will only be somewhat accurate if the machine also obtained a body weight value from you during the setup process. If this wasn't obtained, the calorie estimates are probably based on some reference value of weight and therefore may not be accurate. Table 5 lists estimated METs for different activities, along with calorie estimates (per hour of exercise) for people of different body weights.

A variety of methods can be used to accumulate moderate physical activity for health benefits. Finding 30 minutes or longer for continuous physical activity may be difficult, especially on very busy days. However, the physical activity guidelines emphasize that moderate activity can be accumulated throughout the day. Figure 2 illustrates the

Table 5 ▶ Calories Expended in Lifestyle Physical Activities

Activity Classification / Description	METs[a]	Calories Used per Hour for Different Body Weights					
		100 lb. (45 kg)	120 lb. (55 kg)	150 lb. (70 kg)	180 lb. (82 kg)	200 lb. (91 kg)	220 lb. (100 kg)
Gardening Activities							
Gardening (general)	5.0	227	273	341	409	455	502
Mowing lawn (hand mower)	6.0	273	327	409	491	545	599
Mowing lawn (power mower)	4.5	205	245	307	368	409	450
Raking leaves	4.0	182	218	273	327	364	401
Shoveling snow	6.0	273	327	409	491	545	599
Home Activities							
Child care	3.5	159	191	239	286	318	350
Cleaning, washing dishes	2.5	114	136	170	205	227	249
Cooking / food preparation	2.5	114	136	170	205	227	249
Home / auto repair	3.0	136	164	205	245	273	301
Painting	4.5	205	245	307	368	409	450
Strolling with child	2.5	114	136	170	205	227	249
Sweeping / vacuuming	2.5	114	136	170	205	227	249
Washing / waxing car	4.5	205	245	307	368	409	450
Leisure Activities							
Bocci ball / croquet	2.5	114	136	170	205	227	249
Bowling	3.0	136	164	205	245	273	301
Canoeing	5.0	227	273	341	409	455	501
Cross-country skiing (leisure)	7.0	318	382	477	573	636	699
Cycling (<10 mph)	4.0	182	218	273	327	364	401
Cycling (12–14 mph)	8.0	364	436	545	655	727	799
Dancing (social)	4.5	205	245	307	368	409	450
Fishing	4.0	182	218	273	327	364	401
Golf (riding)	3.5	159	191	239	286	318	350
Golf (walking)	5.5	250	300	375	450	500	550
Horseback riding	4.0	182	218	273	327	364	401
Swimming (leisure)	6.0	273	327	409	491	545	599
Table tennis	4.0	182	218	273	327	364	401
Walking (3.5 mph)	3.8	173	207	259	311	346	387
Occupational Activities							
Bricklaying / masonry	7.0	318	382	477	573	636	699
Carpentry	3.5	159	191	239	286	318	350
Construction	5.5	250	300	375	450	500	550
Electrical work / plumbing	3.5	159	191	239	286	318	350
Digging	7.0	318	382	477	573	636	699
Farming	5.5	250	300	375	450	500	550
Store clerk	3.5	159	191	239	286	318	350
Waiter / waitress	4.0	182	218	273	327	364	401

Note: MET values and caloric estimates are based on values listed in *Compendium of Physical Activities* (see Suggested Readings).

[a]Based on values of those with "good fitness" ratings.

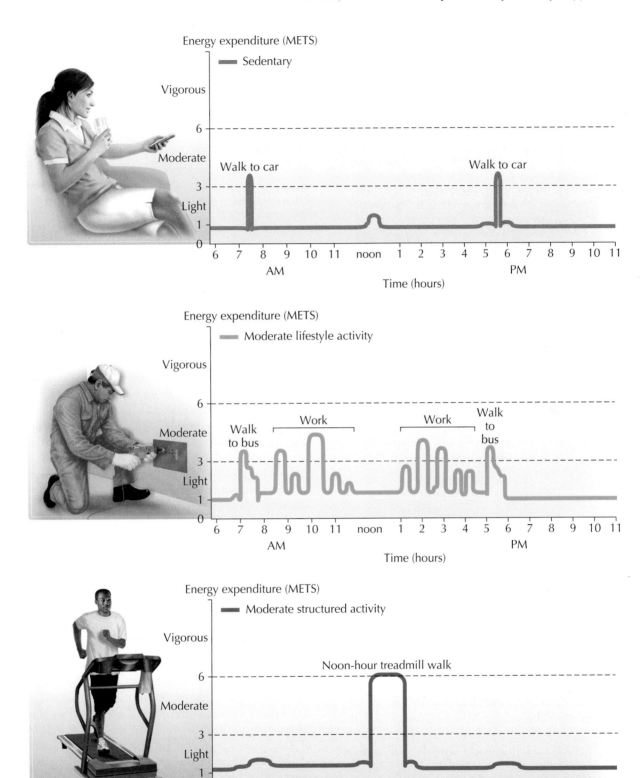

Figure 2 ▶ Comparison of people performing moderate activity in different ways.

activity profiles for three different people. The red line profiles a person who is inactive except for brief walks from the car to the office in the morning and from the office to the car in the evening. This person is sedentary and does not meet the moderate activity guidelines. Because some activity is better than none, the brief walks

Electronic Bikes

The e-bike (electric bike) is a new type of bicycle designed to promote active commuting. Traveling at speeds up to about 15 mph, the e-bike has a small electric engine that gives support to the rider only when he or she is pedaling. It was first developed in Switzerland to encourage people who live in hilly terrains to ride bicycles. A recent study showed that the effort necessary to ride an e-bike to work (about 6 METS) was less than the effort needed to ride a regular bike. Most of the commuters in the study were easily able to use the bike to commute to work. The e-bike is now gaining popularity in other countries because it is comfortable, practical, and contributes to cleaner air. The e-bike also encourages otherwise inactive people to become active.

Would you consider using an e-bike as a way to get more activity? To help the environment?

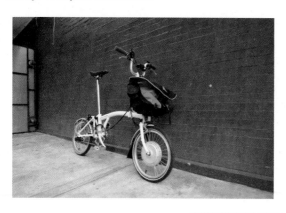

are better than no activity at all. The blue line represents a person who is sedentary most of the day but meets the moderate activity guideline by taking a long walk during the noon hour. The green line represents the activity of a person who meets the moderate activity standard in multiple bouts, including lifestyle activities such as walking to and from work, walking to lunch, and climbing the stairs. You can accumulate activity using the method that you prefer as long as you meet the guidelines outlined in Table 2.

Moderate Activity and the Built Environment

The sedentary nature of our society is due in large part to environmental factors. Many people would like to be more active, but they may not live in an area conducive to activity. Studies have conclusively demonstrated that the physical or **"built environment"** has important influences on physical activity patterns and risk for overweight and obesity. Some early studies had inherent limitations that have made it difficult to determine if the relationship was causal. It is possible, for example, that active people choose to move to environments with less urban sprawl and more access to parks and green spaces. Recent research, however, has demonstrated that *changes* in the environment (e.g., more trails, safer and more accessible walking routes) can lead to *changes* in levels of physical activity. This type of evidence has been important because it indicates that our environment does contribute to our physical activity patterns. The results also help justify expenses to create environments more conducive to physical activity.

Building active community environments has become an important national priority. Many public health organizations have developed awareness campaigns and strong advocacy networks to support the creation of healthier environments. One organization called Active Living by Design is dedicated to promoting more active environments in society. The vision is for neighborhoods that allow physical activity to be built into a person's normal routine (going to the store, visiting friends) and communities with integrated biking and walking paths. These concepts are consistent with other recommendations for urban planning (e.g., Smart Growth Movement). Other groups such as the National Coalition of Walking Advocates, the Alliance for Biking and Walking, and Walkable Communities are positioned to play key roles in promoting awareness and advocating at the state and national levels to improve federal practices and funding decisions that influence biking and walking. These groups encourage community activism since consumers ultimately influence social norms and decision making. See the Web Resources to learn more about these organizations.

Walkability is an important consideration for consumers and homeowners. The national Community Preference Survey conducted by the National Association of Realtors revealed that nearly 60 percent of Americans would prefer to live in neighborhoods that would allow them to easily walk to stores and other businesses. Walkable access to grocery stores was rated as being an important consideration by 75 percent of the respondents.

Built Environment A term used to describe aspects of our created physical environment (e.g., buildings, roads).

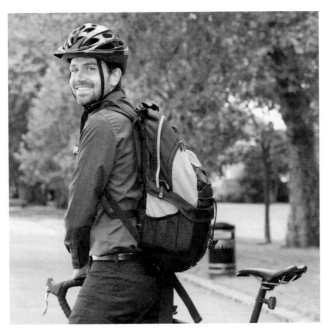

Bike commuting is an effective way to add physical activity to your day.

Distance is one major consideration but researchers have determined that a number of characteristics influence the walkability of an environment. Walking is more likely when the weather is warm, but factors such as availability of sidewalks, good lighting, safe neighborhoods, and aesthetic surroundings are the key factors in making an area walkable. A number of websites now provide tools to rate the walkability of communities (search "walkscore" on the Internet). According to recent rankings, the most walkable of the 50 largest U.S. cities were New York, San Francisco, Boston, and Chicago. In Lab 6B you will evaluate the walkability of your community based on similar criteria.

Consider personal strategies for increasing moderate activity. While the environment has an impact on population levels of physical activity, it does not determine individual behavior. People are autonomous beings and can make decisions about where they go and what they do. The key is to take stock of your lifestyle and your environment and determine ways to integrate more activity into your daily routine.

Active commuting is one way to add physical activity to your lifestyle. It takes additional preparation and the logistics can be challenging, but it is a great way to build activity into your day. In addition to providing beneficial amounts of physical activity, this can save time, reduce gas, save money, and help the environment. Another option is to take a few active trips to the store. Research suggests that the overwhelming majority of our car trips are 1 mile or less. Walking or biking even a few of these trips can have a big impact. The ability to walk or bike to work or to the store may not be possible for you because of the nature of your community or the safety of the roads. However, there are a number of other strategies you can use to get more activity in your day. Consider parking farther away from store entrances, using the stairs rather than the elevator, taking walking breaks, and even standing (instead of sitting) when convenient. Adopting an active lifestyle in a sedentary society is challenging, but it is within your control.

Strategies for Action

A regular plan of moderate physical activity is a good place to start. Moderate physical activity is something that virtually anyone can do. In Lab 6A, you can set moderate physical activity goals and plan a 1-week lifestyle physical activity program. For some, this plan may be the main component of a lifetime plan. For others, it may be only a beginning that leads to the selection of activities from other levels of the physical activity pyramid. Even the most active people should consider regular moderate physical activity because it is a type of activity that can be done throughout life.

Self-monitoring moderate physical activity can help you stick with it. The self-monitoring chart in Lab 6A not only helps you keep a log of moderate activities (or step counts), it also lets you hone your self-management skills. Charts like this can be copied to make a log book for long-term activity self-monitoring.

Environmental factors influence our moderate physical activity patterns. In Lab 6B, you will conduct an evaluation of the walkability of your community and an evaluation of community resources available for physical activity. The purpose of this lab is to increase your awareness of the importance of active, safe environments for promoting physical activity. Becoming an advocate for physical activity in your community is a great way to help promote local change.

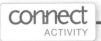

Web Resources

Alliance for Biking and Walking **www.peoplepowered movement.org**

America On the Move **www.americaonthemove.org**

Bike Commute.com **www.bikecommute.com**

Compendium of Physical Activities **http://prevention.sph .sc.edu/tools/compendium.htm**

National Coalition for Promoting Physical Activity **www.ncppa.org**

National Coalition of Walking Advocates **www.americawalks.org/**

The Pedestrian and Bicycle Information Center (PBIC) **www.walkinginfo.org**

Public Broadcasting System/America's Walking Homepage **www.pbs.org/americaswalking**

Walkable Cities (walkscores) **www.walkscore.com**

Walkable Communities Inc **www.walkable.org**

Suggested Readings

ACSM. 2010. *ACSM's Guidelines for Exercise Testing and Prescription.* 8th ed. Philadelphia: Lippincott, Williams & Wilkins, Chapters 2 and 7.

Ainsworth, B. E. 2000. Compendium of physical activities: An update of activity codes and MET intensities. *Medicine and Science in Sports and Exercise* 32 (Suppl):S498–S516.

Chaloupka, F. J., et al. 2010. The association between community physical activity settings and youth physical activity, obesity, and body mass index. *Journal of Adolescent Health.* Published online June 10, 2010, **www.jahonline.org**

Foti, K. K., et al. 2011. Sufficient sleep, physical activity, and sedentary behaviors. *American Journal of Preventive Medicine* 41(6):596–602.

Garber, C. E., et al. 2011. Quantity and quality of exercise for developing and maintaining cardiorespiratory, musculo-skeletal, and neuromotor fitness in apparently healthy adults: Guidance for prescribing exercise. *Medicine and Science in Sports and Exercise* 43(7):1334–1359.

Healy, G. N., et al. 2011. Sedentary times and cardio-metabolic biomarkers in US adults: NHANES 2003-06. *European Heart Journal* 32(5):590–597.

Hyde, A. L., et al. 2012. Unpacking the feel-good effect of free-time physical activity: Between- and within-person associations with pleasant-activated feeling states. *Journal of Sport & Exercise Psychology* 33(6):884–902.

Kohl, H. W., and T. D. Murray. 2012. *Foundations of Physical Activity and Public Health.* Champaign, IL: Human Kinetics.

Matthews, C. E., et al. 2012. Amount of time spent in sedentary behaviors and cause-specific mortality in US adults. *American Journal of Clinical Nutrition* 95(2):437–445.

Mowen, A., and A. Kaczynski. 2008. The potential of parks and recreation in addressing physical activity and fitness. *President's Council on Physical Fitness and Sports Research Digest* 9(1):1–8.

Owen, N., et al. 2010. Too much sitting: The population health science of sedentary behavior. *Exercise and Sport Sciences Reviews* 38(3): 105–113.

Russ, R., and McGuire, K. A. 2011. Incidental physical activity is positively associated with cardiorespiratory fitness. *Medicine and Science in Sports and Exercise* 43(11):2189–2194.

Sattelmair, J., et al. 2011. Dose response between physical activity and risk of coronary heart disease: A meta-analysis. *Circulation* 124(7):789–795.

Healthy People 2020

The objectives listed below are societal goals designed to help all Americans improve their health between now and the year 2020. They were selected because they relate to the content of this concept.

- Reduce proportion of adults who do no leisure-time activity.

- Increase proportion of adults who meet guidelines for aerobic activity.

- Increase proportion of adults who meet guidelines for muscle fitness activity.

- Increase proportion of trips made by walking.

- Increase proportion of youth who meet guidelines for TV viewing and computer use and overuse (overuse is 2 hours a day or more).

- Create social and physical environments that promote good health for all.

- Promote quality of life, healthy development, and healthy behaviors across all stages of life.

A national goal is to increase walking trips (moderate physical activity). Describe three ways that you can increase walking trips during the week and comment on whether you think you are likely to carry out any of these methods as part of your normal routine.

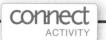

Lab 6A Setting Goals for Moderate Physical Activity and Self-Monitoring (Logging) Program

Name	Section	Date

Purpose: To set moderate activity goals and to self-monitor (log) physical activity

Procedures

1. Read the five stages of change questions below. Place a check by the stage that best represents your current moderate physical activity level. If you are at stages 1–3 (precontemplation, contemplation, or preparation), you may want to set goals below the threshold of 30 minutes per day to get started. Those at the action or maintenance stage should consider goals of 30 minutes or more per day.

2. Determine moderate activity goals for each day of a 1-week period. In the columns (Chart 1) under the heading "Moderate Activity Goals," record the total minutes per day that you expect to perform **OR** the total steps per day that you expect to perform. Record the specific date for each day of the week in the "Date" column.

3. The goals should be realistic for you, but try to set goals that would meet current physical activity guidelines. If you choose step goals, you will need a pedometer. Use Table 4 on page 107 to help you to choose daily step goals.

4. If you choose minutes per day as your goals, use Chart 2 to keep track of the number of minutes of activity that you perform on each day of the 7-day period. Record the number of minutes for each bout of activity of at least 10 minutes in length performed during each day (Chart 2). Determine a total number of minutes for the day and record this total in the last column of Chart 2 and in the "Minutes Performed" column of Chart 1.

5. If you choose steps per day as your goals, determine the total steps per day accumulated on the pedometer and record that number of steps in the "Steps Performed" column for each day of the week (Chart 1).

6. Answer the questions in the Conclusions and Implications section (use full sentences for your answers).

Determine your stage for moderate physical activity. Check only the stage that represents your current moderate activity level.

☐ Precontemplation: I do not meet moderate activity guidelines and have not been thinking about starting.

☐ Contemplation: I do not meet moderate activity guidelines but have been thinking about starting.

☐ Preparation: I am planning to start doing regular moderate activity to meet guidelines.

☐ Action: I do moderate activity, but I am not as regular as I should be.

☐ Maintenance: I regularly meet national goals for moderate activity.

Chart 1 Moderate Physical Activity Goals and Summary Performance Log

Select a goal for each day in a 1-week plan. Keep a log of the activities performed to determine if your goals are met.

	Date:	Moderate Activity Goals		Summary Performance Log	
		Minutes/day	**Steps/day**	**Minutes Performed**	**Steps Performed**
Day 1					
Day 2					
Day 3					
Day 4					
Day 5					
Day 6					
Day 7					

Lab 6A

Setting Goals for Moderate Physical Activity and Self-Monitoring (Logging) Program.

Chart 2 Moderate Physical Activity Log (Daily Minutes Performed)

If you choose minutes per day as goals, write the number of minutes for each bout of moderate activity performed each day. Record a daily total (total minutes of moderate activity per day) in the "Daily Total" column. Record daily totals in Chart 1.

	Date	Moderate Activity Bouts of 10 Minutes or More					Daily Total
		Bout 1	Bout 2	Bout 3	Bout 4	Bout 5	
Day 1							
Day 2							
Day 3							
Day 4							
Day 5							
Day 6							
Day 7							

Did you meet your moderate activity goals for at least 5 days of the week?   Yes   No

Do you think you can consistently meet your moderate activity goals?   Yes   No

What activities did you perform most often when doing moderate activity?
List most common activities in the spaces below.

Conclusions and Interpretations

1. Do you feel that you will use moderate physical activity as a regular part of your lifetime physical activity plan, either now or in the future? Use several sentences to explain your answer.

2. Did setting goals and logging activity make you more aware of your daily moderate physical activity patterns? Explain why or why not.

Lab 6B Evaluating Physical Activity Environments

Name	Section	Date

Purpose: To help you assess community factors that may influence your ability to perform lifestyle physical activity

Procedures

1. Use the community audit forms on the next page to conduct an evaluation of the walkability of your community and the availability of community resources for physical activity. The walkability audit requires that you take a brief walk in your neighborhood to note key features in the environment that may help or hinder walking. The community audit will require you to evaluate the quality of resources and programming available in your community. You can choose your campus community or your hometown.
2. For each question, first use the check boxes to note the presence or absence of key features in the environment. Then base your score for this question on the number of checks and your overall perception.
3. After you have completed both the Walkability Audit and the Community Resource Audit, total the scores for each tool and report the total scores in the bottom. Add up both scores to compute the Combined (physical activity) Environmental Audit.

Results: Record your rating for each of three healthy lifestyles in the following chart.

Environmental Activity Scoring Chart

	Score	Rating
Walkability Audit		
Community Resource Audit		
Combined Environmental Audit		

Rating Chart for Environmental Audits

	Good	Marginal	Poor
Walkability	15–20	11–14	<11
Community	15–20	11–14	<11
Combined	30–40	22–29	<22

Conclusions and Implications

Provide a brief summary of the physical activity environment in your community. Describe your experiences in evaluating the walkability of and resources in your community. If the environment is close to ideal, comment on how this may facilitate active lifestyles. If the environment is not ideal, comment on what needs to be done to improve it.

Comments on Walkability Audit

Comments on Community Resource Audit

Walkability and Community Resource Audits

Directions. Place a check by each box in each questionnaire. Based on the number of boxes checked for each question, place an X over the circle to rate each question (1=poor, 2=marginal, 3=good, 4=very good). Add rating numbers to get walkability scores and community resource scores. Total the two to get a combined environmental score.

Walkability Audit   **Rating**

1. Did you have room to walk?   ① ② ③ ④
   ☐ Sidewalks blocked or not continuous
   ☐ Sidewalks were broken, cracked
   ☐ No sidewalks, paths, or shoulders
   ☐ Too much traffic on sidewalk
   ☐ Other _____

2. Was it easy to cross streets?   ① ② ③ ④
   ☐ Road was too wide
   ☐ Traffic signals were too short/too long
   ☐ Parked cars blocked view of street
   ☐ No striped or designated crosswalks
   ☐ Other _____

3. Was it safe for walking?   ① ② ③ ④
   ☐ Too much traffic
   ☐ Drivers too fast/too close
   ☐ Inadequate lighting
   ☐ Area of high crime
   ☐ Other _____

4. Were there places to go?   ① ② ③ ④
   ☐ No stores in the area
   ☐ No restaurants in the area
   ☐ No friends nearby
   ☐ Nothing interesting to see in area
   ☐ Other _____

5. Was your walk pleasant?   ① ② ③ ④
   ☐ Not enough grass and trees
   ☐ Scary dogs or people
   ☐ Not well lighted
   ☐ Too dirty
   ☐ Other _____

Community Resource Audit   **Rating**

6. Are there walking/biking paths in the area?   ① ② ③ ④
   ☐ Paths are in unsafe areas
   ☐ Paths need to be repaired
   ☐ Paths are too crowded
   ☐ Paths are too far away to be useful
   ☐ Other _____

7. Is there a community fitness/rec center?   ① ② ③ ④
   ☐ Center is too expensive
   ☐ Center is not clean or updated
   ☐ Center is too far away
   ☐ Center has old or limited equipment
   ☐ Other _____

8. Are there bicycle lanes on streets?   ① ② ③ ④
   ☐ Lines not painted well
   ☐ Lines not on all streets
   ☐ Bike lanes not wide enough
   ☐ Cars too close
   ☐ Other _____

9. Are there parks, fields, and playgrounds?   ① ② ③ ④
   ☐ Parks in unsafe areas
   ☐ Equipment/resources in poor repair
   ☐ Too crowded
   ☐ Too far away
   ☐ Other _____

10. Are there community activity programs?   ① ② ③ ④
   ☐ Not enough programs
   ☐ Not the right type of programs
   ☐ Too expensive
   ☐ Too far/inconvenient
   ☐ Other _____

Total Score for Walkability Audit: ☐☐☐   (Sum of Questions 1–5)

Total Score for Community Resources Audit: ☐☐☐   (Sum of Questions 6–10)

Combined Environmental Audit: ☐☐☐   (Sum of Questions 1–10)

Walkability checklist adapted from resources developed by the Partnership for a Walkable America. For information on this organization, visit this website: **www.walkableamerica.org.**

Cardiovascular Fitness

LEARNING OBJECTIVES

After completing the study of this concept, you will be able to:

► Describe the different components of the cardiovascular system.

► List the health benefits of cardiovascular fitness.

► Outline the FIT formula for moderate to vigorous physical activity designed to promote cardiovascular fitness.

► Identify several methods of determining exercise intensity levels for promoting cardiovascular fitness, select the method you think is most useful to you, and explain the reasons for your choice.

► Describe key guidelines for monitoring cardiovascular exercise including self-monitoring heart rate.

► Indicate several self-assessments for cardiovascular fitness, select the self-assessment you feel is most useful to you, and explain the reasons for your choice.

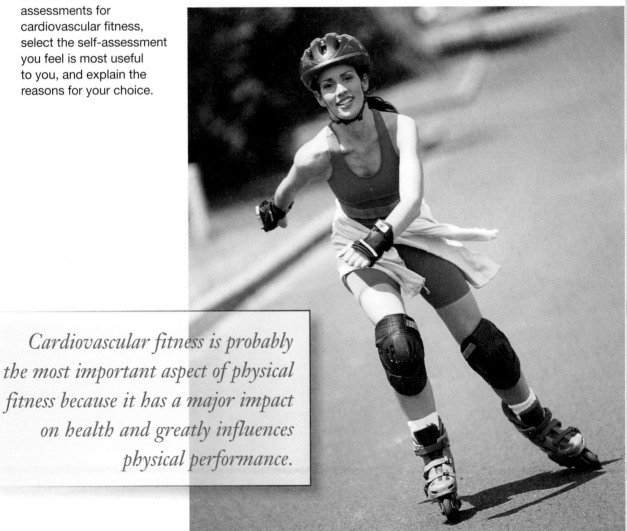

Cardiovascular fitness is probably the most important aspect of physical fitness because it has a major impact on health and greatly influences physical performance.

ardiovascular fitness is generally considered to be the most important aspect of physical fitness. Those who possess reasonable amounts of fitness have a decreased risk for heart disease, reduced risk for premature death, and improved quality of life. Regular cardiovascular exercise promotes fitness and provides additional health and wellness benefits that extend well beyond reducing risks for disease. This concept describes the function of the cardiovascular system and explains how to determine the appropriate intensity of exercise needed to promote cardiovascular fitness.

Elements of Cardiovascular Fitness

The term *cardiovascular fitness* has several synonyms. Cardiovascular fitness is sometimes referred to as *cardiovascular endurance* because a person who possesses this type of fitness can persist in physical activity for long periods without undue fatigue. It has been referred to as *cardiorespiratory fitness* because it requires delivery and utilization of oxygen, which is only possible if the circulatory and respiratory systems are capable of these functions.

The term *aerobic fitness* has also been synonymous with *cardiovascular fitness* because **aerobic capacity**

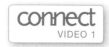

is considered to be the best indicator of cardiovascular fitness, and aerobic physical activity is the preferred method for achieving it. Regardless of the words used to describe it, cardiovascular fitness is complex because it requires fitness of several body systems.

Good cardiovascular fitness requires a fit heart muscle. The heart is a powerful muscle that pumps blood through the body. The heart of a normal individual beats reflexively about 40 million times a year. In a single day, the heart pumps over 4,000 gallons of blood through the body. To keep the cardiovascular system working effectively, it is crucial to have a strong and fit heart.

Like other muscles in the body, the heart becomes stronger if it is exercised. The size and strength of the heart increases, and it can pump more blood with each beat, accomplishing the same amount of work with fewer beats. Typical resting heart rate (RHR) values are around 70–80 beats per minute, but a highly trained endurance athlete may have a resting heart rate in the 40s or 50s. There is some individual variability in RHR, but a decrease in your RHR with training indicates clear improvements in cardiovascular fitness.

Good cardiovascular fitness requires a fit vascular system. The heart has four chambers, which pump and receive blood in a rhythmical fashion to maintain good circulation (see Figure 1). Blood containing a high

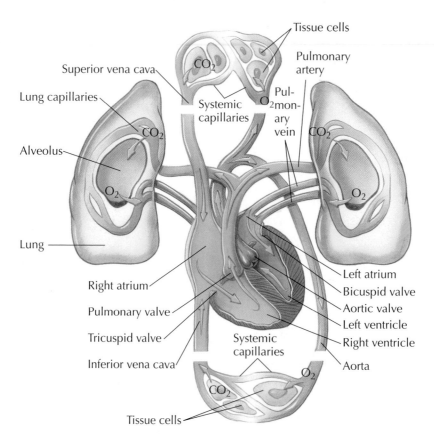

Figure 1 ▶ Cardiovascular system.

concentration of oxygen is pumped by the left ventricle through the aorta (a major artery), where it is carried to the tissues. Blood flows through a sequence of arteries to capillaries and to veins. Veins carry the blood containing lesser amounts of oxygen back to the right side of the heart, first to the atrium and then to the ventricle. The right ventricle pumps the blood to the lungs. In the lungs, the blood picks up oxygen (O_2), and carbon dioxide (CO_2) is removed. From the lungs, the oxygenated blood travels back to the heart, first to the left atrium and then to the left ventricle. The process then repeats itself. A dense network of arteries distributes the oxygenated blood to the muscles, tissues, and organs (see Figure 2).

Healthy arteries are elastic, are free of obstruction, and expand to permit the flow of blood. Muscle layers line the arteries and control the size of the arterial opening upon the impulse from nerve fibers. Unfit arteries may have a reduced internal diameter (atherosclerosis) because of deposits on the interior of their walls, or they may have hardened, nonelastic walls (arteriosclerosis).

The blood in the four chambers of the heart does not directly nourish the heart. Rather, numerous small arteries within the heart muscle provide for coronary circulation. Poor coronary circulation precipitated by unhealthy arteries can be the cause of a heart attack.

Deoxygenated blood flows back to the heart through a series of veins. The veins are intertwined in the skeletal muscle, and this allows normal muscle action to facilitate the return of blood to the heart. When a muscle is contracted, the vein is squeezed, and this pushes the blood back to the heart. Small valves in the veins prevent the backward flow of the blood, but defects in the valves can lead to pooling of blood in the veins. A common condition, known as varicose veins, is associated with the pooling of blood in the leg. Regular physical activity helps reduce pooling of blood in the veins and helps keep the valves of the veins healthy.

Capillaries are the transfer stations where oxygen and fuel are released, and waste products, such as carbon dioxide, are removed from the tissues. The veins receive the blood from the capillaries for the return trip to the heart.

Good cardiovascular fitness requires healthy blood and a fit respiratory system. The process of taking in oxygen (through the mouth and nose) and delivering it to the lungs, where it is picked up by the blood, is called external respiration. External respiration requires fit lungs as well as blood with adequate **hemoglobin.** Hemoglobin carries oxygen through the bloodstream. Lack of hemoglobin reduces oxygen-carrying capacity—a condition known as **anemia.**

Delivering oxygen to the tissues from the blood is called internal respiration. Internal respiration requires an adequate number of healthy capillaries. In addition to delivering oxygen to the tissues, these systems remove carbon dioxide. Good cardiovascular fitness requires fitness of both the external and internal respiratory systems.

Table 1 ► Changes in Cardiovascular Function between Rest and Exercise for a Person with Good Cardiovascular Fitness

		Rest	Maximal Exercise
Lungs	Breathing Rate (# / Minute)	12	30
Heart	Heart Rate (Beats / Minute)	70	190–200
	Stroke Volume (mL / Beat)	75	150
	Cardiac Output[a] (L / Minute)	5.2	28.5
Arteries	Blood Flow Distribution (%)	20%	70%
Muscle	Oxygen Extraction (%)	5%	20%
System	$\dot{V}O_2$ (mL/kg/min.)[b]	3.5	60

[a] Cardiac output = heart rate × stroke volume.
[b] $\dot{V}O_2$ = oxygen consumption = CO × oxygen extraction.

Cardiovascular fitness requires fit muscle tissue capable of using oxygen. Once the oxygen is delivered, the muscle tissues must be able to use oxygen to sustain physical performance (see Figure 2e). Physical activity that promotes cardiovascular fitness stimulates changes in muscle fibers that make them more effective in using oxygen. Outstanding distance runners have high numbers of well-conditioned muscle fibers that can readily use oxygen to produce energy for sustained running. Training in other activities would elicit similar adaptations in the specific muscles used in those activities.

During exercise the performance and function of the cardiovascular system is maximized. During exercise, a number of changes occur to increase the availability of oxygen to the muscles (see Table 1). Breathing rate and depth increase, allowing the body to take in more oxygen. The heart beats faster and pumps more blood with each beat (increased stroke volume). The higher heart rate and larger stroke volume allow

Aerobic Capacity A measure of aerobic or cardiovascular fitness.

Hemoglobin The oxygen-carrying protein (molecule) of red blood cells.

Anemia A condition in which hemoglobin and the blood's oxygen-carrying capacity are below normal.

Major Blood Vessels

Cardiovascular Fitness Characteristics

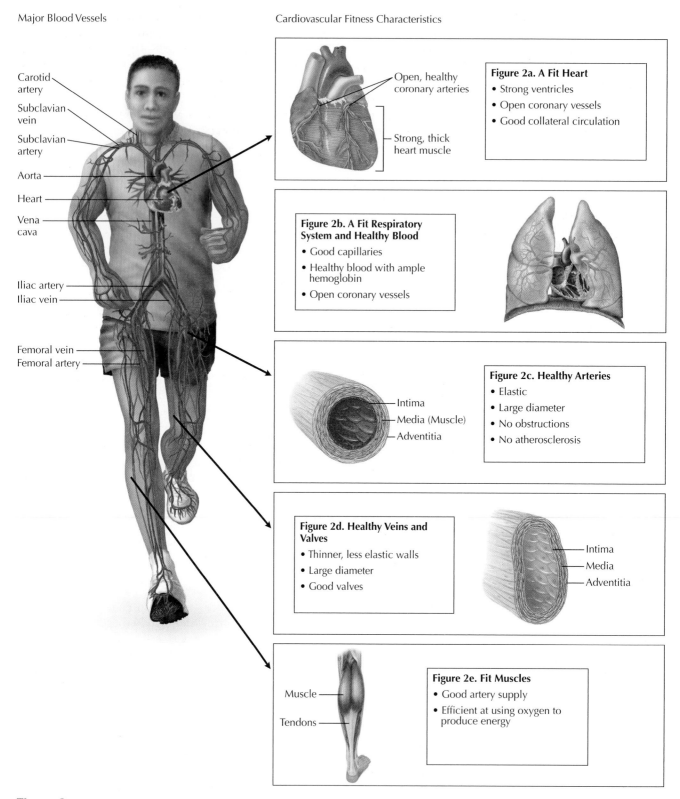

Carotid artery

Subclavian vein

Subclavian artery

Aorta

Heart

Vena cava

Iliac artery
Iliac vein

Femoral vein
Femoral artery

Open, healthy coronary arteries

Strong, thick heart muscle

Figure 2a. A Fit Heart
• Strong ventricles
• Open coronary vessels
• Good collateral circulation

Figure 2b. A Fit Respiratory System and Healthy Blood
• Good capillaries
• Healthy blood with ample hemoglobin
• Open coronary vessels

Intima
Media (Muscle)
Adventitia

Figure 2c. Healthy Arteries
• Elastic
• Large diameter
• No obstructions
• No atherosclerosis

Figure 2d. Healthy Veins and Valves
• Thinner, less elastic walls
• Large diameter
• Good valves

Intima
Media
Adventitia

Muscle

Tendons

Figure 2e. Fit Muscles
• Good artery supply
• Efficient at using oxygen to produce energy

Figure 2 ▶ Major blood vessels and cardiovascular fitness characteristics.

more blood to be pumped each minute (increased cardiac output). During exercise, the blood passing through the lungs picks up more oxygen and distributes it more quickly. Activation of the sympathetic nervous system also leads to a redistribution of the blood flow, so that more of it gets shunted to the working skeletal muscle. During rest, the muscles get about 20 percent of the available blood flow, but this increases to about 70 percent during vigorous exercise. Within the muscles, a larger percentage of the available oxygen is also extracted from the muscles during exercise. Collectively, these changes help provide the muscles with the oxygen needed to maintain aerobic metabolism.

Cardiovascular fitness is often evaluated using an indicator known as maximum oxygen uptake, or $\dot{V}O_2$ max. A person's **maximum oxygen uptake ($\dot{V}O_2$ max),** commonly referred to as aerobic capacity, is determined in a laboratory by measuring how much oxygen a person can use in maximal exercise. The test is usually done on a treadmill using specialized gas analyzers to measure oxygen use. The treadmill speed and grade are gradually increased, and when the exercise becomes very hard, oxygen use reaches its maximum. The test is a good indicator of overall cardiovascular fitness because you cannot take in and use a lot of oxygen if you do not have good fitness throughout the cardiovascular system (heart, blood vessels, blood, respiratory system, and muscles).

Elite endurance athletes can extract 5 or 6 liters of oxygen per minute from the environment, and this high aerobic capacity is what allows them to maintain high speeds in both training and competition without becoming excessively tired. In comparison, an average person typically extracts about 2 to 3 liters per minute. $\dot{V}O_2$ max is typically adjusted to account for a person's body size because bigger people may have higher scores due to their larger size. Values are reported in milliliters (mL) of oxygen (O_2) per kilogram (kg) of body weight per minute (mL/kg/min.).

A number of field tests have been developed to provide estimates of maximum aerobic capacity (see Lab Resource Materials on pages 131–134). These tests are developed and validated based on comparisons with laboratory protocols that directly measure the amount of oxygen that is consumed.

Adaptations to regular aerobic exercise result in improved cardiovascular fitness. Specific adaptations occur within each of the components of the cardiovascular system shown in Figure 2. The heart muscle gets stronger and pumps more blood with each beat, allowing the heart to pump less frequently to deliver the same amount of oxygen. The lungs and blood function more

efficiently in picking up oxygen and delivering it to the muscles. The vessels more effectively deliver the blood and the muscles adapt to use oxygen more efficiently. These adaptations allow a person to take in and use more oxygen during maximal exercise (increased aerobic capacity or $\dot{V}O_2$ max). The adaptations contribute to improved endurance performance as well as health benefits (as described in Concept 4).

Cardiovascular Fitness and Health Benefits

Good cardiovascular fitness reduces risk for heart disease, other hypokinetic conditions, and early death. Numerous studies over the past 30 to 40 years have confirmed that good cardiovascular fitness is associated with a reduced risk for heart disease as well as a number of other chronic, hypokinetic conditions. A recent review of 33 studies involving nearly 200,000 people showed that people with low fitness have had a 70 percent higher death rate from all causes and a 56 percent higher death rate from heart diseases than people of intermediate

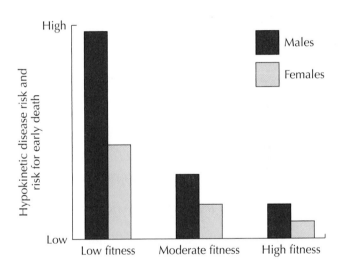

Figure 3 ► Risk reduction associated with cardiovascular fitness.

Source: Adapted from Blair et al.

Maximum Oxygen Uptake ($\dot{V}O_2$ max) A laboratory measure held to be the best measure of cardiovascular fitness. Commonly referred to as $\dot{V}O_2$ max, or the volume (V) of oxygen used when a person reaches his or her maximum (max) ability to supply it during exercise.

fitness. The consensus is that low-fit individuals are three to six times more likely to develop symptoms of metabolic syndrome or diabetes than high-fit individuals. While the specific amount of fitness needed to reduce risks varies by condition and population, evidence clearly supports the need for at least a moderate level of fitness. As shown in Figure 3, there are dramatic reductions in risk in moving from the low fitness category to the moderate fitness category for both males and females. In terms of longevity, studies suggest that individuals with moderate fitness will live 5–6 years longer than low-fit individuals.

The benefits of cardiovascular fitness are independent of its beneficial effect on other risk factors. Physical activity has been shown to have beneficial effects on some other established heart disease risk factors, such as cholesterol, blood pressure, and body fat. It is important to note that the beneficial effects of cardiovascular fitness on risk for heart disease and early death are considered to be independent of these other effects. This means that 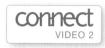 active/fit people would still have lower health risks even if their cholesterol, blood pressure, and body fat levels were identical to a matched set of inactive/unfit people. This evidence contributed to the labeling of physical inactivity as a major, independent risk factor for heart disease. The risk associated with physical inactivity is as large as (or larger than) risks associated with any of the other established risk factors.

Good fitness reduces risks for normal weight, overweight, and obese people. Some people think they cannot be fit if they are overweight or overfat. It is now known that appropriate physical activity can build cardiovascular fitness in all types of people, including those with excess body fat. In fact, numerous studies have demonstrated that a fit, overweight person is at lower risk of chronic disease than an unfit person who is normal weight. These findings demonstrate that for chronic disease prevention, low fitness is a greater risk than excess body fatness. The greatest risk is among people who are both unfit and overfat.

Good cardiovascular fitness enhances the ability to perform various tasks, improves the ability to function, and is associated with a feeling of well-being. Moving out of the low fitness zone is of obvious importance to disease risk reduction. Achieving the good zone on tests further reduces disease and early death risk and promotes optimal wellness benefits, and a position statement by the American College of Sports Medicine shows an improved ability to function among older adults. Other wellness benefits include the ability to enjoy leisure activities and meet emergency situations, as well as

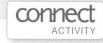
the health and wellness benefits described earlier in this book. Cardiovascular fitness in the high-performance zone enhances the ability to perform in certain athletic events and in occupations that require high performance levels (e.g., firefighters).

The FIT Formula for Cardiovascular Fitness

The FIT formula for cardiovascular fitness varies for people of different activity levels. Adaptations to physical activity are based on the overload principle and the principle of progression. It is important to provide an appropriate challenge to the cardiovascular system (overload), but the challenge should be progressive, increasing gradually as fitness improves. For most people, vigorous physical activity from steps 2 and 3 (see Figure 4) is 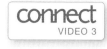 necessary to improve cardiovascular fitness. However, for people with low fitness, moderate physical activity (step 1) produces improvements. Table 2 presents the FIT formulas for people of five different fitness and activity levels. While the *frequency* of exercise is similar for the different levels, the *intensity* and amount of *time* spent in activity vary considerably. The sections that follow provide added information about the FIT formula.

The frequency (F) of physical activity to build cardiovascular fitness ranges from 3 to 5 or more days a week. The new ACSM guidelines for building cardiovascular fitness suggest a frequency of at least 5 days a week for low fit people who do primarily moderate physical activity. Moderate activity can be safely performed every day and can provide additional benefits. For more active people (and those with higher levels of cardiovascular fitness), vigorous physical activity at least 3 days a week is recommended. Vigorous physical activity provides additional benefits (compared to moderate activity), however, it can increase risk for orthopedic injury if it is done too frequently. Therefore, 5 days a week is the maximal recommended dose for most people. Healthy people who are fit and regularly active and have no evidence of joint problems or injuries may train up to 6 days a week, but most experts agree that at least 1 day off a week is beneficial. Use Table 2 to determine the appropriate frequency of exercise for you based on your current activity and fitness level. Complete the fitness assessments at the end of this concept before making your decision. The ACSM guidelines focus on exercise for building cardiovascular fitness but are similar to national guidelines designed to produce health and wellness benefits.

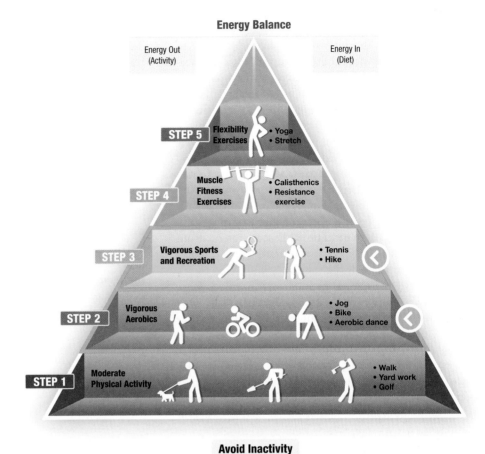

Figure 4 ▶ Select activities from steps 2 and 3 of the pyramid for optimal cardiovascular fitness.
Source: C. B. Corbin

The intensity (I) of physical activity necessary to produce cardiovascular fitness depends on a person's level of fitness. In general, fit people need to exercise at a higher intensity to provide a sufficient challenge to the cardiovascular system. To determine the appropriate intensity, it is important to have some indicator of a person's overall fitness. If the maximal aerobic capacity is known, an appropriate intensity can be set at a percentage of the maximum level. Because these values cannot be calculated without special equipment, other indicators of relative intensity are more commonly used.

Table 2 ▶ FIT Formula for Cardiovascular Fitness for People of Different Fitness and Activity Levels					
Fitness Level	Very Low	Low	Marginal	Good	High Performance
Activity Level	Sedentary	Some light to moderate activity	Sporadic moderate to vigorous activity	Regular moderate to vigorous activity	Habitual moderate to vigorous activity
F = Frequency (days per week)	3–5	3–5	3–5	3–5	3–5
I = Intensity					
Heart Rate Reserve (HRR)	30–40%	40–55%	55–70%	65–80%	70–85%
Max. Heart Rate (max HR)	57–67%	64–74%	74–84%	80–91%	84–94%
Relative Perceived Exertion (RPE)	12–13	12–13	13–14	13–15	14–16
T = Time (minutes per day)	20–30	30–60	30–90	30–90	30–90

Heart rate provides a good indicator of the relative challenge presented by a given bout of exercise. Therefore, guidelines for the intensity of physical activity to build cardiovascular fitness are typically based on percentages of **heart rate reserve (HRR)** or maximal heart rate (maxHR). Current guidelines as outlined in Table 2 specify different intensity levels based on current fitness and activity levels. Calculations of HRR and maxHR will be described in detail later, but the general range for HRR is 30 to 85 percent and for maxHR, 57 to 94 percent.

Ratings of perceived exertion (RPE) refer to the assessment of the intensity of exercise based on how the participant feels; a subjective assessment of effort. RPE has been shown to be useful in assessing the intensity of aerobic physical activity. The RPE scale ranges from 6 (very very light) to 20 (very very hard), with 1-point increments in between. If the values are multiplied by 10, the RPE values loosely correspond to HR values (e.g., 60 = rest HR and 200 = maxHR). Details will be provided later, but the target zone for aerobic activity is from 12 to 16 (see Table 2).

Regardless of what method is used, the important point is that lower intensities provide a cardiovascular fitness benefit for low-fit sedentary people, but higher intensities are needed for more fit people. Use Table 2 to determine the appropriate *intensity of exercise* based on your current activity and fitness level.

The amount of time (T) for building cardiovascular fitness is typically based on minutes of activity per day. Both the ACSM guidelines and the national (DHHS) physical activity guidelines recommend a minimum of 150 minutes of moderate activity per week, or 75 minutes of vigorous activity per week (or a combination of minutes from moderate and vigorous activity). Extending the length time for exercise bouts has additional benefits for health and wellness, as well as cardiovascular fitness. For example, 150 to 300 minutes of moderate activity per week is beneficial in losing body fat and maintaining a healthy body weight. For fit and active people, extending bouts of vigorous activity from 20 up to 90 minutes has both health/wellness benefits and enhanced cardiovascular fitness. Use Table 2 to determine the appropriate length of time for daily exercise for you based on your current activity and fitness level.

Different patterns of activity can be used to achieve the recommended dose of exercise. Some people may prefer to perform regular 30-minute bouts of exercise but others may prefer to accumulate it throughout the day. The ACSM indicates a pattern involving three 10-minute bouts provides similar benefits to one 30-minute session. The amount of physical activity can also vary across days but, as noted in a previous concept, the ACSM discourages a pattern of activity performed by "weekend warriors"—long activity sessions on one day a week with no regular activity in between. The prescriptions in Table 2 are aimed at overall aerobic fitness. Specialized training regimens are typically needed for those interested in aerobic fitness events (e.g., running races, triathlons) and competitive sports (see Concept 12 for suggestions).

Threshold and Target Zones for Intensity of Activity to Build Cardiovascular Fitness

There is a minimum intensity and an optimal intensity range for activity designed to develop cardiovascular fitness. As noted earlier, monitoring heart rate and making ratings of perceived exertion are the most practical methods of determining the intensity of activity necessary to build cardiovascular fitness. The threshold of training (minimum intensity) and the target zone (optimal intensity range) can be determined using several methods. Most methods are based on heart rate so the target zone is typically referred to as *target heart rate zone*. Ratings of perceived exertion (RPE) can also be used to define the target zone for exercise intensity. This section provides details of using these methods.

An estimate of maximal heart rate (maxHR) is needed to determine appropriate target heart rate zones for aerobic exercise. Your maxHR is the highest heart rate attained in maximal exercise. It could be determined using an electrocardiogram while exercising to exhaustion; however, it can also be estimated with formulas. MaxHR is known to decrease with age so one simple and commonly used approach is to subtract your age from 220 (i.e., maxHR = 220 − age). However, studies have shown that this formula leads to inaccurate estimates for most people. A number of more specialized,

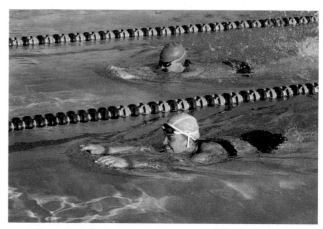

Aerobic activities provide an ideal stimulus for improving cardiovascular fitness.

In the News

Genetics Influence Adaptations to Exercise

One factor over which you have little control is heredity. For years we have known that all people do not respond equally to regular exercise, even when it is done using the correct FIT formula. A recent study published in the *Journal of Applied Physiology* found that about 80 to 85 percent of 423 men and women who participated in a cardiovascular fitness program saw improvements in cardiovascular fitness over a period of 20 weeks. However, 15 to 20 percent of the participants showed little fitness improvement. The researchers found that a genetic profile predicted which people would get the most improvement from exercise.

Some suggested that this was evidence that exercise is of little value to some people. However, researchers who conducted the study suggest that exercise is of value to all, noting that exercise has many benefits in addition to increases in cardiovascular fitness. Even those who do not respond with big gains in CV fitness can have changes in blood pressure, blood sugar, heart rate, and other biological markers.

Would you give up on exercise if you didn't see tangible gains in fitness from your efforts?

connect
ACTIVITY

nonlinear equations have been developed to avoid this problem. For example, a new formula for women was recently developed (MaxHR = 206 × [.88 × age]). However, there is currently no consensus on the most accurate method. In this book, we use a relatively simple nonlinear method known as the Tanaka formula: maxHR = 208 − (.7 × age). Calculations made at a variety of ages show little, if any, differences between the

formulas, so we use the one that makes calculations the easiest (it limits use of fractions). Table 3 illustrates the calculations for determining maxHR for a 22-year-old.

The heart rate reserve (HRR) method is the preferred way to calculate target heart rate zones. Table 2 provides five different intensity ranges for activity designed to build cardiovascular fitness. After you have assessed your fitness using fitness tests (see Lab Resource Materials and Lab 7B), determine which of the five intensity ranges is best for you based on your current activity and fitness. Table 3 provides a worked example for calculating heart rate target zones using the HRR method. The example is for a 22-year-old with good cardiovascular fitness, who does regular moderate-to-vigorous physical activity and who has a resting heart rate of 68 beats per minute. The target heart rate zone for this hypothetical person is 65 to 80 percent.

To determine the threshold of training (minimum heart rate for building cardiovascular fitness), use 65 percent of the working heart rate, and then add that value to the resting heart rate. To determine the upper limit of the target zone, use 80 percent of the working heart rate and add that value to the resting heart rate. Because target zone heart rates vary for people of different fitness and activity levels and because resting

---

Table 3 ▶ Sample Target Heart Zone Calculations for a 22-Year-Old, Using the Percentage of Heart Rate Reserve Method

Calculating Maximal Heart Rate

Maximal heart rate	= 208 − (.7 × age)
	= 208 − (.7 × 22)
	= 208 − 15.4
	193

Calculating Heart Rate Reserve

Maximal heart rate	193 bpm
Minus resting heart rate	− 68 bpm
Equals heart rate reserve (HRR)	125 bpm

Calculating Threshold Heart Rate

HRR	125 bpm
× 65%	× .65
Equals	81 bpm
Plus resting heart rate	+68 bpm
Equals threshold heart rate	149 bpm

Calculating Upper Limit Heart Rate

HRR	125 bpm
× 80%	× .80
Equals	100 bpm
Plus resting heart rate	+68 bpm
Equals upper limit heart rate	168 bpm

Heart Rate Reserve (HRR) The difference between maximum heart rate (highest heart rate in vigorous activity) and resting heart rate (lowest heart rate at rest).

Ratings of Perceived Exertion (RPE) The assessment of the intensity of exercise based on how the participant feels; a subjective assessment of effort.

and maximal heart rates vary, each person will have a unique range of heart rates defining the target heart rate zone. The chart in Figure 5 allows you to look up similar threshold and target heart rate zones based on your resting heart rate and age (up to age 65). Locate your resting heart rate on the left and your age across the top. The values at the point where they intersect represent your target heart rate (based on 65 percent and 80 percent of HR reserve). Look across the columns for a given row to see how the target zone changes with age. Look down the rows for a certain column and see how the target zone changes with fitness. The chart shows that fit individuals (lower rest HR values) have lower target heart rate zones than unfit individuals (higher rest HR values). This may seem somewhat paradoxical but the reason is that fit individuals start exercise with a lower HR value and therefore have a larger HRR.

The percentage of maximum heart rate method is an alternative way to calculate target heart rate zones. The percentage of maxHR method is simpler to use than the HRR method, but it is not as accurate. This procedure takes maximal heart rate into account but does not factor in individual differences in resting heart rate. People with a typical resting HR of 60 to 70 bpm will tend to get similar values with both methods, but the percentage of maxHR method tends to be less accurate for people with high or low resting heart rates.

To use the percentage of maxHR method, first find your maximum HR with the formula ($maxHR = 208 - (.7 \times age)$). Then multiply your maxHR by the appropriate percentages from Table 2. For a person with good fitness and who performs regular moderate-to-vigorous activity, the percentages would be 80 to 91 percent. The maxHR for our hypothetical 22-year-old is 193, so the target heart rate zone would be 154 to 176 using this method ($.80 \times 193 = 154$ and $.91 \times 193 = 176$). As illustrated in Table 3, this procedure yields somewhat similar but higher values for the maxHR method than for the HRR method. The differences between the two methods vary for people of different ages, resting heart rates, and fitness/activity levels. The percentage of maxHR method is considered an acceptable alternative method, but the HRR method is more precise. Threshold and target zone heart rates should be used as general guidelines for cardiovascular exercise. You should check your resting heart rate and learn to calculate your target heart range based on the HRR method. It is important to understand how to make the calculations, since the process explains the relationships.

The target heart ranges should be used as just that, a general target to try for during your exercise session. By bringing your heart rate above the threshold and into the target zone, you will provide an optimal challenge to your cardiovascular system and maintain/improve your cardiovascular fitness. Guidelines for heart rate monitoring are provided in the next section.

Effect of Age and Resting Heart Rate on Target Heart Range											
Rest HR	Threshold	20	25	30	35	40	45	50	55	60	65
50	65%	144	141	139	137	135	132	130	128	125	123
	80%	165	162	160	157	154	151	148	146	143	140
55	65%	145	143	141	139	136	134	132	129	127	125
	80%	166	163	161	158	155	152	149	147	144	141
60	65%	147	145	143	140	138	136	133	131	129	127
	80%	167	164	162	159	156	153	150	148	145	142
65	65%	149	147	144	142	140	137	135	133	131	128
	80%	168	165	163	160	157	154	151	149	146	143
70	65%	151	148	146	144	142	139	137	135	132	130
	80%	169	166	164	161	158	155	152	150	147	144
75	65%	152	150	148	146	143	141	139	136	134	132
	80%	170	167	165	162	159	156	153	151	148	145

Figure 5 ▶ Effect of age and resting heart rate on target heart range.

Table 4 ▶ Ratings of Perceived Exertion (RPE)

Rating	Description
6	
7	Very, very light
8	
9	Very light
10	
11	Fairly light
12	
13	Somewhat hard
14	
15	Hard
16	
17	Very hard
18	
19	Very, very hard
20	

Source: Data from Borg.

Ratings of perceived exertion can be used to monitor the intensity of physical activity. The ACSM suggests that regularly active people can use RPE to determine if they are exercising in the target zone (see Table 4). Ratings of perceived exertion have been shown to correlate well with HRR. For this reason, RPE can be used to estimate exercise intensity, avoiding the need to stop and count heart rate during exercise. A rating of 12 is equal to threshold, and a rating of 16 is equal to the upper limit of the target zone. With practice, most people can recognize when they are in the target zone using ratings of perceived exertion.

Guidelines for Heart Rate and Exercise Monitoring

Learning to count heart rate can help you monitor the intensity of your physical activity. Each time your heart beats, it pumps blood into the arteries. The surge of blood causes a pulse, which can be felt by holding a finger against an artery. The major arteries that are easy to locate and are frequently used for pulse counts are the radial just below the base of 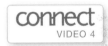 the thumb on the wrist (see Figure 6) and the carotid on either side of the Adam's apple (see Figure 7). Counting the pulse at the carotid is the most popular procedure,

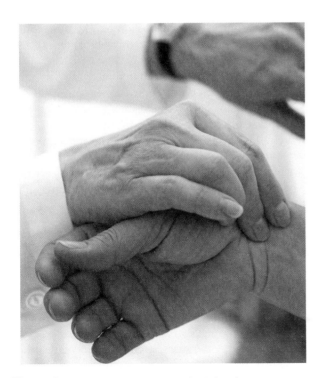
Figure 6 ▶ Counting your radial (wrist) pulse.

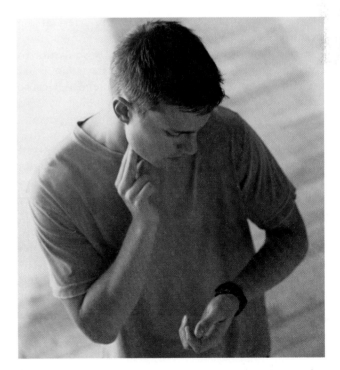
Figure 7 ▶ Counting your carotid (neck) pulse.

TECHNOLOGY UPDATE

New Technology in Activity Monitoring

Physical activity researchers have been using accelerometry-based devices to monitor physical activity behavior for 15 to 20 years. However, the development and deployment of low-cost accelerometers in gaming devices such as the Wii and Kinect made it possible for companies to develop more competitively priced monitoring devices. The monitors are more expensive than standard pedometers but they can capture the intensity of physical activity and most can link wirelessly to the Internet or your cell phone through Bluetooth technology. Some devices also have built-in connections with social media applications, including Facebook, to enable friends to hold each other accountable as virtual exercise buddies. The new devices provide consumers advanced activity monitoring devices to keep track of their exercise sessions.

Would real-time monitoring devices help you stay committed to your exercise goals?

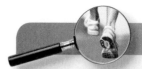

A CLOSER LOOK

Online Fitness Memberships and Consulting

Many people take advantage of employee fitness programs to get advice about exercise. Others prefer to enroll in private gyms where they may contract with a personal trainer. A relatively new option for exercisers is to enroll in an online fitness program. One company offers opportunities for individuals to enroll in the Lifespan Fitness Club to access personalized health and exercise tracking software and exercise tip sheets. Members can also connect with online health coaches who review your status and provide suggestions for programming.

Would you use this type of support to maintain your health status or would you rather do it on your own?

---

probably because the carotid pulse is easy to locate. The radial pulse is a bit harder to find because of the many tendons near the wrist, but it works better for some people.

To count the pulse rate, simply place the fingertips (index and middle finger) over the artery at the wrist or neck location. Move the fingers around until a strong pulse can be felt. Press gently so as not to cut off the blood flow through the artery. Counting the pulse with the thumb is *not* recommended because the thumb has a relatively strong pulse of its own, and it could be confusing when counting another person's pulse.

Counting heart rates during exercise presents some additional challenges. To obtain accurate exercise heart rate values, it is best to count heart beats or pulses while moving; however, this is difficult during most activities.

The most practical method is to count the pulse immediately after exercise. During physical activity, the heart rate increases, but immediately after exercise, it begins to slow and return to normal. In fact, the heart rate has already slowed considerably within 1 minute after activity ceases. Therefore, you must locate the pulse quickly and count the rate for a short period in order to obtain accurate results. For best results, keep moving while quickly

locating the pulse; then stop and take a 15-second count. Multiply the number of pulses by 4 to convert heart rate to beats per minute.

You can also count the pulse for 10 seconds and multiply by 6, or count the pulse for 6 seconds and multiply by 10 to estimate a 1-minute heart rate. The latter method allows you to calculate heart rates easily by adding 0 to the 6-second count. However, short-duration pulse counts increase the chance of error because a miscount of 1 beat is multiplied by 6 or 10 beats rather than by 4 beats.

The pulse rate should be counted after regular activity, not after a sudden burst. Some runners sprint the last few yards of their daily run and then count their pulse. Such a burst of exercise will elevate the heart rate considerably. This gives a false picture of the actual exercise heart rate. Everyone should learn to determine resting heart rate accurately and to estimate exercise heart rate by quickly and accurately making pulse counts after activity (see Lab 7A).

Declines in resting heart rate and exercise heart rate signal improvements in cardiovascular fitness. As described in this concept, the heart beats to provide the body (and working muscles) with oxygen. Oxygen is used to produce energy using aerobic metabolism. During rest, the heart can beat relatively slowly to provide sufficient oxygen to the body. During exercise, the demand for energy increases, so the body increases heart rate (and respiration) to help distribute more oxygen to the body. Changes in resting heart rate and exercise heart rate provide good indicators of improvements in fitness because they indicate that the heart can pump fewer times to provide the same amount of blood flow to the body. A fit individual has a stronger heart and can pump more blood with each beat.

A comparison of resting and exercise heart rates for three hypothetical individuals performing the same bout of exercise is shown in Figure 8. The column labeled "A" shows the response of an unfit person. This person has a high resting heart rate of 90, and this increases to 160 during the exercise. This intensity would feel pretty hard, so an RPE would likely be about 17. Compare this response to the results for a moderately or highly fit person. Both have a lower resting heart rate and a lower exercise heart rate, so exercise is easier and can be maintained more easily.

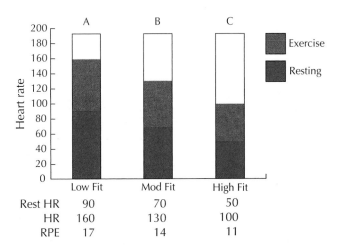

	Low Fit	Mod Fit	High Fit
Rest HR	90	70	50
HR	160	130	100
RPE	17	14	11

Figure 8 ▶ Comparison of resting and exercise heart for three 22-year-old individuals (maxHR = 193) with different levels of fitness (A = low fitness, B = moderate fitness, C = high fitness).

Strategies for Action

An important first step in developing and maintaining cardiovascular fitness is assessing your current status. For an activity program to be most effective, it should be based on personal needs. Some type of testing is necessary to determine your personal need for cardiovascular fitness. The best measure of cardiovascular fitness is a laboratory assessment of $\dot{V}O_2$ max, but this is not possible for most people. To provide alternatives, researchers have developed other tests that give reasonable estimates. Commonly used tests are the step test, the swim test, the 12-minute run, the Astrand-Ryhming bicycle test, and the walking test. These tests are developed 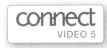 based on comparisons with measured $\dot{V}O_2$ max and are good general indicators of cardiovascular fitness. In Lab 7B you will be able to compare estimates from several tests.

The self-assessment you choose depends on your current fitness and activity levels, the availability of equipment, and other factors. The walking test is probably best for those at beginning levels because more vigorous forms of activity may cause discomfort and discourage future participation. The step test is somewhat less vigorous than the running test and takes only a few minutes to complete. The bicycle test is also submaximal or relatively moderate in intensity. It is quite accurate but requires more equipment and expertise than the other tests. You may need help from a fitness expert to do this

test properly. The swim test is especially useful to those with musculoskeletal problems and other disabilities. The running test is the most vigorous and for this reason may be best for more advanced exercisers with high levels of motivation.

Results on the walking, running, and swimming tests are greatly influenced by the motivation of the test taker. If the test taker does not try hard, fitness results are underestimated. The bicycle and step tests are influenced less by motivation because one must exercise at a specified workload and at a regular pace. Because heart rate can be influenced by emotional factors, by exercise prior to the test, and other factors, tests using heart rate can sometimes give incorrect results. Thus, do your self-assessments when you are relatively free from stress and are rested.

Prior to performing any of these, be sure that you are physically and medically ready. Prepare yourself by doing some regular physical activity for 3 to 6 weeks before actually taking the tests. If possible, take more than one test and use the summary of your test results to make a final assessment of your cardiovascular fitness. In Lab 7B, you 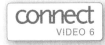 will have the opportunity to self-assess your cardiovascular fitness using one or more tests. A nonexercise estimate of cardiovascular fitness is also provided for comparison. Although this self-report tool has limitations, it is increasingly being used as a screening tool in physicians' offices to determine if patients have risks associated with poor fitness.

Web Resources

American College of Sports Medicine **www.acsm.org**
American Heart Association **www.americanheart.org**
The Cooper Institute **www.cooperinst.org**
Fitnessgram Youth Fitness Test **www.fitnessgram.net**
Plugout Fitness **www.plugoutfitness.com**

Suggested Readings

ACSM. 2010. *ACSM's Guidelines for Exercise Testing and Prescription*. 8th ed. Philadelphia: Lippincott, Williams & Wilkins, Chapters 4 and 7.

Ding, E. L., and F. B. Hu. 2010. Commentary: Relative importance of diet vs. physical activity for health. *International Journal of Epidemiology* 39(1):209–211.

Garber, C. E., et al. 2011. Quantity and quality of exercise for developing and maintaining cardiorespiratory, musculoskeletal, and neuromotor fitness in apparently healthy adults: Guidance for prescribing exercise. *Medicine and Science in Sports and Exercise* 43(7):1334–1359.

Gulati, M., et al. Heart rate response to exercise stress testing in asymptomatic women. The St. James Women Take Heart Project. *Circulation*. Published online June 28, 2010, **http://circ.ahajournals.org**

Heroux, M., et al. 2010. Dietary patterns and the risk of mortality: Impact of cardiorespiratory fitness. *International Journal of Epidemiology* 39(1):197–209.

Kodama, S., et al. 2009. Cardiorespiratory fitness as a quantitative predictor of all-cause mortality and cardiovascular events in healthy men and women: A Meta-analysis. *Journal of the American Medical Association* 301(19):2024–2035.

Kohl, H. W., and T. D. Murray. 2012. *Foundations of Physical Activity and Public Health*. Champaign, IL: Human Kinetics.

Liu, R. et al. (2012). Cardiorespiratory fitness as a predictor of dementia mortality in men and women. *Medicine and Science in Sports and Exercise*. 44(2): 253–259.

Healthy People 2020

The objectives listed below are societal goals designed to help all Americans improve their health between now and the year 2020. They were selected because they relate to the content of this concept.

- Increase overall cardiovascular health, reduce heart disease, stroke, high blood pressure, and high blood cholesterol, increase screening, and increase emergency treatment by professionals or bystanders.

- Increase proportion of adults who meet guidelines for moderate to vigorous aerobic activity.

- Increase percentage of college students receiving risk factor information.

- Increase counseling about physical activity by physicians.

- Increase weight-control efforts and activity levels of adults with high LDL.

- Increase young adult awareness of CHD signs and symptoms.

- Attain high-quality, longer lives free of preventable disease, injury, and premature death.

A national goal is to promote and encourage counseling about physical activity by physicians. Many physicians suggest that people get more exercise, but often offer few specifics. What type of information do you think physicians should provide? Suggest cost-effective ways they can provide information to their patients.

Lab Resource Materials: Evaluating Cardiovascular Fitness

The Walking Test

- Warm up; then walk 1 mile as fast as you can without straining. Record your time to the nearest second.

- Immediately after the walk, count your heart rate for 15 seconds; then multiply by four to get a 1-minute heart rate. Record your heart rate.

- Use your walking time and your postexercise heart rate to determine your rating using Chart 1.

Chart 1 Walking Ratings for Males and Females

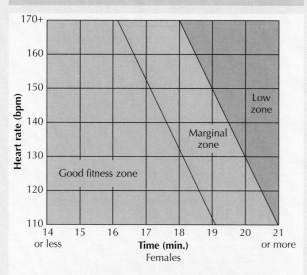

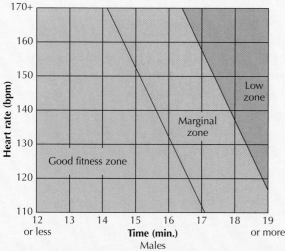

Source: James M. Rippe, M.D.

The ratings in Chart 1 are for ages 20 to 29. They provide reasonable ratings for people of all ages.

Note: The walking test is not a good indicator of high performance; the running and bicycle tests are recommended.

Step Test

- Step up and down on a 12-inch bench for 3 minutes at a rate of 24 steps per minute. One step consists of four beats—that is, "up with the left foot, up with the right foot, down with the left foot, down with the right foot."

- Immediately after the exercise, sit down on the bench and relax. Don't talk.

- Locate your pulse or have someone locate it for you.

- Five seconds after the exercise ends, begin counting your pulse. Count the pulse for 60 seconds.

- Your score is your 60-second heart rate. Locate your score and your rating on Chart 2.

Chart 2 Step Test Rating Chart

Classification	60-Second Heart Rate
High-performance zone	84 or less
Good fitness zone	85–95
Marginal zone	96–119
Low zone	120 and above

Source: Kasch and Boyer.

As you grow older, you will want to continue to score well on this rating chart. Because your maximal heart rate decreases as you age, you should be able to score well if you exercise regularly.

The Astrand-Ryhming Bicycle Test

- Ride a stationary bicycle ergometer for 6 minutes at a rate of 50 pedal cycles per minute (one push with each foot per cycle). Cool down after the test.

- Set the bicycle at a workload between 300 and 1,200 kpm. For less fit or smaller people, a setting in the range of 300 to 600 is appropriate. Larger or fitter people will need to use a setting of 750 to 1,200. The workload should be enough to elevate the heart rate to at least 125 bpm but no more than 170 bpm during the ride. The ideal range is 140–150 bpm.

- During the sixth minute of the ride (if the heart rate is in the correct range—see previous step), count the heart rate for the entire sixth minute. The carotid or radial pulse may be used.

- Use Chart 3 (males) or 4 (females) to determine your predicted oxygen uptake score in liters per minute. Locate your heart rate for the sixth minute of the ride in the left column and the work rate in kp·m/min. across the top. The number in the chart where the heart rate and work rate intersect represents your predicted O_2 uptake in liters per minute. The bicycle you use must allow you to easily and accurately determine the work rate in kp·m/min.

- Ratings are typically assigned based on milliliters per kilogram of body weight per minute. To convert your score to milliliters per kilogram per minute (mL/kg/min.), the first step is to multiply your score from Chart 3 or 4 by 1,000. This converts your score from liters to milliliters. Then divide your weight in pounds by 2.2. This converts your weight to kilograms. Then divide your score in milliliters by your weight in kilograms. This gives you your score in mL/kg/min.

- Example: An oxygen uptake score of 3.5 liters is equal to a 3,500-milliliter score (3.5 × 1,000). If the person with this score weighed 150 pounds, his or her weight in kilograms would be 68.18 kilograms (150 divided by 2.2). The person's oxygen uptake would be 51.3 mL/kg/min. (3,500 divided by 68.18).

- Use your score in mL/kg/min. to determine your rating (Chart 5).

Chart 3 Determining Oxygen Uptake Using the Bicycle Test—Men (Liters O_2/min.)

Heart Rate	Work Rate (kp·m/min.)				Heart Rate	Work Rate (kp·m/min.)					Heart Rate	Work Rate (kp·m/min.)				
	450	600	900	1,200		450	600	900	1,200	1,500		450	600	900	1,200	1,500
123	3.3	3.4	4.6	6.0	139	2.5	2.6	3.6	4.8	6.0	155	2.0	2.2	3.0	4.0	5.0
124	3.3	3.3	4.5	6.0	140	2.5	2.6	3.6	4.8	6.0	156	1.9	2.2	2.9	4.0	5.0
125	3.2	3.2	4.4	5.9	141	2.4	2.6	3.5	4.7	5.9	157	1.9	2.1	2.9	3.9	4.9
126	3.1	3.2	4.4	5.8	142	2.4	2.5	3.5	4.6	5.8	158	1.8	2.1	2.9	3.9	4.9
127	3.0	3.1	4.3	5.7	143	2.4	2.5	3.4	4.6	5.7	159	1.8	2.1	2.8	3.8	4.8
128	3.0	3.1	4.2	5.6	144	2.3	2.5	3.4	4.5	5.7	160	1.8	2.1	2.8	3.8	4.8
129	2.9	3.0	4.2	5.6	145	2.3	2.4	3.4	4.5	5.6	161	1.7	2.0	2.8	3.7	4.7
130	2.9	3.0	4.1	5.5	146	2.3	2.4	3.3	4.4	5.6	162	1.7	2.0	2.8	3.7	4.6
131	2.8	2.9	4.0	5.4	147	2.3	2.4	3.3	4.4	5.5	163	1.7	2.0	2.8	3.7	4.6
132	2.8	2.9	4.0	5.3	148	2.2	2.4	3.2	4.3	5.4	164	1.6	2.0	2.7	3.6	4.5
133	2.7	2.8	3.9	5.3	149	2.2	2.3	3.2	4.3	5.4	165	1.6	1.9	2.7	3.6	4.5
134	2.7	2.8	3.9	5.2	150	2.2	2.3	3.2	4.2	5.3	166	1.6	1.9	2.7	3.6	4.5
135	2.7	2.8	3.8	5.1	151	2.2	2.3	3.1	4.2	5.2	167	1.5	1.9	2.6	3.5	4.4
136	2.6	2.7	3.8	5.0	152	2.1	2.3	3.1	4.1	5.2	168	1.5	1.9	2.6	3.5	4.4
137	2.6	2.7	3.7	5.0	153	2.1	2.2	3.0	4.1	5.1	169	1.5	1.9	2.6	3.5	4.3
138	2.5	2.7	3.7	4.9	154	2.0	2.2	3.0	4.0	5.1	170	1.4	1.8	2.6	3.4	4.3

Chart 4 Determining Oxygen Uptake Using the Bicycle Test—Women (Liters O_2/min.)

Heart Rate	Work Rate (kp·m/min.)					Heart Rate	Work Rate (kp·m/min.)					Heart Rate	Work Rate (kp·m/min.)			
	300	450	600	750	900		300	450	600	750	900		400	600	750	900
123	2.4	3.1	3.9	4.6	5.1	139	1.8	2.4	2.9	3.5	4.0	155	1.9	2.4	2.8	3.2
124	2.4	3.1	3.8	4.5	5.1	140	1.8	2.4	2.8	3.4	4.0	156	1.9	2.4	2.8	3.2
125	2.3	3.0	3.7	4.4	5.0	141	1.8	2.3	2.8	3.4	3.9	157	1.8	2.3	2.7	3.2
126	2.3	3.0	3.6	4.3	5.0	142	1.7	2.3	2.8	3.3	3.9	158	1.8	2.3	2.7	3.1
127	2.2	2.9	3.5	4.2	4.8	143	1.7	2.2	2.7	3.3	3.8	159	1.8	2.3	2.7	3.1
128	2.2	2.8	3.5	4.2	4.8	144	1.7	2.2	2.7	3.2	3.8	160	1.8	2.2	2.6	3.0
129	2.2	2.8	3.4	4.1	4.8	145	1.6	2.2	2.7	3.2	3.7	161	1.8	2.2	2.6	3.0
130	2.1	2.7	3.4	4.0	4.7	146	1.6	2.2	2.6	3.2	3.7	162	1.8	2.2	2.6	3.0
131	2.1	2.7	3.4	4.0	4.6	147	1.6	2.1	2.6	3.1	3.6	163	1.7	2.2	2.5	2.9
132	2.0	2.7	3.3	3.9	4.6	148	1.6	2.1	2.6	3.1	3.6	164	1.7	2.1	2.5	2.9
133	2.0	2.6	3.2	3.8	4.5	149	1.5	2.1	2.6	3.0	3.5	165	1.7	2.1	2.5	2.9
134	2.0	2.6	3.2	3.8	4.4	150	1.5	2.0	2.5	3.0	3.5	166	1.7	2.1	2.5	2.8
135	2.0	2.6	3.1	3.7	4.4	151	1.5	2.0	2.5	3.0	3.4	167	1.6	2.0	2.4	2.8
136	1.9	2.5	3.1	3.6	4.3	152	1.4	2.0	2.5	2.9	3.4	168	1.6	2.0	2.4	2.8
137	1.9	2.5	3.0	3.6	4.2	153	1.4	2.0	2.4	2.9	3.3	169	1.6	2.0	2.4	2.8
138	1.8	2.4	3.0	3.5	4.2	154	1.4	2.0	2.4	2.8	3.3	170	1.6	2.0	2.4	2.7

Chart 5 Bicycle Test Rating Scale (mL/O$_2$/kg/min.)

Men					
Age	17–26	27–39	40–49	50–59	60–69
High-performance zone	50+	46+	42+	39+	35+
Good fitness zone	43–49	35–45	32–41	29–38	26–34
Marginal zone	35–42	30–34	27–31	25–28	22–25
Low zone	<35	<30	<27	<25	<22

Women					
Age	17–26	27–39	40–49	50–59	60–69
High-performance zone	46+	40+	38+	35+	32+
Good fitness zone	36–45	33–39	30–37	28–34	24–31
Marginal zone	30–35	28–32	24–29	21–27	18–23
Low zone	<30	<28	<24	<21	<18

The 12-Minute Run Test

- Locate an area where a specific distance is already marked, such as a school track or football field, or measure a specific distance using a bicycle or automobile odometer.
- Use a stopwatch or wristwatch to accurately time a 12-minute period.
- For best results, warm up prior to the test; then run at a steady pace for the entire 12 minutes (cool down after the test).
- Determine the distance you can run in 12 minutes in fractions of a mile. Depending upon your age, locate your score and rating in Chart 6.

Chart 6 Twelve-Minute Run Test Rating Chart

	Men (Age)							
	17–26		27–39		40–49		50+	
Classification—Men	Miles	Km	Miles	Km	Miles	Km	Miles	Km
High-performance zone	1.80+	2.90+	1.60+	2.60+	1.50+	2.40+	1.40+	2.25+
Good fitness zone	1.55–1.79	2.50–2.89	1.45–1.59	2.35–2.59	1.40–1.49	2.25–2.39	1.25–1.39	2.00–2.24
Marginal zone	1.35–1.54	2.20–2.49	1.30–1.44	2.10–2.34	1.25–1.39	2.00–2.24	1.10–1.24	1.75–1.99
Low zone	<1.35	<2.20	<1.30	<2.10	<1.25	<2.00	<1.1	<1.75

	Women (Age)							
	17–26		27–39		40–49		50+	
Classification—Women	Miles	Km	Miles	Km	Miles	Km	Miles	Km
High-performance zone	1.45+	2.35+	1.35+	2.20+	1.25+	2.00+	1.15+	1.85+
Good fitness zone	1.25–1.44	2.00–2.34	2.20–1.34	1.95–2.19	1.15–1.24	1.85–1.99	1.05–1.14	1.70–1.84
Marginal zone	1.15–1.24	1.85–1.99	1.05–1.19	1.70–1.94	1.00–1.14	1.60–1.84	.95–1.04	1.55–1.69
Low zone	<1.15	<1.85	<1.05	<1.70	<1.00	<1.60	<.95	<1.55

Source: Based on data from Cooper.

The 12-Minute Swim Test

- Locate a swimming area with premeasured distances, preferably 20 yards or longer.
- After a warm-up, swim as far as possible in 12 minutes using the stroke of your choice.

- For best results, have a partner keep track of your time and distance. A degree of swimming competence is a prerequisite for this test.
- Determine your score and rating using Chart 7.

Chart 7 Twelve-Minute Swim Rating Chart

	Men (Age)							
	17–26		27–39		40–49		50+	
Classification—Men	Yards	Meters	Yards	Meters	Yards	Meters	Yards	Meters
High-performance zone	700+	650+	650+	600+	600+	550+	550+	500+
Good fitness zone	600–699	550–649	550–649	500–599	500–599	475–549	450–549	425–499
Marginal zone	500–599	450–549	450–459	400–499	400–499	375–475	350–449	325–424
Low zone	Below 500	Below 450	Below 450	Below 400	Below 400	Below 375	Below 350	Below 325

	Women (Age)							
	17–26		27–39		40–49		50+	
Classification—Women	Yards	Meters	Yards	Meters	Yards	Meters	Yards	Meters
High-performance zone	600+	550+	550+	500+	500+	450+	450+	400+
Good fitness zone	500–599	450–549	450–549	400–499	400–499	375–449	350–449	325–400
Marginal zone	400–499	350–449	350–449	325–399	300–399	275–375	250–349	225–324
Low zone	Below 400	Below 350	Below 350	Below 325	Below 300	Below 275	Below 250	Below 225

Source: Based on data from Cooper.

Chart 8 Non-Exercise Fitness Assessment Rating Chart

Rating	Score
Needs Improvement	1–4
Marginal	5–9
Good Conditioning	10–13
Highly Conditioned	13+

Lab 7A Counting Target Heart Rate and Ratings of Perceived Exertion

Name	**Section**	**Date**

Purpose: To learn to count heart rate accurately and to use heart rate and/or ratings of perceived exertion (RPE) to establish the threshold of training and target zones

Procedure

1. Practice counting the number of pulses felt for a given period of time at both the carotid and radial locations. Use a clock or watch to count for 15, 30, and 60 seconds. To establish your heart rate in beats per minute, multiply your 15-second pulse by four, and your 30-second pulse by two.
2. Practice locating your carotid and radial pulses quickly. This is important when trying to count your pulse after exercise.
3. Run a quarter mile; then count your heart rate at the end of the run. Try to run at a rate you think will keep the rate of the heart above the threshold of training and in the target zone. Use 15-second pulse counts (choose either carotid or radial) and multiply by four to get heart rate in beats per minute (bpm). Record the bpm in the Results section.
4. Rate your perceived exertion (RPE) for the run (see RPE chart below). Record your results.
5. Repeat the run a second time. Try to run at a speed that gets you in the heart rate and RPE target zone. Record your heart rate and RPE results.

Results: Record your *resting* heart rates in the boxes below.

Carotid Pulse   **Heart Rate per Minute**   **Radial Pulse**   **Heart Rate per Minute**

	15 seconds × 4 =			15 seconds × 4 =	
	30 seconds × 2 =			30 seconds × 2 =	
	60 seconds × 1 =			60 seconds × 1 =	

Record your heart rate and rating of perceived exertion for run 1.

Pulse Count   **Heart Rate per Minute**

| | 15 seconds × 4 = | |

Rating of Perceived Exertion

Record your heart rate and rating of perceived exertion for run 2.

Pulse Count   **Heart Rate per Minute**

| | 15 seconds × 4 = | |

Rating of Perceived Exertion

Ratings of Perceived Exertion (RPE)	
Rating	**Description**
6	
7	Very, very light
8	
9	Very light
10	
11	Fairly light
12	
13	Somewhat hard
14	
15	Hard
16	
17	Very hard
18	
19	Very, very hard
20	

Source: Data from Borg, G.

Answer the following questions:

Which pulse-counting technique did you use after the runs?   Carotid ◯   Radial ◯

What is your heart rate target zone (to calculate, see pages 125 and 126) [   ] bpm

Was your heart rate for run 1 enough to get in the heart rate target zone?   Yes ◯   No ◯

Was your RPE for run 1 enough to get in the target zone (12–16)?   Yes ◯   No ◯

Was your heart rate for run 2 enough to get in the heart rate target zone?   Yes ◯   No ◯

Was your RPE for run 2 enough to get in the target zone (12–16)?   Yes ◯   No ◯

Conclusions and Implications: In several sentences, discuss your results, including which method you would use to count heart rate and why. Also discuss heart rate versus RPE (Rating of Perceived Exertion) for determining the target zone.

Lab Supplement:* You may want to keep track of your exercise heart rate over a week's time or longer to see if you are reaching the target zone in your workouts. Shade your target zone with a highlight pen and plot your exercise heart rate for each day of the week (see sample).

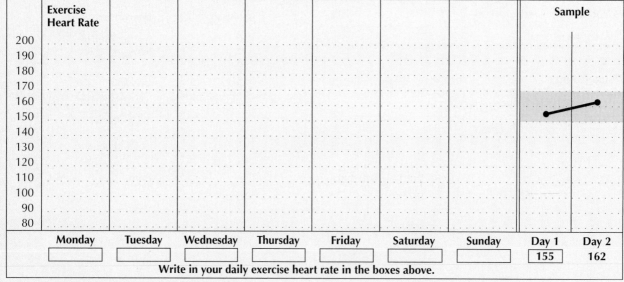

Write in your daily exercise heart rate in the boxes above.

*Thanks to Ginnie Atkins for suggesting this lab supplement.

Lab 7B Evaluating Cardiovascular Fitness

Name	Section	Date

Purpose: To acquaint you with several methods for evaluating cardiovascular fitness and to help you evaluate and rate your own cardiovascular fitness

Procedure

1. Perform one or more of the four cardiovascular fitness tests and determine your ratings using the information in the Lab Resource Materials.
2. Perform each of the four steps for the Non-Exercise Estimate of Cardiovascular Fitness using the information on the back of this page. Learning this technique will allow you to estimate your fitness when you are injured or for some other reason cannot do a performance test.

Results

1. Record the information from your cardiovascular fitness test(s) in the spaces provided.
2. After you have completed the four steps for the Non-Exercise Estimate of Cardiovascular Fitness, use Chart 8 in Lab Resource Materials (page 134) to determine your fitness rating.

Walking Test

Time ☐ minutes

Heart rate ☐ bpm

Rating ☐ (see Chart 1, page 131)

Bicycle Test

Workload ☐ kpm

Heart rate ☐ bpm

Weight ☐ pounds

Weight in kg* ☐

mL/O$_2$/kg ☐

Rating ☐ (see Chart 5, page 133)

Non-Exercise Test

Score ☐

Rating ☐ (see Chart 8, page 134)

*Weight in lb. ÷ 2.2.

Step Test

Heart rate ☐ bpm

Rating ☐ (see Chart 2, page 131)

12-Minute Run Test

Distance ☐ miles

Rating ☐ (see Chart 6, page 133)

12-Minute Swim Test

Distance ☐ yards

Rating ☐ (see Chart 7, page 134)

Non-Exercise Cardiovascular Fitness Rating

Record your scores and do the calculations to determine scores for A to E below.

- Look up your activity score on Chart 1 (below). Record score in box A. [_____] (A)

- Record your gender (female = 0/male = 1) _____ × 2.77 = [_____] (B)

- Determine your resting heart rate (Lab 7A), record here _____ × 0.03 = [_____] (C)

- Calculate your BMI (see Lab 13B), record here _____ × 0.17 = [_____] (D)

- Record your age in years. _____ × 0.10 = [_____] (E)

Use the following formula to calculate your score. Use Chart 8 on page 134 to get your rating.

| 18.07 | + | A | + | B | – | C | – | D | – | E | = | **Estimated Cardiovascular Fitness (METs)** |

18.07 + [____] + [____] – [____] – [____] – [____] = [_____]

Chart 1 Self-Reported Activity Score (for Step 1 Above)	

Activity Score	Choose the Score That Best Describes Your Physical Activity Level
0.00	I am inactive or do little activity other than usual daily activities.
0.32	I regularly (> 5 d/wk) participate in physical activities requiring low levels of exertion that result in slight increases in breathing and heart rate for at least **10 minutes** at a time.
1.06	I participate in aerobic exercises such as brisk walking, jogging, or running, cycling, swimming, or vigorous sports at a comfortable pace, or activities requiring similar levels of exertion for **20 to 60 minutes per week.**
1.76	I participate in aerobic exercises such as brisk walking, jogging, or running at a comfortable pace, or other activities requiring similar levels of exertion for **1 to 3 hours per week.**
3.03	I participate in aerobic exercises such as brisk walking, jogging, or running at a comfortable pace, or other activities requiring similar levels of exertion for **over 3 hours per week.**

Conclusions and Implications

1. In several sentences, explain why you selected the tests you selected. Discuss your current level of cardiovascular fitness and steps you will need to take to maintain or improve it. Comment on the effectiveness of the tests you selected.

2. In several sentences, explain your results from the non-exercise assessment by comparing the results with the other test(s). Did the self-report version classify you into the same fitness category? Try to explain any differences you noted.

Vigorous Aerobics, Sports, and Recreational Activities

LEARNING OBJECTIVES

After completing the study of this concept, you will be able to:

▶ Explain the difference between moderate and vigorous physical activity and describe the unique benefits of vigorous physical activity.

▶ Identify several different types of vigorous aerobic activities and describe the advantages of each as possible activities in a personal activity program.

▶ Identify several different types of vigorous sports activities, describe the advantages of sports activities in a personal activity program, and explain the importance of skill learning to sports performance.

▶ Identify several different types of vigorous recreational activities and explain how they differ from vigorous aerobic and sports activities.

▶ Plan and self-monitor a vigorous physical activity program, and evaluate the factors that will help you adhere to it.

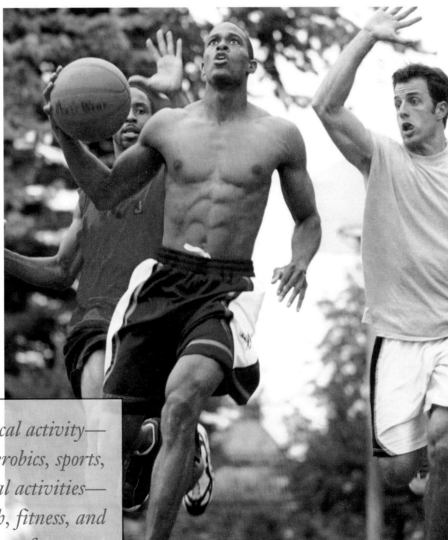

Vigorous physical activity—including vigorous aerobics, sports, and recreational activities—promotes health, fitness, and enhanced performance.

In Concept 6, you learned the many values of moderate physical activity. In this concept, you learn the value of vigorous physical activity as shown in steps 2 and 3 of the physical activity pyramid (see Figure 1). The threshold of training and target zones described in Concept 7 for building cardiovascular fitness help define the nature of vigorous physical activity. Except for those with low fitness or who are sedentary, activities intense enough to build cardiovascular fitness are considered to be vigorous in nature.

We look at three different types of vigorous physical activity: vigorous aerobics, sports, and recreational activities. In the past, vigorous physical activity was recommended for people who wanted to build cardiovascular fitness and for enhancing performance, but it was not included as a method of meeting the national physical activity guidelines. The new activity guidelines explicitly include vigorous physical activity. In other words, people can choose moderate activity or vigorous activity to meet the guidelines, depending on

the activities of preference. The ACSM and AHA also indicate that moderate and vigorous physical activities can be combined to meet the guidelines.

Physical Activity Pyramid: Steps 2 and 3

A variety of popular vigorous *aerobic* activities are included at step 2 of the pyramid. The word aerobics literally means "with oxygen." Aerobic activity is generally defined as activity that is rhythmical, uses the large muscles, and is performed in a continuous manner. Many activities meet these criteria, including walking, doing housework, and performing many other light to moderate physical activities.

Dr. Ken Cooper of the Cooper Institute in Dallas popularized the term aerobics in his book, *Aerobics*, published in 1968. His book featured **vigorous aerobic activities** such as those in step 2 of the physical activity pyramid (see Figure 1). The activities included in step 2 of the pyramid are at least 6 METs (six times more intense than resting) and significantly elevate the heart rate. Examples include jogging, aerobic dance, and cycling.

An advantage of these vigorous aerobic activities is that they provide a good cardiovascular workout in a short time and can often be done by oneself. A disadvantage (or barrier) for some people is that they are generally more vigorous and fast paced than other forms of activity. The more vigorous nature is the most likely explanation for the age-related patterns that exist for participation in vigorous aerobic activity. Young adults are far more likely to participate in vigorous aerobic activity than are older adults. Most statistics report three- to five-fold differences in participation rates for young adults and older adults (40 to 60). The declining interest in vigorous activity for older adults is a concern to public health officials only if older adults fail to substitute moderate physical activity when they discontinue more vigorous activity.

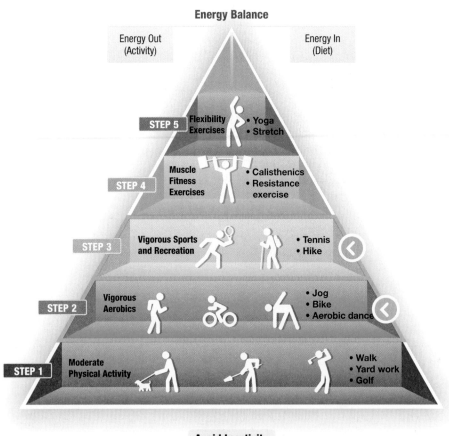

Figure 1 ▶ Vigorous aerobics, sports, and recreational activities are included at the second and third steps of the physical activity pyramid.

Source: C. B. Corbin

Vigorous sports and recreation at step 3 of the pyramid can provide the same benefits as vigorous aerobic activities. Vigorous sports are not always continuous in nature. These activities involve intermittent activity with bursts of activity and short periods of rest but typically are at an intensity that provides benefits similar to vigorous aerobic activities. Examples of vigorous sports include rowing, racquetball, soccer, and hockey. Swimming and cycling are also popular activities that can be considered sports. However, most people do these activities noncompetitively, so they are considered as vigorous aerobics in this book. Sports such as golf, bowling, and billiards/pool are aerobic but are light to moderate in intensity. For this reason, they are classified as moderate physical activities.

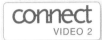

Activities such as hiking, boating, fishing, horseback riding, and other such outdoor activities are generally classified as recreation. Because many of these activities can be performed at intensities suitable for building cardiovascular fitness, some can be categorized as **vigorous recreational activities.** Hiking, skiing, kayaking, canoeing, hunting, and rock climbing are examples of recreation activities that may involve a considerable amount of activity. Recreation activities such as fishing and boating are typically done at lower intensities and can be considered as moderate activities.

Physical activities at steps 2 and 3 of the pyramid produce improvements in cardiovascular fitness and health in addition to those produced by moderate physical activities. Participation in moderate activity provides important health benefits, but vigorous aerobic activity results in additional health benefits, such as improved cardiovascular fitness and improved performance (see Table 1). The guidelines call for performing vigorous activity at least 3 days a week for 20 minutes at the appropriate target intensity. The ACSM/AHA guidelines indicate that "physical activity above the recommended minimum provides even greater health benefits" than meeting only minimum standards. The guidelines further indicate that "the point of maximum benefits for most health benefits has not yet been established . . . but exceeding the minimum recommendation further reduces the risk of inactivity-related chronic disease."

Moderate and vigorous physical activity can be combined to meet national guidelines. National guidelines specify the total amount of activity that should be performed rather than having separate recommendations for moderate and vigorous activity. This approach helps people incorporate both moderate and vigorous activity into their lifestyle. The guidelines are based on tracking

Table 1 ▶ Benefits of Vigorous Physical Activity*
• Vigorous activity meets national guidelines for reducing risk of chronic disease and early death.
• Vigorous activity provides disease risk reduction in addition to moderate activity alone (even when calorie expenditure is the same).
• Vigorous activity provides disease risk reduction in addition to moderate activity when done in addition to moderate physical activity.
• Vigorous activity improves cardiovascular fitness.
• Vigorous activity enhances ability to perform activities that require good cardiovascular fitness.

*Benefits depend on regular participation (at least 3 days a week) and appropriate intensity and duration (at least 20 minutes at target intensity).

the total "MET-minutes" of physical activity performed. Because vigorous activity is performed at higher intensities (higher MET values), it makes a larger contribution to total activity than moderate-intensity activity performed for the same time. To determine MET-minutes, you multiply the MET value of an activity by the number of minutes that you perform it. For example, if a person walked for 10 minutes at 4 mph (4 METs), the MET-minutes would be 40 (4 METs × 10 minutes). If the person also jogged for 20 minutes at 5 mph (8 METs), the MET-minutes for jogging would be 160 (8 METs × 20 minutes); the total MET-minutes for the day would be 200.

To meet the new physical activity guidelines, a person must accumulate a minimum of 500 MET-minutes per week. These are considered to be minimal levels and the physical activity guidelines encourage people to move toward the target of 1,000 MET-minutes per

Vigorous Aerobic Activities Aerobic activities of an intensity at least six times that of resting (6 METs), commonly defined as activities with enough intensity to produce improvements in cardiovascular fitness.

Vigorous Sports Sports are competitive activities that have an organized set of rules, along with winners and losers. Vigorous sports are those of similar intensity to vigorous aerobic activities.

Vigorous Recreational Activities Recreational activities are those that are done during leisure time that do not meet the characteristics of sports. Vigorous recreational activities are of similar intensity to vigorous aerobics.

week for additional benefits. Activity should be done at least 3 days a week when the combined method is used, even though the MET-minute standard could be met with large amounts of activity performed on 1 or 2 days. Bouts of activity must be at least 10 minutes in length to be counted toward the recommendation. MET values for a variety of moderate activities are included in Concept 6 (Table 5) on page 108. A complete list of the MET values for a variety of activities can be found at **http://prevention.sph.sc.edu/tools/compendium.htm.** In Lab 8C you will learn more about how to combine moderate and vigorous activity to meet national goals.

Not all activities at level 2 and 3 of the pyramid are equally safe. Sports medicine experts indicate that certain types of physical activities are more likely than others to result in injury. Walking and low-impact dance aerobics are among the least risky activities. Skating, an aerobic activity, is the most risky, followed by basketball and competitive sports. Among the most popular aerobic activities, running has the greatest risk, with cycling, high-impact dance aerobics, and step aerobics having moderate risk for injury. Swimming and water aerobics are among those least likely to cause injuries because they do not involve impact, falling, or collision. In general, activities that require high-volume training (aerobics and jogging), collision (football, basketball, and softball), falling (biking, skating, cheerleading, and gymnastics), the use of specialized equipment that can fail (biking), and repetitive movements that stress the joints (tennis and high-impact aerobics) increase risk for injury. These

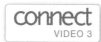

statistics reinforce the importance of using proper safety equipment, proper performance techniques, and proper training techniques.

Vigorous Aerobic Activities

A variety of vigorous aerobic activities are available for meeting individual needs and interests. Because there are so many choices, many beginning exercisers want to know which type of aerobic exercise is best. The best form of exercise is clearly whatever form you enjoy and will do regularly. Some people tend to be very consistent in performing their favorite form of activity, while others stay active by participating in a variety of activities. Seasonal differences are also common with physical activity participation. Many people choose to remain indoors during very hot or very cold weather and perform outdoor activities when temperatures are more moderate.

Vigorous aerobics can be done either continuously or intermittently. We generally think of vigorous aerobics as being continuous. Jogging, swimming, and cycling at a steady pace for long periods are classic examples. Experts have shown that aerobic exercise can be done intermittently as well as continuously. Both **continuous** and **intermittent aerobic activities** can build cardiovascular fitness. For example, studies have shown that three 10-minute exercise sessions in the target zone are as effective as one 30-minute exercise session. Still, experts recommend bouts of 20 to 60 minutes in length, with several 10- to 15-minute bouts being an acceptable alternative when longer sessions are not possible.

Vigorous aerobic activities are often rhythmical and typically involve the large muscle groups of the legs. The rhythmical nature of aerobic activity allows it to be performed continuously and in a controlled manner. The activation of a large muscle mass is important in providing an appropriate challenge to the cardiovascular system.

Descriptions of the most common individual forms of vigorous aerobic activity are provided below:

- *Fitness Walking: A safe and popular aerobic activity.* Walking is generally considered a moderate physical activity, but it is effective in promoting metabolic fitness and overall health. To achieve cardiovascular fitness, walking must be done intensely enough to elevate the heart rate to target zone levels.

- *Running (jogging): The prototypical aerobic activity.* Running is convenient and the intensity can be easily modified to suit individual needs. Some people view running as the only way they can truly challenge their

HELP   Health is available to Everyone for a Lifetime, and it's Personal

Former Olympic swimmer Diana Nyad has pushed the limits of endurance and perseverance. In her 60s, Nyad has embarked on some of the boldest and most challenging open water swims in history. Her main quest has been to swim 100+ miles from Cuba to Florida. If it weren't for the battles with sharks and jellyfish, she would likely be able to pull it off. The commitment and impressive performance of Nyad are certainly inspirational. Regular exercisers often become hooked and enjoy challenging the limits of endurance. Imagine the mental toughness it would take to train for and persevere through this extreme challenge.

What lessons can people take away from this example of commitment if they are struggling to maintain motivation for exercise?

cardiovascular system. However, many others may be limited in their ability to run due to previous injuries (e.g., knee problems) or gait problems.

- *Bicycling: An excellent vigorous aerobic activity requiring special equipment and time.* Cycling is a very popular activity and there are different types of bikes to fit the needs and interests of almost any rider. Road bikes are most common, but mountain bikes are also popular. Many people prefer a versatile bike suitable for different conditions and select a "city bike" or "hybrid bike" that is good for a variety of conditions. Cycling is more efficient than running and some other aerobic activities because of the mechanical efficiency of a bike (a pace of 13 mph might correspond to a running speed of 5 mph). 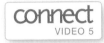 Speed is not a good indicator of exertion on a bike, so heart rate or a rating of perceived exertion (RPE) should be used. Biking may need to be performed for longer periods of time than jogging to get the same benefit.

- *Swimming: An outstanding whole body conditioning activity.* Most people know how to swim but a relatively small number have the skill and technique required to swim efficiently. Swimming provides a great cardiovascular workout but a person must be able to swim long enough to benefit. Even highly trained athletes can be exhausted after a few hundred yards if they do not have good skills. Because of the water environment and the non-weight-bearing status, the heart rate response to swimming is typically lower for the same intensity of exercise. The heart rate does not increase as rapidly in response to swimming, so target heart rates should be set about 5 to 10 beats lower than for other aerobic activities.

- *Cross-country skiing: A low-impact, whole body exercise that challenges the cardiovascular system.* Cross-country skiing is one of the more popular aerobic activities in colder climates and it can be done for transportation, recreation, or sport. There are two main techniques: classic, or diagonal stride, and skating. Each requires a different type of ski and technique. Classic skiing is more common since it can be done at various paces and in various settings and on tracked or untracked snow. Skate skiing is faster, but more technical as it requires a variety of sub-techniques for different terrain. Because skiing involves both the arms and legs in a coordinated movement, cross-country skiing is one of the most effective types of cardiovascular fitness exercises. The downside is that it requires some degree of skill to perform the movements correctly.

- *Inline skating: A popular, low-impact aerobic activity.* Inline skating, or "rollerblading," offers speed and freedom of movement, but the risk of injury is greater than most other activities. Special equipment is recommended,

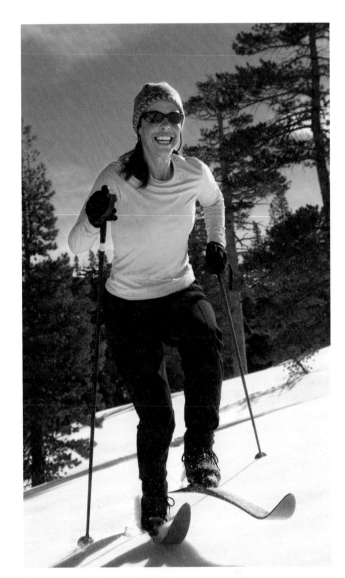

Vigorous physical activity builds cardiovascular fitness.

including a helmet, knee and elbow pads, wrist supporters, and hand protectors. Some degree of skill is necessary to perform skating safely and effectively, so it is wise to practice in a controlled environment before taking to the streets. Like cycling, rollerblading is mechanically very efficient. A person may need to work out longer to derive the same benefit from rollerblading.

Continuous Aerobic Activities Aerobic activities that are slow enough to be sustained for relatively long periods without frequent rest periods.

Intermittent Aerobic Activities Aerobic activities, relatively high in intensity, alternated with frequent rest periods.

Cardiovascular exercise machines provide an engaging indoor alternative to traditional aerobic exercises. The popularity of exercise machines has increased in recent years, due perhaps to increased access, ease of use, safety, and convenience. Treadmills are the most commonly used exercise machine, followed by stationary bikes and stair climbers. Elliptical trainers have increased in popularity, leading to reductions in the use of other equipment, such as rowing machines and ski machines. Most machines have modes that allow users to specify different types and intensities of exercise. Newer machines feature feedback systems, which provide continuous readouts of total exercise time, distance traveled, target and goal intensity, and estimates of calories burned. The estimates of calories expended may not be accurate unless it incorporates your body weight. These numbers should not be considered especially accurate.

A drawback of exercise machines is that interest and novelty may wear off over time. Many new features have been developed to enhance interest and ease of use. Some clubs have personalized key systems, which automatically track personal preferences and settings and record time spent on each machine. This information can then be downloaded onto computers for automatic logging. Newer machines have started to utilize gaming technology to further enhance the user experience. Interactive displays in these machines allow you to feel like you are exercising outdoors and you can compete against virtual or real opponents. Through wireless computer networks, it is now possible for users to save their data on websites and/or share their results through social media applications (see Technology Update*)*.

TECHNOLOGY UPDATE

Interactive Gaming in Exercise Equipment
Interactive games are popular on platforms such as Wii, Kinect, and PlayStation 3, but interactive *exergames* are making their way into fitness centers. The Expresso Interactive Gaming bikes are designed to combine a realistic indoor biking experience with gaming and associated social media applications. The user chooses a course and then navigates through the virtual terrain by turning the handlebars and shifting the gears. The display provides updates of your progress and completed workouts can be saved on the Internet or sent to an associated smartphone app. If you want competition, you can try to set the course record or share your workout and performance on Facebook to challenge your friends.

The technology may make the workout more engaging but is this enough to keep you motivated long-term?

Vigorous exercise in a group setting provides a social exercise experience. Although most vigorous aerobics can be done individually, many people prefer the social interactions and challenge of group exercise classes. Many fitness centers and community recreation centers offer group exercise classes.

An advantage of group exercise classes is that there is a social component, which helps to increase motivation and promote consistency. A disadvantage is that all participants are generally guided through the same exercise. A vigorous routine can cause unfit people to overextend themselves, while an easy routine may not be intense enough for experienced exercisers. A well-trained group exercise leader can help participants adjust the exercise to their own level and ability. Check the qualifications of the exercise leader to be sure that he or she is certified to lead group exercise. Descriptions of the most common individual forms of aerobic activity are provided below:

- *Dance aerobics: A choreographed series of movements done to music.* A variety of forms of dance aerobics accommodate different interests and abilities. Traditional dance aerobic classes are characterized as "high impact" aerobics because both feet leave the ground simultaneously for a good part of the routine. While this provides a good workout, it may not be ideal for everyone. "Low-impact" aerobics reduce the risk for injury or soreness. In this form, one foot stays on the floor at all times. Low-impact is an especially wise choice for beginners or older exercisers. Step aerobics, also known as bench stepping and step training, is another adaptation in which the performer steps up and down on a bench when performing various dance steps. In most cases, step aerobics is considered to be low impact, but it is higher in intensity than many forms of aerobics due to the stepping.

- *Rhythmic dance: A more fluid dance-oriented form of aerobics.* Rhythmic dance evolved naturally out of the aerobic dance movement and there are many examples of dance-based classes. Jazzercise is one of the more long-lasting and well-known forms. Jazzercise classes developed a unique style that paved the way for more hybridized group exercise classes, incorporating a variety of exercises and movements including yoga, Pilates, kickboxing, and resistance training. Classes in Hip Hop Aerobics were popular for a while but the new craze is Zumba® and other Latin-based dance classes. This type of dance aerobics incorporates Latin moves with a party or club-like atmosphere (see A Closer Look on page 146).

- *Martial arts: Popular, vigorous aerobic activities.* In addition to traditional martial arts, such as karate and tae kwon do, a number of other alternative forms have been developed, including kickboxing, aerobic boxing,

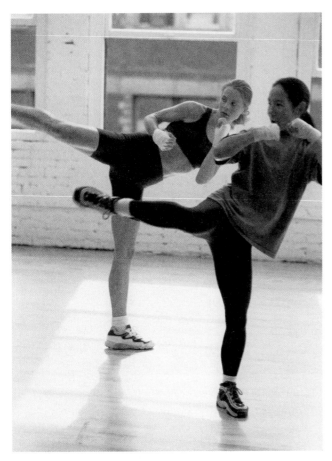

Kickboxing and martial arts are popular ways to stay in shape.

cardio karate, box fitness, and tae bo. These activities involve intermittent bouts of high-intensity movements and lower-intensity recovery. Because martial arts involve a lot of arm work, they can be effective in promoting good overall fitness. Some activities are more intense than others, so consider the alternatives to find the best fit for you.

- *Spinning classes: Attracting new people to the benefits of bicycling exercise.* A spinning class is a group cycling class performed on specialized indoor bike trainers. A group leader typically instructs participants on what pace, gear, and/or cadence to use. In most cases, the routines involve intermittent bursts of high-intensity intervals followed by spinning at lower resistance to recover. The instructor may help riders simulate hill climbing or extended sprints to simulate competitive biking conditions. Although the class relates most directly to cycling, the format has appealed to a broader set of fitness enthusiasts who just enjoy the challenge it provides.

- *Water-based classes: Taking advantage of the resistive properties of water.* Water walking and water exercise classes are popular alternatives to swimming. Although these

activities can be done alone, they are typically conducted in group settings to provide access to pools and certified instructors trained in water safety. Water aerobics are especially good for people with arthritis or other musculoskeletal problems and for people relatively high in body fat. The body's buoyancy in water assists the participant and reduces injury risk. The resistance of the water provides an overload that helps the activity promote health and cardiovascular benefits. Exercises done in shallow water tend to be low in impact, while deeper-water exercises are considered to be higher-impact activities. An advantage of water walking and water exercise is that neither requires the ability to swim. Many classes include activities designed to promote flexibility and muscle fitness development, as well as cardiovascular benefits. Many injured athletes use water activity as a way to rehabilitate from injuries without losing too much fitness.

- *Hybridized "combo" classes: Cross-training applications.* Most fitness centers now offer "combo" classes designed to combine aerobic movements with resistance exercise movements, plyometrics, or calisthenic exercises. An advantage of these **cross-training** classes is that a person can get a complete workout in a structured and engaging group environment. The classes typically use customized names to reflect the nature of the activities involved (e.g., CardioPump, PowerPump, Cardio Sculpt. BodyJam, BodyAttack, etc.). These hybridized classes have become increasingly popular and there are a number of certification programs and leadership models being developed to ensure consistency and quality of programming in fitness centers all over the world.

- *Individualized small group fitness centers: A personal focus.* Large commercial fitness centers remain popular but many small private fitness centers provide an appealing alternative for some people. An example is the Curves franchise that provides a structured group exercise format, allowing people to exercise in a more convenient, small group setting. A similar line of centers branded under the name Kosama offer shorter enrollments and personalized attention over a set period of time rather than an ongoing membership.

Cross Training A term used to describe the performance of a variety of activities to meet exercise goals (e.g., performing a variety of activities from different steps of the physical activity pyramid).

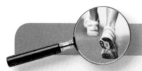

A CLOSER LOOK

The Zumba® Craze

Zumba® is an incredibly popular dance aerobics activity that started from a rather fortunate accident. According to the Zumba® website, the founder (a Colombian fitness leader named Beto Perez) forgot his traditional aerobics dance music and improvised using his own music and creativity. His experimentation led to a form of "dance fitness" that has captured the imagination of millions of people across the world. Zumba® classes are offered in over 110,000 locations in more than 125 countries.

What elements make Zumba® such a popular fitness program?

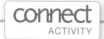
ACTIVITY

Vigorous Sport and Recreational Activities

Some sports are more vigorous than others. Some sports require many muscles from different parts of the body and are more vigorous than those that involve fewer muscles. Some are of high intensity and others are less intense. When done vigorously, tennis and basketball involve many different muscle groups and are high in intensity. Soccer involves many muscle groups and is high in intensity but does not emphasize the use of the arms. Golf, on the other hand, is less intense and relies more on skill and technique. The action in basketball, tennis, and soccer involves bursts of activity followed by rest but requires persistent, vigorous activity over a relatively long time. Golf requires little vigorous activity. Sports that have characteristics similar to those of basketball, tennis, and soccer have benefits like those of vigorous aerobic activities. Of course, any sport can be more or less active, depending on how you perform it. Shooting baskets or even playing half-court basketball is not as vigorous as playing a full-court game.

The most popular sports share characteristics that contribute to their popularity. The most popular sports are often considered to be lifetime sports because they can be done at any age. The characteristics that make these sports appropriate for lifelong participation probably contribute significantly to their popularity. Often, the popular sports are adapted so people without exceptional skill can play them. For example, bowling uses a handicap system to allow people with a wide range of abilities to compete. Slow-pitch softball is much more popular than fast-pitch softball or baseball because it allows people of all abilities to play successfully.

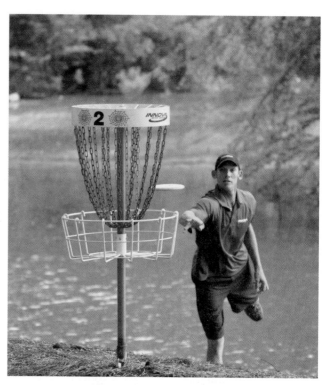

Disc golf is a popular recreational activity but it would not be classified as a vigorous activity.

One of the primary reasons sports participation is so popular is that sports provide a challenge. For the greatest enjoyment, the challenge of the activity should be balanced by the person's skill in the sport. If you choose to play against a person with lesser skill, you will not be challenged. On the other hand, if you lack skill or your opponent has considerably more skill, the activity will be frustrating. For optimal challenge and enjoyment, the skills of a given sport should be learned before competing. Likewise, choose an opponent who has a similar skill level.

Some recreational activities can also be classified as vigorous. Activities that you do in your free time for personal enjoyment or to "re-create" yourself are considered recreational activities. Recreational activities that exceed threshold intensity for cardiovascular fitness are considered vigorous. They are more vigorous than activities such as fishing, bowling, and golf, which are typically classified as lifestyle or moderate-level activities (step 1 in the pyramid). Examples of vigorous recreational activities include common snow activities (downhill skiing, snowboarding), water activities (surfing, wakeboarding, kayaking, canoeing), and mountain activities (hiking, mountain biking). These are simply examples as there are many other recreational activities. As with sports, recreational activities can be done at different intensities. If done for a sufficient length of time, vigorous recreational activities can provide the same benefits

In the News

Vigorous Exercise Boosts Metabolism for up to 14 Hours

The benefits of exercise persist even after the workout is over. A recent study reported that a single 45-minute bout of vigorous exercise helps you burn calories long after the exercise session is over. Study participants lived and exercised in an enclosed metabolic chamber in order to quantify this effect. The vigorous 45-minute bike workout burned approximately 330 calories, but participants expended an extra 190 calories (37 percent of the total energy expenditure) long after the workout was done (up to 14 hours). This extra boost to the metabolism can have important implications for energy balance and weight control.

How does this information influence your perception about the importance of vigorous exercise?

as vigorous sports or other vigorous activities. Note that vigorous activities such as cycling, jogging, and skiing, could be classified in the vigorous recreation as well as in the vigorous aerobics section. Sports can also be considered vigorous recreational activities, depending on how the individual views them. Many people view recreation as simply time to relax and be outdoors, and find the resulting improvements in fitness to be just an additional benefit. This is a healthy attitude since activities pursued purely for enjoyment are easier to maintain than activities pursued purely for fitness.

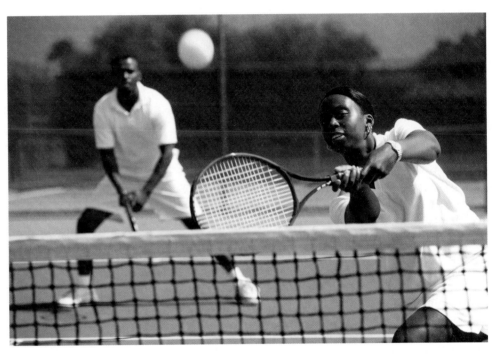

Learning new skills can be challenging but rewarding.

Becoming skillful will help you enjoy sports and recreation. Improving your skill can increase the probability that you will do sports for a lifetime. The following self-management guidelines can help you improve your sport performance:

- *When learning a new activity, concentrate on the general idea of the skill first; worry about details later.* For example, a diver who concentrates on pointing the toes and keeping the legs straight at the end of a flip may land flat on his or her back. To make it all the way over, the diver should concentrate on merely doing the flip. When the general idea is mastered, then concentrate on details.

- *The beginner should be careful not to emphasize too many details at one time.* After the general idea of the skill is acquired, the learner can begin to focus on the details, one or two at a time. Concentration on too many details at one time may result in **paralysis by analysis.** For example, a golfer who is told to keep the head down, the left arm straight, and the knees bent cannot possibly concentrate on all of these details at once. As a result, neither the details nor the general idea of the golf swing is performed properly.

Paralysis by Analysis An overanalysis of skill behavior. This occurs when more information is supplied than a performer can use or when concentration on too many details results in interference with performance.

- *Once the general idea of a skill is learned, a skill analysis of the performance may be helpful.* Be careful not to overanalyze; it may be helpful to have a knowledgeable person help you locate strengths and weaknesses. Movies and videotapes of skilled performances can be helpful to learners.

- *In the early stages of learning a lifetime sport or physical activity, it is not wise to engage in competition.* Beginners who compete are likely to concentrate on beating their opponent rather than on learning a skill properly. For example, in bowling, the beginner may abandon the newly learned hook ball in favor of the sure-thing straight ball. This may make the person more successful immediately, but is not likely to improve the person's bowling skills for the future.

- *To be performed well, sports skills must be overlearned.* Often, when you learn a new activity, you begin to play the game immediately. The best way to learn a skill is to overlearn it, or practice it until it becomes habit. Frequently, games do not allow you to overlearn skills. For example, during a tennis match is not a good time to learn how to serve because there may be only a few opportunities to do so. For the beginner, it is much more productive to hit many serves (overlearn) with a friend until the general idea of the serve is well learned. Further, the beginner *should not* sacrifice speed to concentrate on serving for accuracy. Accuracy will come with practice of a properly performed skill.

- *When unlearning an old (incorrect) skill and learning a new (correct) skill, a person's performance may get worse before it gets better.* For example, a golfer with a baseball swing may want to learn the correct golf swing. It is important for the learner to understand that the score may worsen during the relearning stage. As the new skill is overlearned, skill will improve, as will the golf score.

- *Mental practice may aid skill learning.* Mental practice (imagining the performance of a skill) may benefit performance, especially if the performer has had previous experience in the skill. Mental practice can be especially useful in sports when the performer cannot participate regularly because of weather, business, or lack of time.

- *For beginners, practicing in front of other people may be detrimental to learning a skill.* An audience may inhibit the beginner's learning of a new sports skill. This is especially true if the learner feels that his or her performance is being evaluated by someone in the audience.

- *There is no substitute for good instruction.* Getting good instruction, especially at the beginning level, will help you learn skills faster and better. Instruction will help you apply these rules and use practice more effectively.

Patterns and Trends in Physical Activity Participation

The popularity of different forms of physical activities changes over time. The Sporting Goods Manufacturers Association (SGMA) conducts regular surveys to monitor changes in consumer preferences related to physical activity. While the surveys are designed primarily for marketing purposes, they provide useful data to evaluate trends in physical activity and sports participation. The results suggest that consumers are motivated by aerobic fitness as 8 of the top 20 activities were aerobic in nature, including walking (1st), treadmill (3rd), running (4th), biking (7th), elliptical machines (14th), aerobics (16th), indoor cycling (19th), and home exercise (20th). Four resistance training activities—calisthenics (5th), machines (9th), dumbbells (10th), barbells (15th), and stretching (11th)—also made the top 20. The remaining activities include 3 popular outdoor activities—fishing (8th), hiking (12th), and camping (13th)—and four sports—bowling (2nd), billiards (6th), basketball (17th), and golf (18th). It may surprise you that only four sports made the top 20 list, but it is important to remember that this survey asked whether people had participated in the activity at least once in the past year.

Because the focus of this concept is on aerobic activities, the specific rates of participation in common aerobic activities are shown in Figure 2. The figures are scaled to reflect the percentage of the population in the various activities (participation was indicated by performing it at least once). Walking for fitness is by far the most popular aerobic activity with over 40 percent of the population indicating some participation. Activities with the largest growth trajectories were high-impact aerobics (41 percent), spinning/cycling (41 percent), cardio kickboxing (37 percent), step aerobics (32 percent), low-impact aerobics (21 percent), running/jogging (20 percent), and elliptical motion training (19 percent). The trend toward efficient (value-oriented) activities was attributed in part to the weak economy as consumers seemed to favor accessible, low-cost, and "efficient" sports and fitness options.

Participation in physical activity is different than "regular" participation in physical activity. The participation rates in Figure 2 show overall popularity but results vary when tracking "regular" participation. While over 40 percent of the population reported walking for fitness at least once, a smaller number can be considered regular walkers. Over 10 million women and 6 million men walk for exercise more than 100 days a year, but not all likely walk in bouts long enough to meet national activity guidelines. Similarly, over 25 million Americans report jogging/running for exercise,

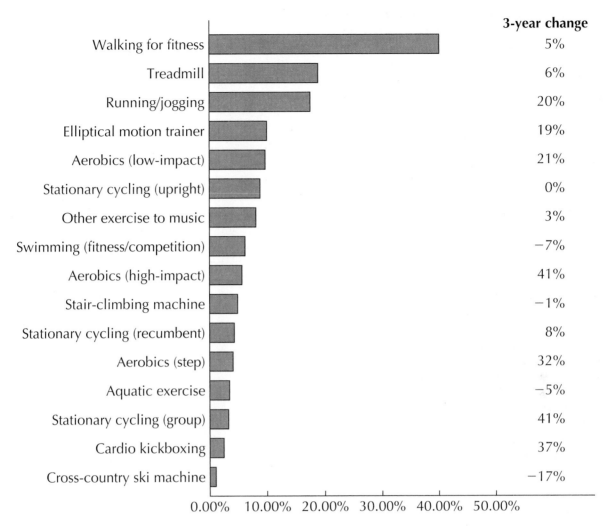

3-year change

Activity	3-year change
Walking for fitness	5%
Treadmill	6%
Running/jogging	20%
Elliptical motion trainer	19%
Aerobics (low-impact)	21%
Stationary cycling (upright)	0%
Other exercise to music	3%
Swimming (fitness/competition)	−7%
Aerobics (high-impact)	41%
Stair-climbing machine	−1%
Stationary cycling (recumbent)	8%
Aerobics (step)	32%
Aquatic exercise	−5%
Stationary cycling (group)	41%
Cardio kickboxing	37%
Cross-country ski machine	−17%

Figure 2 ▶ U.S. Adult Participation in Primary Aerobic Activities (%) and 3-year Change Rates.

Source: The Sporting Goods Manufacturers Association, 2010

but only 10 million report running regularly (about 6 million males and 4 million females). Distinctions in participation and regular participation are even more evident for other activities. An estimated 50 million Americans report riding their bike for recreation but approximately 15 million report frequent recreational bike riding, and a still smaller segment of the population (about 2 million) participates in regular fitness bicycling. Nearly 100 million people report participating in "recreational swimming"; however, the number of people that report regular fitness swimming is only about 2.5 million.

Rates of participation in vigorous activity change during college years. Activity levels tend to be high in young adults, but a recent study indicated that significant declines occur between high school and college. The study, conducted on a representative sample of college students from 119 schools, found declines in participation between high school and college. Approximately 48 percent of college students met the recommended criteria for vigorous physical activity, a sharp decline from the percentage of the same students who met the criteria when they were in high school. Participation in high school athletics was associated with higher participation rates in vigorous activity in college. A concern to public health researchers is the decline in participation with age in college and the lower levels of participation for college students over age 25.

A trend for declining activity was also evident in the SGMA reports referenced above. The report indicated that over 30 percent of Americans said they were not participating in a single physical activity and over 30 percent of these inactive respondents were under the age of 34. The percentage of inactive 18- to 24-year-olds has increased in the past 3 years of this report while the percentage of inactive people 65 and older actually decreased. Many students presume they will be able to establish regular exercise habits once they finish college, but results from these studies suggest that regular involvement in vigorous physical activity is important for establishing a lifelong pattern.

There is increased interest in group exercise programming. According to a separate SGMA report (*Tracking the Fitness Movement*), participation in group exercise has seen the greatest growth of any other fitness activity. The popularity of aerobics was fueled in large part by the explosion of interest in Zumba® and other cultural dancing activities. However, there has been an overall interest in classes that fuse traditional aerobic movements with other movement activities (e.g., pilates, yoga, dance) and resistance activities. As reported in Figure 2, there were dramatic increases in the popularity of high-impact aerobics, step aerobics, low-impact aerobics, cardio kickboxing, and spinning classes.

Consumer experts from SGMA attribute much of the changes to different generational interests (see Figure 3). Based on the report, Generation X (born 1965 to 1979) is more likely to do activities outside (biking, fishing, hiking, running, etc.); however, this generation is also more likely to belong to health clubs, exercise with machines, and use personal trainers. Generation Y (born 1980 to 1999) was characterized as having interest in strength (i.e., working out with weights, etc.) and social activities (i.e., fitness classes, etc.). The fun and engaging environment of hybridized group fitness classes seems to be meeting the needs of Gen X and Gen Y consumers.

Vigorous recreation and extreme sports are popular with some segments of the population. Vigorous recreation provides ways to experience new things, to socialize, and to obtain important health benefits. Some "extreme" sports have become popularized through the

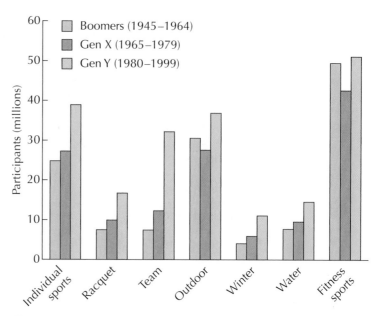

Figure 3 ▶ Patterns and Trends in Physical Activity Preference by Generation.

Source: The Sporting Goods Manufacturers Association

X Games and other media outlets, and there have been corresponding increases in participation for some of these activities. For example, activities such as surfing, snowboarding, and skateboarding had had some of the highest increases in reported participation. Other activities highlighted in the SGMA survey with strong growth over the past 10 to 15 years are mountain biking, kayaking, and wakeboarding. These may or may not be "extreme," but they are typically more appealing to individuals interested in outdoor adventures.

Self-Promoting Activities Activities that do not require a high level of skill to be successful.

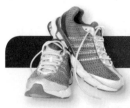

Strategies for Action

Use self-management skills to enjoy activities at the second and third steps of the pyramid.

- *Select self-promoting activities.* **Self-promoting activities** require relatively little skill and can be done in a way that avoids comparison with other people. They allow you to set your own standards of success and can be done

individually or in small groups that are suited to your personal needs. Examples include wheelchair distance events, jogging, resistance training, swimming, bicycling, and dance exercise.

- *Find activities that you enjoy.* There is no best form of activity! The key for long-term exercise adherence is to find exercises that you enjoy and that fit

connect
VIDEO 6

into your lifestyle. Sports are a common form of activity for younger people, but other aerobic and recreational activities have become more common among adults. This is partially because of changing interests, but also because of changing opportunities and lifestyles. In Lab 8A, you will evaluate predisposing, enabling, and reinforcing factors that may help you identify the types of activity best suited to you.

- *Self-monitor your activity to help you stick with your plan.* Self-monitoring encourages long-term activity adherence. A self-monitoring chart is provided in Lab 8B to help you plan and log the activities you perform in a 1-week period. This is a short-term record sheet, but you can copy it and make a log book for long-term self-monitoring.

- *Consider combining moderate and vigorous physical activity to meet activity guidelines.* Cross training is a term used to describe the performance of a variety of activities to meet exercise goals. For example, on different days you can do a moderate activity such as walking, a vigorous aerobic activity such as jogging on a treadmill, a vigorous sport such as tennis, and a vigorous recreational activity such as mountain biking. As discussed on page 141, these activities from different levels on the activity pyramid can be combined to meet activity guidelines. Lab 8C will help you learn and use this MET-minute system.

- *Improve your performance skills and technique.* Consider taking lessons and practice the skills you want to learn. Also, work to try to improve your technique. Better skills and better technique can make exercise more enjoyable (and safer).

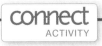

Web Resources

American Council on Exercise **www.acefitness.org**
Disabled Sports USA **www.dsusa.org**
National Academy of Podiatric Sports Medicine **www.aapsm.org**
National Athletic Trainers Association **www.nata.org**
National Center on Physical Activity and Disability
    www.ncpad.org and **www.ncpad.org/newsletter**
President's Council on Fitness, Sports, and Nutrition
    www.fitness.gov
Special Olympics International **www.specialolympics.org**
Sporting Goods Manufacturers Association **www.sgma.com**
US Product Safety Commission **www.cpsc.gov**
X Sports **www.expn.com**

Suggested Readings

ACSM. 2010. *ACSM's Guidelines for Exercise Testing and Prescription.* 8th ed. Philadelphia: Lippincott, Williams & Wilkins.

Berg, K. 2010. Sports and games: Fitness, function and fun. *ACSM's Health and Fitness Journal* 14(2):9–15.

Bishop, J. G. 2010. *Fitness Through Aerobics.* 8th ed. San Francisco: Benjamin Cummings.

Cooper, K. H. 1982. *The Aerobics Program for Total Well-Being.* New York: M. Evans.

Dong-Chul, D., and M. Torabi. 2007. Differences in vigorous and moderate physical activity by gender, race/ethnicity, age, education and income among U.S. adults. *American Journal of Health Education* 38(3):122–129.

Garber, C. E., et al. 2011. Quantity and quality of exercise for developing and maintaining cardiorespiratory, musculoskeletal, and neuromotor fitness in apparently healthy adults: Guidance for prescribing exercise. *Medicine and Science in Sports and Exercise* 43(7):1334–1359.

Kahn, L. K., et al. 2009. Recommended community strategies and measurements to prevent obesity in the United States. *Morbidity and Mortality Weekly Reports* 58(RR07):1–26.

Khan, K. M., et al. 2012. Sport and exercise as contributors to the health of nations. *Lancet.* 380(9836):59–64.

Knab, A. M., et al. 2011. 45-minute vigorous exercise bout increases metabolic rate for 14 hours. *Medicine and Science in Sports and Exercise* 43(9):1643–1648.

Kohl, H. W., and T. D. Murray. 2012. *Foundations of Physical Activity and Public Health.* Champaign, IL: Human Kinetics.

Magill, R. A. 2010. *Motor Learning and Control: Concepts and Applications.* 8th ed. New York: McGraw-Hill.

Montgomery, J., and M. Chambers. 2009. *Mastering Swimming.* Champaign, IL: Human Kinetics.

Pappas-Baun, M. 2008. *Fantastic Water Workouts.* Champaign, IL: Human Kinetics.

Schurman, C., and D. Schurman. 2009. *The Outdoor Athlete.* Champaign, IL: Human Kinetics.

Thompson, W. R. 2009. Worldwide survey reveals fitness trends for 2010. *ACSM's Health and Fitness Journal* 13(6):9–16.

Healthy People 2020

The objectives listed below are societal goals designed to help all Americans improve their health between now and the year 2020. They were selected because they relate to the content of this concept.

- Increase proportion of adults who meet guidelines for moderate to vigorous aerobic activity.

- Reduce proportion of adults who do no leisure-time activity.

- Increase access to employee-based exercise facilities and programs.

- Create social and physical environments that promote good health for all.

- Attain high-quality, longer lives free of preventable disease, injury, and premature death.

A national goal is to increase moderate to vigorous physical activity. Vigorous activity provides added benefits to those from moderate activity. For some people, vigorous activity is not as appealing as moderate activity. Why do some enjoy the challenge of pushing their body to this level while others do not?

Lab 8A The Physical Activity Adherence Questionnaire

Name	Section	Date

Purpose: To help you understand the factors that influence physical activity adherence and to see which factors you might change to improve your chances of achieving the action or maintenance level for physical activity

Procedures

1. The factors that predispose, enable, and reinforce adherence to physically active living are listed below. Read each statement. Place an X in the circle under the most appropriate response for you: very true, somewhat true, or not true.
2. When you have answered all of the items, determine a score by summing the four numbers for each type of factor. Then sum the three scores (predisposing, enabling, reinforcing) to get your total score.
3. Record your scores in the Results section and answer the questions in the Conclusions and Implications section.

	Very True	Somewhat True	Not True	
Predisposing Factors				
1. I am very knowledgeable about physical activity.	3	2	1	
2. I have a strong belief that physical activity is good for me.	3	2	1	
3. I enjoy doing regular exercise and physical activity.	3	2	1	
4. I am confident of my abilities in sports, exercise, and other physical activities.	3	2	1	
			Predisposing Score =	
Enabling Factors				
5. I possess good sports skills.	3	2	1	
6. I know how to plan my own physical activity program.	3	2	1	
7. I have a place to do physical activity near my home or work.	3	2	1	
8. I have the equipment I need to do physical activities I enjoy.	3	2	1	
			Enabling Score =	
Reinforcing Factors				
9. I have the support of my family for doing my regular physical activity.	3	2	1	
10. I have many friends who enjoy the same kinds of physical activities that I do.	3	2	1	
11. I have the support of my boss and my colleagues for participation in activity.	3	2	1	
12. I have a doctor and/or an employer who encourages me to exercise.	3	2	1	
			Reinforcing Score =	
			Total Score (Sum 3 Scores) =	

153

Results: Record your scores in the "Score" column. Use your score and the Physical Activity Adherence Rating Chart to determine your ratings. Record your ratings in the "Rating" column below.

Physical Activity Adherence Ratings

Adherence Category	Score	Rating
Predisposing		
Enabling		
Reinforcing		
Total		

Physical Activity Adherence Ratings Chart

Classification	Predisposing Score	Enabling Score	Reinforcing Score	Total Score
Adherence likely	11–12	11–12	11–12	33–36
Adherence possible	9–10	9–10	9–10	25–32
Adherence unlikely	<9	<9	<9	<25

Conclusions and Implications: In several sentences, discuss your ratings from this questionnaire. Also discuss the predisposing, enabling, and reinforcing factors you may need to alter in order to increase your prospects for lifetime activity.

In several sentences, discuss what type of activity you find most enjoyable (vigorous aerobics, vigorous recreation, or vigorous sports). Comment on *why* you enjoy the activities that you have selected.

Lab 8B Planning and Logging Participation in Vigorous Physical Activity

Name	Section	Date

Purpose: To set 1-week vigorous physical activity goals, to prepare a plan, and to self-monitor progress in your 1-week vigorous aerobics, vigorous sports, and recreation plan

Procedures

1. Consider your current stage of change for vigorous activity using the questions provided below. Read the five stages of change questions below and place a check by the stage that best represents your current vigorous physical activity level.
2. Determine vigorous activity (active aerobics, active sports, or active recreation) goals for each day of a 1-week period. In the columns (Chart 1) under the heading "Vigorous Activity Goals," record the total minutes per day that you expect to perform. Record the specific date for each day of the week in the "Date" column and the activity or activities that you expect to perform in the "Activity" column.
3. Only bouts of 10 minutes or longer should be considered when selecting your daily minutes goals. The daily goals should be at least 20 minutes a day in the target zone for vigorous activity for at least 3 days of the week.
4. Use Chart 2 to keep track of the number of minutes of activity that you perform on each day of the 7-day period. Record the number of minutes for each bout of activity of at least 10 minutes in length performed during each day in Chart 2. Determine a total number of minutes for the day and record this total in the last column of Chart 2 and in the "minutes performed" column of Chart 1.
5. After completing Charts 1 and 2, answer the questions and complete the Conclusions and Implications section (use full sentences for your answers).

Determine your stage for vigorous physical activity. Check only the stage that represents your current vigorous activity level.

☐ Precontemplation. I do not meet vigorous activity guidelines and have not been thinking about starting.

☐ Contemplation. I do not do vigorous activity guidelines but have been thinking about starting.

☐ Preparation. I am planning to start doing regular vigorous activity to meet guidelines.

☐ Action. I do vigorous activity, but I am not as regular as I should be.

☐ Maintenance. I regularly meet national goals for vigorous activity.

Results

Chart 1 Vigorous Physical Activity Goals and Summary Performance Log

Select a goal for each day in a 1-week plan. Keep a log of the activities performed to determine if your goals are met (see Chart 2), and record total minutes performed in the chart below.

	Date	Vigorous Activity Goals		Summary Performance Log Total Minutes Peformed/Day
		Minutes/Day	Activity	
Day 1				
Day 2				
Day 3				
Day 4				
Day 5				
Day 6				
Day 7				

Chart 2 Vigorous Physical Activity Log (Daily Minutes Performed)

Record the number of minutes for each bout of vigorous activities performed each day. Add the minutes in each column for the day and record a daily total (total minutes of vigorous activity per day) in the "Daily Total" column. Record your daily totals in the last column of Chart 1.

	Date	Vigorous Activity Bouts of 10 Minutes or More					Daily Total
		Bout 1	Bout 2	Bout 3	Bout 4	Bout 5	
Day 1							
Day 2							
Day 3							
Day 4							
Day 5							
Day 6							
Day 7							

Did you meet your vigorous activity goals for at least 3 days of the week? (Yes) (No)

Do you think that you can consistently meet your vigorous activity goals? (Yes) (No)

What activities did you perform most often when doing vigorous activity? List the most common activities that you performed in the spaces below.

Vigorous Aerobics   Vigorous Sports   Vigorous Recreation

_____   _____   _____

_____   _____   _____

_____   _____   _____

Conclusions and Interpretations

Are the activities that you listed above ones that you think you will perform regularly in the future? (Yes) (No)

Did setting goals and logging activity make you more aware of your daily vigorous physical activity patterns? Explain why or why not.

Lab 8C Combining Moderate and Vigorous Physical Activity

Name	**Section**	**Date**

Purpose: To learn about MET-minutes and how to combine moderate and vigorous physical activity to meet physical activity guidelines and goals

Procedures

1. National guidelines recommend at least 150 minutes of moderate or 75 minutes of vigorous physical activity as the minimum amount per week. The guidelines indicate that you can combine the two forms to meet your activity goal. When combining moderate and vigorous activities, MET-minutes are used. The minimum goal for beginners is 500 MET-minutes and 1,000 MET-minutes is the minimum goal for a reasonably fit and active person. Consider this information as you complete the rest of this lab.
2. In Chart 1 below list several moderate activities and several vigorous activities for each day of one week. Next to the activities indicate the number of minutes you plan to perform each activity. Be sure to choose both moderate and vigorous activities.
3. Use the information in Chart 2 to determine a MET value for each activity or use the compendium of activities website to determine values for those not listed in Chart 2. Record the MET value in the space provided for each activity.
4. Multiply the MET values for each activity by the number of minutes you plan to perform each activity to determine MET-minutes for each activity.
5. Total the MET-minute columns for both moderate and vigorous activities to be performed during the week.
6. Answer the questions in the Conclusions and Implications Section.

Results

Chart 1 Moderate and vigorous activity plan for one week

Day	Date	Moderate Activity				Vigorous Activity			
		Activity	Min.	METs	MET-min.	Activity	Min.	METS	MET-min.
1									
2									
3									
4									
5									
6									
7									
Totals							+		=

Total MET-minutes for the Week

Did you meet the 500 MET-minute recommendation for beginners? (Yes) (No)

Did you meet the 1,000 MET-minute recommendation for more active people? (Yes) (No)

Which is your weekly activity plan most likely to include?

☐ Moderate activity only

☐ Vigorous activity only

☐ Both moderate and vigorous activity

Chart 2 MET Values for Selected Moderate and Vigorous Physical Activities

Moderate Activities	METs		Vigorous Activities	METs
Vacuuming/Mopping	3.0		Shoveling Snow	6.0
Walking (3 mph)	3.0		Walking (4.5 mph)	6.3
Bowling	3.0		Aerobic Dance	6.5
Child Care	3.5		Bricklaying	7.0
Golf (riding)	3.5		Cross-Country Skiing (leisure)	7.0
Biking (10 mph flat)	4.0		Soccer (leisure)	7.0
Fishing (moving, not stationary)	4.0		Basketball (game)	8.0
Raking Leaves	4.0		Biking (12–17 mph)	8.0
Table Tennis	4.0		Hiking Terrain (pack)	8.0
Volleyball (non-comp.)	4.0		Jogging (5 mph)	8.0
Waitress	4.0		Tennis (singles)	8.0
Ballroom (social)	4.5		Volleyball (games)	8.0
Basketball (shooting)	4.5		Step Aerobics	8.5
Mowing Lawn (power)	4.5		Digging Ditches	8.5
Painting	4.5		Cross-Country Skiing (fast-5–7 mph)	9.0
Tennis Doubles	5.0		Swimming Laps (varies with strokes)	9.0
Walking (4 mph)	5.0		Jogging (6 mph)	10.0
Construction	5.5		Racquetball (games)	10.0
Farming	5.5		Soccer (competitive)	10.0
Golf (walking)	5.5		Running (11.5 mph)	11.5
Softball (games)	5.5		Handball (games)	12.0
Swimming (leisure)	5.5			

MET values based on the Compendium of Physical Activities (available at **http://prevention.sph.sc.edu/tools/docs/documents_compendium.pdf).**

Conclusions and Implications: In the space provided below discuss the MET-minute method of combining activities to meet goals. Do you think that this method will be useful to you? Explain why or why not using full sentences.

Muscle Fitness and Resistance Exercise

LEARNING OBJECTIVES

After completing the study of this concept, you will be able to:

▶ Identify and explain the factors that influence strength and muscular endurance.

▶ List the health benefits of fitness and resistance exercise.

▶ Describe the types of progressive resistance exercise (PRE) and their advantages and disadvantages, including some basic exercises for each type of PRE.

▶ Describe different types of PRE equipment and the advantages and disadvantages of each.

▶ Determine the amount of exercise necessary to improve muscle fitness and explain the FIT formulas for the different types of PRE.

▶ Describe how to design PRE programs for optimal effectiveness.

▶ Evaluate facts and fallacies about PRE and the risks of performance-enhancing drugs, supplements, and steroids.

▶ Describe several self-assessments for muscle fitness, understand the self-assessments that help you identify personal needs, and plan (and self-monitor) a personal PRE program.

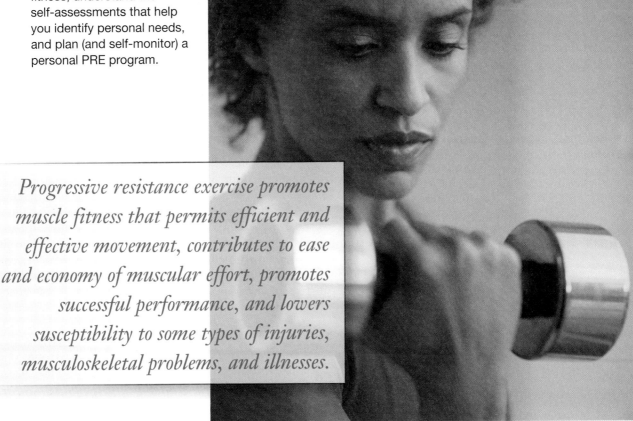

Progressive resistance exercise promotes muscle fitness that permits efficient and effective movement, contributes to ease and economy of muscular effort, promotes successful performance, and lowers susceptibility to some types of injuries, musculoskeletal problems, and illnesses.

There are two components of muscle fitness: strength and muscular endurance. Strength is the amount of force you can produce with a single maximal effort of a muscle group. Muscular endurance is the capacity of the skeletal muscles or group of muscles to continue contracting over a long period of time. You need both strength and muscular endurance to increase work capacity, to decrease chance of injury, to prevent poor posture and back pain, to improve athletic performance, and to prepare for emergencies.

Muscle power (strength × speed) is typically referred to as a skill-related component of fitness, but there is increasing evidence that power is health-related (see page 163). Because power is dependent on strength, it can be enhanced through resistance training. **Progressive resistance exercise (PRE)** is the type of physical activity done with the intent of improving muscle fitness. *Weight training* and *progressive resistance training (PRT)* are often used as synonyms for *PRE*, but they should not be confused with the various competitive events related to resistance exercise. Weight lifting is a competitive sport that involves two lifts: the snatch and the clean and jerk. Powerlifting, also a competitive sport, includes three lifts: the bench press, the squat, and the dead lift. Bodybuilding is a competition in which participants are judged on the size and **definition** of their muscles. Participants in these competitive events rely on highly specialized forms of PRE to optimize their training. Individuals interested in general muscular fitness also rely on PRE but do not need to follow the same routines or regimens to achieve good results. This concept covers the scientific basis of muscular fitness and provides guidelines and principles that can be used to establish an appropriate PRE program.

connect
VIDEO 1

Factors Influencing Strength and Muscular Endurance

There are three types of muscle tissue. The three types of muscle tissue—smooth, cardiac, and skeletal—have different structures and functions. Smooth muscle

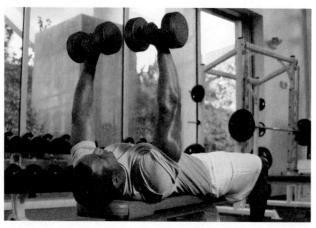

Progressive resistance exercises are used in programs designed to build muscle fitness.

tissue consists of long, spindle-shaped fibers, with each fiber containing only one nucleus. The fibers are involuntary and are located in the walls of the esophagus, stomach, and intestines, where they move food and waste products through the digestive tract. Cardiac muscle tissue is also involuntary and, as its name implies, is found only in the heart. These fibers contract in response to demands on the cardiovascular system. The heart muscle contracts at a slow, steady rate at rest but contracts more frequently and forcefully during physical activity. Skeletal muscle tissues consist of long, cylindrical, multinucleated fibers. They provide the force needed to move the skeletal system and can be controlled voluntarily.

Leverage is an important mechanical principle that influences strength. The body uses a system of levers to produce movement. Muscles are connected to bones via tendons, and some muscles (referred to as "primary movers") cross over a particular joint to produce movement. The movement occurs because when a muscle contracts it physically shortens and pulls the two bones connected by the joint together. Figure 1 shows the two heads of the biceps muscle inserting on the forearm. When the muscle contracts, the forearm is pulled up toward the upper arm (elbow flexion). A person with long arms and legs has a mechanical advantage in most movements, since the force that is exerted can act over a longer distance. Although it is not possible to change the length of your limbs, it is possible to learn to use your muscles more effectively. The ability of elite golfers, to hit a golf ball 350 yards, for example, is due primarily to the ability to generate torque and power rather than due to strength.

Skeletal muscle tissue consists of different types of fibers that respond and adapt differently to training. Three distinct types of muscle fibers are slow-twitch (Type I), fast-twitch (Type IIb), and intermediate (Type IIa). The slow-twitch fibers are generally red in color and are well suited to produce energy with aerobic metabolism. Slow-twitch fibers generate less tension but are more resistant to fatigue. Endurance training leads to adaptations in the slow-twitch fibers that allow them to produce energy more efficiently and to better resist fatigue. Fast-twitch fibers are generally white in color and are well suited to produce energy with anaerobic processes. They generate greater tension than slow-twitch fibers, but they fatigue more quickly. These fibers are particularly well suited to fast, high-force activities, such as explosive weight-lifting movements, sprinting, and jumping. Resistance exercise enhances strength primarily by increasing the size (muscle **hypertrophy**) of fast-twitch fibers, but cellular adaptations also take place to enhance various metabolic properties. Intermediate fibers have biochemical and physiological properties that are between those of the slow-twitch and fast-twitch fibers. A distinct property of these intermediate fibers is

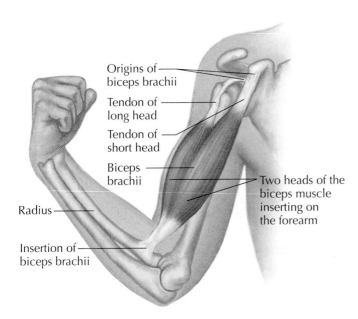

Origins of
biceps brachii

Tendon of
long head

Tendon of
short head

Biceps
brachii

Two heads of the
biceps muscle
inserting on
the forearm

Radius

Insertion of
biceps brachii

Figure 1 ▶ Muscle action on body levers.

that they are highly adaptable, depending on the type of training that is performed.

An example of fast-twitch muscle fiber in animals is the white meat in the flying muscles of a chicken. The chicken is heavy and must exert a powerful force to fly a few feet up to a perch. A wild duck that flies for hundreds of miles has dark meat (slow-twitch fibers) in the flying muscles for better endurance.

People who want large muscles will use PRE designed to build strength (fast-twitch fibers). People who want to participate in activities for a long period of time without fatigue will want to use PRE programs designed to build muscular endurance (slow-twitch fibers).

Though strength and muscular endurance are developed in different ways, they are part of the same continuum. Absolute strength is the maximal force that can be exerted at one time, while **absolute endurance** reflects the ability to sustain a submaximal force over an extended period of time. Most activities rely on various combinations of strength and endurance; thus it is important to have sufficient amounts of strength and endurance. Studies show that a person who is strength-trained will fatigue as much as four times faster than a person who is endurance-trained. However, there is a modest correlation between strength and endurance. A person who trains for strength will develop some endurance, and a person who trains for endurance will develop some strength.

Genetics, gender, and age affect muscle fitness performance. Each person inherits a certain percentage of fast-twitch and slow-twitch muscle fibers. This allocation influences the potential a person has for muscle

fitness activities. Individuals with a larger percentage of fast-twitch fibers will generally increase muscle size and strength more readily than individuals endowed with a larger percentage of slow-twitch fibers. People with a larger percentage of slow-twitch fibers have greater potential for muscular endurance performance. Regardless of genetics, all people can improve their strength and muscular endurance with proper training.

Women have smaller amounts of the anabolic hormone testosterone and, therefore, have less muscle mass than men. Because of this, women typically have 60 to 85 percent of the absolute strength of men. When expressed relative to lean body weight, women have **relative strength** similar to that of men. For example, a 150-pound female who lifts 150 pounds has relative strength equivalent to that of a 250-pound male who lifts 250 pounds, even though she has less absolute strength. Absolute muscular endurance is also greater for males, but the difference again is negated if **relative muscular endurance** is considered. Relative strength and endurance are better indicators of muscle fitness, since they take into account differences in size and muscle mass, but, for some activities, absolute strength and endurance are more important.

Maximum strength is usually reached in the 20s and typically declines with age. Muscle loss is estimated to be approximately 3 percent per decade, accounting for decreases in strength. Because of muscle loss with age, muscular endurance also typically declines as people grow older, but the decrease is less dramatic for

Progressive Resistance Exercise (PRE) The type of physical activity done with the intent of improving muscle fitness.

Definition The detailed external appearance of a muscle.

Hypertrophy Increase in the size of muscles as a result of strength training; increase in bulk.

Absolute Strength The maximum amount of force one can exert—e.g., the maximum number of pounds or kilograms that can be lifted on one attempt.

Absolute Endurance Muscular endurance measured by the maximum number of repetitions one can perform against a given resistance—e.g., the number of times you can bench press 50 pounds.

Relative Strength Amount of force that one can exert in relation to one's body weight or per unit of muscle cross section.

Relative Muscular Endurance Endurance measured by the maximum number of repetitions one can perform using a given percentage of absolute strength—e.g., the number of times you can lift 50 percent of your absolute strength.

muscular endurance than for strength. As people grow older, regardless of gender, PRE helps prevent muscle loss and, as would be expected, strength and muscular endurance are better among people who train than people who do not. This suggests that PRE is one antidote to premature aging.

Muscular endurance is related to cardiovascular endurance, but it is not the same thing. Cardiovascular endurance depends on the efficiency of the heart muscle, circulatory system, and respiratory system. It is developed with activities that stress these systems, such as running, cycling, and swimming. Muscular endurance depends on the efficiency of the local skeletal muscles and the nerves that control them. Most forms of cardiovascular exercise, such as running, require both cardiovascular and muscular endurance. For example, if your legs lack the muscular endurance to continue contracting for a sustained period of time, it will be difficult to perform well in running and other aerobic activities.

Health Benefits of Muscle Fitness and Resistance Exercise

Good muscle fitness helps prevent chronic lifestyle diseases and early death. Recent physical activity recommendations have placed considerable emphasis on muscle fitness exercises. Both the ACSM/AHA and DHHS guidelines indicate that muscle fitness exercises aid in chronic disease prevention. A separate document prepared by the American Heart Association Council on Clinical Cardiology and Council on Nutrition, Physical Activity and Metabolism notes that resistance training has benefits for younger adults, older adults, and even those with a previous history of heart disease (with proper medical supervision). Research has documented the benefits of resistance training in lowering risk for heart disease, high blood pressure, diabetes, rehabilitation from some forms of cancer, and reducing risk of metabolic syndrome. A very recent study 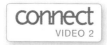 showed that women with breast cancer experienced fewer symptoms after performing resistance training. In addition, resistance exercise can reduce risk for other conditions described in the sections that follow.

Good muscle fitness is associated with reduced risk for injury. People with good muscle fitness are less likely to suffer joint injuries (e.g., neck, knee, ankle) than those with poor muscle fitness. Weak muscles are more likely to be involuntarily overstretched than are strong muscles.

Muscle balance is important in reducing the risk for injury. Resistance training should build both **agonist**

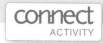
and **antagonist muscles.** For example, if you do resistance exercise to build the quadriceps muscles (front of the thigh), you should also exercise the hamstring muscles (back of the thigh). In this instance, the quadriceps are the agonist (muscle being used), and the hamstrings are the antagonist. If the quadriceps become too strong relative to the antagonist hamstring muscles, the risk for injury increases (see Figure 2).

Good muscle fitness is associated with good posture and reduced risk for back problems. When muscles in specific body regions are weak or overdeveloped, poor posture can result. Lack of fitness of the abdominal and low back muscles is particularly related to poor posture and potential back problems. Excessively strong hip flexor muscles can lead to swayback. Poor balance in muscular development can also result in postural problems. For example, the muscles on the sides of the body must be balanced to maintain an erect posture.

Good muscle fitness contributes to weight control. Regular PRE results in muscle mass increases. Muscle or lean body mass takes up less space than fat, contributing to attractive appearance. Further, muscle burns calories at rest, so extra muscle built through PRE can contribute to increased resting and basal metabolism. For each pound of muscle gained, a person can burn approximately 35 to 50 calories more per day. A typical strength training program performed at least three times a week can lead to 2 additional pounds of muscle after 8 weeks, so this can amount to an expenditure of an additional 100 calories a day, or 700 a week. Conversely, muscle mass tends to decrease with age, and this can slow metabolism by a similar amount and contribute to gradual increases in body fatness. PRE can help people retain muscle mass as they grow older.

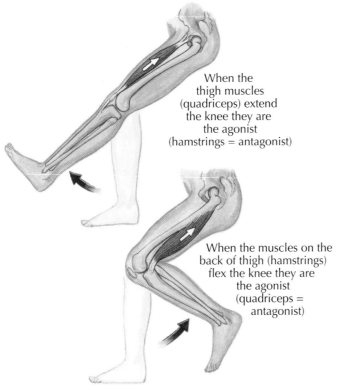

When the thigh muscles (quadriceps) extend the knee they are the agonist (hamstrings = antagonist)

When the muscles on the back of thigh (hamstrings) flex the knee they are the agonist (quadriceps = antagonist)

Figure 2 ▶ Agonist and antagonist muscles.

Good muscle fitness is associated with wellness and quality of life. A person with muscle fitness is able to perform for long periods without undue fatigue. As a result, the person has energy to perform daily work efficiently and effectively and has reserve energy to enjoy leisure time. Among older people, maintenance of strength is associated with increased balance, less risk for falling, and greater ability to perform the tasks of daily living independently. Muscle fitness also contributes to looking one's best and improved athletic performance. The ACSM indicates that one of the major goals of a resistance training program should be to make activities of daily living less stressful physiologically.

Resistance exercise is associated with reduced risk for osteoporosis. Resistance exercises provide a positive stress on the bones. Together with good diet, including adequate calcium intake, this stress on the bones reduces the risk for osteoporosis. Evidence suggests that young people who do PRE develop a high bone density. As we grow older, bone mass decreases, so people who have a high bone density when they are young have a "bank account" from which to draw as they grow older. These people have bones that are less likely to fracture or be injured. Injuries to the bones, particularly the hip and back, are common among older adults. Regular PRE can reduce the risk for these conditions. Postmenopausal women are especially at risk for osteoporosis (see Concept 4).

Core strength is an important health parameter. Core strength refers to strength of the abdominal, paraspinal (back), and gluteal muscles. Core strength has been emphasized by athletes to reduce injuries and improve sports performance. However, it is now viewed as being important for good health for everyone. Core strength contributes most directly to health by improving posture and reducing risk of back pain and injuries. Core strength is developed using very specific exercises and movements that isolate the core musculature.

Power is emerging as a health-related fitness component. Power has been typically classified as a skill-related component of physical fitness. However, evidence is accumulating that power is important for health, especially in youth and at older ages. A recent review indicated that activities such as jumping are especially important to building bone mass in children and teens. The standing long jump, a common test of power, is included in a European Youth Fitness Test because it is related to bone mass and muscle strength. Because of this, the American College of Sports Medicine now lists power as a component of health-related fitness. Further, it indicates that muscle fitness can "slow or even reverse" bone loss among adults. The ACSM notes that muscular power is more associated with risk of falling and bone fractures among older adults than muscular strength. (See Table 3 on page 169.)

Types of Progressive Resistance Exercise

There are different types of PRE, and each has its advantages and disadvantages. The main types of PRE are isotonic, isometric, and isokinetic. These terms refer to the way in which a load or stimulus is provided to the muscles. The advantages of each type are summarized in Table 1.

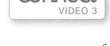

- **Isotonic** exercises are the most common type of PRE. They include calisthenics resistance machine exercises, free weight exercises, and exercises using

Agonist Muscles Muscle or muscle group that contracts to cause movement during an isotonic exercise.

Antagonist Muscles Muscle or muscle group on the opposite side of the limb from the agonist muscles (e.g., biceps are the antagonist when the triceps contract as an agonist to extend the arm).

Isotonic Type of muscle contraction in which the muscle changes length, either shortening (concentrically) or lengthening (eccentrically).

Table 1 ▶ Advantages and Disadvantages of Isotonic, Isometric, and Isokinetic Exercises

	Advantages	Disadvantages
Isotonic	• Can effectively mimic movements used in sport skills • Enhance dynamic coordination • Promote gains in strength	• Do not challenge muscles through the full range of motion • Require equipment or machines • May lead to soreness
Isometric	• Can be done anywhere • Require only low-cost/little equipment • Can rehabilitate an immobilized joint	• Build strength at only one position • Cause less muscle hypertrophy • Are a poor link or transfer to sport skills
Isokinetic	• Build strength through a full range of motion • Are beneficial for rehabilitation and evaluation • Are safe and less likely to promote soreness	• Require specialized equipment • Cannot replicate natural acceleration found in sports • Are more complicated to use and cannot work all muscle groups

other types of resistance such as exercise bands. The defining feature of isotonic exercise is that the muscle shortens and lengthens to cause movement. Isotonic exercise allows for the use of resistance through a full range of joint motion and provides an effective stimulus for muscle development.

When performing isotonic exercise, both **concentric** (shortening) and **eccentric** (lengthening) contractions are important. For example, in a standard biceps curl, the biceps contract concentrically to lift the weight and then eccentrically to lower the weight back down to the starting position. Many people only emphasize the lifting (concentric) phase, but isotonic exercises are most effective when weights are lowered in a slow and controlled manner. Depending on the resistance used, isotonic exercises can build both **dynamic strength** and **dynamic muscular endurance.** *Dynamic* refers to movement, so strength and muscular endurance that causes movement are referred to as dynamic.

• **Isometric** exercises are those in which no movement takes place while a force is exerted against an immovable object. When properly done, isometric exercise can build **static strength** or **static endurance.** Isometric exercises are not emphasized in most exercise programs because the gains are only evident at the angle of the joint used in the exercise.

• **Isokinetic** exercises are isotonic-concentric muscle contractions performed on machines that keep the velocity of the movement constant through the full range of motion. Isokinetic devices essentially match the resistance to the effort of the performer, permitting maximal tension to be exerted throughout the range of motion. Isokinetic exercises are effective, but they are typically only found in sport training or rehabilitation settings.

Core training uses different types of resistance training to build the core muscles of the body. **Core training** is not a specific type of resistance training such as isotonics, isokinetics, or isometrics. It can be

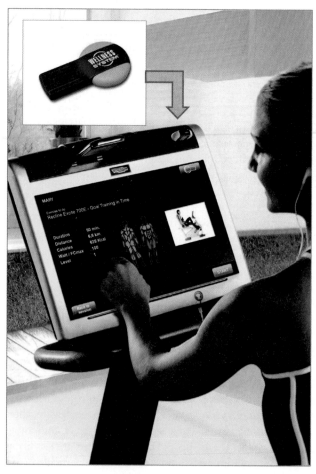

Innovative technology in modern resistance equipment can store personal settings as well as weight used and repetitions performed. (Image provided courtesy of Technogym Inc.)

done with a variety of methods. However, specific types of exercises are used to more effectively engage the core musculature. Inadequate development of these muscles has been shown to be a risk factor for back pain, so it is important to incorporate specialized core exercises into a resistance training program.

The plank is one of the most common isometric core training exercises as it effectively activates a number of stabilizing core muscles. In the front plank, a person holds a horizontal push-up position, bearing the body weight on the forearms, elbows, and toes. The plank strengthens primarily the abdominals, back, and shoulders, but a variety of stabilizing muscles are engaged to resist the pull of gravity and keep the body horizontal (see Figure 3 on page 166). Many variations of the plank exist and they can be modified to fit different fitness levels. Specialized core training exercises are discussed in detail in Concept 11.

Functional fitness training focuses on improving movements used in real life. The importance of the core musculature for posture and back health has increased attention on functional tasks and movements. Simple everyday movements such as lifting a box use multiple muscle groups and require a complex set of coordinated movements. Functional fitness training emphasizes movements that challenge these systems. Movements can be set up with varying degrees of difficulty and with varying amounts of resistance. Adaptations can occur in the core musculature, in individual muscle groups, as well as in motor systems that influence coordination, balance, and agility. Functional fitness training can be incorporated

into an overall PRE program to ensure good levels of muscular fitness.

Plyometrics is a form of isotonic exercise that promotes athletic performance. **Plyometrics** involves sets of high-intensity hops, jumps, and bounding-type movements. A common plyometric exercise involves jumping off of a box and explosively leaping up into the air (or onto another box). The loading phase stretches the muscle before it contracts, allowing the muscle to contract with greater force. Plyometric exercise trains the muscular system for explosive speed and power. Many

---

Concentric Contractions Isotonic muscle contractions in which the muscle gets shorter as it contracts, such as when a joint is bent and two body parts move closer together.

Eccentric Contractions Isotonic muscle contractions in which the muscle gets longer as it contracts—that is, when a weight is gradually lowered and the contracting muscle gets longer as it gives up tension. Eccentric contractions are also called negative exercise.

Dynamic Strength A muscle's ability to exert force that results in movement. It is typically measured isotonically.

Dynamic Muscular Endurance A muscle's ability to contract and relax repeatedly. This is usually measured by the number of times (repetitions) you can perform a body movement in a given period. It is also called isotonic endurance.

Isometric Type of muscle contraction in which the muscle remains the same length. Also known as static contraction.

Static Strength A muscle's ability to exert a force without changing length; also called isometric strength.

Static Muscular Endurance A muscle's ability to remain contracted for a long period. This is usually measured by the length of time you can hold a body position.

Isokinetic Isotonic-concentric exercises done with a machine that regulates movement velocity and resistance.

Core Training A specialized training regimen designed to improve the strength and functionality of core muscles.

Plyometrics A training technique used to develop explosive power. It consists of isotonic-concentric muscle contractions performed after a prestretch or an eccentric contraction of a muscle.

TECHNOLOGY UPDATE

Technogym Wellness System Key

A new line of fitness equipment by Technogym provides a comprehensive solution to personalized fitness center equipment. The basis for the programming is a personalized "key" that is inserted into each machine prior to starting, much like a flash drive is inserted into a computer. (See photo at left.) The key loads the most recently used position and resistance and tracks the resistance, reps, and sets completed on each machine. The key also tracks duration and intensity on aerobic exercise resistance and can be clipped to the individual's waist to record activity while not at the gym.

Would this type of technology get you to join a new gym? How could it help you to stay committed to exercise?

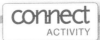

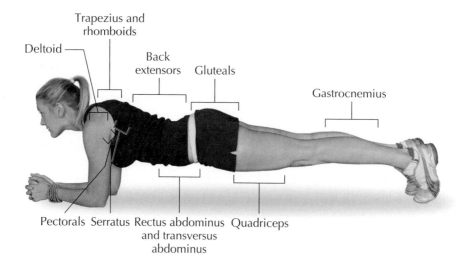

Trapezius and rhomboids

Deltoid

Back extensors

Gluteals

Gastrocnemius

Pectorals Serratus Rectus abdominus Quadriceps
and transversus
abdominus

Figure 3 ▶ The plank is a core exercise that strengthens the abdominals, back, shoulders, and a number of other stabilizing muscles of the core.

sports require quick changes in direction and bursts of power, so plyometric exercises are commonly used by athletes. They have less value for people interested in general health benefits, but plyometric exercises are now included in many functional fitness programs (e.g., P90X program). Beginners should use these exercises with caution due to the increased risk of injury. For more information on plyometrics, refer to Concept 12.

Functional balance training can improve core strength and balance. Balance tends to deteriorate with age, partly due to corresponding declines in muscle strength, range of motion, and a lower ability to coordinate muscle movements. Functional balance training can help improve balance and mobility in the elderly. It is also used in rehabilitation and in specialized training regimens for sports. This type of training is typically conducted with specialized devices, such as exercise balls (Swiss balls), BOSU platforms, and balance boards. Because these devices challenge you to remain balanced, they recruit muscles that are not typically worked in most strength training regimens.

Resistance Training Equipment

Free weights are the most commonly used equipment for resistance exercise. Free weight equipment consists of weights that are typically loaded onto a barbell or a dumbbell. They have often been considered to be the domain of serious weight lifters, but now they are widely used by more casual fitness enthusiasts. Based on 3-year-trend data from the Sporting Goods Manufacturers Association, use of free weight equipment has increased by 5 to 15 percent while use

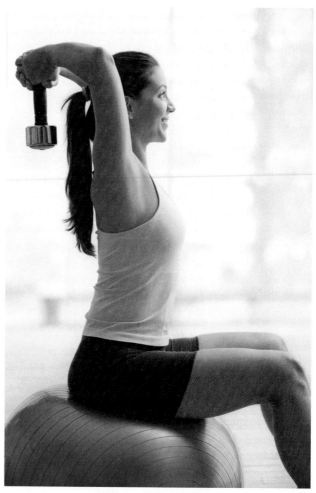

Exercise balls can be used to enhance or facilitate resistance exercises.

of machines has decreased by 2 to 5 percent. Factors that contribute to their popularity are their versatility, the ability to change weight in gradual increments, and

Table 2 ▶ Advantages (+) and Disadvantages (−) of Free Weights and Machine Weights

		Free Weights		Machine Weights
Isolation of Major Muscle Groups	−/+	Movements require balance and coordination; more muscles are used for stabilization.	+/−	Other body parts are stabilized during lift, allowing isolation, but muscle imbalances can develop.
Applications to Real-Life Situations	+	Movements can be developed to be truer to real life.	−	Movements are determined by the paths allowed on the machine.
Risk for Injury	−	There is more possibility for injury because weights can fall or drop on toes.	+	They are safer because weights cannot fall on participants.
Needs for Assistance	−	Spotters are needed for safety with some lifts.	+	No spotters are required.
Time Requirement	−	More time is needed to change weights.	+	It is easy and quick to change weights or resistance.
Number of Available Exercises	+	Unlimited number of exercises is possible.	−	Exercise options are determined by the machine.
Cost	+	They are less expensive, but good (durable) weights are still somewhat expensive.	−	They are expensive; access to a club is usually needed, since multiple machines are usually needed.
Space Requirement	+/−	Equipment can be moved, but loose weights may clutter areas.	−/+	Machines are stationary but take up large spaces.

the ability to modify exercises for specific muscles or movements (see Table 2). Because free weights require balance and technique, they may be more difficult for beginners to use.

Resistance training machines offer many advantages for overall conditioning. Resistance training machines can be effective in developing strength and muscular endurance if used properly. They can save time because, unlike free weights, the resistance can be changed easily and quickly. They may be safer because you are less likely to drop weights. A disadvantage is that the kinds of exercises that can be done on these machines are more limited than free weight exercises. They also may not promote optimal balance in muscular development, since a stronger muscle can often make up for a weaker muscle in the completion of a lift. Some machines have mechanisms that provide variable, or accommodating, resistance. These features allow the machine to provide a more appropriate resistance across the full range of motion. New lines of equipment allow for more natural movements (e.g., lines of Free Motion fitness machines). These features allow the arms to work more independently and enable the exercises to better simulate free living movements.

A variety of resistance devices are available to aid in functional fitness training. To improve functional fitness, it is important to mimic movements that occur in real life. Kettlebells, for example, are now widely available in fitness centers. While kettlebells are not really different from a traditional dumbbell, the handles make them more versatile for more dynamic, functional fitness movements. Other simple resistance devices used in functional fitness training include weighted "medicine balls," weighted bars (e.g., Bodybar), and sand/water bag resistance cords.

In the News

Reebok CrossFit—"The new sport of fitness"

Cross training has been well supported by science but now it is becoming popularized as a sport of its own. Reebok has put considerable attention on building interest in the "CrossFit" movement. Prominent ads on TV promote CrossFit by referring to it as the "sport of fitness." Reebok also sponsors CrossFit training at affiliated fitness centers as well as the national CrossFit Games. Specific CrossFit exercises and events focus on functional movements rather than the non-functional movements involved in traditional resistance exercises.

Is the interest on functional fitness just a new fad or is it a sound transition to a more balanced and functional concept of fitness?

connect ACTIVITY

Many resistance training exercises can be done with little or no equipment. Calisthenics are among the most popular forms of muscle fitness exercise among adults. Calisthenics, such as curl-ups and push-ups, are suitable for people of different ability levels and can be used to improve both strength and muscular endurance. Many variations can be added to increase the difficulty of various calisthenic exercises. For example, push-ups can be made more challenging by elevating your feet. Performing regular calisthenics can help build and maintain good muscular fitness.

Other alternatives to expensive resistance training machines or commercially made free weights are homemade weights and elastic exercise bands. Homemade weights can be constructed from pieces of pipe or broom sticks and plastic milk jugs filled with water. Elastic tubes or bands available in varying strengths may be substituted for the weights and for the pulley device used in many resistance training machines to impart resistance.

Progressive Resistance Exercise: How Much Is Enough?

PRE is the best type of training for muscle fitness. PRE is the most common type of training for building muscle fitness—and the most effective. It is sometimes referred to as progressive resistive training (PRT). The word *progressive* is used because the frequency, intensity, and length of time of muscle overload are gradually, or progressively, increased as muscle fitness increases.

There is a FIT formula for each type of PRE. The FIT formula varies for each type of isotonic PRE, depending on the expected benefit. Days of exercise per week are used to determine frequency (F). Intensity (I) is determined using a percentage of your **1 repetition maximum (1RM)** for a given exercise (see below). Time (T) is determined by the number of sets and repetitions of an exercise. Table 3 illustrates the FIT formulas for PRE designed primarily to build strength, muscular endurance, and general muscle fitness (combination of strength and endurance). The FIT formula for isometric PRE is also included in Table 3.

There is an optimal frequency of PRE for building muscle fitness. As illustrated in Table 3, exercise for muscle strength should be done 2 to 3 days per week. The ACSM recommends 48 hours of rest between exercise sessions to provide appropriate time for recovery. The great proportion of potential strength gains can be accomplished with 2 days of training per week. Exercise done on a third day results in additional increases, but the amount of gain is relatively small, compared with gains resulting from 2 days of training per week. For people interested in health benefits rather than performance benefits, 2 days a week saves time and may result in greater adherence to a strength training program. For people interested in performance benefits, more frequent training may be warranted. Rotating exercises so that certain muscles are exercised on one day and other muscles are exercised the next allows for more frequent training. For example, the total-body workout can be split so that upper body exercises are performed on 2 days of the week and lower body exercises are performed on 2 different days.

There is an optimal intensity of PRE for building muscle fitness. The amount of resistance (intensity of exercise) used in a PRE program is based on a percentage of your 1 repetition maximum (1RM)—the maximum amount of resistance you can move (or weight you can lift) one time. The 1RM value provides

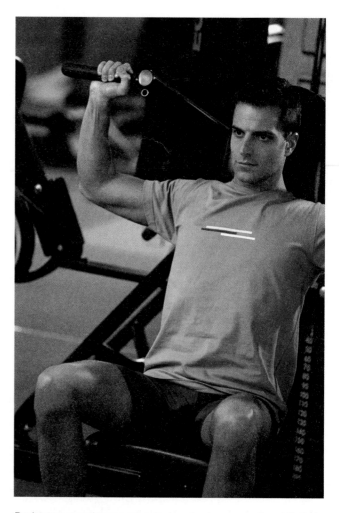

Resistance exercise can promote lean body mass and contribute to a healthy appearance.

Table 3 ▶ Threshold of Training and Fitness Target Zones for Muscular Fitness		
	Threshold of Training	**Fitness Target Zones**
Muscular Strength		
Frequency	2 days a week for each muscle group	2–3 days per week for each muscle group
Intensity		
Beginners/intermediates*	60% of 1RM	60–70% of 1RM
Experienced	vary by schedule**	80% of 1RM**
Older people	40% of 1RM	50% of 1RM
Time (sets and repetitions)		
Most people	2 sets of 8–12 reps	2–4 sets of 8–12 reps
Experienced	2 sets, reps vary by schedule**	2–4 sets, reps vary by schedule**
Older people, beginners	1 set, 10–15 reps	1–2 sets, 10–15 reps
Muscular Endurance		
Frequency	2 days a week for each muscle group	2–3 days per week for each muscle group
Intensity	<50% of 1RM	50% of 1RM
Time (sets and repetitions)	1 set of 15–20 reps	1–4 sets of 15–20 reps
General Muscle Fitness (combined strength and muscular endurance)		
Frequency	2 days a week for each muscle group	2–3 days per week for each muscle group
Intensity		
Young adults	40% of 1RM	60% of 1RM
>50 years old	20% or 1RM***	50% of 1RM
Time		
Most people	1 sets of 8–12 reps	1–3 sets of 8–12 reps
Older adults	1 set of 10–15 reps	1–3 sets 0f 10–15 reps
Rest Intervals		2–3 minutes between sets
		48 hours between sessions

*40% may be beneficial for sedentary beginners.
**Experienced strength trainers often use varied schedules of varied exercise intensity.
***Power is important to older adults and 20–50% of 1RM can increase power.

an indicator of your maximum strength, but desired levels of resistance are determined using percentages of the 1RM value. The specific prescription depends on the program goals. For strength, the percentages typically vary 60 to 80 percent of the 1RM value depending on experience. For older adults, the percentage of 1RM is less (40 to 50 percent). For muscular endurance, the percentages are 50 percent or less. Older people typically use a lower percentage of 1RM (40 to 50 percent).

Evidence suggests that very strong people interested in high-level performance can train at 80 percent of 1RM (see Table 3).

1 Repetition Maximum (1RM) The maximum amount of resistance you can move a given number of times—for example, 1RM = maximum weight lifted one time; 6RM = maximum weight lifted six times.

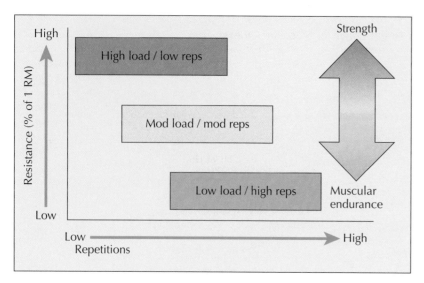

Figure 4 ▶ Comparison of muscular endurance with muscle strength by different repetitions and resistance.

Sets and repetitions are typically used for determining the optimal amount of time for building muscle fitness. Unlike cardiovascular fitness where the time (T) of exercise sessions is determined in minutes, the time for a PRE session is determined in sets and repetitions. As illustrated in Table 3, the number of sets is similar for all forms of PRE (2 to 4). Each set should be performed to muscle fatigue, but not to muscle failure as this can result in increased injury risk and muscle soreness that reduces adherence to regular training.

The number of repetitions varies with the type or PRE. The stimulus for strength is high-level exertion. Because resistance for strength is relatively high, the number of reps for strength is relatively low (compared to muscular endurance): 8 to 12 for most people and 10 to 15 for older people; for experienced strength trainers, the number of reps varies. For muscular endurance, the resistance is lower, so the repetitions are typically higher (15 to 20). Rest intervals vary depending on the goals of the program but would generally be 2 to 3 minutes per set for general fitness.

The graph in Figure 4 illustrates the relationship between strength and muscular endurance. Training that requires high resistance and low repetitions (top bar) results in the least gain in endurance but the greatest gain in strength. Training with moderate resistance and moderate repetitions (second bar) results in moderate gains in both strength and endurance. Training that requires a high number of repetitions and a relatively low resistance (third bar) results in small gains in strength but large increases in muscular endurance.

Circuit resistance training (CRT) is an effective way to build muscular endurance as well as cardiovascular endurance. CRT consists of the performance of high repetitions of an exercise with low to moderate resistance, progressing from one station to another, performing a different exercise at each station. The stations are usually placed in a circle to facilitate movement. CRT typically uses about 20 to 25 reps against a resistance that is 30 to 40 percent of 1RM for 45 seconds. Fifteen seconds of rest is provided while changing stations. Approximately 10 exercise stations are used, and the participant repeats the circuit two to three times (sets). Because of the short rest periods, significant cardiovascular benefits have been reported in addition to muscular endurance gains.

CRT strategies are commonly used in new hybridized group fitness classes aimed at building both muscular fitness and aerobic fitness. CRT strategies are also commonly used in functional fitness training programs since various real-world movement tasks can be easily added to a base of aerobic activity. Thus, CRT can be broadly viewed as a method of integrating resistance exercise with aerobic exercise.

Programs intended to slim the figure/physique should be of the muscular endurance type. Many men and women are interested in exercises designed to decrease girth measurements. High-repetition, low-resistance exercise is suitable for this because it usually brings about some strengthening and may decrease body fatness, which in turn changes body contour. Exercises do not spot-reduce fat, but they do speed up metabolism, so more calories are burned. However, if weight or fat reduction is desired, aerobic (cardiovascular) exercises are best. To increase girth, use strength exercises.

Endurance training may have a negative effect on strength and power. Some studies have shown that for athletes who rely primarily on strength and power in their sport too much endurance training can cause a loss of strength and power because of the modification of different muscle fibers. Strength and power athletes need some endurance training, but not too much, just as endurance athletes need some strength and power training, but not too much.

Designing PRE Programs for Optimal Effectiveness

Apply the overload principle to determine appropriate workloads. For the body to adapt and improve, the muscles and systems of the body must be challenged. As noted earlier, the concept behind PRE

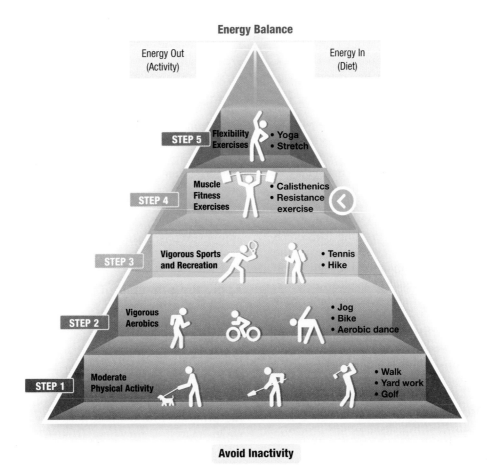

Energy Balance

Energy Out
(Activity)

Energy In
(Diet)

STEP 5 | Flexibility Exercises | • Yoga
• Stretch

STEP 4 | Muscle Fitness Exercises | • Calisthenics
• Resistance exercise

STEP 3 | Vigorous Sports and Recreation | • Tennis
• Hike

STEP 2 | Vigorous Aerobics | • Jog
• Bike
• Aerobic dance

STEP 1 | Moderate Physical Activity | • Walk
• Yard work
• Golf

Avoid Inactivity

Figure 5 ▶ To build muscle fitness, activities should be selected from step 4 of the physical activity pyramid.
Source: C.B. Corbin

is that the frequency, intensity, and duration of lifts are progressively increased to maintain an effective stimulus as the muscle fitness improves. It was in the area of muscle fitness development that the overload principle was first clearly outlined. Legend holds that centuries ago a Greek named Milo of Crotona became progressively stronger by repeatedly lifting his calf. As the calf grew into a bull, its weight increased, and Milo's strength increased as well.

The increasing weight of the growing calf provided the overload to promote continued improvement. As applied to modern life, neither lifestyle tasks nor aerobic exercise provide an appropriate stimulus to maintain or improve muscular fitness. Therefore, specific exercises from step 4 of the pyramid are needed to improve this dimension of fitness (see Figure 5).

Apply the principle of progression to adapt and change the program. An effective PRE program should build progressively over time as your fitness level improves. Many beginning resistance trainers experience soreness after the first few days of training. The reason for

the soreness is that the principle of progression has been violated. Soreness can occur with even modest amounts of training if the volume of training is considerably more than normal. In the first few days or weeks of training, the primary adaptations in the muscle are due to motor learning factors rather than to muscle growth. Because these adaptations occur no matter how much weight is used, start your program slowly with light weights. After these adaptations occur and the rate of improvement slows down, the intensity and volume of training can increase to achieve proper overload.

The most common progression used in resistance training is the double progressive system, so-called because this system periodically adjusts both the resistance and the number of repetitions of the exercise performed. For example, if you are training for strength, you may begin with three repetitions in one set. As the repetitions become easy, additional repetitions are added. When you have progressed to eight repetitions, increase the resistance and decrease the repetitions in each set back to three and begin the progression again.

Apply the principle of specificity to get specific results. The adaptations resulting from exercise are specific to the type and intensity of exercise performed. Training programs should therefore be customized to suit personal goals or to target personal needs. Factors that can be varied in your program are the type of muscle contraction (isometric or isotonic), the speed or cadence of the movement, and the amount of resistance being moved. For example, if you want strength in the elbow extensor muscles (e.g., triceps) so that you can more easily lift heavy boxes onto a shelf, you can train using isotonic contractions, at a relatively slow speed, with a relatively high resistance. If you want muscle fitness of the fingers to grip a heavy bowling ball, much of your training should be done isometrically using the fingers the same way you normally hold the ball. If you are training for a skill that requires explosive power, such as in throwing, striking, kicking, or jumping, your strength exercises should be done with less resistance and greater speed. If you are training for a skill that uses both concentric and eccentric contractions, you should perform exercises using these characteristics (e.g., plyometrics).

If you are not training for a specific task, but merely wish to develop muscle fitness for daily living, consider a general fitness program or a functional fitness program. You may wish to use a variety of methods.

Apply the principle of diminishing returns for program efficiency. To get optimal strength gains from progressive resistance training, several sets of exercise repetitions should be performed. Some high-level performers use as many as five sets of a particular exercise. Research indicates that considerable fitness and health benefits, however, can be achieved in one set. In fact, one set can produce approximately 50 percent of the available gain. Each additional set produces additional benefits, but not as great as the benefits for the preceding set(s). For those interested in high level performance, the extra benefits from additional sets are worth the effort. However, for many people this may not be the case. Because compliance with resistance training programs is less likely as the time needed to complete the program increases, performing one or two sets is better than performing none, especially if performing fewer sets increases adherence. There is no doubt that more sets provide greater benefits, but something is better than nothing.

Apply the principle of rest and recovery to avoid overtraining. Rest is an important part of the body's adaptation to exercise. The frequency guidelines proposed in Table 3 are based on the need for rest following vigorous resistance training exercise. For most people, 3 days of resistance training provides an appropriate amount of overload and rest. If PRE is done more often than this, injuries and overtraining are more likely.

While often not appreciated, an adequate rest period between workouts ensures that there is appropriate time for cellular adaptations to occur. The repeated repetitions in a PRE workout create some minor damage to the outer layers of the contracting muscle fibers. With adequate rest, these muscle fibers rebuild and become stronger. The cycle of catabolic and anabolic processes is critical for effective adaptation to PRE. Some advanced lifters may work out more than 3 days a week, but the ACSM recommends at least 48 hours separating exercise training sessions for the same muscle groups.

Apply the principle of periodization to optimize program effectiveness. Periodization refers to a systematic effort to maintain a novel and challenging training stimulus. The principle of periodization integrates many of the preceding principles (most notably overload, progression, and rest-recovery) to help athletes optimize the effectiveness of their training. The most common periodization plan divides a training program into distinct periods called macrocycles which may last anywhere from 6 months to 1 year. The macrocycles are divided into monthly mesocycles and weekly microcycles. The intensity of individual weeks may build up progressively over 3 weeks with a lighter load on the fourth week to facilitate rest and recovery. The overall progression across the macrocycle moves from lower intensity (lower workloads) to higher intensity (higher workloads) with total volume following the opposite progression, from high to low. A diagram depicting the general progression leading up to a competition or event is shown in Figure 6. Additional detail on periodization is provided in Concept 12.

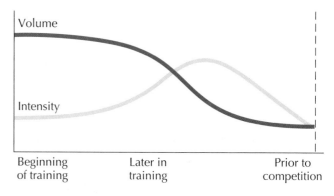

Figure 6 ▶ Volume and intensity of training during periodization.

Table 4 ▶ Adverse Effects of Anabolic Steroids

On Both Males and Females:

Negative Effects on Behavior

- Hostile and aggressive behavior
- Violent behavior
- Depression and mood swings
- Sleep disturbances
- Personality changes and apathy
- Addiction

Negative Effects on the Body

- Reduced aerobic capacity
- Premature stoppage of bone growth
- Brittle connective tissue
- Increased risk of muscle/bone injury
- Immune system suppression
- Sterility

Negative Impacts on Health

- Increased cancer risk (liver)
- Increased stroke risk
- Increased heart attack risk
- Increased early death risk

Negative Effects on Appearance

- Edema (puffy face)
- Headache and fever
- Acne (face, chest, back, thighs)
- Oily skin
- Hair loss / baldness
- Nose bleeds

On Males Only:

- Testicular atrophy/impotence
- Decreased sperm count
- Breast enlargement
- Prostate enlargement
- Baldness

On Females Only:

- Menstrual irregularity
- Decreased breast size
- Deepened voice
- Uterine atrophy
- Clitoral enlargement

Guidelines for Safe and Effective Resistance Training

There are no (safe) shortcuts to strength development or muscular fitness. The use of **anabolic steroids** in sports has received considerable media attention, but more concerning are reports of use among high school youth and young adults. It is important to understand that they are illegal and extremely dangerous. Steroid use directly increases risk for heart disease, liver disease, and early death. It leads to a variety of negative psychological outcomes (e.g., hostility, violence, depression, mood swings, apathy, and addiction) and undesirable body changes such as hair loss, acne, breast enlargement (males), and breast reduction (females). Perhaps more salient to young adults is the fact that steroids lead to adverse sexual/reproductive effects in both males (e.g., testicular atrophy, impotence, and sterility) and females (e.g., uterine atrophy, menstrual irregularities, and sterility). The serious consequences of steroid use are summarized in Table 4.

A number of other dietary supplements are on the market (either legally or illegally) to capitalize on interest in muscular development and sports performance. Contrary to popular belief, they are typically ineffective or dangerous (often both). Details on several common supplements are provided here:

- Prohormone nutritional supplements are marketed as testosterone "prohormones" because they are thought to lead to the production of testosterone and testosterone analogs. Studies have found that these compounds did not produce anabolic or ergogenic effects, and many were found to increase the risk of negative health consequences.

- Androstenedione (andro) is a precursor of naturally occurring testosterone and estrogen. Early studies suggested that andro use did not lead to increases in testosterone levels, but more recent evidence suggests that andro would probably have anabolic effects at the high doses most likely used by athletes. Andro has been found to be associated with most of the same health risks as conventional steroids and has been banned by the FDA.

- Tetrahydrogestrinone (THG) is a chemically engineered steroid that, until recently, has been undetectable by standard drug tests. It is a purely synthetic

Anabolic Steroids Synthetic hormones similar to the male sex hormone testosterone. They function androgenically to stimulate male characteristics and anabolically to increase muscle mass, weight, bone maturation, and virility.

steroid, which exhibits the same properties (and risks) of other anabolic steroids.

- Human growth hormone (HGH) is produced by the pituitary gland but is also made synthetically. Athletes often use growth hormone in combination with anabolic steroids so they can increase bone strength (the main effect of HGH) along with muscle mass. Athletes assume this will protect them from some of the bone injuries that occur among steroid users. However, these athletes are compounding their health risks, as the use of HGH only adds to the health risks of steroid use.

- Creatine is a nutrient involved in the production of energy during short-term, high-intensity exercise, such as resistance exercise. The body produces creatine naturally from foods containing protein, but some athletes take creatine supplements (usually a powder dissolved into a liquid) to increase the amounts available in the muscle. The concept behind supplementation is that additional creatine intake enhances energy production and therefore increases the body's ability to maintain force and delay fatigue. Some studies have shown improvements in athletic

performance with creatine, but reviews indicate that the supplement may be effective only for athletes who are already well trained. Studies have been more consistent with regard to the performance-enhancing effects of creatine on muscle strength. It is important to recognize, though, that the benefits are due to the ability to work the muscles harder during an exercise session, not to the supplement itself. Increases in body weight may result, but this is likely due to water retention. At present, creatine usage hasn't been linked to any major health problems, but the long-term effects are unknown.

There are many fallacies, superstitions, and myths associated with resistance training. Some common misconceptions about resistance training are described in Table 5. The following are guidelines for safe and effective resistance training.

There is a proper way to perform. Although PRE offers considerable health benefits, there are also some risks if the exercises are not performed correctly or if

Table 5 ▶ Fallacies and Facts about Resistance Training

Fallacies	Facts
Resistance training will make you muscle-bound and cause you to lose flexibility.	Normal resistance training will not reduce flexibility if exercises are done through the full range of motion and with proper technique. Powerlifters who do highly specific movements have been shown to have poorer flexibility than other weight lifters.
Women will become masculine-looking if they gain strength.	Women will not become masculine-looking from resistance exercise. Women have less testosterone and do not bulk up from resistance training to the same extent as men. Women and men can make similar relative gains in strength and hypertrophy from a resistance training program, however. The greater percentage of fat in most women prevents the muscle definition possible in men and camouflages the increase in bulk.
Strength training makes you move more slowly and look uncoordinated.	Strength training, if done properly, can enhance sport-specific strength and increase power. There are no effects on coordination from having high levels of muscular fitness.
No pain, no gain.	It is not true that you have to get to the point of soreness to benefit from resistance exercise. It may be helpful to strive until you can't do a final repetition, but you should definitely stop before it is painful. Slight tightness in the muscles is common 1 to 2 days following exercise but is not necessary for adaptations.
Soreness occurs because lactic acid builds up in the muscles.	Lactic acid is produced during muscular work but is converted back into other substrates within 30 minutes after exercising. Soreness is due to microscopic tears or damage in the muscle fibers, but this damage is repaired as the body builds the muscle. Excessive soreness occurs if you violate the law of progression and do too much too soon.
Strength training can build cardiovascular fitness and flexibility.	Resistance exercise can increase heart rate, but this is due primarily to a pressure overload rather than a volume overload on the heart that occurs from endurance (aerobic) exercise. Gains in muscle mass do cause an increase in resting metabolism that can aid in controlling body fatness.
Strength training is beneficial only for young adults.	Studies have shown that people in their 80s and 90s can benefit from resistance exercise and improve their strength and endurance. Most experts would agree that resistance exercise increases in importance with age rather than decreases.

safety procedures are not followed. Before using unfamiliar equipment get instruction in proper use.

Beginners should emphasize lighter weights and progress their program gradually. When beginning a resistance training program, start with light weights so that you can learn proper technique and avoid soreness and injury. Most of the adaptations that occur in the first few months of a program are due to improvements in the body's ability to recruit muscle fibers to contract effectively and efficiently. These neural adaptations occur in response to the movement itself and not the weight that is used. Therefore, beginning lifters can achieve significant benefits from lighter weights. As experience and fitness levels improve, use heavier loads and more challenging sets to continually challenge the muscles.

Use proper technique to reduce the risks for injury and to isolate the intended muscles. An important consideration in resistance exercise is to complete all lifts through the full range of motion using only the intended muscle groups. A common cause of poor technique is using too heavy of a weight. If you have to jerk the weight up or use momentum to lift the weight, it is too heavy. Using heavier weights will provide a greater stimulus to your muscles only if your muscles are actually doing the work. Therefore, it is best to use a weight that you can control safely. By lifting through the full range of motion, you increase the effectiveness of the exercise and maintain good flexibility. Some safety tips are presented in Table 6.

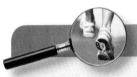

A CLOSER LOOK

P90X

There are many infomercials about new fitness equipment and exercises, but the P90X program has emerged as perhaps the most successful online workout regimen. Developed by fitness guru Tony Horton, the P90X system includes a DVD series of workouts that guide a person through a 90-day functional fitness program. The basis for the program is the idea of "muscle confusion," suggesting that muscles need novel challenges and stimuli to continue adapting. The daily workouts (approximately 60 minutes each) emphasize strength training, but they incorporate cardio, yoga, plyometrics, and stretching into a highly structured circuit training routine. The program employs periodization principles with daily workout grouped into weeks that build across 4-week cycles.

Would this type of program work for you? Who might best benefit from this kind of program?

ACTIVITY

Table 6 ▶ How to Prevent Injury

- Warm up 10 minutes before the workout and stay warm.

- Do not hold your breath while lifting. This may cause blackout or hernia.

- Avoid hyperventilation before lifting a weight.

- Avoid dangerous or high-risk exercises.

- Progress slowly.

- Use good shoes with good traction.

- Avoid arching the back. Keep the pelvis in normal alignment.

- Keep the weight close to the body.

- Do not lift from a stoop (bent over with back rounded).

- When lifting from the floor, do not let the hips come up before the upper body.

- For bent-over rowing, lay your head on a table and bend the knees, or use one-arm rowing and support the trunk with your free hand.

- Stay in a squat as short a time as possible and do not do a full squat.

- Be sure collars on free weights are tight.

- Use a moderately slow, continuous, controlled movement and hold the final position a few seconds.

- Overload but don't overwhelm! A program that is too intense can cause injuries.

- Do not allow the weights to drop or bang.

- Do not train without medical supervision if you have a hernia, high blood pressure, a fever, an infection, recent surgery, heart disease, or back problems.

- Use chalk or a towel to keep your hands dry when handling weights.

Perform lifts in a slow, controlled manner to enhance both effectiveness and safety. Lifting at a slow cadence provides a greater stimulus to the muscles and increases strength gains. A good recommendation is to take 2 seconds on the lifting phase (concentric) and 3 to 4 seconds on the lowering (eccentric) phase.

Provide sufficient time to rest during and between workouts. The body needs time to rest in order to allow beneficial adaptations to occur. Choose an exercise sequence that alternates muscle groups so muscles have a chance to rest before another set. Lifting every other day or alternating muscle groups (if lifting more than 3 or 4 days per week) provides rest for the muscles.

Include all body parts and balance the strength of antagonistic muscle groups. A common mistake made by many beginning lifters is to perform only a few different exercises or to emphasize a few body parts. Training the biceps without working the triceps, for example, can lead to muscle imbalances that can compromise flexibility and increase risks for injury. In some cases, training must be increased in certain areas to compensate for stronger antagonist muscle groups. Many sprinters, for example, pull their hamstrings because the

quadriceps are so overdeveloped that they overpower the hamstrings. The recommended ratio of quadriceps to hamstring strength is 60:40.

Customize your training program to fit your specific needs. Athletes should train muscles the way they will be used in their skill, using similar patterns, range of motion, and speed (the principle of specificity). If you wish to develop a particular group of muscles, remember that the muscle group can be worked harder when isolated than when worked in combination with other muscle groups.

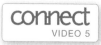

Strategies for Action

Choose exercises that build muscle fitness in the major muscle groups of the body. Table 7 (page 178) provides eight basic exercises for free weights. Table 8 (page 180) presents eight basic exercises for resistance machines. For additional options in resistance training, see the eight calisthenic exercises in Table 9 (page 182) and the eight core strength exercises in Table 10 (page 184). Since good muscular fitness in the abdominals is important, it is recommended that some abdominal or core training be performed as part of any program.

An important step in taking action for developing and maintaining muscle fitness is assessing your current status. A 1RM test of isotonic strength is described in *Lab Resource Materials*. This test allows you to determine absolute and relative strength for the arms and legs. In addition, the 1RM values can be used to help you select the appropriate resistance for your muscle fitness training program. A grip strength test of isometric strength is also provided in *Lab Resource Materials* for Lab 9A.

Three tests of muscular endurance are described in the *Lab Resource Materials* for Lab 9B. It is recommended that you perform the assessments for both strength and muscular

endurance before you begin your progressive resistance training program. Periodically reevaluate your muscle fitness using these assessments.

Many factors other than your own basic abilities affect muscle fitness test scores. If muscles are warmed up before lifting, more force can be exerted and heavier loads can be lifted. Muscle endurance performance may also be enhanced by a warm-up. Do not perform your self-assessments after vigorous exercise because that exercise can cause fatigue and result in suboptimal test results. It is appropriate to practice the techniques in the various tests on days preceding the actual testing. People who have good technique achieve better scores and are less likely to be injured when performing tests than those without good technique. It is best to perform the strength and muscular endurance tests on different days.

Keeping records of progress will help you adhere to a PRE program. Labs 9C and 9D provide activity logging sheets to help you keep records of your progress as you regularly perform PRE to build and maintain good muscle fitness. A guide to the major muscle groups is presented in Figure 7, page 186.

Web Resources

American College of Sports Medicine **www.acsm.org**

Free Motion fitness equipment **www.freemotionfitness.com**

Growing Stronger: Strength Training for Older Adults
www.cdc.gov/physicalactivity/growingstronger/index.html

National Athletic Trainers Association **www.nata.org**

National Health Interview Survey—Strength Activities **www.cdc.gov/mmwr/preview/mmwrhtml/mm5834a6.htm**

National Strength and Conditioning Association **www.nsca-cc.org**

P90X Program **www.beachbody.com/P90X**

Reebok CrossFit Games **games.crossfit.com**

Technogym **www.technogym.com**

Suggested Readings

ACSM. 2010. *ACSM's Guidelines for Exercise Testing and Prescription.* 8th ed. Philadelphia: Lippincott, Williams & Wilkins, Chapter 7.

Baechle, T. R., and R. W. Earle. 2010. *Weight Training: Steps to Success.* Champaign, IL: Human Kinetics.

Bompa, T., and G. G. Haff. 2009. *Periodization.* 5th ed. Champaign, IL: Human Kinetics.

Brumitt, J. 2010. *Core Assessment and Training.* Champaign, IL: Human Kinetics.

Delavier, F. 2010. *Strength Training Anatomy.* 3rd ed. Champaign, IL: Human Kinetics.

Garber, C. E., et al. 2011. Quantity and quality of exercise for developing and maintaining cardiorespiratory, musculoskeletal, and neuromotor fitness in apparently healthy adults: Guidance for prescribing exercise. *Medicine and Science in Sports and Exercise* 43(7):1334–1359.

Gunter, K. B., et al. 2012. Physical activity in childhood may be key to optimizing lifespan skeletal health. *Exercise and Sports Sciences Reviews* 40(1):13–21.

Lewis-McCormick, I. (2012). *A Woman's Guide to Muscle and Strength.* Champaign, IL: Human Kinetics.

Morbidity and Mortality Weekly Reports (MMWR). 2010. National health interview survey strength activities by 18+. *Morbidity and Mortality Weekly Reports* 58(34):955. **www.cdc.gov/mmwr/preview/mmwrhtml/ mm5834a6.htm.**

National Strength and Conditioning Association. 2011. *NSCA's Exercise Techniques.* Champaign, IL: Human Kinetics. (IPad version with video)

Nelson, M. E., et al. 2007. Physical activity and public health in older adults: Recommendation from the American College of Sports Medicine and the American Health Association. *Medicine and Science in Sports and Exercise* 39(8):1435–1445.

Ratamess, N. 2012. *ACSM's Foundations of Strength Training and Conditioning.* Philadelphia: Lippincott, Williams & Wilkins.

Ruiz, J. R., et al. 2011. Field-based fitness assessment in young people. The ALPHA health-related fitness test battery for children and adolescents. *British Journal of Sports Medicine* 45(6):518–524.

Sandler, D. 2010. *Fundamental Weight Training.* Champaign, IL: Human Kinetics.

Schmidt, K. H., et al. 2009. Weight lifting in women with breast-cancer-related lymphedema. *New England Journal of Medicine* 361(7):664–673.

Westcott, W. 2009. ACSM strength training guidelines: Role in body composition and health enhancement. *ACSM's Health and Fitness Journal* 13(4):14–22.

Willardson, J. M. 2008. A periodized approach to core training. *ACSM's Health and Fitness Journal* 12(1):7–13.

Williams, M. A., et al. 2007. Resistance exercise in individuals with and without cardiovascular disease: 2007 update: A scientific statement from the American Heart Association Council on Clinical Cardiology and Council on Nutrition, Physical Activity, and Metabolism. *Circulation* 116(5):572–584.

Healthy People 2020

The objectives listed below are societal goals designed to help all Americans improve their health between now and the year 2020. They were selected because they relate to the content of this concept.

- Increase proportion of people who regularly perform muscle fitness exercises.

- Reduce sports and recreation injuries.

- Reduce percentage of adults who do no leisure-time activity.

- Increase access to employee-based exercise facilities and programs.

- Reduce osteoporosis and hip fractures among older adults.

- Reduce activity limitations due to chronic back pain.

A national goal is to increase the proportion of people who regularly perform muscle fitness exercises. Will it be easier to get people performing resistance exercise or aerobic activity? Which do you find easier to maintain over time?

connect
ACTIVITY

Table 7 The Basic Eight for Free Weights

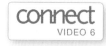

1. Bench Press

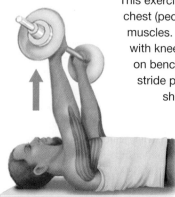

This exercise develops the chest (pectoral) and triceps muscles. Lie supine on bench with knees bent and feet flat on bench or flat on floor in stride position. Grasp bar at shoulder level. Push bar up until arms are straight. Return and repeat. Do not arch lower back. Note: Feet may be placed on floor if lower back can be kept flattened. Do not put feet on the bench if it is unstable.

Pectoralis major

Triceps

2. Overhead (Military) Press

This exercise develops the muscles of the shoulders and arms. Sit erect, bend elbows, palms facing forward at chest level with hands spread (slightly more than shoulder width). Have bar touching chest; spread feet (comfortable distance). Tighten your abdominal and back muscles. Move bar to overhead position (arms straight). Lower bar to chest position. Repeat. Caution: Keep arms perpendicular and do not allow weight to move backward or wrists to bend backward. Spotters are needed.

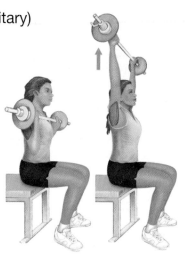

Deltoid

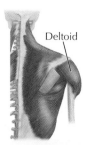

3. Biceps Curl

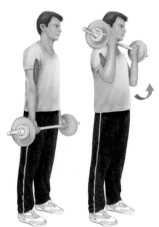

This exercise develops the muscles of the upper front part of the arms (biceps). Stand erect with back against a wall, palms forward, bar touching thighs. Spread feet in comfortable position. Tighten abdominals and back muscles. Do not lock knees. Move bar to chin, keeping body straight and elbows near the sides. Lower bar to original position. Do not allow back to arch. Repeat. Spotters are usually not needed. Variations: Use dumbbell and sit on end of bench with feet in stride position; work one arm at a time. Or use dumbbell with the palm down or thumb up to emphasize other muscles.

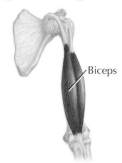

Biceps

4. Triceps Curl

This exercise develops the muscles on the back of the upper arms (triceps). Sit erect, elbows and palms facing up, bar resting behind neck on shoulders, hands near center of bar, feet spread. Tighten abdominal and back muscles. Keep upper arms stationary. Raise weight overhead, return bar to original position. Repeat. Spotters are needed. Variation: Substitute dumbbells (one in each hand, or one held in both hands, or one in one hand at a time).

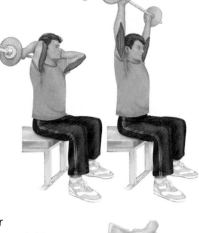

Triceps

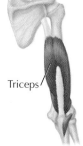

5. Wrist Curl

This exercise develops the muscles of the fingers, wrist, and forearms. Sit astride a bench with the back of one forearm on the bench, wrist and hand hanging over the edge. Hold a dumbbell in the fingers of that hand with the palm facing forward. To develop the flexors, lift the weight by curling the fingers then the wrist through a full range of motion. Slowly lower and repeat. To strengthen the extensors, start with the palm down. Lift the weight by extending the wrist through a full range of motion. Slowly lower and repeat. Note: Both wrists may be exercised at the same time by substituting a barbell in place of the dumbbell.

Wrist flexors

7. Half Squat

This exercise develops the muscles of the thighs and buttocks. Stand erect, feet shoulder-width apart and turned out 45 degrees. Rest bar behind neck on shoulders. Spread hands in a comfortable position. Begin squat by first moving hips backwards, keeping back straight, eyes ahead. By moving first at the hips and then bending knees, shins will remain vertical. Bend knees to approximately 90 degrees. Pause; then stand. Repeat. Spotters are needed. Variations: Substitute dumbbell in each hand at sides.

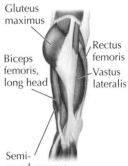

Gluteus maximus
Rectus femoris
Biceps femoris, long head
Vastus lateralis
Semimembranosus

6. Dumbbell Rowing

This exercise develops the muscles of the upper back. It is best performed with the aid of a bench or chair for support. Grab a dumbbell with one hand and place opposite hand on the bench to support the trunk. Slowly lift the weight up until the elbow is parallel with the back. Lower the weight and repeat to complete the set. Switch hands and repeat with the opposite arm. The exercise can also be performed with one leg kneeling on the bench.

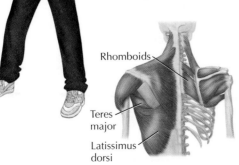

Rhomboids
Teres major
Latissimus dorsi

8. Lunge

This exercise develops the thigh and gluteal muscles. Place a barbell (with or without weight) behind your head and support with hands placed slightly wider than shoulder-width apart. In a slow and controlled motion, take a step forward and allow the leading leg to drop so that it is nearly parallel with the ground. The lower part of the leg should be nearly vertical and the back should be maintained in an upright posture. Take stride with opposite leg to return to standing posture. Repeat with other leg, remaining stationary or moving slowly in a straight line with alternating steps.

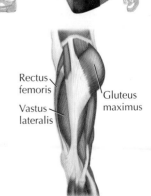

Rectus femoris
Gluteus maximus
Vastus lateralis

Table 8

Table 8 The Basic Eight for Resistance Machine Exercises

connect
VIDEO 7

1. Chest Press

This exercise develops the chest (pectoral) and tricep muscles. Position seat height so that arm handles are directly in front of chest. Position backrest so that hands are at a comfortable distance away from the chest. Push handles forward to full extension and return to starting position in a slow and controlled manner. Repeat. Note: Machine may have a foot lever to help position, raise, and lower the weight.

Pectoralis major

Triceps

2. Overhead Press

This exercise develops the muscles of the shoulders and arms. Position seat so that arm handles are slightly above shoulder height. Grasp handles with palms facing away and push lever up until arms are fully extended. Return to starting position and repeat. Note: Some machines may have an incline press.

Deltoid

3. Biceps Curl

This exercise develops the elbow flexor muscles on the front of the arm, primarily the biceps. Adjust seat height so that arms are fully supported by pad when extended. Grasp handles palms up. While keeping the back straight, flex the elbow through the full range of motion.

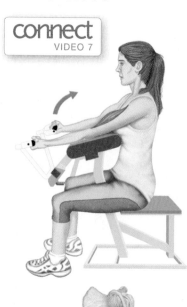

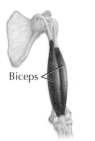

Biceps

4. Triceps Press

This exercise develops the extensor muscles on the back of the arm, primarily the triceps. Adjust seat height so that arm handles are slightly above shoulder height. Grasp handles with thumbs toward body. While keeping the back straight, extend arms fully until wrist contacts the support pad (arms straight). Return to starting position and repeat.

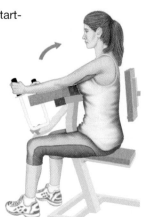

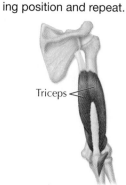

Triceps

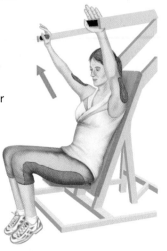

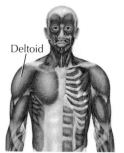

5. Lat Pull Down

This exercise primarily develops the latissimus dorsi, but the biceps, chest, and other back muscles may also be developed. Sit on the floor. Adjust seat height so that hands can just grasp bar when arms are fully extended. Grasp bar with palms facing away from you and hands shoulder-width (or wider) apart. Pull bar down to chest and return. Repeat.

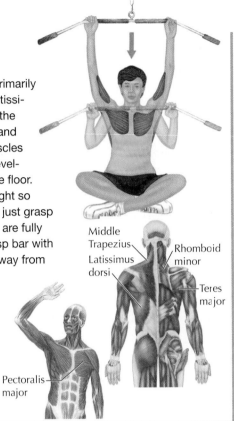

Middle Trapezius
Latissimus dorsi
Rhomboid minor
Teres major
Pectoralis major

7. Knee Extension

This exercise develops the thigh (quadriceps) muscles. Sit on end of bench with ankles hooked under padded bar. Grasp edge of table. Extend knees. Return and repeat. Alternative: Leg press (similar to half-squat).

Note: The knee extension exercise isolates the quadriceps but places greater stress on the structures of the knee than the leg press or half squat.

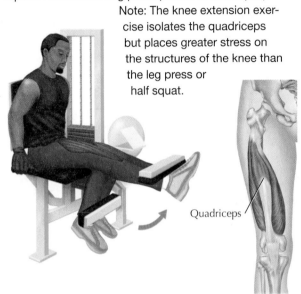

Quadriceps

6. Seated Rowing

This exercise develops the muscles of the back and shoulder. Adjust the machine so that arms are almost fully extended and parallel to the ground. Grasp handgrip with palms turned down and hands shoulder-width apart. While keeping the back straight, pull levers straight back to chest. Slowly return to starting position and repeat.

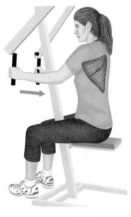

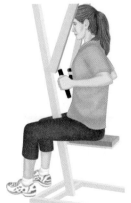

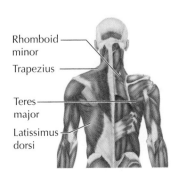

Rhomboid minor
Trapezius
Teres major
Latissimus dorsi

8. Hamstring Curl

This exercise develops the hamstrings (muscles on back of thigh) and other knee flexors. Sit on bench with legs over padded bar, pads contracting lower leg or calf just above the ankles. Grasp handles or edge of seat. Bend knees as far as possible. Return slowly and repeat.

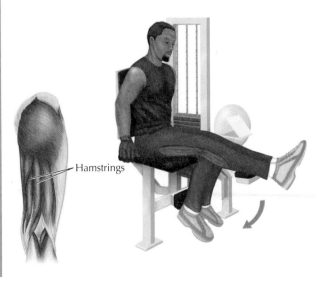

Hamstrings

Table 9

Table 9 The Basic Eight for Calisthenics

1. Bent Knee Push-Ups and Let-Down

This exercise develops the muscles of the arms, shoulders, and chest. Lie on the floor, face down with the hands under your shoulders. Keep your body straight from the knees to the top of the head. Push up until the arms are straight. Slowly lower chest (let-down) to floor. Repeat. Variation: full push-up and let-down performed the same way except body is straight from the toes to the top of head.

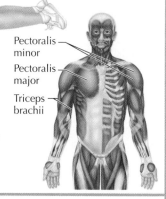

Variation: Start from the up position and lower until the arm is bent at 90 degrees; then push up until arms are extended. Caution: Do not arch back.

Pectoralis minor
Pectoralis major
Triceps brachii

2. Modified Pull-Ups

This exercise develops the muscles of the arms and shoulders. Hang (palms forward and shoulder-width apart) from a low bar (may be placed across two chairs), heels on floor, with the body straight from feet to head. Bracing the feet against a partner or fixed object is helpful. Pull up, keeping the body straight; touch the chest to the bar; then lower to the starting position. Repeat. Note: This exercise becomes more difficult as the angle of the body approaches horizontal and easier as it approaches the vertical. Variation: Perform so that the feet do not touch the floor (full pull-up). Variation: Perform with palms turned up.

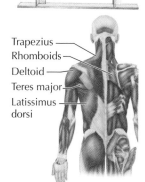

Trapezius
Rhomboids
Deltoid
Teres major
Latissimus dorsi

When palms are turned away from the face, pull-ups tend to use all the elbow flexors. With palms facing the body, the biceps are emphasized more.

3. Dips

connect VIDEO 8

This exercise develops the latissimus dorsi, deltoid, rhomboid, and tricep. Start in a fully extended position with hands grasping the bar (palms facing in). Slowly drop down until the upper part of the arm is horizontal or parallel with the floor. Extend the arms back up to the starting position and repeat. Note: Many gyms have a dip/pull-up machine with accommodating resistance that provides a variable amount of assistance to help you complete the exercise.

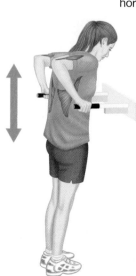

Rhomboid major
Deltoid
Triceps
Latissimus dorsi

4. Crunch (Curl-Up)

This exercise develops the upper abdominal muscles. Lie on the floor with the knees bent and the arms extended or crossed with hands on shoulders or palms on ears. If desired, legs may rest on bench to increase difficulty. For less resistance, place hands at side of body (do not put hands behind head or neck). For more resistance, move hands higher. Curl up until shoulder blades leave floor; then roll down to the starting position. Repeat. Note: Twisting the trunk on the curl-up develops the oblique abdominals.

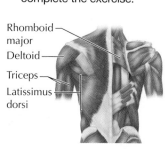

Internal abdominal oblique
External abdominal oblique
Rectus abdominis

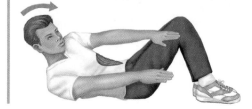
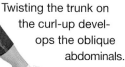

5. Trunk Lift

This exercise develops the muscles of the upper back and corrects round shoulders. Lie face down with hands clasped behind the neck. Pull the shoulder blades together, raising the elbows off the floor. Slowly raise the head and chest off the floor by arching the upper back. Return to the starting position; repeat. For less resistance, hands may be placed under thighs. Caution: Do not arch the lower back. Lift only until the sternum (breastbone) clears the floor. Variations: arms down at sides (easiest), hands by head, arms extended (hardest).

Back extensors

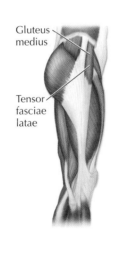

7. Lower Leg Lift

This exercise develops the muscles on the inside of thighs. Lie on the side with the upper leg (foot) supported on a bench. Note: If no bench is available, bend top leg and cross it in front of bottom leg for support. Raise the lower leg toward the ceiling. Repeat. Roll to opposite side and repeat. Keep knees pointed forward. Variation: An ankle weight may be added for greater resistance.

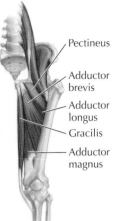

Pectineus

Adductor brevis

Adductor longus

Gracilis

Adductor magnus

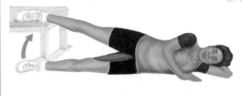

6. Side Leg Raises

This exercise develops the muscles on the outside of thighs. Lie on your side. Point knees forward. Raise the top leg 45 degrees; then return. Do the same number of repetitions with each leg. Caution: Keep knees and toes pointing forward. Variation: Ankle weights may be added for greater resistance.

Gluteus medius

Tensor fasciae latae

8. Alternate Leg Kneel

This exercise develops the muscles of the legs and hips. Stand tall, feet together. Take a step forward with the right foot, touching the left knee to the floor. The knees should be bent only to a 90-degree angle. Return to the starting position and

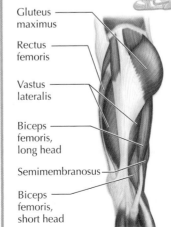

Gluteus maximus

Rectus femoris

Vastus lateralis

Biceps femoris, long head

Semimembranosus

Biceps femoris, short head

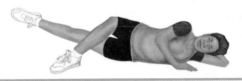

step out with the other foot. Repeat, alternating right and left. Variation: Dumbbells may be held in the hands for greater resistance.

Table 10

Table 10 Exercises for Core Strength

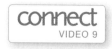

1. Crunch (Curl-Up)

This exercise develops the upper abdominal muscles. Lie on the floor with the knees bent and the arms extended or crossed with hands on shoulders or palms on ears. If desired, legs may rest on bench to increase difficulty. For less resistance, place hands at side of body (do not put hands behind neck). For more resistance, move hands higher. Curl up until shoulder blades leave floor; then roll down to the starting position. Repeat. Note: Twisting the trunk on the curl-up develops the oblique abdominals.

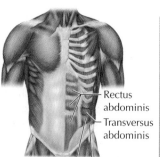

Rectus abdominis
Transversus abdominis
Internal oblique (cut)
External oblique (cut)

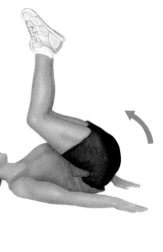

2. Reverse Curl

This exercise develops the lower abdominal muscles. Lie on the floor. Bend the knees, place the feet flat on the floor, and place arms at sides. Lift the knees to the chest, raising the hips off the floor. Do not let the knees go past the shoulders. Return to the starting position. Repeat.

Rectus abdominis

3. Crunch with Twist (on Bench)

This exercise strengthens the oblique abdominals and helps prevent or correct lumbar lordosis, abdominal ptosis, and backache. Lie on your back with your feet on a bench, knees bent at 90 degrees. Arms may be extended or on shoulders or hand on ears (the most difficult). Same as crunch except twist the upper trunk so the right shoulder is higher than the left. Reach toward the left knee with the right elbow. Hold. Return and repeat to the opposite side.

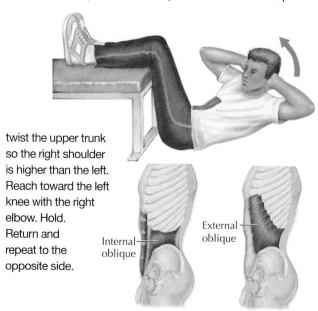

Internal oblique
External oblique

4. Sitting Tucks

This exercise strengthens the lower abdominals, increases their endurance, improves posture, and prevents backache. (This is an advanced exercise and is not recommended for people who have back pain.) Sit on floor with feet raised, arms extended for balance. Alternately bend and extend legs without letting back or feet touch floor.

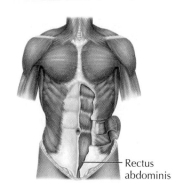

Rectus abdominis

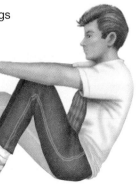

5. Hands and Knees Balance

Begin with both hands and knees placed on Bosu®. Place hands directly below shoulders and knees directly below hips. Look straight down at floor. Draw in lower abdomen. Extend one leg and raise opposite arm to a horizontal position. Keep spine in neutral position. Hold. Relax. Repeat with opposite arm and leg. Do 10 or more repetitions on each side.

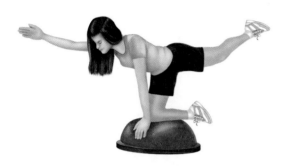

6. Marching

Stand in the middle of the Bosu® with shoulders back and lower abdomen drawn in. March in place, swinging arms in opposite directions—forward and backward—while maintaining spine in neutral position. Progress to jogging in place. Continue for 1 to 2 minutes or longer.

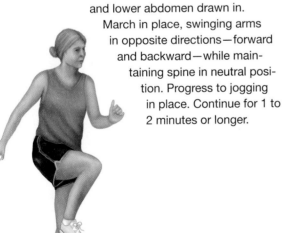

7. Side Step

Begin standing on the floor with Bosu® on your left. Step up onto the center of Bosu® with left foot. Tap right foot on top; then step back to the floor with first the right foot and then the left. Repeat for 60 seconds. Switch to the opposite side.

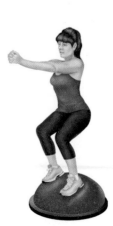

8. Squatting

Stand with feet apart on Bosu®. With knees angled outward slightly, draw abdomen in. Reach forward with hands clasped. Draw shoulder blades down and back. Squat up and down by moving hips backward and then bending knees. (Imagine the movement pattern involved in sitting back on a stool.) Repeat for 1 to 2 minutes.

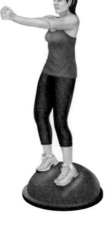

Lab Resource Materials: Muscles in the Body

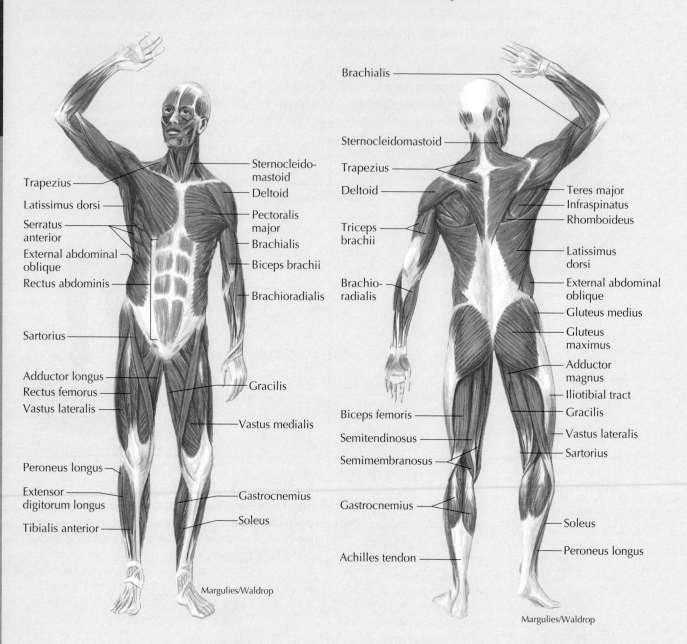

Trapezius

Latissimus dorsi

Serratus anterior

External abdominal oblique

Rectus abdominis

Sartorius

Adductor longus

Rectus femorus

Vastus lateralis

Peroneus longus

Extensor digitorum longus

Tibialis anterior

Sternocleido-mastoid

Deltoid

Pectoralis major

Brachialis

Biceps brachii

Brachioradialis

Gracilis

Vastus medialis

Gastrocnemius

Soleus

Margulies/Waldrop

Brachialis

Sternocleidomastoid

Trapezius

Deltoid

Triceps brachii

Brachio-radialis

Biceps femoris

Semitendinosus

Semimembranosus

Gastrocnemius

Achilles tendon

Teres major

Infraspinatus

Rhomboideus

Latissimus dorsi

External abdominal oblique

Gluteus medius

Gluteus maximus

Adductor magnus

Iliotibial tract

Gracilis

Vastus lateralis

Sartorius

Soleus

Peroneus longus

Margulies/Waldrop

Lab Resource Materials: Muscle Fitness Tests

Evaluating Isotonic Strength: 1RM

1. Use a weight machine for the leg press and seated arm press (or bench press) for the evaluation.
2. Estimate how much weight you can lift two or three times. Be conservative; it is better to start with too little weight than too much. If you lift the weight more than 10 times, the procedure should be done again on another day when you are rested.
3. Using correct form, perform a leg press with the weight you have chosen. Perform as many times as you can up to 10.
4. Use Chart 1 to determine your 1RM for the leg press. Find the weight used in the left-hand column and then find the number of repetitions you performed across the top of the chart.
5. Your 1RM score is the value where the weight row and the repetitions column intersect.
6. Repeat this procedure for the seated arm press.
7. Record your 1RM scores for the leg press and seated arm press in the Results section on page 191.
8. Next, divide your 1RM scores by your body weight in pounds to get a "strength per pound of body weight" (str/lb./body wt.) score for each of the two exercises.
9. Finally, determine your strength rating for your upper body strength (arm press) and lower body (leg press) using Chart 2 (page 188).

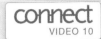

Chart 1 Predicted 1RM Based on Reps-to-Fatigue

Wt.	1	2	3	4	5	6	7	8	9	10	Wt.	1	2	3	4	5	6	7	8	9	10
30	30	31	32	33	34	35	36	37	38	39	170	170	175	180	185	191	197	204	211	219	227
35	35	37	38	39	40	41	42	43	44	45	175	175	180	185	191	197	203	210	217	225	233
40	40	41	42	44	46	47	49	50	51	53	180	180	185	191	196	202	209	216	223	231	240
45	45	46	48	49	51	52	54	56	58	60	185	185	190	196	202	208	215	222	230	238	247
50	50	51	53	55	56	58	60	62	64	67	190	190	195	201	207	214	221	228	236	244	253
55	55	57	58	60	62	64	66	68	71	73	195	195	201	206	213	219	226	234	242	251	260
60	60	62	64	65	67	70	72	74	77	80	200	200	206	212	218	225	232	240	248	257	267
65	65	67	69	71	73	75	78	81	84	87	205	205	211	217	224	231	238	246	254	264	273
70	70	72	74	76	79	81	84	87	90	93	210	210	216	222	229	236	244	252	261	270	280
75	75	77	79	82	84	87	90	93	96	100	215	215	221	228	235	242	250	258	267	276	287
80	80	82	85	87	90	93	96	99	103	107	220	220	226	233	240	247	255	264	273	283	293
85	85	87	90	93	96	99	102	106	109	113	225	225	231	238	245	253	261	270	279	289	300
90	90	93	95	98	101	105	108	112	116	120	230	230	237	244	251	259	267	276	286	296	307
95	95	98	101	104	107	110	114	118	122	127	235	235	242	249	256	264	273	282	292	302	313
100	100	103	106	109	112	116	120	124	129	133	240	240	247	254	262	270	279	288	298	309	320
105	105	108	111	115	118	122	126	130	135	140	245	245	252	259	267	276	285	294	304	315	327
110	110	113	116	120	124	128	132	137	141	147	250	250	257	265	273	281	290	300	310	321	333
115	115	118	122	125	129	134	138	143	148	153	255	256	262	270	278	287	296	306	317	328	340
120	120	123	127	131	135	139	144	149	154	160	260	260	267	275	284	292	302	312	323	334	347
125	125	129	132	136	141	145	150	155	161	167	265	265	273	281	289	298	308	318	329	341	353
130	130	134	138	142	146	151	156	161	167	173	270	270	278	286	295	304	314	324	335	347	360
135	135	139	143	147	152	157	162	168	174	180	275	275	283	291	300	309	319	330	341	354	367
140	140	144	148	153	157	163	168	174	180	187	280	280	288	296	305	315	325	336	348	360	373
145	145	149	154	158	163	168	174	180	186	193	285	285	293	302	311	321	331	342	354	366	380
150	150	154	159	164	169	174	180	186	193	200	290	290	298	307	316	326	337	348	360	373	387
155	155	159	164	169	174	180	186	192	199	207	295	295	303	312	322	332	343	354	366	379	393
160	160	165	169	175	180	186	192	199	206	213	300	300	309	318	327	337	348	360	372	386	400
165	165	170	175	180	186	192	198	205	212	220	305	305	314	323	333	343	354	366	379	392	407

Source: JOPERD.

Chart 2 Fitness Classification for Relative Strength in Men and Women (1RM/Body Weight)

Age:	Leg Press			Arm Press		
	30 or Less	31–50	51+	30 or Less	31–50	51+
Ratings for Men						
High-performance zone	2.06+	1.81+	1.61+	1.26+	1.01+	.86+
Good fitness zone	1.96–2.05	1.66–1.80	1.51–1.60	1.11–1.25	.91–1.00	.76–.85
Marginal zone	1.76–1.95	1.51–1.65	1.41–1.50	.96–1.10	.86–.90	.66–.75
Low fitness zone	1.75 or less	1.50 or less	1.40 or less	.95 or less	.85 or less	.65 or less
Ratings for Women						
High-performance zone	1.61+	1.36+	1.16+	.76+	.61+	.51+
Good fitness zone	1.46–1.60	1.21–1.35	1.06–1.15	.66–.75	.56–.60	.46–.50
Marginal zone	1.31–1.45	1.11–1.20	.96–1.05	.56–.65	.51–.55	.41–.45
Low fitness zone	1.30 or less	1.10 or less	.95 or less	.55 or less	.50 or less	.40 or less

Evaluating Muscular Endurance

1. Curl-Up (Dynamic)

Sit on a mat or carpet with your legs bent more than 90 degrees so your feet remain flat on the floor (about halfway between 90 degrees and straight). Make two tape marks 4½ inches apart or lay a 4½-inch strip of paper or cardboard on the floor. Lie with your arms extended at your sides, palms down and the fingers extended so that your fingertips touch one tape mark (or one side of the paper or cardboard strip). Keeping your heels in contact with the floor, curl the head and shoulders forward until your fingers reach 4½ inches (second piece of tape or other side of strip). Lower slowly to beginning position. Repeat one curl-up every 3 seconds. Continue until you are unable to keep the pace of one curl-up every 3 seconds.

Two partners may be helpful. One stands on the cardboard strip (to prevent movement) if one is used. The second assures that the head returns to the floor after each repetition.

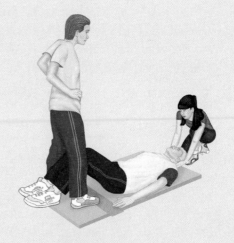

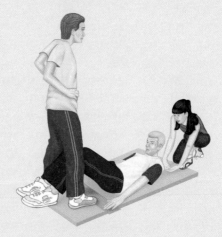

Evaluating Isometric Strength

Test: Grip Strength

Adjust a hand dynamometer to fit your hand size. Squeeze it as hard as possible. You may bend or straighten the arm, but do not touch the body with your hand, elbow, or arm. Perform with both right and left hands. *Note:* When not being tested, perform the basic eight isometric strength exercises, or squeeze and indent a new tennis ball (*after* completing the dynamometer test).

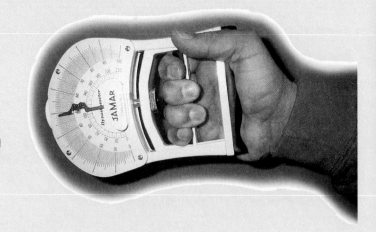

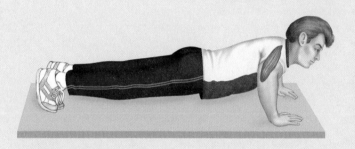

2. Ninety-Degree Push-Up (Dynamic)

Support the body in a push-up position from the toes. The hands should be just outside the shoulders, the back and legs straight, and toes tucked under. Lower the body until the upper arm is parallel to the floor or the elbow is bent at 90 degrees. The rhythm should be approximately 1 push-up every 3 seconds. Repeat as many times as possible up to 35.

3. Flexed-Arm Support (Static)

Women: Support the body in a push-up position from the knees. The hands should be outside the shoulders, the back and legs straight. Lower the body until the upper arm is parallel to the floor or the elbow is flexed at 90 degrees.

Men: Use the same procedure as for women except support the push-up position from the toes instead of the knees. (Same position as for 90-degree push-up.) Hold the 90-degree position as long as possible, up to 35 seconds.

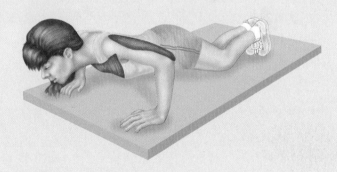

Chart 3 Isometric Strength Rating Scale (Pounds)

Classification	Left Grip	Right Grip	Total Score
Ratings for Men			
High-performance zone	125+	135+	260+
Good fitness zone	100–124	110–134	210–259
Marginal zone	90–99	95–109	185–209
Low fitness zone	<90	<95	<185
Ratings for Women			
High-performance zone	75+	85+	160+
Good fitness zone	60–74	70–84	130–159
Marginal zone	45–59	50–69	95–129
Low fitness zone	<45	<50	<95

Suitable for use by young adults between 18 and 30 years of age. After 30, an adjustment of 0.5 of 1 percent per year is appropriate because some loss of muscle tissue typically occurs as you grow older.

Chart 4 Rating Scale for Dynamic Muscular Endurance

Age:	17–26		27–39		40–49		50–59		60+	
Classification	Curl-Ups	Push-Ups	Curl-Ups	Push-Ups	Curl-Ups	Push-Ups	Curl-Ups	Push-Ups	Curl-Ups	Push-Ups
Ratings for Men										
High-performance zone	35+	29+	34+	27+	33+	26+	32+	24+	31+	22+
Good fitness zone	24–34	20–28	23–33	18–26	22–32	17–25	21–31	15–23	20–30	13–21
Marginal zone	15–23	16–19	14–22	15–17	13–21	14–16	12–20	12–14	11–19	10–12
Low fitness zone	<15	<16	<14	<15	<13	<14	<12	<12	<11	<10
Ratings for Women										
High-performance zone	25+	17+	24+	16+	23+	15+	22+	14+	21+	13+
Good fitness zone	18–24	12–16	17–23	11–15	16–22	10–14	15–21	9–13	14–20	8–12
Marginal zone	10–17	8–11	9–16	7–10	8–15	6–9	7–14	5–8	6–13	4–7
Low fitness zone	<10	<8	<9	<7	<8	<6	<7	<5	<6	<4

Chart 5 Rating Scale for Static Endurance (Flexed-Arm Support)

Classification	Score in Seconds
High-performance zone	30+
Good fitness zone	20–29
Marginal zone	10–19
Low fitness zone	<10

Lab 9A Evaluating Muscle Strength: 1RM and Grip Strength

Name _Jason Herrin_ Section _____ Date _3/6/16_

Purpose: To evaluate your muscle strength using 1RM and to determine the best amount of resistance to use for various strength exercises

Procedures: 1RM is the maximum amount of resistance you can lift for a specific exercise. Testing yourself to determine how much you can lift only one time using traditional methods can be fatiguing and even dangerous. The procedure you will perform here allows you to estimate 1RM based on the number of times you can lift a weight that is less than 1RM.

Evaluating Strength Using Estimated 1RM

1. Use a resistance machine for the leg press and arm or bench press for the evaluation part of this lab.
2. Estimate how much weight you can lift two or three times. Be conservative; it is better to start with too little weight than too much. If you lift a weight more than 10 times, the procedure should be done again on another day when you are rested.
3. Using correct form, perform a leg press with the weight you have chosen. Perform as many times as you can up to 10.
4. Use Chart 1 in *Lab Resource Materials* to determine your 1RM for the leg press. Find the weight used in the left-hand column and then find the number of repetitions you performed across the top of the chart.
5. Your 1RM score is the value where the weight row and the repetitions column intersect.
6. Repeat this procedure for the arm or bench press using the same technique.
7. Record your 1RM scores for the leg press and bench press in the Results section.
8. Next divide your 1RM scores by your body weight in pounds to get a "strength per pound of body weight" (1RM/body weight) score for each of the two exercises.
9. Determine your strength rating for your upper body strength (arm press) and lower body (leg press) using Chart 2 in *Lab Resource Materials.* Record in the Results section. If time allows, assess 1RM for other exercises you choose to perform (see Lab 9C).
10. If a grip dynamometer is available, determine your right-hand and left-hand grip strength using the procedures in *Lab Resource Materials.* Use Chart 3 in *Lab Resource Materials* to rate your grip (isometric) strength.

Results

Arm press: Wt. selected | 140 | Reps | 10 | Estimated 1RM | 180 |
(or bench press)

(Chart 1, *Lab Resource Materials,* page 187)

Strength per lb. body weight | .947 | Rating | Good |

(1RM ÷ body weight) (Chart 2, *Lab Resource Materials,* page 188)

Leg press: Wt. selected | 240 | Reps | 6 | Estimated 1RM | 279 |

(Chart 1, *Lab Resource Materials,* page 187)

Strength per lb. body weight | 1.46 | Rating | high |

(1RM ÷ body weight) (Chart 2, *Lab Resource Materials,* page 188)

Grip strength: Right grip score | | Right grip rating | |

Left grip score | | Left grip rating | |

Total score | | Total rating | |

(Chart 3, *Lab Resource Materials,* page 190)

Seated Press (Arm Press)

This test can be performed using a seated press (see below) or using a bench press machine. When using the seated press, position the seat height so that arm handles are directly in front of the chest. Position backrest so that hands are at comfortable distance away from the chest. Push handles forward to full extension and return to starting position in a slow and controlled manner. Repeat. Note: Machine may have a foot lever to help position, raise, and lower the weight.

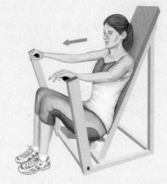

Leg Press

To perform this test, use a leg press machine. Typically, the beginning position is with the knees bent at right angles with the feet placed on the press machine pedals or a foot platform. Extend the legs and return to beginning position. Do not lock the knees when the legs are straightened. Typically, handles are provided. Grasp the handles with the hands when performing this test.

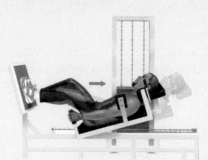

Conclusions and Implications: In several sentences, discuss your current strength, whether you believe it is adequate for good health, and whether you think that your "strength per pound of body weight" scores are representative of your true strength.

> Overall, I feel that my arm strength is reasonable but I have a lot of area to improve. I feel that my leg strength is good but I would like to focus more effort on glute workouts so I can protect myself from back problems

Lab 9B Evaluating Muscular Endurance

Name	**Section**	**Date**

Purpose: To evaluate the dynamic muscular endurance of two muscle groups and the static endurance of the arms and trunk muscles

Procedures

1. Perform the curl-up, push-up, and flexed-arm support tests described in *Lab Resource Materials* (pp. 188–189).
2. Record your test scores in the Results section. Determine and record your rating in Chart 1 below, based on Charts 4 and 5 in *Lab Resource Materials* (page 190).

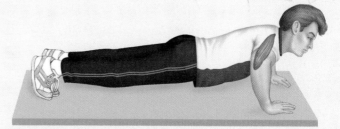

2. Ninety-degree push-up (dynamic)

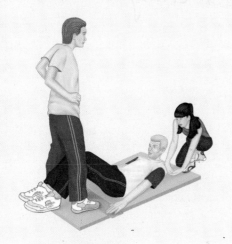

1. Curl-up (dynamic)

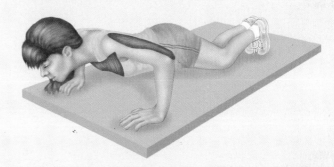

3. Flexed-arm support (static): women in knee position and men in full support position

Results

Record your scores below.

Curl-up [25]   Push-up [30]   Flexed-arm support (seconds) [35]

Check your ratings in Chart 1.

Chart 1	Rating Scale		
	Curl-Up	**Push-Up**	**Flexed-Arm Support**
High	○	⊗	⊗
Good	⊗	○	○
Marginal	○	○	○
Poor	○	○	○

On which of the tests of muscular endurance did you score the lowest?

Curl-up ⊗ Push-up ◯ Flexed-arm support ◯

On which of the tests of muscular endurance did you score the best?

Curl-up ◯ Push-up ⊗ Flexed-arm support ◯

Conclusions and Implications: In several sentences, discuss your current level of muscular endurance and whether this level is enough to meet your health, work, and leisure-time needs in the future.

I need to work on my core strength more. I posted adequate marks but relative to the rest of my body my core and abs are lacking.

Lab 9C Planning and Logging Muscle Fitness Exercises:
Free Weights or Resistance Machines

Name	**Section**	**Date**

Purpose: To set lifestyle goals for muscle fitness exercise, to prepare a muscle fitness exercise plan, and to self-monitor progress for the 1-week plan

Procedures

1. Using Chart 1, provide some background information about your experience with resistance exercise, your goals, and your plans for incorporating these exercises into your normal exercise routine.

2. Using Chart 2, select at least eight muscle fitness exercises by circling the name of the exercises or writing in the name of the exercises. Perform the exercises for 2 or 3 days. Record the weight, reps, and sets performed on each day. Be sure that you plan your exercise program so it fits with the goals you described in Chart 1. If you are just starting out, it is best to start with light weights and more repetitions, e.g., 12–15. For best results, take the log with you during your workout, so you can remember the weights, reps, and sets you performed.

3. Describe your experiences with your resistance exercise program. Be sure to comment on your plans for future resistance exercise.

Chart 1 Muscle Fitness Survey

1. Determine your current stage for resistance exercise. Check only the stage that represents your current activity level.

   ◯ Precontemplation. I do not meet resistance exercise guidelines and have not been thinking about starting.

   ◯ Contemplation. I do not do resistance exercises but have been thinking about starting.

   ◯ Preparation. I am planning to start doing regular resistance exercises to meet guidelines.

   ⊗ Action. I do resistance exercises, but I am not as regular as I should be.

   ◯ Maintenance. I regularly meet guidelines for resistance exercises.

2. What are your primary goals for resistance exercise?

   ◯ General conditioning   ⊗ Improved appearance   ◯ Other_____

   ◯ Sports training   ◯ Avoidance of back pain

3. Are you currently involved in a regular resistance exercise program?

   ⊗ Yes   ◯ No

4. Describe your current program or your future goals.

   • What days and times do you lift weights (or when can you lift)?
   • Where do you lift (or where can you lift)?
   • Describe your goals (or plans) for resistance exercise:

   > I am semi consistent with my work out plan.
   > On one day, I do biceps, back, and abs. The
   > next day I do triceps, pectorals, shoulders and
   > legs. I alternate for the 3-4 days per week
   > I go to the gym

Chart 2 Muscle Fitness Exercise Log

Check the exercises you performed and the days you performed them. You can do all free weights, all machines, or some of both. List others that you added.

Exercises	Day 1 (date)			Day 2 (date)			Day 3 (date)		
	Wt.	Reps	Sets	Wt.	Reps	Sets	Wt.	Reps	Sets
Free Weight Exercises									
1 Bench press	120	10	3				120	10	3
2 Overhead press				45	15	3			
3 Biceps curl				35	10	3			
4 Triceps curl									
5 Wrist curl									
6 Dumbbell rowing									
7 Half squat				~~190~~ 200	12	3			
8 Lunge									
9 Crunches	20	20	3				20	20	3
10									
Machine Exercises									
11 Chest press	115	8	3				110	8	3
12 Overhead press									
13 Biceps curl									
14 Triceps press									
15 Lat pull-down									
16 Seated rowing				45	10	3			
17 Knee extension									
18 Hamstring curl									
19									
20									

Results

Were you able to do your basic eight exercises at least 2 days in the week?   Yes Ⓧ   No ◯

Conclusions and Implications: Do you feel that you will use muscle fitness exercises as part of your regular lifetime physical activity plan, either now or in the future? Comment on what modifications you would make in your program in the future. Use several sentences to answer.

I will continue to use muscle fitness. I like how I feel when I do muscle exercises. I need to mix up the exercises to get more complex movement.

Lab 9D Planning and Logging Muscle Fitness Exercises: Calisthenics or Core Exercises

Name   **Section**   **Date**

Purpose: To set lifestyle goals for muscle fitness exercises that can easily be performed at home, to prepare a muscle fitness exercise plan, and to self-monitor progress for a 1-week plan

Procedures

1. Using Chart 1, provide some background information about your experience with calisthenic or core exercise, your goals, and your plans for incorporating these exercises into your normal exercise routine.
2. Using Chart 2, select at least eight calisthenics or core exercises by circling the name of the exercises or writing in the name of the exercises. Perform the exercises for 2 or 3 days. Record the reps and sets performed on each day.
3. Describe your experiences with your resistance exercise program. Be sure to comment on your plans for future resistance exercise.

Chart 1 Muscle Fitness Survey

1. Determine your current stage for calisthenics or core exercise. Check only the stage that represents your current activity level.

- ( ) Precontemplation. I do not do calisthenics or core exercises and have not been thinking about starting.
- ( ) Contemplation. I do not do calisthenics or core exercises but have been thinking about starting.
- ( ) Preparation. I am planning to start doing calisthenics or core exercises.
- (✗) Action. I do calisthenics or core exercises, but I am not as regular as I should be.
- ( ) Maintenance. I regularly perform calisthenics or core exercises.

2. What is your level of experience with core exercises (refer to Table 10 on pages 185 and 186)? Check the box that best describes you.

- ( ) I have done abdominal exercises but have never done the other core exercises.
- (✗) I have done abdominal exercises and have tried core exercises with the Bosu® or similar devices.
- ( ) I regularly perform core exercises and am very experienced with the Bosu® or similar devices.

3. What are your primary reasons for doing calisthenic or core exercise?
- ( ) General conditioning
- ( ) Sports training
- (✗) Improved appearance
- ( ) Avoidance of back pain

4. Describe your current program or your present or future goals.
- What days and times do you exercise (or when can you exercise)?
- Where do you perform these exercises (or where can you exercise)?
- Describe your goals/plans:

I exercise 3-4 times per week in the morning when I wake up. I work out at the gym or at my home.

Chart 2 Muscle Fitness Exercise Log

Check the exercises you performed and the days you performed them. List others that you added.

Exercises	Day 1 (date)		Day 2 (date)		Day 3 (date)	
	Reps	Sets	Reps	Sets	Reps	Sets
Calisthenic Exercises						
1 Bent knee push-ups						
2 Modified pull-ups	12	3			12	3
3 Dips			15	3		
4 Crunch (curl-up)			30	3		
5 Trunk lift						
6 Side leg raise						
7 Lower leg lift						
8 Alternate leg kneel						
9						
10						
Core Exercises						
11 Crunch						
12 Reverse curl						
13 Crunch with twist						
14 Sitting tucks						
15 Hands and knees balance			15	3		
16 Marching						
17 Side step						
18 Squatting			10	3		
19						
20						

Results

Were you able to do your planned exercises at least 2 days in the week?　　Yes ⊗　　No ◯

Conclusions and Implications: Do you feel that you will use these muscle fitness exercises as part of your regular lifetime physical activity plan, either now or in the future? Discuss the exercises you feel benefited you and the ones that did not. What modifications would you make in your program for it to work better for you?

I will likely use these exercises in my regular fitness. I really like the core workouts. I will probably not have a set regiment every day but rather mix it up day by day

Flexibility

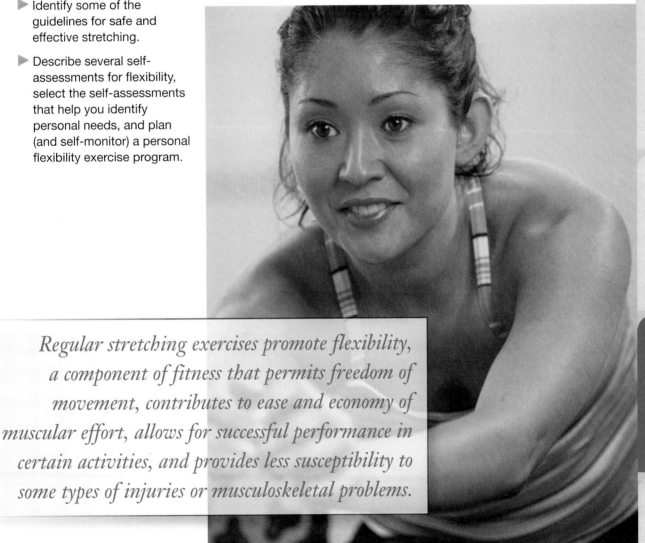

Regular stretching exercises promote flexibility, a component of fitness that permits freedom of movement, contributes to ease and economy of muscular effort, allows for successful performance in certain activities, and provides less susceptibility to some types of injuries or musculoskeletal problems.

Concept 10

Flexibility refers to the amount of motion that is possible at a given joint or series of joints. A joint with limited ability to bend or straighten is said to be tight or stiff, while joints with a high degree of flexibility are loose-jointed, or hypermobile. A reasonable amount of flexibility is needed to perform efficiently and effectively in daily life, but excessive flexibility is not desirable.

Flexibility is important for good health because it helps with the maintenance of good posture and the prevention of back and neck problems. It directly contributes to wellness as it enables people to move more freely and perform daily tasks more effectively, which is especially important for maintaining independence and function later in life. Lastly, flexibility contributes to improved performance in sports. Good flexibility is obvious in sports such as gymnastics, figure skating, diving, wrestling, and swimming, but it contributes to dynamic movement and performance in many other sports as well.

While these points are widely accepted, there are a number of misconceptions about flexibility, stemming largely from confusion about differences between flexibility and stretching. *Flexibility* is a state of being and something that can be measured. *Stretching*, in contrast, is a behavior that can improve flexibility if performed regularly. The effects of stretching and of flexibility must be considered independently to interpret research in this area. For example, research has shown that stretching may have little impact on injuries during a bout of physical activity, but this does not discount the benefits of good flexibility (and broader indicators of functional fitness) on injury prevention. Similarly, research now indicates that stretching prior to exercise may (in some circumstances) reduce performance in some speed and power activities. This has caused some athletes to erroneously assume that stretching (and flexibility) is not important and even detrimental to their performance. Stretching should still be an important part of a training program for athletes, but, as described later in this concept, the timing and length of stretches are critical for optimal results.

This concept will further clarify the distinctions between flexibility and stretching. The initial sections explain the factors influencing flexibility and how flexibility impacts health and wellness. We look at various stretching methods for improving flexibility and the recommended amounts to perform. The final section covers flexibility-based activities and guidelines for incorporating stretching into your fitness program.

Flexibility Fundamentals

The range of motion in a joint or joints is a reflection of the flexibility at that joint. Clinically, the **range of motion (ROM)** of a joint is the extent *and* direction of movement that is possible. The extent of movement is described by the arc through which a joint moves and is typically measured in degrees using a tool called a goniometer. The direction of movement at a specific joint is determined by the shapes of the bony surfaces that are in contact. Certain types of joints allow for greater movement than others. In fact, flexibility is highly joint specific. An individual may demonstrate optimal flexibility in one region of the body but not in others. For example, a person may have good flexibility of the spine, hips, and legs in order to reach down and touch the toes, but is unable to clasp both hands behind the back due to stiffness of the shoulder joints.

Medical professionals use a specific vocabulary to describe the movement of joints. Figure 1 illustrates some of these movement terms as they relate to hip, knee, or ankle motion. Similar terms are applied in describing movement of the spine and upper body. Note that the same terms (such as *flexion/extension*) can be applied to different joints, while other terms (such as *dorsiflexion/plantar flexion*) are unique to a specific joint such as the ankle.

The shape, size, and orientation of a joint greatly influence the amount of motion available. The circular surface of the ball-and-socket joint of the hip, for example, allows for considerable mobility, including movement to the side (adduction and abduction), forward and backward (flexion and extension), and in

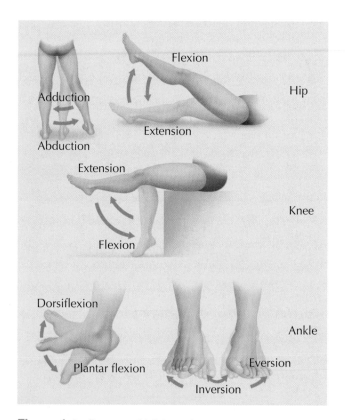

Figure 1 ▶ Ranges of joint motion.

and out (internal and external rotation). The hinge joint of the knee is more restrictive and limits movement to primarily forward and backward (flexion and extension). Motion at other joints, such as the ankle, involves the combined movements of numerous bony surfaces. A hinge-type portion permits the up and down motion of the foot (dorsiflexion and plantar flexion), while a separate planar-type joint allows the side-to-side motion (inversion and eversion) of the foot. A basic understanding of this terminology is important in understanding principles of flexibility and stretching.

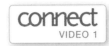

Flexibility is influenced by the extensibility of soft tissues such as muscles, tendons, and ligaments. Soft tissues are made up of a number of substances, including fibers called collagen and elastin. These structural building blocks influence the degree of extensibility of tissues such as **ligaments, tendons,** and muscles. Tissues with a greater proportion of collagen fibers tend to be stiffer while those with more elastin tend to bend and stretch more readily. Ligaments contain a greater proportion of collagen and this enhances their function in providing rigidity and stability to a joint and their role in restricting excessive joint motion. Damage to ligaments from repeated sprains can lead to excessive joint **laxity** and increased risk for injuries. Tendons contain a greater proportion of elastin than ligaments but muscles contain even more and this contributes to their relatively high degree of flexibility. Together, the muscles and tendons are referred to as a **muscle-tendon unit (MTU)** and due to their connection, they are both stretched together. In this book we will generally refer to muscles or tissues rather than the MTU.

The short-term gains in range of motion immediately following stretching are commonly attributed to changes in the "viscoelastic" properties of muscle. Viscosity refers to a property that allows tissues to undergo slow changes in length over time (like taffy) while elasticity refers to a property that allows tissues to return to normal shape after being stretched (like a rubber band). When a muscle is stretched, there are changes in muscle length as well as a decline in muscle **stiffness.** However, due to the elastic nature of the MTU, these changes are short-lived. In fact, studies have shown that the beneficial effects of a 30- or 45-second static stretch can disappear in less than 30 seconds. Thus, changes in viscoelasticity contribute to small temporary changes in muscle length and stiffness rather than long-term changes in flexibility.

Some regions of the body are more prone to tightness than others. A number of muscles in the body have a predictable tendency toward tightness. Clinicians refer to these muscles as "tonic" or "postural" muscles because of their tendency to tighten or shorten.

A characteristic of these muscles is that they tend to cross more than one joint. Included in the list are the upper trapezius, the muscles at the base of the skull, the pectoralis, hip flexors, low back extensors, hamstrings, adductors, and calf muscles. These muscles typically benefit the most from stretching and therefore are often targeted by common stretching exercises. Specific exercises for these muscle groups are provided at the end of the concept.

Static flexibility is different from dynamic flexibility. A joint's flexibility can be described differently depending on how it is assessed. Static flexibility is the maximum range a joint can achieve under stationary conditions. An example is the hip ROM achieved during a hamstring stretch. Static flexibility is limited by passive viscous and elastic properties of the muscles. Dynamic flexibility is the maximum range a joint can achieve under active conditions. An example is the maximum height and position of a hurdler's lead leg. While it may seem logical that dynamic flexibility would be greater than static, the opposite is true. This is because dynamic flexibility is influenced by both passive and dynamic properties of the tissues. A hurdler's performance, for example, depends on the passive muscle and tendon extensibility as well as the ability to move against gravity, at fast speeds, and without elicitation of a stretch reflex. While good static flexibility is necessary for good dynamic flexibility, it does not ensure it. Athletes must train both static and dynamic flexibility for optimal performance.

Factors Influencing Flexibility

Flexibility varies considerably across the lifespan. Flexibility is generally high in children but declines during adolescence because of the rapid changes in

---

Range of Motion (ROM) The full motion possible in a joint or series of joints.

Ligaments Bands of tissue that connect bones. Unlike muscles and tendons, overstretching ligaments is not desirable.

Tendons Fibrous bands of tissue that connect muscles to bones and facilitate movement of a joint.

Laxity Motion in a joint outside the normal plane for that joint, due to loose ligaments.

Muscle-Tendon Unit (MTU) The skeletal muscles and the tendons that connect them to bones. Stretching to improve flexibility is associated with increased length of the MTU.

Stiffness Elasticity in the MTU; measured by force needed to stretch.

growth—essentially, the bones grow faster than the soft tissues. In early adulthood, the muscles and tendons catch up to the skeletal system, causing flexibility to peak in the mid- to late 20s. With increasing age, range of motion tends to decline again. Reduced flexibility is due to a loss of elasticity in the MTU and cross-linkages within collagen fibers of the tendons, ligaments, and joint capsules. Over the span of their working lives, adults typically lose 3 to 4 inches of lower back flexibility as measured by the common "sit-and-reach" test. Research studies have confirmed that declines in flexibility are not as evident in individuals who maintain regular patterns of physical activity. The use of planned stretching programs has also been shown to help maintain flexibility with age.

Gender differences exist in flexibility. Girls tend to be more flexible than boys at young ages, but the gender difference decreases for adults. Greater flexibility of females is generally attributed to anatomical differences (e.g., wider hips) and hormonal influences.

Genetic factors can explain some individual variability in flexibility. In some families, the trait for loose joints is passed from generation to generation. This **hypermobility** is sometimes referred to as joint looseness. Studies show that people with this trait may be more prone to joint dislocation. There is not much research evidence, but some experts believe that those with hypermobility may also be more susceptible to athletic or dance injuries, especially to the knee, ankle, and shoulder, and may be more apt to develop premature osteoarthritis.

TECHNOLOGY UPDATE

Software Facilitates Stretching at Work
Millions of people have sedentary office jobs that require them to be at their desk all day, which isn't good for your body. New computer software may help address this problem. One commercially available program generates a series of pop-up reminders that prompt you to periodically move or take stretching breaks during the day. The user can control the frequency of the prompts; but if you skip the recommended prompt, an animated avatar delivers a stronger message encouraging you to take a break. The theory behind these tools is that the periodic prompts and reminders will help encourage workers to take brief stretch breaks to break up computer/sedentary time and reduce risk of repetitive motion injuries and fatigue,.

What impact would this type of tool have on your daily activity pattern?

connect
ACTIVITY

Lack of use or misuse can cause reductions in flexibility. Lack of physical activity is one of the major factors contributing to poor flexibility. When muscles are moved as part of normal daily activities or during structured physical activity, the muscles and tendons get stretched. Without this regular stimulation, flexibility will decrease.

Improper exercise can lead to muscle imbalances that may negatively impact flexibility. The most common example is when body builders overdevelop their biceps in comparison to their triceps. This leads to a *muscle-bound* look characterized by a restricted range of motion in the elbow joint. To avoid this, it is important to exercise muscles through the full range of motion.

Health Benefits of Flexibility and Stretching

Adequate flexibility is necessary for achieving and maintaining optimal posture and movement patterns. Good posture implies that the body's segments are well-aligned for efficient function and the least amount of strain. Poor posture, on the other hand, places body segments at a biomechanical disadvantage, adding stress and strain to the body with eventual wear and tear on the joints and tendons. In many cases, poor posture occurs over time due to poor habits. Sensory receptors in the skin and joints appear to maintain poor posture through feedback loops within the nervous system. The nervous system keeps some muscles overly active and "tight" and others overly quiet or "weak." This feedback loop reinforces the muscle imbalance and the poor posture—long/weak muscles on one side of the body are countered by muscles on the opposite side of the body which are too short/tight. Postural correction begins by improving the flexibility of the shortened muscles, followed by strengthening of the "weak" muscles, and finally use of improved body awareness.

Good flexibility and posture are also important for optimal movement patterns of the limbs and trunk. When good flexibility and posture are sacrificed, movement patterns can be adversely affected, resulting in joint motion that is either too restricted or too excessive. Poor movement patterns add stress and strain to adjoining joint structures, leading to possible damage of the joints or tendons. For example, motion of the shoulder is adversely affected by a slouched posture. The arm can be raised further over the head from an upright posture than a slouched posture. To develop and maintain good posture and movement patterns, muscles must have sufficient flexibility and appropriate levels of strength. Additional information on posture and back care is presented in Concept 11.

Flexibility contributes to functional fitness, which has been shown to provide protection against risks for injury. Many people stretch before exercise because they believe it is important for reducing the likelihood of getting injured. A good warm-up probably helps to prepare the body for exercise, but the consensus in the literature is that stretching does not reduce the risks for musculotendinous injuries. However, this may be an oversimplification. A recent study showed considerable individual variability in effects. People that currently stretched were at greater risk of injury if they stopped stretching. People that never stretched were at greater risk of injury if they started stretching. (See In the News for details on this study).

While stretching may not directly impact risk of injury, research is accumulating on the importance of flexibility for overall injury prevention. In this recent work, flexibility is a key contributor to a broader construct of functional fitness which also incorporates core strength, balance, and agility. Several different *functional movement* batteries have been developed to identify individuals that may have poor levels of functional fitness. The screening assessments typically score individuals based upon the quality of motion during basic functional movement tasks, each requiring a combination of strength, balance, dynamic, and/or static flexibility. The screening movements are used to identify asymmetries and functional limitations that may predispose people to injury. Studies have shown the utility of these tests for predicting risks of injuries in football players, firefighters, and military personnel. They have not been widely used for preventive health screens, but this will likely follow. Detailed information about functional fitness would allow clinicians and health and fitness professionals to design effective interventions and track progress over time.

Stretching is used to assist in rehabilitation from injuries and for prevention. Physical therapists and athletic trainers frequently prescribe stretching to help patients regain normal range of motion or function or to reduce pain after injury. Typical injuries include muscle strains, ligamentous sprains, and open wounds. Joint stiffness is also a common problem following surgery to the shoulder, knee, and ankle or following immobilization of any fracture in a cast or walking boot. In each case, gentle stretching and range of motion exercises are used to stimulate the healing process and add strength to the healing tissues. Prior to stretching, tissues are warmed up through the use of active exercise, massage techniques, or modalities such as moist heat or ultrasound. Stretching is followed by exercises to increase strength within

HELP **Health is available to Everyone for a Lifetime, and it's Personal**

The concept of *functional fitness* has generated considerable interest among health and fitness professionals. Many fitness centers offer group classes focused on improving functional fitness and these courses typically involve flexibility and functional movement tasks.

Do you believe that flexibility and functional fitness provide important benefits to your health now or do you think the benefits may be more relevant as you age? How does this influence your current views about stretching and flexibility exercise?

Hypermobility Looseness or slackness in the joint and of the muscles and ligaments (soft tissue) surrounding the joint.

In the News

Changing Your Stretching Routine May Impact Your Injury Risk

You may think that stretching prior to exercise reduces the risk of injury, but research doesn't necessarily support this. A recent study followed more than 2,000 runners to examine the impact of stretching on injury. Participants were assigned to one of four groups: those who *continued* with their normal pre-run routine (maintaining an existing pattern of either stretching or nonstretching) and those who *altered* their normal pre-run routine (adding or deleting stretching to the existing routine). Interestingly, the groups that were asked to alter their normal

pre-run routines (performing or not performing stretching) demonstrated an increased risk of injury by 40 percent. Those that continued their normal pre-run routine (whatever it was) had no increased risk for injury. This suggests that people may accommodate to stretching and that need for (and response to) pre-exercise stretching may vary across individuals.

Does this finding change your opinion of whether you should stretch prior to exercise? Why or why not?

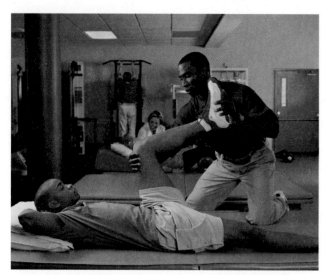

Physical therapists and athletic trainers use carefully planned stretching exercise for treatment.

the newly-gained range of motion and neuromuscular activities to restore functional movement patterns. Physical therapists and athletic trainers prescribe stretching to assist in rehabilitation and recovery, but it is up to the patient to perform the recommended stretching exercises.

Stretching may contribute to treatment of musculoskeletal pain. Stretching is often one component of a larger treatment plan for addressing low back and neck pain, muscle strains, and joint stiffness post surgery or following immobilization. Because it is rarely used as the sole treatment approach, it is difficult to isolate its effectiveness from other treatments commonly provided. However, it has been shown to be as effective as strengthening or massage in the treatment of chronic neck pain. Additionally, movement-based activities such as tai chi have been shown to facilitate movement and reduce low back pain.

Stretching may help relieve muscle cramps and pain associated with myofascial trigger points. Many people experience some form of muscle cramping during exercise. A muscle spasm or cramp may result for various reasons, including overexertion, dehydration, and heat stress. Stretching a cramped (but not a strained) muscle will often help relieve the cramp. We have less understanding of myofascial **trigger points,** but they are typically more painful than cramps. They are characterized by taut bands within skeletal muscle that have a nodular texture. They are sensitive to touch and can produce a radiating pain in specific regions of the body when touched. Trigger points can be caused by trauma, or occur after overuse or from prolonged spasm in the muscles. The application of direct pressure on myofascial trigger points followed by stretching has been shown to help relieve pain. However, stretching has less effect on relieving nonspecific areas of soft tissue tenderness in the body (often referred to as tender points).

Stretching is probably *ineffective* in preventing muscle soreness. In the past, it was suggested that stretching during a cool-down will *prevent* muscular soreness. In a controlled study, however, muscle soreness was deliberately induced in a group of subjects. When half of the group stretched immediately afterward and at intervals for 48 hours, they had as much soreness as the group who did not stretch. While studies have shown limited effects of stretching on reducing soreness, it is still a useful part of an overall cool-down routine following exercise.

Good flexibility can be beneficial to one's ability to function effectively at work and in daily life. Lack of joint range of motion can negatively affect one's ability to perform tasks at work and daily activities such as driving a car. It is well documented that as people grow older their range of motion in the neck decreases resulting in reduced ability to turn the head and effectively anticipate movements to the side and rear of the car. 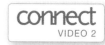 Reduced range of motion can also increase risk of accidents in automobiles and around the home. Regular stretching is important to everyday functioning in a variety of settings.

Stretching Methods

Static stretching is the safest and most commonly used method of stretching. Static stretching is done slowly and held for a period of several seconds. The probability of tearing the soft tissue is low if performed properly. Static stretches can be performed with **active assistance** or with **passive assistance**. When active

---

Trigger Points Especially irritable spots, usually tight bands or knots in a muscle or fascia (a sheath of connective tissue that binds muscles and other tissues together). Trigger points often refer pain to another area of the body.

Active Assistance An assist to stretch from an active contraction of the opposing (antagonist) muscle.

Passive Assistance Stretch imposed on a muscle with the assistance of a force other than the opposing muscle.

Contrasting Three Methods of Stretching

I. Static Stretch

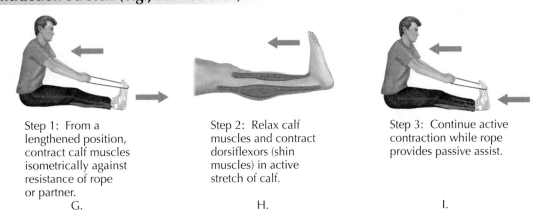

Active
A.

Passive
(Self Assisted)
B.

Passive
(Gravity Assisted)
C.

II. Dynamic Stretch

Active
D.

Passive
(Partner Assisted)
E.

Passive
(Gravity Assisted)
F.

III. Pre-Contraction Stretch (e.g., PNF Stretch)

Step 1: From a lengthened position, contract calf muscles isometrically against resistance of rope or partner.
G.

Step 2: Relax calf muscles and contract dorsiflexors (shin muscles) in active stretch of calf.
H.

Step 3: Continue active contraction while rope provides passive assist.
I.

Figure 2 ▶ Examples of static, dynamic, and pre-contraction stretches of the calf muscles (gastronemius and soleus). Muscles shown in dark pink are the muscles being contracted. Muscles shown in light pink are those being stretched.

assistance is used, the opposing muscle group is contracted to produce a reflex relaxation **(reciprocal inhibition)** in the muscle being stretched. This enables the muscle to be more easily stretched. For example, when doing a calf stretch exercise (see Figure 2A, page 205), the muscles on the front of the shin are contracted to assist in the stretch of the muscles of the calf. However, active assistance to static stretching has one problem. It is almost impossible to produce adequate overload by simply contracting the opposing muscles.

When passive assistance (see Figure 2B, C) is used, an outside force, such as a partner, aids in the stretching. For example, in the calf stretch, passive assistance can be provided by another person, another body part (Figure 2B), or gravity (Figure 2C). This type of stretch does not create the relaxation in the muscle associated with active assisted stretch. An unrelaxed muscle cannot be stretched as far, and injury may happen. Therefore, it is best to combine the active assistance with a passive assistance when performing a static stretch. This gives the advantage of a relaxed muscle and a sufficient force to provide an overload to stretch it.

A good way to begin static stretching exercises is to stretch until tension is first felt, back off slightly and hold the position several seconds, and then gradually stretch a little farther, back off, and hold. Decrease the stretch slowly after the hold.

Dynamic stretching can be safe and effective if performed properly. Dynamic stretching uses gradual and controlled movement of body parts up to the limit of a joint's range of motion. Stretches may involve arm or leg swings of increasing reach or increasing speed. The key is to perform the movement in a controlled manner through the normal range of motion. This approach allows dynamic stretching to be a safe and efficient means

of using active stretching techniques. As with static stretching, the movement can be provided either actively or passively. For example, in the calf stretch shown in Figure 2D, E, and F, the foot is actively bounced forward by the antagonist muscle force or passively by an assist from another person or gravity. Dynamic stretching movements are common in many functional fitness programs and hybrid exercise classes.

Ballistic stretching is a specific type of dynamic stretching but it presents risks if not done properly. A **ballistic stretch** uses momentum to stretch the muscles up to (and beyond) their normal range of motion. Momentum is produced by a more vigorous body motion, such as flinging a body part (bobbing) or rocking it back and forth to create a bouncing movement. The inherent problem with most ballistic stretching is lack of control over the force and range of movement. The forceful movement in ballistic stretching may increase risks for injury. Ballistic stretching may be useful for some athletes who do sports that involve ballistic movements; however, this form of stretching is not recommended for most people.

Pre-contraction stretching activities such as PNF have proven to be most effective at improving flexibility. Proprioceptive neuromuscular facilitation (PNF) stretching utilizes techniques to stimulate muscles to contract more strongly (and relax more fully) in order to enhance the effectiveness of stretching. The contract-relax-antagonist-contract (CRAC) technique is the most popular. CRAC PNF involves three specific steps: (1) Move the limb so the muscle to be stretched is elongated initially; then contract it (agonist muscle) isometrically for several seconds (against an immovable object or the resistance of a partner); (2) relax the muscle; and (3) immediately stati- 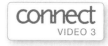 cally stretch the muscle with the active assistance of the antagonist muscle and an assist from a partner, gravity, or another body part. Figure 2G, H, and I provide a detailed illustration of how this technique is applied to the calf stretch. Research shows that this and other types of PNF stretch are more effective than a simple static stretch.

How Much Stretch Is Enough?

The appropriate amount of flexibility for health is not known. Flexibility is joint specific, so the amount of flexibility varies by joint. Norms are available for the amount of flexibility for males and females of different ages, but it is not clear how much is needed for health. For example, there is little scientific evidence to indicate that a person who can reach 2 inches past his or her toes on a sit-and-reach test is less fit (or healthy) than a person who

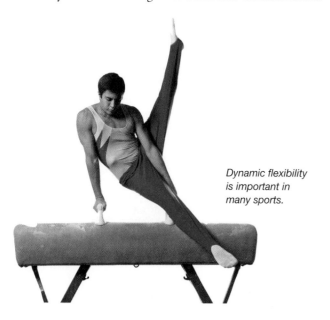

Dynamic flexibility is important in many sports.

can reach 8 inches past the toes. The standards presented in the *Lab Resource Materials* are based on the best available evidence.

Too much flexibility (hyperflexibility) in a joint may increase susceptibility to injury. While an appropriate amount of flexibility is beneficial, too much flexibility can compromise the integrity of the joint and make it less stable and prone to injury. Most muscles and tendons can lengthen (extensibility) and return to their normal length after appropriate stretching (elasticity). However, short, tight muscles and tendons can be easily overstretched (strained). Even more likely to be injured are the ligaments that connect bone to bone. Ligaments and the joint capsule lack the elasticity and tensile strength of the muscles and tendons. When involuntarily overstretched, they may remain in a lengthened state or become ruptured (sprained). If this occurs, the joint loses stability and is susceptible to chronic dislocation, repeated sprains, and excessive wear and tear of the joint surface. This is particularly true of weight-bearing joints, such as the hip, knee, and ankle. Appropriate

stretching techniques can increase flexibility without leading to hyperflexibility.

Specific FIT guidelines are established for safe and effective stretching. Lifestyle and cardiovascular activity do little to develop flexibility. To build this important part of fitness, stretching exercises from step 5 of the pyramid are essential (see Figure 3). The American College of Sports Medicine (ACSM) recently released new guidelines for effective stretching. The guidelines indicate that stretching can be done using static stretches

Reciprocal Inhibition Reflex relaxation in stretched muscle during contraction of the antagonist.

Ballistic Stretch Bouncing or bobbing to facilitate lengthening of the muscle-tendon unit.

Proprioceptive Neuromuscular Facilitation (PNF) A stretching technique that incorporates muscle contraction prior to stretch.

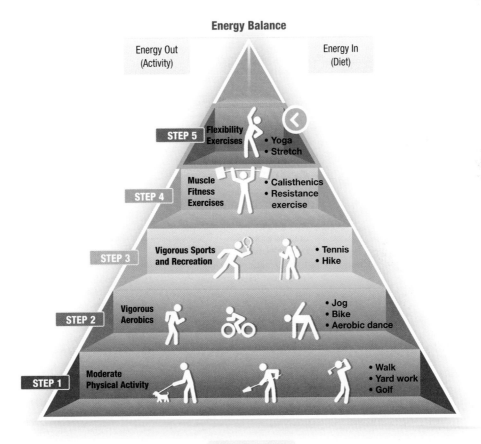

Figure 3 ▶ Flexibility or stretching exercises should be selected from step 5 of the physical activity pyramid.
Source: C. B. Corbin

(active or passive), dynamic stretches, or pre-contraction stretches. The recommended threshold and target zones for safe and effective stretching are provided in Table 1. The threshold of training refers to the minimum amount of stretching required to make gains and/or maintain a level of flexibility. Target zone refers to the overload needed to make significant gains in flexibility or to progress one's level of flexibility following a plateau.

Stretching should ideally be performed at least 2 to 3 days a week (frequency). The ACSM guidelines suggest that 2 to 3 days are effective for increasing range of motion, but they point out that gains are greater if performed daily. However, like other forms of exercise, 1 day a week is still better than none. The ACSM guidelines emphasize that stretching is most effective when the muscles are warm. Performing a light to moderate aerobic warm-up activity prior to stretching can increase internal muscle temperature and the extensibility of soft tissues, allowing for a more effective stretch. Since some people do not want to interrupt their workout in the middle, they prefer to stretch at the end. Stretching at the end of the workout serves a dual purpose—building flexibility and cooling down. It is, however, appropriate to stretch at any time in the workout after the muscles

have been active and are warm. If you prefer to include it at the beginning of a workout, ease into the stretching gradually.

To increase the length of a muscle, stretch it more than its normal length but do not overstretch it (intensity). The best evidence suggests that muscles should be stretched to about 10 percent beyond their normal length to bring about an improvement in flexibility. More practical indicators of the intensity of stretching are to stretch just to the point of tension or just before discomfort. Exercises that do not cause an overload will not increase flexibility. Once adequate flexibility has been achieved, **range of motion (ROM) exercises** that do not require stretch greater than normal can be performed to maintain flexibility and joint range of motion.

To increase flexibility, stretch and hold muscles beyond normal length for an adequate amount of time (intensity). When a muscle is stretched (lengthened), the stretch reflex acts to resist the stretch (see Figure 4). Sensory receptors (A) in the muscle-tendon unit send a signal to the sensory neurons (B), and these neurons signal the motor neurons (C) to contract (shorten) the muscles (D). This reflex restricts initial

Table 1 ▶ FIT Formula for Stretching—Thresholds and Target Zones

	Static		Ballistic		PNF (CRAC)	
	Threshold	Target	Threshold	Target	Threshold	Target
Frequency	At least 2 to 3 days a week (threshold)	2–7 days a week	At least 2 to 3 days a week (threshold)	2–7 days a week	At least 2 to 3 days a week (threshold)	2–7 days a week
Intensity	Stretch to the point of feeling tightness or slight discomfort. Holding a static stretch for 10–30 seconds is recommended for most adults. In older persons, holding a stretch for 30–60 seconds may give greater benefit.	Add passive assistance. Avoid overstretching or pain.	Stretch beyond normal length with gentle bounce or swing. Do not exceed 10% of static range of motion.	Same as ballistic threshold	Use a 3- to 6-second contraction at 20%–75% maximum voluntary contraction followed by a 10- to 30-second assisted stretch.	Perform 4–5 reps with 6-second contractions, each followed by a 10–30-second assisted stretch. Thirty seconds between reps.
Time	Perform 2 repetitions. Hold each for 15 seconds. Rest 30 seconds between reps.	Perform 3-4 repetitions. Hold each for 15–60 seconds. Rest 30 seconds between reps.	Perform 1 set involving 30 continuous seconds.	Perform 2–3 sets of 30 consecutive seconds of motion. Rest 1 minute between sets.	Perform 2 repetitions. Thirty seconds between reps.	Perform 3-4 repetitions. Rest 30 seconds between reps. Rest 1 minute between sets.

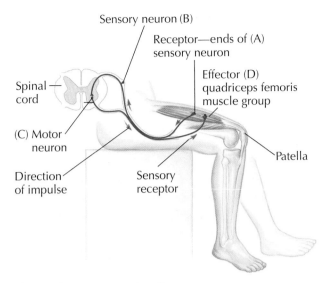

Figure 4 ▶ The stretch reflex.
Source: Shier, Butler, and Lewis.

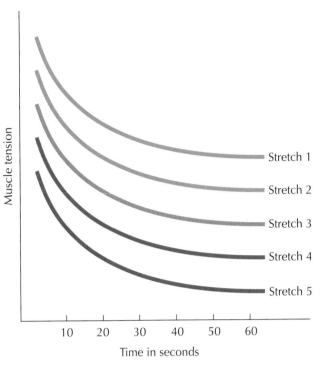

Figure 5 ▶ Typical responses to a stretched muscle during a series of stretches.

efforts at stretching; however, if the stretch is held and maintained over time, the stretch reflex subsides and allows the muscle to lengthen (this phase is called the development phase because this is when improvements occur). Neurological evidence documenting the activation of the stretch reflex during stretching is not available, but the reflex mechanism clearly explains why it is important to hold a stretch for an extended period of time. Attempts to stretch for shorter durations are limited by the opposing action of the opposing muscles (see Figure 4). Guidelines suggest that to get the most benefit for the least effort stretches should be held between 10 and 30 seconds. The ACSM suggests that 10 seconds may be an adequate threshold when performing PNF (stretch after muscle contraction).

To increase flexibility, repeat stretching exercises an adequate number of times (time). Figure 5 shows the typical responses to a stretched muscle during a series of stretches. Tension in a muscle decreases as the stretch is held. Most of the decrease occurs in the first 15 seconds. The tension curves are lower with each successive repetition of stretching, which is why multiple sets of stretching are recommended. The ACSM recommends 2–4 reps but, as shown in Figure 5, up to 5 reps can be beneficial.

Principles of overload and progression can be applied to a regular stretching program to both improve and maintain flexibility. Threshold of training refers to the minimum amount of stretching required to make gains and/or maintain a level of flexibility. Target zone refers to the overload needed to make significant

gains in flexibility or to progress one's level of flexibility following a plateau. There are no accepted guidelines for scientifically progressing stretching exercises, but the principles of overload and specificity described for muscle fitness would apply. Principles of threshold and target zones are presented in Table 1 for each type of stretching.

Regular stretching exercise (based on the FIT guidelines) leads to improved range of motion, but the mechanisms of action are not completely understood. As previously described, the increases in muscle length and reductions in stiffness immediately following stretching are temporary. However, regular stretching does lead to improvements in flexibility. Many scientists believe that the resulting gains in motion following stretching are due as much to sensory changes in the nervous system as to increased muscle length or reduced muscle stiffness. According to the theory, stretching leads to increases in **stretch tolerance** which causes people to perceive discomfort at greater ranges of motion.

Range of Motion (ROM) Exercises Exercises used to maintain existing joint mobility (to prevent loss of ROM).

Stretch Tolerance Greater stretch for the same pain level.

For example, an individual that regularly performs stretches for tight hamstring muscles may see improvements in range of motion during a straight leg raise. The sensory theory explains that much of the improvement in range of motion is due to a change in sensation. In other words, the perceived onset of pain is now further toward the end range of motion. The sensory theory has also been used to explain individual differences in flexibility. Persons that are hypermobile or very flexible may not have longer muscles or looser joints but rather perceive the physical limits later in the arc of motion.

Flexibility-Based Activities

The popularity of flexibility-based activity has increased in recent years. A recent survey of Worldwide Fitness Trends indicates that of the 20 top trends, 6 relate to flexibility. Included are yoga, functional fitness training, special training for older adults, core training, Pilates, and sport-specific training. Data from the Sporting Goods Manufacturers Association (SGMA) also indicates that yoga and tai chi are among the fastest growing activities. The popularity of these activities suggests that people may be more interested in flexibility-related activity when it is presented in an engaging and interactive format. Some of the growth may also be attributed to increased acceptance of these activities by medical professionals. Distinctions between these activities are provided below.

Tai chi is one of the safest and more established movement disciplines. Tai chi (often translated as Chinese shadow boxing) is considered a martial art but involves the execution of slow, flowing movements called "forms." Numerous studies have supported the benefits of tai chi on a variety of health-related parameters, including flexibility, muscular strength, balance, posture, pain relief, stress, weight reduction, and cardiovascular fitness. Recent studies have shown that tai chi can be particularly useful for people with arthritis, strengthening muscles by using both isometric (holding) and isotonic (moving) muscle contractions. Studies have shown strength gains of 15 to 20 percent in elderly tai chi participants. This improved strength translates into joint protection and stability, as well as increased strength for daily living tasks. The highly cited FICSIT study demonstrated significant benefits of tai chi on balance and risk of falls in the elderly. Young participants can benefit as well.

Yoga is a diverse and controversial movement discipline. *Yoga* is an umbrella term that refers to a number of yoga traditions. The foundation for most

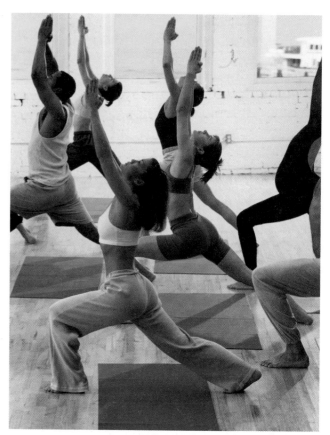

Yoga and other movement classes involving stretching are increasingly popular.

yoga traditions is hatha yoga, which incorporates a variety of asanas (postures). Iyengar yoga is another popular variation. It uses similar asanas as hatha yoga but uses props and cushions to enhance the movements. Emphasis is placed on balance through coordinated breathing and precise body alignment. Most forms of yoga are considered to be safe, but positions in some of the extreme yoga disciplines have been criticized by movement specialists and physical therapists as causing more harm than good, so care should be used when performing some movements. Evidence for health benefits of yoga are not as established as those for tai chi.

Pilates classes are a popular offering at many fitness centers and health clubs. Pilates is a therapeutic exercise regimen that combines strength and flexibility movements. It was originally developed as more of a therapeutic form of exercise, but it is increasingly being promoted as an overall form of conditioning. Emphasis in Pilates exercise is on core stabilization movements and enhanced body awareness, but classes typically include some stretching activities as well.

Check the qualifications of instructors conducting flexibility-related classes. The popularity of flexibility exercise has led to an increasing array of classes, videos, and resources available for tai chi, yoga, and Pilates. When reviewing these programs and materials, keep in mind that presently there is not a strong scientific basis for yoga and Pilates programming. When performed safely with a qualified instructor, they probably can be beneficial. However, many of the positions and movements may be contraindicated exercises that could increase risk for injuries. If you choose to participate in these activities, seek qualified instructors and progress gradually. See Concept 11 for more information about safe and contraindicated exercises.

Guidelines for Safe and Effective Stretching Exercise

There is a correct way to perform flexibility exercises. Remember that stretching can *cause* muscle soreness, so "easy does it." Start at your threshold if you are unaccustomed to stretching a given muscle group; then increase within the target zone. The list in Table 2 will help you gain the most benefit from your exercises.

Stretching is specific to each muscle or muscle group. No single exercise can produce total flexibility. For example, stretching tight hamstrings can increase the length of these muscles but will not lengthen the muscles in other areas of the body. For total flexibility, it is important to stretch each of the major muscle groups and to use the major joints of the body through full range of normal motion.

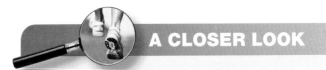

A CLOSER LOOK

Potent Health Benefits from Tai Chi

Tai chi can improve flexibility, improve balance, improve lower leg strength, improve immune capacity, build bone density, reduce fall risk, improve cardiovascular function, reduce stress, and improve quality of life. The evidence for most health outcomes has been substantiated in well-controlled clinical trials. Interestingly, scientists really don't have a good sense of how tai chi works to improve these outcomes. The movements are very slow and controlled, so it is likely that the effects are related in part to the concentration and focus required to execute the various movements rather than the movements themselves.

In what ways could you benefit from tai chi?

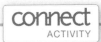
connect ACTIVITY

Table 2 ▶ Do and Don't List for Stretching

Do	Don't
Do warm muscles before you attempt to stretch them.	Don't stretch to the point of pain. Remember, you want to stretch muscles, not joints.
Do stretch with care if you have osteoporosis or arthritis.	Don't use ballistic stretches if you have osteoporosis or arthritis.
Do use static or PNF stretching rather than ballistic stretching if you are a beginner.	Don't perform ballistic stretches with passive assistance unless you are under the supervision of an expert.
Do stretch weak or recently injured muscles with care.	Don't ballistically stretch weak or recently injured muscles.
Do use great care in applying passive assistance to a partner; go slowly and ask for feedback.	Don't overstretch a muscle after it has been immobilized (such as in a sling or cast) for a long period.
Do perform stretching exercises for each muscle group and at each joint where flexibility is desired.	Don't bounce muscles through excessive range of motion. Begin ballistic stretching with gentle movements and gradually increase intensity.
Do make certain the body is in good alignment when stretching.	Don't stretch swollen joints without professional supervision.
Do stretch muscles of small joints in the extremities first; then progress toward the trunk with muscles of larger joints.	Don't stretch several muscles at one time until you have stretched individual muscles. For example, stretch muscles at the ankle, then the knee, then the ankle and knee simultaneously.

A flexibility workout should be done when the body is warmed up and when adequate time is available to perform stretching exercises. As noted in Concept 3, stretching can be done as one part of a comprehensive warm-up routine. While a warm-up may have benefits, stretching before exercise is not a substitute for a regular stretching program to build flexibility. If you are not flexible and have short muscles, a single warm-up cannot make you flexible. Regular stretching is needed to see improvements in flexibility.

connect
VIDEO 4

The consensus is that stretching exercise is most effective when the body is already warmed up. For this reason, some people prefer to perform their stretching routine at the end of a workout when muscles are warm. Others prefer to perform their flexibility workout at a time when they can concentrate specifically on building flexibility. In either case, sufficient time should be allowed to ensure that the exercises are done correctly.

Specialized equipment may help improve the effectiveness and ease of stretching exercise. One advance in equipment technology for flexibility training is the development of "stretching ropes." These ropes have multiple loops, which enable individuals to change the length of the rope and perform a variety of different exercises. This feature provides an easy way to put muscles on stretch and to vary the degree of stretch. Because you can apply resistance through the elastic straps, it is even possible to perform PNF stretching without the assistance of a partner. A variety of stretching ropes are available on the market, and they all provide similar functionality.

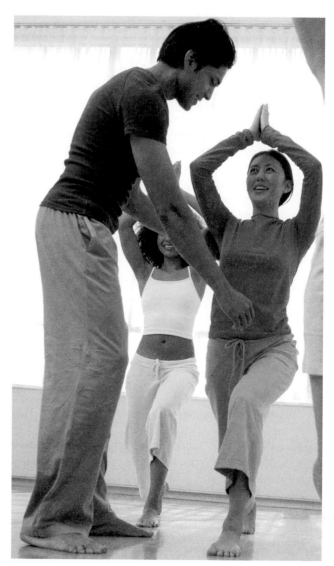

To get the most out of yoga, tai chi, and Pilates classes, find a qualified instructor.

Strategies for Action

An important step for developing and maintaining flexibility is assessing your current status. There are dozens of tests of flexibility. Four tests that assess range of motion in the major joints of the body, that require little equipment, and that can be easily administered are presented in the *Lab Resources Materials* at the end of this concept. In Lab 10A, you will get an opportunity to try these self-assessments. Perform these assessments before you begin your regular stretching program and use these assessments to reevaluate your flexibility periodically.

Scores on flexibility tests may be influenced by several factors. Your range of motion at any one time may be influenced by your motivation to exert maximum effort, warm-up preparation, muscular soreness, tolerance for pain, room temperature, and ability to relax. Recent studies have found a relationship between leg or trunk length and the scores made on the sit-and-reach test. The sit-and-reach test used in this book is adapted to allow for differences in body build.

Select exercises that promote flexibility in all areas of the body. For total body flexibility, 8 to 10 stretching exercises for the major muscle groups of the body are recommended. Table 3 describes some of the most effective exercises for a basic flexibility routine. Individual stretching needs may vary, but the most common areas to target are the trunk, the legs, and the arms. A variety of stretches for these areas are described in Tables 3, 4, and 5. Most are designed for static stretching, but the pectoral stretch and back-saver hamstring stretch use PNF techniques. Ballistic stretching exercises are discussed in more detail in Concept 12.

Keeping records of progress will help you adhere to a stretching program. An activity logging sheet is provided in Lab 10B to help you keep records of your progress as you regularly perform stretching exercises to build and maintain good flexibility.

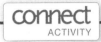

Web Resources

Functional Movement.com (functional fitness information)
www.Functionalmovement.com
Gray Institute (information on functional fitness) **www .Grayinstitute.com**
National Center for Complementary and Alternative Medicine
http://nccam.nih.gov/

Suggested Readings

ACSM. 2010. *ACSM's Guidelines for Exercise Testing and Prescription.* 8th ed. Philadelphia: Lippincott, Williams & Wilkins, Chapter 7.

Kay, A. D., and A. Blazevich. J. 2011. Effect of acute static stretch on maximal muscle performance: A systematic review. *Medicine and Science in Sports and Exercise.* Available at **www.ncbi.nlm.nih.gov/pubmed/21659901**

Kiesel, K., P. Plisky, and M. Voight. 2007. Can serious injury in professional football be predicted by a preseason functional movement screen? *North American Journal of Sports and Physical Therapy* 2(3):147–150.

Kovacs, M. 2009. *Dynamic Stretching: The Revolutionary New Warm-up Method to Improve Power, Performance and Range of Motion.* Berkeley, CA: Ulysses Press.

McAttee, R., and J. Charland. 2011. *Facilitated Stretching.* 4th ed. Champaign, IL: Human Kinetics. (iPad version with video)

O'Connor, F. G., et al. 2011. Functional Movement Screening: Predicting Injuries in Officer Candidates. *Medicine and Science in Sports and Exercise* 43(12):2224–2230.

Page, P. 2012. Current concepts in muscle stretching for exercise and rehabilitation. *The International Journal of Sports Physical Therapy* 7(1):109–118.

Pereles, D., A. Roth, and D. J. S. Thompson. 2010. A large, randomized, prospective study of the impact of a pre-run stretch on the risk of injury in teenage and older runners. *USA Track and Field.* **http://www.usatf.org/stretchStudy/StretchStudyReport.pdf**

Thompson, W. R. (2011). Worldwide survey of fitness trends for 2012. *ACSM's Health and Fitness Journal* 15(6):9–18.

Weppler, C. H., and S. P. Magnusson. 2010. Increasing muscle extensibility: A matter of increasing length or modifying sensation? *Physical Therapy* 90(3):438–450.

Yeh, G. Y., et al. 2011. Tai chi exercise in patients with chronic heart failure: A randomized clinical trial. *Archives of Internal Medicine* 171(8):750–757.

Healthy People 2020

The objectives listed below are societal goals designed to help all Americans improve their health between now and the year 2020. They were selected because they relate to the content of this concept.

- Increase proportion of people who regularly perform exercises for flexibility.

- Reduce sports and recreation injuries.

- Reduce percentage of adults who do no leisure-time activity.

- Increase access to employee-based exercise facilities and programs.

A national goal is to increase the proportion of people who regularly perform flexibility exercises. Why is flexibility exercise often not prioritized in an exercise program, even by regular exercisers? What specific benefits would you gain from flexibility exercise?

Table 3 The Basic Eight for Trunk Stretching Exercises

1. Upper Trapezius/Neck Stretch

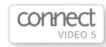

This exercise stretches the muscles on the back and sides of the neck. To stretch the right trapezius, place left hand on top of your head. Gently look down toward your left underarm, tucking your chin toward your chest. Let the weight of your arm gently draw your head forward. Hold. Repeat to the opposite side.

Variations: The stretch above may be modified to stretch the muscles on the front and sides of the neck. Start from the stretch position described above. Keep your left ear near your left shoulder. Turn your head slightly and look up toward the ceiling, lifting your chin 2–3″. Hold.

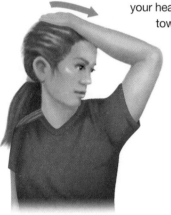

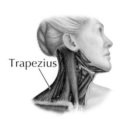

Trapezius

2. Chin Tuck

This exercise stretches the muscles at the base of the skull and reduces headache symptoms. Sit up straight, with chest lifted and shoulders back. Gently tuck in the chin by making a slight motion of nodding "yes." Imagine a string attached to the back of your head, which is pulling your head upward, like a puppet. As your chin draws inward, attempt to lengthen the back of your neck. Hold.

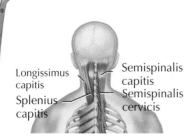

Longissimus capitis
Splenius capitis
Semispinalis capitis
Semispinalis cervicis

3. Pectoral Stretch

This exercise stretches the chest muscles (pectorals).

1. Stand erect in doorway, with arms raised 45 degrees, elbows bent, hands grasping the doorjamb, and feet in front-stride position. Press out on door frame, contracting your arms maximally for 6 seconds. Relax and shift weight forward on legs. Lean into doorway, so that the muscles on the front of your shoulder joint and chest are stretched. Hold.
2. Repeat with your arms raised 90 degrees.
3. Repeat with your arms raised 135 degrees. This exercise is useful to prevent or correct round shoulders and sunken chest.

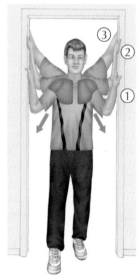

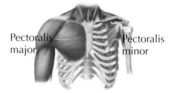

Pectoralis major
Pectoralis minor

4. Lateral Trunk Stretch

This exercise stretches the trunk muscles. Sit on the floor. Stretch the left arm over your head, to the right. Bend to the right at the waist, reaching as far to the right as possible with your left arm and as far as possible to the left with your right arm; hold. Do not let your trunk rotate. Repeat on the opposite side. For less stretch, your overhead arm may be bent at the elbow. This exercise can be done in the standing position, but is less effective.

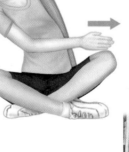

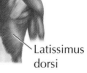

Latissimus dorsi

214

5. Leg Hug

This exercise stretches the hip and back extensor muscles. Lie on your back. Bend one leg and grasp your thigh under the knee. Hug it to your chest. Keep the other leg straight and on the floor. Hold. Repeat with the opposite leg.

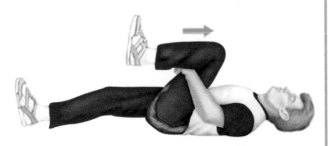

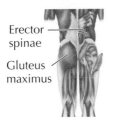

Erector
spinae

Gluteus
maximus

7. Trunk Twist

This exercise stretches the trunk muscles and the muscles on the outside of the hip. Sit with your right leg extended, left leg bent and crossed over the right knee. Place your right arm on the left side of the left leg and push against that leg while turning the trunk as far as possible to the left. Place the left hand on the floor behind the buttocks. Stretch and hold. Reverse position and repeat on the opposite side.

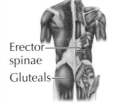

Erector
spinae
Gluteals

6. Heel Sit

This exercise stretches the muscles of the lower back. Begin on hands and knees with eyes looking down toward the floor. Keep your hands on the floor directly below your shoulders. Rock backwards, bringing your buttocks toward your heels. Gently round the lower back outward. Hold.

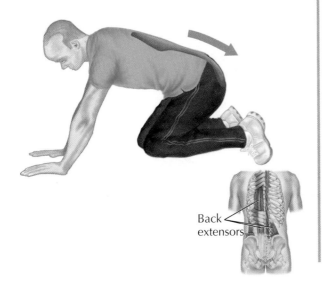

Back
extensors

8. Spine Twist

This exercise stretches the trunk rotators and lateral rotators of the thighs. Start in hook-lying position, arms extended at shoulder level. Cross your left knee over the right. Push the right knee to the floor, using the pressure of the left knee and leg. Keep your arms and shoulders on the floor while touching your knees to the floor on the left. Stretch and hold. Reverse leg position and lower your knees to right.

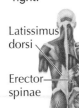

Latissimus
dorsi

Erector
spinae

Gluteus
maximus

Table 3

Table 4 The Basic Eight for Leg Stretching Exercises

Table 4

1. Calf Stretch

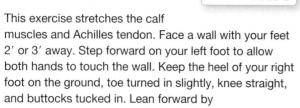

This exercise stretches the calf muscles and Achilles tendon. Face a wall with your feet 2′ or 3′ away. Step forward on your left foot to allow both hands to touch the wall. Keep the heel of your right foot on the ground, toe turned in slightly, knee straight, and buttocks tucked in. Lean forward by bending your front knee and arms and allowing your head to move nearer the wall. Hold. Bend your right knee, keeping your heel on floor. Stretch and hold. Repeat with the other leg.

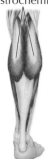

Gastrocnemius

2. Shin Stretch

This exercise relieves shin muscle soreness by stretching the muscles on the front of the shin. Kneel on both knees, turn to the right, and press down and stretch your right ankle with your right hand. Move your pelvis forward. Hold. Repeat on the opposite side. Except when they are sore, most people need to strengthen rather than stretch these muscles.

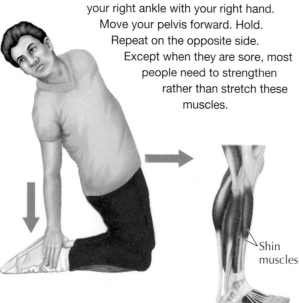

Shin muscles

3. Back-Saver Hamstring Stretch

This exercise stretches the hamstrings and calf muscles and helps prevent or correct backache caused in part by short hamstrings. Sit on the floor with the feet against the wall or an immovable object. Bend left knee and bring foot close to buttocks. Clasp hands behind back. Contract the muscles on the back of the upper leg (hamstrings) by pressing the heel downward toward the floor; hold; relax. Bend forward from hips, keeping lower back as straight as possible. Let bent knee rotate outward so trunk can move forward. Lean forward keeping back flat; hold and repeat on each leg.

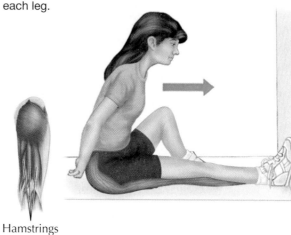

Hamstrings

4. Hip and Thigh Stretch

This exercise stretches the hip (iliopsoas) and thigh muscles (quadriceps) and is useful for people with lordosis and back problems. Place your right knee directly above your right ankle and stretch your left leg backward so your knee touches the floor. If necessary, place your hands on floor for balance.

1. Tilt the pelvis backward by tucking in the abdomen and flattening the back.
2. Then shift the weight forward until a stretch is felt on the front of the thigh; hold. Repeat on the opposite side. Caution: Do not bend your front knee more than 90 degrees.

Iliopsoas

Quadriceps

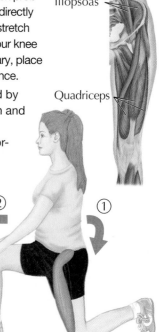

5. Sitting Stretch

This exercise stretches the muscles on the inside of the thighs. Sit with the soles of your feet together; place your hands on your knees or ankles and lean your forearms against your knees; resist (contract) by attempting to raise your knees. Hold. Relax and press the knees toward the floor as far as possible; hold. This exercise is useful for pregnant women and anyone whose thighs tend to rotate inward, causing backache, knock-knees, and flat feet.

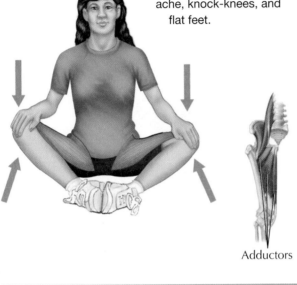

Adductors

6. Lateral Thigh and Hip Stretch

This exercise stretches the muscles and connective tissue on the outside of the legs (iliotibial band and tensor fascia lata). Stand with your left side to the wall, left arm extended and palm of your hand flat on the wall for support. Cross the left leg behind the right leg and turn the toes of both feet out slightly. Bend your left knee slightly and shift your pelvis toward the wall (left) as your trunk bends toward the right. Adjust until tension is felt down the outside of the left hip and thigh. Stretch and hold. Repeat on the other side.

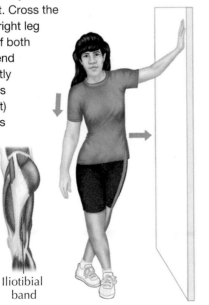

Iliotibial band

7. Inner Thigh Stretch

This exercise stretches the muscles of the inner thigh. Stand with feet spread wider than shoulder-width apart. Shift weight onto the right foot and bend the right knee slightly. Straighten left knee and raise toes of left foot off the floor. Lean forward slightly from the waist keeping back straight/shoulders back. Shift weight back over the right foot by moving hips diagonally away from the left foot. Hold. Repeat in the opposite direction.

Adductors

8. Deep Buttock Stretch

This exercise stretches the deep buttock muscles, such as the piriformis. Lie on your back with knees bent and one ankle crossed over opposite knee. Hold thigh of bottom leg and pull gently toward your chest. Hold. Repeat on the other side.

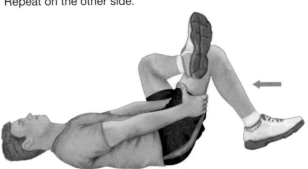

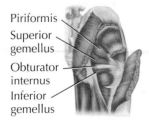

Piriformis
Superior gemellus
Obturator internus
Inferior gemellus

217

Table 5

Table 5 The Basic Four for Arm Stretching Exercises

1. Forearm Stretch

This exercise stretches the muscles on the front and back sides of the lower arm. It is particularly useful in relieving stress from excessive keyboarding activity. Hold your right arm straight out in front, with your palm facing down. Use your left hand to gently stretch the fingertips of your right hand toward the floor. Hold. Turn your right arm over with your palm facing up. Use your left hand to gently stretch the fingertips of your right hand toward the floor. Hold. Repeat on the opposite side.

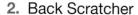

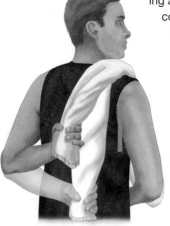

Forearm flexor or extensors

3. Overhead Arm Stretch

This exercise stretches the triceps and latissimus dorsi muscles. Stretch your arms up overhead. Grasp your right elbow with your left hand. Pull your right elbow back behind your head. Hold. Repeat on opposite side.

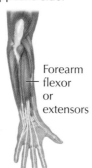

Triceps

Latissimus dorsi

2. Back Scratcher

Stand straight with back of left hand held flat against back. With right hand, throw one end of a towel over right shoulder from front to back. Grab end of towel with left hand. Pull down gently on the towel with right hand, raising arm in back as high as is comfortable. Hold. Repeat to opposite side.

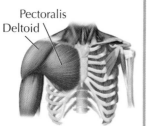

Pectoralis
Deltoid

4. Arm Pretzel

This exercise stretches the shoulder muscles (lateral rotators). Stand or sit with your elbows flexed at right angles, palms up. Cross your right arm over your left; grasp your right thumb with your left hand and pull gently downward, causing your right arm to rotate laterally. Stretch and hold. Reverse arm position and repeat on your left arm.

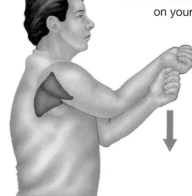

Posterior Cuff

Lab Resource Materials: Flexibility Tests

 VIDEO 7

Directions: To test the flexibility of all joints is impractical. These tests are for joints used frequently. Follow the instructions carefully. Determine your flexibility using Chart 1.

Test

1. *Modified Sit-and-Reach* (Flexibility Test of Hamstrings)

    a. Remove shoes and sit on the floor. Place the sole of the foot of the extended leg flat against a box or bench. Bend opposite knee and place the head, back, and hips against a wall with a 90-degree angle at the hips.

    b. Place one hand over the other and slowly reach forward as far as you can with arms fully extended. Keep head and back in contact with the wall. A partner will slide the measuring stick on the bench until it touches the fingertips.

    c. With the measuring stick fixed in the new position, reach forward as far as possible, three times, holding the position on the third reach for at least 2 seconds while the partner records the distance on the ruler. Keep the knee of the extended leg straight (see illustration).

    d. Repeat the test a second time and average the scores of the two trials.

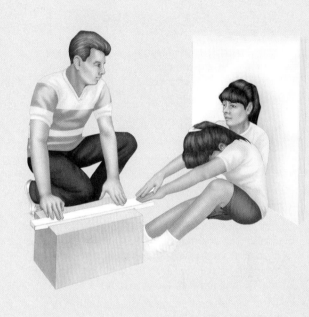

Test

2. *Shoulder Flexibility* ("Zipper" Test)

    a. Raise your arm, bend your elbow, and reach down across your back as far as possible.

    b. At the same time, extend your left arm down and behind your back, bend your elbow up across your back, and try to cross your fingers over those of your right hand as shown in the accompanying illustration.

    c. Measure the distance to the nearest half-inch. If your fingers overlap, score as a plus. If they fail to meet, score as a minus; use a zero if your fingertips just touch.

    d. Repeat with your arms crossed in the opposite direction (left arm up). Most people will find that they are more flexible on one side than the other.

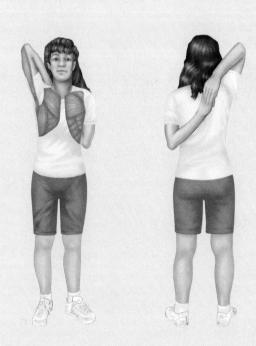

Test

3. *Hamstring and Hip Flexor Flexibility*

   a. Lie on your back on the floor beside a wall.

   b. Slowly lift one leg off the floor. Keep the other leg flat on the floor.

   c. Keep both legs straight.

   d. Continue to lift the leg until either leg begins to bend or the lower leg begins to lift off the floor.

   e. Place a yardstick against the wall and underneath the lifted leg.

   f. Hold the yardstick against the wall after the leg is lowered.

   g. Using a protractor, measure the angle created by the floor and the yardstick. The greater the angle, the better your score.

   h. Repeat with the other leg.*

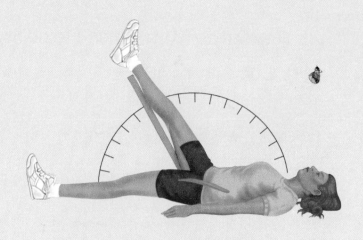

*Note: For ease of testing, you may want to draw angles on a piece of posterboard, as illustrated. If you have goniometers, you may be taught to use them instead.

Test

4. *Trunk Rotation*

   a. Tape two yardsticks to the wall at shoulder height, one right side up and the other upside down.

   b. Stand with your left shoulder an arm's length (fist closed) from the wall. Toes should be on the line, which is perpendicular to the wall and even with the 15-inch mark on the yardstick.

   c. Drop the left arm and raise the right arm to the side, palm down, fist closed.

   d. Without moving your feet, rotate the trunk to the right as far as possible, reaching along the yardstick, and hold it 2 seconds. Do not move the feet or bend the trunk. Your knees may bend slightly.

   e. A partner will read the distance reached to the nearest half-inch. Record your score. Repeat two times and average your two scores.

   f. Next, perform the test facing the opposite direction. Rotate to the left. For this test, you will use the second yardstick (upside down) so that, the greater the rotation, the higher the score. If you have only one yardstick, turn it right side up for the first test and upside down for the second test.

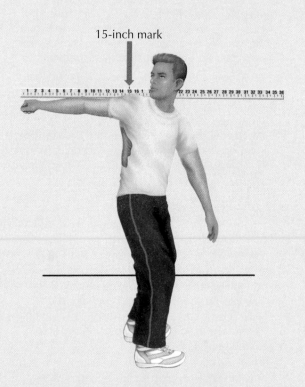

15-inch mark

Chart 1 Flexibility Rating Scale for Tests 1–4

Classification	Men					Women				
	Test 1	Test 2		Test 3	Test 4	Test 1	Test 2		Test 3	Test 4
		Right Up	Left Up				Right Up	Left Up		
High performance*	16+	5+	4+	111+	20+	17+	6+	5+	111+	20.5 or >
Good fitness zone	13–15	1–4	1–3	80–110	16–19.5	14–16	2–5	2–4	80–110	17–20
Marginal zone	10–12	0	0	60–79	13.5–15.5	11–13	1	1	60–79	14.5–16.5
Low zone	<9	<0	<0	<60	<13.5	<10	<1	<1	<60	<14.5

*Though performers need good flexibility, hypermobility may increase injury risk.

Lab 10A Evaluating Flexibility

Name: Jason Herrin   Section: ____   Date: 3/12/16

Purpose: To evaluate your flexibility in several joints

Procedures

1. Take the flexibility tests outlined in *Lab Resource Materials,* pages 219–220.
2. Record your scores in the Results section.
3. Use Chart 1 in *Lab Resource Materials* (page 218) to determine your ratings on the self-assessments; then place an X over the circle for the appropriate rating.

Results

Flexibility Scores and Ratings

Record Scores			High Performance	Good Fitness	Marginal	Low
Modified sit-and-reach						
Test 1	Left	15	○	⊗	○	○
	Right	15	○	⊗	○	○
Zipper						
Test 2	Left	5	⊗	○	○	○
	Right	5	⊗	○	○	○
Hamstring/hip flexor						
Test 3	Left	90	○	⊗	○	○
	Right	92	○	⊗	○	○
Trunk rotation						
Test 4	Left	16	○	⊗	○	○
	Right	17	○	⊗	○	○

Do any of these muscle groups need stretching? Check yes or no for each muscle group.

	Yes	No
Back of the thighs and knees (hamstrings)	⊗	○
Calf muscles	⊗	○
Lower back (lumbar region)	⊗	○
Front of right shoulder	○	⊗
Back of right shoulder	○	⊗
Front of left shoulder	○	⊗
Back of left shoulder	○	⊗
Most of the body	⊗	○
Trunk muscles	○	⊗

Conclusions and Implications: In several sentences, discuss your current flexibility and your flexibility needs for the future. Include comments about your current state of flexibility, need for improvement in specific areas, and special flexibility needs for sports or other special activities.

My flexibility is fairly good. I have always been reasonably flexible. I do stretch before workouts to prevent injury. Stretching also helps me feel better in general.

Lab 10B Planning and Logging Stretching Exercises

Name _Jason Herrin_

Section _____

Date _____

Purpose: To set 1-week lifestyle goals for stretching exercises, to prepare a stretching for flexibility plan, and to self-monitor progress in your 1-week plan

Procedures

1. Using Chart 1, provide some background information about your experience with stretching exercise, your goals, and your plans for incorporating these exercises into your normal exercise routine.

2. In Chart 2, keep a log of your actual participation in stretching exercise. You can choose from any of the stretching exercises described in Table 3, 4, or 5. Try to pick at least eight exercises and perform them at least 3 days in the week (ideally every day).

3. Describe your experiences with your stretching exercise program. Be sure to comment on your plans for future stretching exercise.

Chart 1 Stretching Exercise Survey

1. Determine your current stage for flexibility exercise. Check only the stage that represents your current activity level.

( ) Precontemplation. I do not meet flexibility exercise guidelines and have not been thinking about starting.

( ) Contemplation. I do not meet flexibility exercise guidelines but have been thinking about starting.

( ) Preparation. I am planning to start doing regular flexibility exercises to meet guidelines.

(X) Action. I do flexibility exercises, but I am not as regular as I should be.

( ) Maintenance. I regularly meet guidelines for flexibility exercises.

2. What are your primary goals for flexibility exercise?

( ) General conditioning

( ) Sports improvement (specify sport:_____)

(X) Health benefits

3. Are you currently involved in a regular stretching program? If yes, describe your program. If no, describe barriers that have prevented you from stretching.

(X) Yes

( ) No

I stretch all parts of my body before workouts regardless of if my exercise will target the muscle group.

Results

	Yes	No
Did you do eight exercises at least 3 days in the week?	X	( )
Did you do eight exercises more than 3 days in the week?	X	( )

Chart 2 Stretching Exercise Log

List the stretching exercises you actually performed and the days on which you performed them.	Day 1 Date:	Day 2 Date:	Day 3 Date:	Day 4 Date:	Day 5 Date:	Day 6 Date:	Day 7 Date:
1. sit and reach	3/6	3/7	3/8	3/9	3/10	3/11	3/12
2. zipper							
3. across arm							
4. trunk							
5. hamstring							
6. calf stretch							
7.							
8.							

Conclusions and Interpretations

1. Do you feel that you will use stretching exercises as part of your regular lifetime physical activity plan, either now or in the future? Use several sentences to explain your answer.

> I already stretch a lot as part of my daily routine. Stretching is one area that I feel is a strength. When I do not stretch I find I am more prone to injury and discomfort.

2. Discuss the exercises you feel benefited you and the ones that did not. What exercises would you continue to do and which ones would you change? Use several sentences to explain your answer.

> All of the exercises were beneficial. I will likely use some form of the stretches.

Body Mechanics: Posture, Questionable Exercises, and Care of the Back and Neck

LEARNING OBJECTIVES

After completing the study of this concept, you will be able to:

▶ Identify and describe the anatomy and function of the spine.

▶ Identify and describe the anatomy and function of core muscles.

▶ Clarify the causes and consequences of back and neck pain.

▶ Describe how to prevent and rehabilitate back and neck problems.

▶ Explain why posture is important to neck and back health and ways to improve posture.

▶ Explain why good body mechanics is important to neck and back health and ways to improve body mechanics.

▶ Indicate the exercise guidelines for back health and ways to implement the guidelines.

▶ Name questionable exercises and safer alternatives.

▶ Determine self-assessments to identify potential back, neck, and posture problems and risks, and plan a self-monitored personal program that includes exercises for reducing these problems.

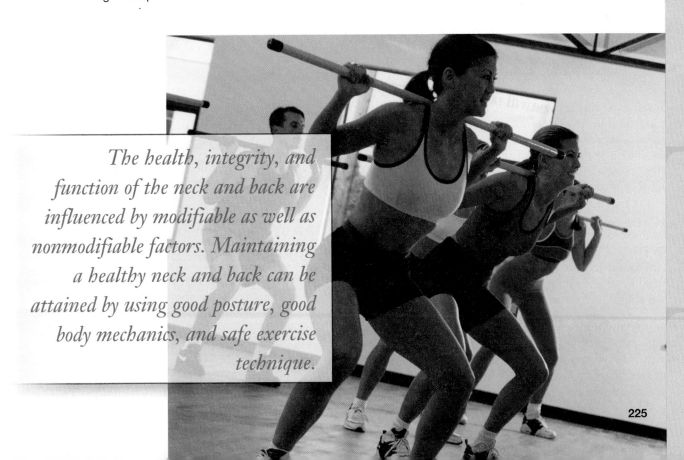

The health, integrity, and function of the neck and back are influenced by modifiable as well as nonmodifiable factors. Maintaining a healthy neck and back can be attained by using good posture, good body mechanics, and safe exercise technique.

The neck and back serve vital roles in supporting the weight of the head and body, producing movement, carrying loads, and protecting the spinal cord and nerves. These roles are facilitated by optimal alignment of the vertebrae and a balance between muscular strength and flexibility. Impairment of one or more of these functions can lead to injuries to the muscles, vertebrae, discs, ligaments, or nerves of the spine. Neck and back pain are common in today's society, with nearly 80 percent experiencing an episode of low back pain sometime in life. Back pain is second only to headache as a common medical complaint, and an estimated 30 to 70 percent of Americans have recurring back problems. The multiple functions of the spinal column may predispose this area to injuries. The spine helps to produce an array of movements while bearing significant loads.

Chronic back and neck pain are associated with many personal health problems. Some cases of back pain are "idiopathic" (no known cause), but some are clearly preventable. This concept provides information about the interrelated function of the spine and trunk musculature. Specific information about core training, posture, body mechanics, and safe exercise performance will help you adopt preventive measures that may reduce your risk for back and neck problems. As this information is intended to provide a basic foundation of knowledge, persons with neck or back pain should always seek direction from their own medical provider.

Anatomy and Function of the Spine

The spinal column is arranged for movement. The bones that make up the spine are called vertebrae. There are 33 vertebrae in the spine, and most are separated from one another by an **intervertebral disc** (see Figure 1). The vertebrae are divided into three main regions commonly referred to as cervical (neck), thoracic (upper back), and lumbar (low back). The fused vertebrae that form the tailbone are called the sacrum and coccyx. The connections among the vertebrae of the cervical, thoracic, and lumbar spine allow the trunk to move in complex ways. The spine is capable of flexion (forward bending), extension (backward bending), side bending, and rotation, but functionally, these movements often occur in combination. For example, in executing a tennis serve, the spine both extends and rotates. The spine is at risk for injury when movements are performed repetitively, performed beyond a joint's healthy range of motion, or performed under conditions of heavy or inefficient lifting.

The spinal column has an important role in bearing loads and protecting the neck and back from injury. The widest portion of each vertebra articulates with the intervertebral disc to form a strong pillar of support extending from the skull to the pelvis. The

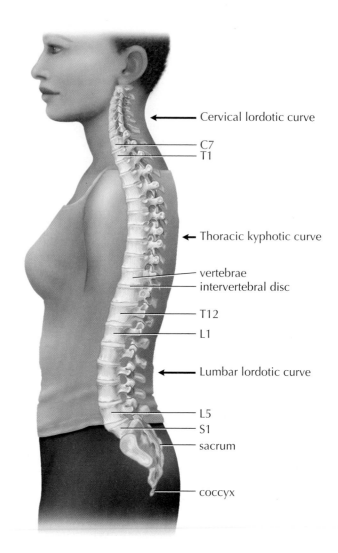

Figure 1 ▶ Curvatures of the spinal column.

- Cervical lordotic curve
- C7
- T1
- Thoracic kyphotic curve
- vertebrae
- intervertebral disc
- T12
- L1
- Lumbar lordotic curve
- L5
- S1
- sacrum
- coccyx

unique structure of the intervertebral discs is critical in distributing force and absorbing shock. The bony structure of the spine bears loads and provides protection to the spinal cord and spinal nerves. Poor posture and poor body mechanics can damage discs and vertebrae, resulting in pain and disability.

Anatomy and Function of the Core Musculature

The core is part of an integrated system that provides stability to the spine. The core includes musculature of the abdominals, back extensors, lateral trunk flexors, diaphragm, pelvic floor, and hips. A few of the more familiar muscles of the core include the lumbar multifidus, transversus abdominis, and internal oblique. There is no definitive list of muscles belonging to the core. Some sources may describe the core in terms of 6 or fewer key

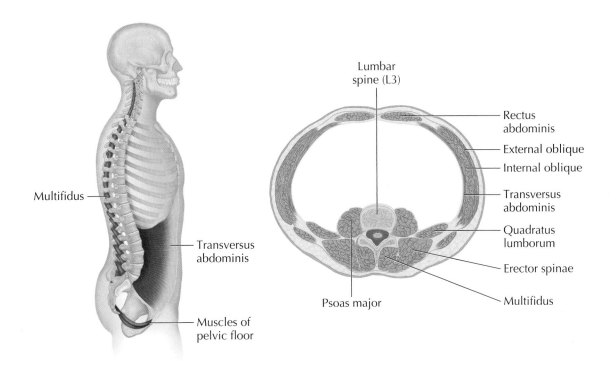

Figure 2 ▶ Cross section showing layers of core musculature.

muscle groups, while other sources may include as many as 20 different muscle groups. Regardless, muscles of the core all share a common anatomical trait: their location and attachment to either the spine, pelvis, or rib cage. Collectively, the core musculature form a three-dimensional cylinder that encompasses the body's center of gravity. This three-dimensional cylinder is inclusive of the lumbar spine, pelvis, and hips (see Figure 2).

Core stability refers to the body's ability to maintain the spine in a "neutral" postural zone, one in which the physiologic load on the spine is minimized. The overall function of the spinal stabilization system depends on the contribution of three components: a passive restraint system (ligaments, discs, vertebrae, and joints), active restraint system (muscle-tendon units), and neural control system (proprioception and feed-forward mechanisms of the nervous system). Core muscles incorporate functions of both the active restraint and neural control systems to maintain ideal postural alignment, thereby minimizing excessive stress and strain to the spine.

Muscles of the core are commonly classified as either mobilizers or stabilizers. In general, the mobilizers are those muscles that are more superficial and contract concentrically to produce trunk movements. The stabilizers are muscles that are more deeply located and contract isometrically or eccentrically to stabilize the trunk during arm and leg movements. The stabilizer

group is further divided into two categories, local and global. These groups are distinguished by differences in anatomy and function.

The **local core stabilizers** provide stiffness and stability to the spine. They include muscles that possess a small cross-sectional area, are deeply located, and may span just one or two vertebral levels at a time. Functionally, these muscles provide local spinal support, control motion between adjacent vertebrae, increase intra-abdominal pressure, and provide proprioceptive input to the body to avoid injury. The most notable example of a local core stabilizer is the lumbar multifidus. Also included in the group are muscles that indirectly influence the stability of the spine due to their role in increasing intra-abdominal pressure and their supportive attachment to the fascia of the back. These muscles include the transversus abdominis, internal oblique, diaphragm, and pelvic floor muscles. The local core muscles are believed to maintain the spine in "neutral" via isometric co-contractions, thereby minimizing excessive loading of the spine.

Intervertebral Discs Spinal discs; cushions of cartilage between the bodies of the vertebrae. Each disc consists of a fibrous outer ring (annulus fibrosus) and a pulpy center (nucleus pulposus).

Local Core Stabilizers Deep core muscles that provide stiffness and stability to the spine.

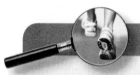

A CLOSER LOOK

Functional Fitness Predicts Injury Risk

Being physically fit provides many health benefits but studies have typically not shown that fitness can reduce risk of injuries. This is because many injuries often happen dynamically and acutely. However, several recent studies demonstrate the utility of a specific screening protocol—the Functional Movement Screen (FMS)—that can diagnose limitations and imbalances that may predispose a person to injury. To address these problems, functional fitness training tends to rely on large, multi-planar movements of the limbs that indirectly target core muscles. The deep core muscles are known to contract in anticipation of most arm and leg movements. By contracting prior to arm or leg movement, the deep core muscles act as a brace around the trunk and a solid anchor from which powerful arm and leg movements can occur. By utilizing functional fitness training techniques, the core musculature can be better prepared to handle the forces, postures, and actions involved in real-life activities and sports.

Do you think you have sufficient functional fitness for your lifestyle? Why or Why not?

connect ACTIVITY

The **global core stabilizers** function to produce trunk motion as well as trunk stability based on their attachments to the pelvis. These muscles tend to have a larger cross-sectional area, are more superficially located, often span multiple vertebral levels, and possess attachments to the pelvis, rib cage, and/or thoracic spine. Examples include the rectus abdominis, external oblique, quadratus lumborum, and erector spinae. Also included are muscles of the hip, which indirectly influence lumbar stability by altering tilt of the pelvis. Functionally the global core stabilizers generate movement of the trunk as well as provide stabilization.

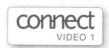

connect VIDEO 1

Causes and Consequences of Back and Neck Pain

Most back and neck pain stems from lifestyle choices or life experiences. The original cause (or causes) of back and neck pain are typically hard to identify. Although back and neck problems can result from an acute injury (e.g., a diving accident or car accident), most are caused by accumulated stresses over a lifetime. These factors include the avoidable effects of poor posture and body mechanics as well as questionable exercises that put the back at risk. (Exercises to avoid are discussed later in the concept.) Musculoskeletal injuries and degenerative changes to the discs, vertebrae, joint surfaces, muscles, or ligaments can predispose you to back and neck problems. Depression, cancer, infections, and some visceral diseases (kidney, pelvic organs) can also contribute to back problems. Although people have some control over these causes, some back pain stems directly from structural or functional disorders that a person is born with. Inherited causes include anomalies of the spine and some forms of **scoliosis.**

To reduce risk for back pain, reduce the risk factors that you have control over. Modifiable risk factors (factors you can change) include regular heavy labor, use of vibrational tools, routines of prolonged sitting, smoking, a hypokinetic lifestyle, coronary artery disease, and obesity. Nonmodifiable risk factors include a family history of joint disease, age, congenital anomalies, and direct trauma (e.g., a fall or rough athletic activity when young). Lab 11A provides a questionnaire for assessing your potential risk for back and neck pain.

The nervous system and various pain-sensitive structures contribute to back pain. Back pain can result from direct or indirect causes. Direct causes are typically the result of tissue trauma to areas in or around the spinal column. The most common sources of pain are ligaments, intervertebral discs, nerve roots, spinal joints, and muscles. Indirect causes stem from the release of pain-causing chemicals from injured tissues. These

 Health is available to Everyone for a Lifetime, and it's Personal

Is Back Pain in Your Future?
According to the National Institutes of Health, the most common medical problem in the United States is back pain, which is very often caused by degeneration of the disks in the spine. Preventative measures include maintaining a healthy weight over the lifespan, using proper lifting techniques, and engaging in regular exercise, particularly strength training and flexibility exercises.

What steps are you taking today to help prevent back problems later in life?

connect ACTIVITY

chemicals cause nerves in the area to remain irritated and sensitive. Processes within the brainstem, spinal cord, and peripheral nerves can also modulate the sensation of pain, either increasing or decreasing it. For example, some back pain can be caused by abnormal feedback loops that enhance or maintain the perception of pain—even when the original cause or problem is corrected.

The integrity of the neck and back are jeopardized by excessive stress and strain.

Forces are constantly at work to bend, twist, shear, compress, or lengthen tissues of the body. Stress on these tissues may eventually create strain, a change in the tissue's size or dimension. Healthy tissues typically return to their normal state once the force is removed. Injury occurs when excessive stress and strain prevent the tissue from returning to its normal state. A number of factors can contribute to stress and strain on the back.

- *Poor posture can cause body segments to experience stress and strain.* When body segments are in poor alignment (e.g., slouching or forward head positions), the muscles in the back and neck must work hard to compensate. This creates excessive stress and strain in the affected area(s). Over time, tension in these muscles can lead to **myofascial trigger points,** causing headache or **referred pain** in the face, scalp, shoulder, arm, and chest. The chronic stress from poor alignment can also lead to other postural deviations and degenerative changes in the neck.

- *Prolonged sitting contributes to back problems.* Sitting, by itself, is not a risk factor for the development of back pain. However, when prolonged sitting (more than half the work day) is combined with exposure to vibration and awkward postures at work, an individual has four times the risk of developing back pain. Occupations with the highest risk based on these three factors include helicopter pilots and truck drivers.

- *Bad body mechanics and improper lifting techniques contribute to stress and strain on the spine.* The lumbar vertebrae and the sacrum are most vulnerable to this type of injury due to the significant weight they support and the thinner ligamentous support at this level.

- *Being overweight or obese increases the risk of back pain.* Those who are obese are on average 20 percent more likely to have back pain than those of normal weight. Obesity and overweight status are hard on the body because they overload the bones, discs, tendons, and ligaments of the body. Added wear and tear on joint surfaces can lead to osteoarthritis. Postural changes accompany weight gain and create additional stress and strain on joints. For example, a large protruding abdomen often causes forward tipping of the pelvis and excessive arching of the low back that can lead to back pain.

Some exercises and movements can produce microtrauma, which can lead to back and neck pain.

Most people are familiar with acute injuries, such as ankle sprains. These injuries are associated with immediate onset of pain and swelling. **Microtrauma** is a "silent injury"—a subtle form of injury that results from accumulated damage over time. It can result from repetitive motion, repeated forceful exertion, long-term vibration or working with awkward postures. When microtrauma occurs as the result of activities at work, it is often referred to by the medical terms Repetitive Stress Injury (RSI) or Cumulative Trauma Disorder (CTD). One common example is carpal tunnel syndrome, a painful irritation of the median nerve at the wrist, often brought on by repetitive motion of the wrist during long and extended periods of typing, assembly line tasks, or construction work.

Microtrauma can also result from the repetitive performance of unsafe exercises or contraindicated movements. For example, regular performance of full deep knee squats or full neck circles may irritate the joint surfaces and eventually cause knee or neck pain. Repeated overhead lifting with excessive loads can irritate and damage the rotator cuff tendon of the shoulder. The initial wear and tear of microtrauma is not something typically noticed. However, over many years, microscopic changes occur in the joint. Examples include swelling, fibrosis of the synovial lining, abnormal thickening of the surrounding joint capsule, calcifications in the tendons, and thinning and roughening of the cartilage cushioning the joint surfaces. Because these changes are unseen and often unfelt, the offending exercise or activity is often viewed as harmless. However, later in life the effects from the microtrauma become more apparent, manifesting in tendonitis, bursitis, arthritis, or nerve compression. Chances are, when the injury reaches a painful stage, the cause is not identified and it gets attributed to aging.

Global Core Stabilizers Superficial core muscles that produce motion and aid in stabilization.

Scoliosis A curvature of the spine that produces a sideways curve with some rotation; while typically mild, this condition can sometimes be painful.

Myofascial Trigger Points Tender spots in the muscle or muscle fascia that refer pain to a location distant to the point.

Referred Pain Pain that appears to be located in one area, though it actually originates in another area.

Microtrauma Injury so small it is not detected at the time it occurs.

The lumbar intervertebral discs are particularly susceptible to injury and herniation. The intervertebral discs located between the vertebrae of the spine are composed of a tirelike outer ring (annulus fibrosus) surrounding a gel-like center (nucleus pulposus). The greatest risk for injury to the discs occurs during excessive loading and twisting motions of the spine. While most people think that disc injuries occur from an acute injury, disc herniation typically reflects a degenerative process that takes place over time. With repeated microtrauma, small tears begin to occur in the inner fibers of the annulus. The nucleus begins to move outward (**herniated disc**), much like toothpaste moving within a squeezed tube. Disc herniation is termed *incomplete* or *contained* as long as the migrating edge of the nucleus remains within the fibers of the annulus. As damage continues (often the result of years of cumulative microtrauma), the annular fibers may reach a point of rupture at their periphery (see Figure 3). At this point (termed *disc extrusion*), the nucleus pulposus moves into the space around the spinal cord or nerve root. At this stage, herniation is termed *complete* or *noncontained*.

The risk of disc herniation is greater for younger adults. Disc herniation is frequently listed as a cause of back pain, but studies show that only 5 to 10 percent of persons with herniated discs experience pain. The reason for this is that pain is often not experienced until complete herniation occurs. Pain is felt as the nuclear material begins to press on pain-sensitive structures in its path. Interestingly, the risk for disc herniation is greatest for individuals in their 30s and 40s. Risk decreases with age as the disc degenerates and becomes less soft and pliable.

Degenerative disc disease is a common part of aging and a source of back pain. Many elderly adults get shorter as they age, often due to degenerative changes within the vertebral bodies and discs. One notable change is flattening of the discs as a result of lost water content. This reduces the space between vertebrae and increases the compressive forces on the small facet joints and the large vertebral bodies. This results in a decrease in the size of the spinal canal, which in turn increases the likelihood of nerve impingement, bone spur development, and arthritis, all of which can contribute to back pain and disability (see Figure 4).

Injury to the spine negatively affects the function of the core musculature. One of the more important core muscles, the lumbar multifidus, is adversely affected by back pain. Studies demonstrate that with low back pain, the muscle becomes inhibited (exhibiting decreased levels of activation and increased fatigability), is subject to atrophy, and becomes infiltrated with fatty deposits. In the healthy individual, the multifidus is believed to be responsible for providing more than two-thirds of the dynamic rigidity to the lumbar spine and serves an important role in proprioception and kinesthetic awareness. Research studies have shown specific spinal stabilization exercises to be effective in reversing some of the adverse changes to the multifidus, including positive

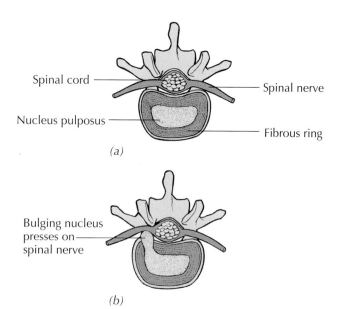

Figure 3 ▶ Normal disc (*a*) and herniated disc (*b*).

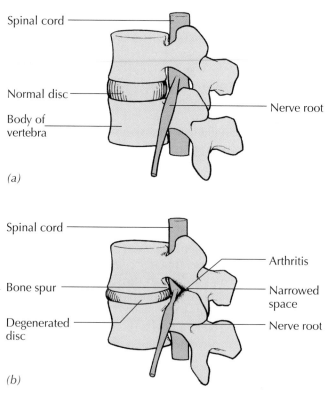

Figure 4 ▶ Normal disc (*a*) and degenerated disc with nerve impingement and arthritic changes (*b*).

gains in cross-sectional area/muscle bulk and improved neural recruitment. More importantly, participation in a program of core training exercise has also been shown to improve pain tolerance and function. Rehabilitation of the lumbar multifidus appears critical in the recovery period following back pain.

Medical intervention is sometimes needed for neck or back pain. Most cases of back pain resolve spontaneously, with 70 percent having no symptoms at the end of 3 weeks and 90 percent recovered after 2 months. However, medical approaches have been shown to speed up recovery from acute back/neck pain and to improve pain tolerance and function in chronic cases. Conservative treatment typically involves the use of anti-inflammatory medications, muscle relaxants, heat, cryotherapy, traction, or electrical stimulation. It can also include therapeutic exercise, massage, and joint mobilization. When this treatment is unsuccessful, referral to an alternative therapy, such as acupuncture, or to a pain clinic for steroidal anti-inflammatory injections may occur. As a last measure, surgery may be needed for removal of a herniated portion of a disc.

Prevention of and Rehabilitation from Back and Neck Problems

Exercise is a frequently prescribed treatment for back or neck pain. Exercise, such as resistance and aerobic exercises, has been found to be helpful in treating many types of chronic pain. Exercises that are selected specifically to help correct pain-related problems are classified as therapeutic. These exercises are aimed at correcting the underlying cause of neck or back pain by strengthening weak muscles, stretching short ones, and improving circulation to and nourishment of tissues of the body. Both therapeutic and health-related fitness exercises may be considered preventive. Done faithfully, and with the appropriate FIT formula, they improve the health of the musculoskeletal system, allowing greater efficiency of function and reduced incidence of injury.

Use of specific core stabilization exercises may reduce low back pain and functional disability. The integrity of individual vertebral segments of the spine is often compromised with injury to the neck or back. One or more components of the passive restraint system (ligaments, discs, vertebrae, or joints) may be damaged, creating a weak link in the stabilization system. In addition, optimal function of the dynamic and neural control systems is often adversely affected by injury. This may make a specific segment of the spine more vulnerable to delayed healing or further injury. Core training may enhance stability to the injured area by improving the function of the dynamic and neural control systems. Core training programs are also effective in treating low back pain. Studies have shown significant improvements in pain level and functional status following a program of spinal stabilization exercises, but positive results have also been obtained from more general exercise interventions. Future research may help identify subsets of people who may benefit from one type of exercise program over another.

Core stability training and core strengthening training can promote good back health. As described in Concept 9, building **core strength** is important for overall muscular fitness. However, to reduce the risks for back and neck problems, you need to train the muscles involved in core stabilization. There are two main types of core training programs, and each requires somewhat different methods.

   Core stability training refers to the training of the deeper ("local") core musculature. Physiologically, the local core stabilizers are slow-twitch endurance muscles that are poorly recruited, demonstrate low force production, and often sag/lengthen due to weakness. Training

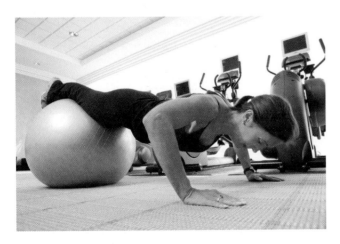

Core stability training can help maintain a healthy back.

Herniated Disc The soft nucleus of the spinal disc that protrudes through a small tear in the surrounding tissue; also called prolapse.

Core Strength Strength of muscles that demonstrate optimal firing patterns and tension-generating capabilities to create movement of the trunk.

Core Stability Strength of muscles that demonstrate optimal firing patterns and tension-generating capabilities to "brace" the trunk in anticipation of, and during, movement of the head, arms, or legs.

principles for the local core stabilizers are based on the respective physiology of the muscles. In general, exercises should involve slow and controlled movements and be held for long durations. The focus should be on improving trunk muscle endurance, since endurance of the trunk musculature appears to be more important than strength for reducing the risk of low back pain. Therefore, exercises should emphasize lower resistance and involve more repetitions. Sets of 8 to 12 repetitions at very light to moderate intensity are appropriate for improving the endurance of core stabilizers. Exercises for improving local core stability are described and illustrated in the exercise section at the end of the concept.

Core strength training refers to the training of the more superficial "global" core musculature. Physiologically, these muscles are fast-twitch in nature, contract at higher resistance levels, possess greater potential for force production, work in a noncontinuous fashion, and are preferentially recruited over the local stabilizers. They are often in a shortened (tight) position. Based on the physiologic function of the global core muscles, recommended training principles include shorter duration holds, faster speeds of concentric contractions, greater resistance, and fewer numbers of repetitions. Several sets of exercise (2 to 4 sets of 8 to 12 repetitions at moderate to hard intensity) are recommended to improve the core strength of the global core stabilizers. Traditional abdominal and trunk extensor strengthening exercises are included in the exercise section at the end of the concept.

TECHNOLOGY UPDATE

New Training Aids for Core Training

Core training is an immensely popular concept across the fields of sport, fitness, and rehabilitation. The popularity of core training programs and classes has led to an expanding array of core-training devices and functional fitness classes. One category of devices includes those that provide an unstable surface for challenging balance and stability. Rocker boards, air-filled domes, therapy balls, foam rollers, and sliding disks are a few examples. Participants creatively position themselves on these devices in various postures—standing, lunging, kneeling, or on hands and knees. A second category of devices includes equipment that provides a dynamic challenge to the arms or legs. Elastic tubing, stretch cords, vibrating wands, kettle bells, and medicine balls are used to overload the extremities and elicit a corresponding and supportive contraction of the core stabilizers. Creative new devices enter the fitness market on a monthly basis, giving exercise participants fresh new ideas for their workout regimen.

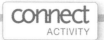

Resistance exercise can often correct muscle imbalance, the underlying cause of many postural and back problems. If the muscles on one side of a joint are stronger than the muscles on the opposite side, the body part is pulled in the direction of the stronger muscles. Corrective exercises are usually designed to strengthen the long, weak muscles and to stretch the short, strong ones in order to have equal pull in both directions. For example, people with lumbar lordosis may need to strengthen the abdominals and gluteal muscles and also stretch the lower back and hip flexor muscles.

Although general resistance training may help improve the strength and endurance of the back muscles, the exercises may not be specific enough to target the areas that contribute to risk for low back pain. Because of this, increased attention has been given to the development of back exercise machines that can more effectively rehabilitate and/or strengthen back musculature. The machines help isolate the muscles by restraining or preventing other muscles from assisting. For example, pelvic muscles are restrained in a back extension machine to help isolate the lumbar muscles. This isolation helps strengthen the lumbar muscles, an important target for reducing risks for back problems.

Good Posture Is Important for Neck and Back Health

Good posture has aesthetic benefits. Posture is an important part of nonverbal communication. The first impression a person makes is usually a visual one, and

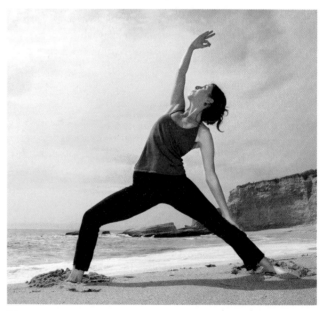

Movement disciplines like yoga and tai chi can promote body awareness and contribute to back health.

good posture can help convey an impression of alertness, confidence, and attractiveness.

Proper posture allows the body segments to be balanced. Segments of the human body (i.e., the head, shoulder girdle, pelvic girdle, rib cage, and spine) are balanced in a vertical column by muscles and ligaments. Proper posture helps maintain an even distribution of force across the body, improve shock absorption, and minimize the degree of active muscle tension required to maintain upright posture. When viewed from the side, three normal curvatures of the spine are present, causing the vertebral column to appear S-shaped. These curvatures are created by the **lordotic (inward) curve** of the cervical and lumbar spines and the **kyphotic (outward) curve** of the thoracic spine (see Figure 1). The curves help balance forces on the body and minimize muscle tension. They are also responsible for humans' unique ability to walk upright on two legs while maintaining a forward gaze.

The degree of curvature is influenced by the tilt of the pelvis. A forward pelvic tilt increases curvature in the neck and lower back, whereas a backward pelvic tilt flattens the lower back. The most desirable position is a **neutral spine** in which the spine has neither too much nor too little lordotic curvature. The forces across the spine are balanced and muscular tension is at a minimum.

Awareness of good standing posture is important to a healthy spine. In the standing position, the head should be centered over the trunk with forward gaze, the shoulders should be down and back but relaxed, with the chest high and the abdomen flat. The spine should have gentle curves when viewed from the side but should be straight when seen from the back. When the pelvis is tilted properly, the pubis falls directly underneath the lower tip of the sternum. The knees should be relaxed, with the kneecaps pointed straight ahead. The feet should point straight ahead or slightly outward, and the weight should be borne over the heel, on the outside border of the sole, and across the ball of the foot and toes (see Figure 5).

Awareness of good seated posture is important to a healthy spine. A large percentage of our days are spent sitting as we attend class, commute to work, sit at a computer, dine out, or relax in front of the television. Good seated posture decreases pressure within the discs of the lower back and reduces fatigue of lower back muscles. In sitting, the head should be centered over the trunk, the shoulders down and back. If one is using a computer, the monitor should be at eye level with the screen 18 to 24 inches from the eyes. The seat of the chair should be at an angle that allows the knees to be positioned slightly lower than the hips. The back should firmly rest against the chair, with support to the lumbar spine. The feet

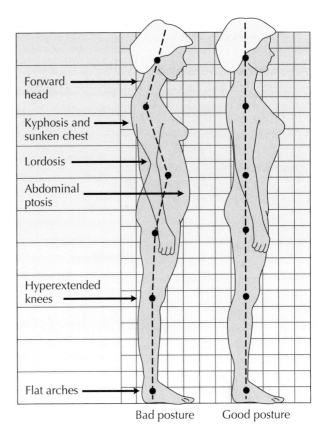

Forward head

Kyphosis and sunken chest

Lordosis

Abdominal ptosis

Hyperextended knees

Flat arches

Bad posture   Good posture

Figure 5 ▶ Comparison of bad and good posture.

should be supported on the floor and arms supported on armrests for ideal unloading of the spine (see Figure 6).

Poor posture contributes to a variety of health problems. When posture deviates from neutral, weight distribution becomes uneven and tissues are at risk for injury. Examples of common postural deviations are described in Table 1, along with associated health problems. Two of those highlighted are lumbar lordosis (excessive

Posture The relationship among body parts, whether standing, lying, sitting, or moving. Good posture is the relationship among body parts that allows you to function most effectively, with the least expenditure of energy and with a minimal amount of stress and strain on the body.

Lordotic Curve The normal inward curvature of the cervical and lumbar spine.

Kyphotic Curve The normal outward curvature of the thoracic spine.

Neutral Spine Proper position of the spine to maintain a normal lordotic curve. The spine has neither too much nor too little lordotic curve.

Table 1 ▶ Health Problems Associated with Poor Posture

Posture Problem	Definition	Health Problem
Forward head	The head aligned in front of the center of gravity	Headache, dizziness, and pain in the neck, shoulders, or arms
Kyphosis	Excessive curvature (flexion) in the upper back; also called humpback	Impaired respiration as a result of sunken chest and pain in the neck, shoulders, and arms
Lumbar lordosis	Excessive curvature (hyperextension) in the lower back (sway back), with a forward pelvic tilt	Back pain and/or injury, protruding abdomen, low back syndrome, and painful menstruation
Flat back	Reduced curvature in the lower back	Back pain, increased risk for injury due to reduced shock absorption
Abdominal ptosis	Excessive protrusion of abdomen	Back pain and/or injury, lordosis, low back syndrome, and painful menstruation
Hyperextended knees	The knees bent backward excessively	Greater risk for knee injury and excessive pelvic tilt (lordosis)
Pronated feet	The longitudinal arch of the foot flattened with increased pressure on inner aspect of foot	Decreased shock absorption, leading to foot, knee, and lower back pain

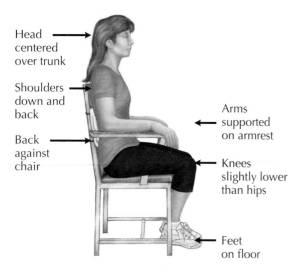

Head centered over trunk

Shoulders down and back

Back against chair

Arms supported on armrest

Knees slightly lower than hips

Feet on floor

Figure 6 ▶ Good sitting posture.

curvature of the lower back) and flat back (reduced curvature of the lower back).

Lumbar lordosis posture occurs when the pelvis is tipped forward from a position of neutral tilt. With this posture, the hip flexor muscles become shortened and tight, while the abdominal muscles become weak and long (with a reduced ability to "hold" within inner range). This muscle imbalance shifts body segment alignment toward a position of uneven loading, increasing pressure on the facet joints of the vertebrae. Over time, degenerative changes may occur, including a narrowing of the openings where spinal nerves exit, thus increasing risk for pain.

Flat back posture, on the other hand, occurs when the pelvis is tipped backward from a position of neutral tilt.

With this posture, the lumbar spine is flexed, the lower back muscles are in a lengthened (weak) position, and the hamstring muscles are shortened and tight. A reduced lumbar curvature increases pressure on the intervertebral bodies and decreases shock absorption capabilities. Relative differences in flexibility between tight hamstring and long trunk muscles may also increase risk for injury. Laws of physics demonstrate that the body takes the path of least resistance during a chain of movement (e.g., forward bending), with the most flexible segment (i.e., the back) providing a greater contribution to the total range of movement. It follows that regions of greater movement will experience greater tissue strain. In the case of flat back posture, tight hamstrings may limit the contribution of hip motion during forward bending tasks, thus predisposing the lower back to become the fulcrum for movement and the site of injury.

Correcting postural deviations begins with restoring adequate muscle fitness and muscle length. Most of us have a natural tendency to sit or stand with poor posture. For the most part, we can correct our posture with conscious effort. However, if poor posture is maintained for very long or very frequent periods of time, the body loses resiliency. With poor posture, muscles on one side of a joint or body segment can become shortened or tight while muscles on the opposite side can become lengthened and weak. Poor posture can also result following muscle injury. This may manifest itself in guarded postures or muscle dysfunction, which eventually leads to muscles on one side of the joint becoming inflexible due to facilitation and muscles on the opposite side becoming weak due to inhibition. Postural correction can be achieved by improving body awareness, increasing flexibility of tight muscles, and improving strength of weak (inhibited) muscles. For example, a slouched posture with rounded and forward shoulders can be improved by elongating the pectoralis (chest) muscles and strengthening muscles of the upper back. A lumbar lordosis posture can be improved by stretching the hip flexors and back extensors that keep the top of the pelvis tipped forward, followed by strengthening of the abdominal and gluteal muscles that help tip the pelvis backward (see Figure 7).

Hereditary, congenital, and disease conditions, as well as certain environmental factors, can also cause poor posture. Some environmental factors that contribute to poor posture include ill-fitting clothing and shoes, chronic fatigue, improperly fitting furniture (including poor chairs, beds, and mattresses), emotional and personality problems, poor work habits, poor physical fitness due to inactivity, and lack of knowledge relating to good posture. Some posture problems, such as scoliosis, may be congenital, hereditary, or acquired but can be improved with exercise, braces, and/or other medical procedures. Early detection is critical in treating scoliosis.

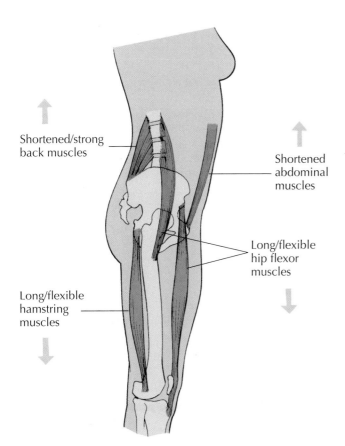

Shortened/strong back muscles

Shortened abdominal muscles

Long/flexible hip flexor muscles

Long/flexible hamstring muscles

Figure 7 ▶ Balanced muscle strength and length permit good postural alignment.

Good Body Mechanics Is Important for Neck and Back Health

Proper body mechanics can help prevent back and neck injury. Biomechanics is a discipline that applies mechanical laws and principles to study how the body performs more efficiently and with less energy. Good body mechanics, as applied to back care, implies maintaining a neutral spine during activities of daily living. A neutral spine maintains the normal curvature of the spine, thus allowing an optimal balance of forces across the spine, reducing compressive forces, and minimizing muscle tension. In the following sections, specific recommendations and examples of good body mechanics are provided for a variety of body positions.

Ergonomics is a discipline that uses biomechanical principles to develop tools and workplace settings that put the least amount of strain on the body. Many employers take an active interest in ergonomic principles, since repetitive motion injuries and other musculoskeletal conditions are the leading cause of work-related ill health. Back pain contributes to reduced job productivity, with workers losing an average of 4.6 hours per week of productive time during each episode of back pain. Back pain has societal costs as well. It is the sixth most costly medical condition in the United States, burdening the country with $85.9 billion worth of work expenses each year related to health care, lost income, and lost work productivity. One application of ergonomics (also known as human factors engineering) is the design of effective workstations for computer users. Properly fitting desks and chairs and the effective positioning of computer screens and keyboards can minimize problems such as carpal tunnel syndrome.

Good lifting technique focuses on using the legs. Keep in mind that the muscles of the legs are relatively large and strong, compared with the back muscles. Likewise, the hip joint is well designed for motion. It is less likely to suffer the same amount of wear and tear as the smaller joints of the spine. When lifting an object from the floor, straddle the object with a wide stance; squat down by hinging through the hips and bending the knees; maintain a slight arch to the lower back by sticking out the buttocks; test the load and get help if it is too heavy or awkward; rise by tightening the leg muscles, not the back; keep the load close to the waist; don't pivot or twist.

Poor body mechanics can increase risks for back pain. A common cause of backache is muscle strain, frequently precipitated by poor body mechanics in daily activities, such as lifting or exercising. If lifting is done improperly, great pressure is exerted on the lumbar discs,

Lifting

Do:
- Keep a slight arch in the lower back, bend with the knees, straddle and test the load, keep load close to body, tighten abdominals, and lift using legs.
- Lower a load using the same principles in reverse.

Don't:
- Bend at the waist.
- Twist.
- Lift more than you can handle.
- Hyperextend the neck or back.

Reaching

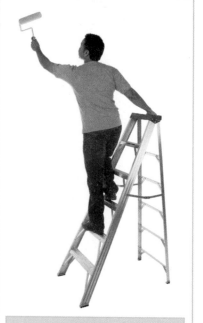

Do:
- Use a stool or ladder when working with arms above head level.
- Keep tools within easy reach.
- Choose tools with extended handles.

Don't:
- Keep arms extended out in front or out to side for long periods of time without rest.
- Hyperextend your neck.

Elements of Good Body Mechanics

Pushing & Pulling

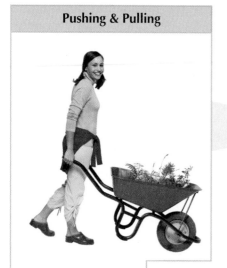

Do:
- Push or pull heavy objects.
- Push rather than pull, if given a choice.

Do:
- Keep load midline and close to the body.
- Divide the load if possible, carrying half in each arm/hand.
- Alternate load from one side of the body to the other when it cannot be divided.
- Carry light-moderate loads in a backpack with straps.

Carrying

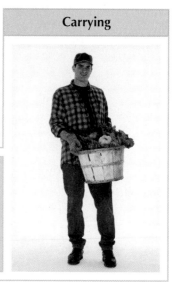

Figure 8 ▶ Characteristics of good body mechanics for different lifestyle tasks.

and excessive stress and strain are placed on the lumbar muscles and ligaments (see Figure 8). Many popular exercises involve poor body mechanics and should be viewed with caution. Poor postures (e.g., sleeping on a soft mattress or slouching in a chair) can also cause back strain (see Figure 9). Descriptions and examples of unsafe exercises and postures are provided later in the concept.

connect VIDEO 2

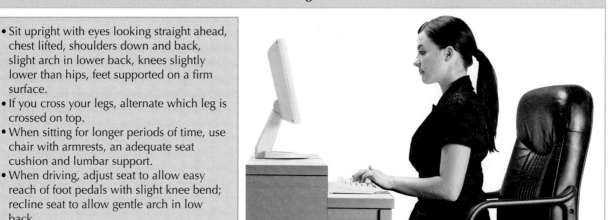

Sitting

- Sit upright with eyes looking straight ahead, chest lifted, shoulders down and back, slight arch in lower back, knees slightly lower than hips, feet supported on a firm surface.
- If you cross your legs, alternate which leg is crossed on top.
- When sitting for longer periods of time, use chair with armrests, an adequate seat cushion and lumbar support.
- When driving, adjust seat to allow easy reach of foot pedals with slight knee bend; recline seat to allow gentle arch in low back.
- Reading material should be elevated or supported at eye level.
- The office desk should be about 29 to 30 inches high for the average man and about 27 to 29 inches high for the average woman. The computer screen should be about 20 to 40 inches away from your eyes with the top of the screen at or slightly below eye level.

Elements of Good Posture

Standing

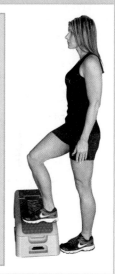

- Stand upright with forward gaze, shoulders down and back, chest raised, stomach pulled up and in, slight arch in the lower back, slight bend in the knees, feet shoulder width apart, and toes pointing straight ahead or slightly outward.
- If you stand with weight shifted to one side, alternate which leg you lean on.
- If you stand in one place for a prolonged time, prop one foot on small step stool.
- Height of work surface should be about 2 to 4 inches below the waist.

Lying

- Use a pillow between the knees when lying on your side and under the knees when lying on the back.
- Choose a pillow that supports the head and neck in neutral alignment.
- Avoid reading in bed.

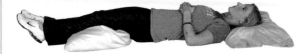
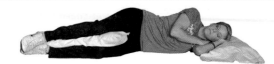

Figure 9 ▶ Characteristics of good posture for sitting, standing, and lying.

Exercise Guidelines for Back Health

Some exercises and movements may put the back and neck at risk. The human body is designed for motion. Nevertheless, certain movements can put the joints and musculoskeletal system at risk and should therefore be avoided. With respect to care of the spine, many **contraindicated** movements involve the extremes of hyperflexion and hyperextension. Hyperflexion causes increased pressure in the discs, potentially leading to disc herniation. Hyperextension causes compressive wear and tear on the facet joints that join vertebral segments (see Figure 10). Hyperextension of the spine also causes narrowing of the intervertebral canal, potentially causing nerve impingement. Extremes of motion can be harmful to other joints as well. For example, knee hyperextension places excessive stress on structures at the back of the knee, whereas hyperflexion increases compressive forces under the kneecap (patello-femoral joint).

Following established exercise guidelines is important for safe exercise. "Safe" exercises are defined as those performed with normal body posture, mechanics, and movement in mind. They don't compromise the integrity or stability of one body part to the detriment of another. "Questionable" exercises, on the other hand, are exercises that may violate normal body mechanics and place the joints, ligaments, or muscles at risk for injury. No harm may occur from doing the exercise once, but repeated use over time can lead to injury. A number of commonly used exercises are regarded as poor choices (contraindicated) for nearly everyone in the general population due to the reasonable risk for injury over time. A separate category of questionable exercises are poor choices for certain segments of the population because of a specific health issue or known physical problem.

Differentiating exercises as "safe" or "questionable" can be difficult—even experts in the field have different opinions on the subject. These views change over time as new knowledge and research findings reshape our understanding of the effect of exercise on the human body.

When considering the merits and risks of different exercises, it may be necessary to consult an expert. Professionals such as athletic trainers, biomechanists, physical educators, physical therapists, and certified strength and conditioning specialists typically have college degrees and 4 to 8 years of study in such courses as anatomy, physiology, kinesiology, preventive and therapeutic exercise, and physiology of exercise. On-the-job training, a good physique or figure, and good athletic or dancing ability are not sufficient qualifications for teaching or advising about exercise. Most fitness centers hire instructors and personal trainers with appropriate certifications. Unfortunately, certification is not always a requirement. When searching for advice on training or exercise, inquire about an individual's qualifications.

Exercises prescribed for a particular individual differ from those that are good for everyone (mass prescription). In a clinical setting, a therapist works with one patient. A case history is taken and tests made to determine which muscles are weak or strong, short or long. Exercises are then prescribed for that person. For example, a wrestler with a recent history of shoulder dislocation would probably be prescribed specific shoulder-strengthening exercises to regain stability in the joint. Common shoulder stretching exercises would likely be contraindicated for this individual. In this case, the muscles and joint capsule on the front of the shoulder are already quite lax to have allowed dislocation to occur in the first place.

Exercises prescribed or performed as a group cannot typically take individual needs into account. For example, when a physical educator, an aerobics instructor, or a coach leads a group of people in exercise, there is little (if any) consideration for individual differences, except for some allowance made in the number of repetitions or in the amount of weight or resistance used. Some of the exercises performed in this type of group setting may not be

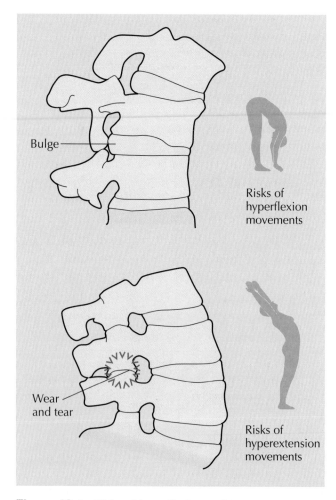

Figure 10 ▶ Risks of hyperflexion and hyperextension.

Table 2 ▶ Controllable Variables in Reducing Risk for Injury

Variables	Activity Examples	Potential Injury	Modifications to Reduce Risk
Frequency	• Repeated back hyperextension in a gymnast • Repeated wrist movement in an assembly-line worker	Microtrauma to the joints undergoing repeated motions	• Maintain a balance of flexibility and strength in the vulnerable regions of the body. • Provide rest/rotate workstations. • Use ergonomic modifications to the worksite.
Duration	• Sustained position of a deep squat in a baseball catcher • Forward head posture of an office worker	Stress and strain to the muscles and ligaments used to hold the posture	• Strengthen the muscles of the knees and maintain leg muscle flexibility in the catcher. • Take regular posture breaks in the office worker and modify computer station for good seated posture.
Intensity	Excessive loads and reaction forces experienced by a • Power lifter • Runner • Construction worker	Stress and strain to the musculoskeletal system, especially the weaker portions of the back and shoulders	• Do a proper warm-up and correct training progression. • Wear supportive shoes and clothing. • Be aware of personal limits, seeking help or a spot when needed.
Speed	High-velocity movement of • A 50-yd sprinter • The rapid fingering of a concert pianist	• Motions applied over a short time under conditions of high tension predispose the muscles and tendons to injury. • With fast-paced motions, precision is often sacrificed (particularly with fatigue), possibly leading to faulty movement patterns.	• Follow activity-specific training protocols to optimize recruitment of appropriate muscle fiber types. • Maintain balance of flexibility and strength. • Use deep muscles for stability and superficial muscles for mobility.
Movement quality	• Extended range of motion during ballistic shoulder stretching of swimmers • Poor body mechanics when shoveling snow	• Movement through extreme ranges or at the limit of normal motion can lead to instability or wear/tear of joints. • Poor balance of forces throughout the body increases risk for stress and strain.	• Balance flexibility with strength and respect pain, the body's signal of injury. • Use good posture and body mechanics in recreational and lifestyle activities to balance forces.

appropriate for all individuals. Similarly, an exercise that is appropriate for a certain individual may not be appropriate for all members of a group. Since it is not always practical to prescribe individual exercise routines for everyone, it is often necessary to provide general recommendations that are appropriate for most individuals. The classification of exercises in this concept should be viewed in this context.

The risks associated with physical activity can be reduced by modifying the variables or conditions under which the activity is performed. While some exercises are contraindicated, it is almost always possible to find safer (or modified) alternatives. The variables that are typically under the direct control of the participant include exercise frequency (the number of repetitions performed in a given time span), duration (the length of time activity is sustained), intensity (the amount of resistance), speed (the velocity of activity, or rate, at which resistance is applied), and quality (the posture and mechanics of the body parts involved in the movement). Table 2 highlights these five activity variables, illustrates how each might be involved in potential injury, and provides suggestions for

modifying the variable to reduce the risk for injury. In some cases, changing a single variable may significantly reduce risk, but in other cases, multiple factors may need to be changed. In many cases, the best strategy is to look for a safer exercise. A variety of contraindicated exercises and safer alternatives are presented in Table 3 (pages 242–248) at the end of the concept.

Risks from exercise can't be completely avoided. Variables that are not always under the direct control of the participant include environmental conditions, such as temperature, humidity, or exercise surface. Likewise, the demands of sport and certain occupations may require individuals to train or work to the maximal limit of these variables (up to or just short of injury). Circumstances may not always permit every variable to be modified to suit an individual. However, making an active effort to adjust variables that are modifiable will make a difference in reducing injury risk.

Contraindicated Not recommended because of the potential for harm.

In the News

Clinical Applications (and Implications) of New Gaming Technology

Gaming technology has spawned a variety of sport and clinical applications since it creates an engaging and motivational climate for medical rehabilitation. Many physical therapy clinics now use the Wii to promote interest and motivation in patients. The games can be set up to require similar postures and body movements needed for traditional therapy exercises. Patients may tire of repetitive exercise but become engrossed in the task of the game and forget that they are exercising. The potential of the tools for rehabilitation is clearly a positive application but new studies report some clinical problems associated with excessive gaming—prompting some to characterize new conditions of Wii-itis and Nintendin-itis.

Do you see more advantages or disadvantages associated with the increased availability of gaming technology in society?

Some additional general guidelines will help prevent postural, back, and neck problems. In addition to the suggestions for improving body mechanics noted in the previous sections, the following guidelines should be helpful:

- Do exercises to strengthen abdominal and hip extensors and to stretch the hip flexors and lumbar muscles if they are tight (see Tables 3 to 10).

- Avoid hazardous exercises.

- Do regular physical activity for the entire body, such as walking, jogging, swimming, and bicycling.

- Choose an appropriate warm-up before strenuous activity.

- Sleep on a moderately firm mattress or place a 3/4-inch-thick plywood board under the mattress.

- Avoid sudden, jerky back movements, especially twisting.

- Maintain a healthy weight. The smaller the waistline, the less the strain on the lower back.

- Use appropriate back and seat supports when sitting for long periods.

- Maintain good posture when carrying heavy loads; do not lean forward, sideways, or backward.

- Adjust sports equipment to permit good posture; for example, adjust a bicycle seat and handle bars to permit good body alignment.

- Avoid long periods of sitting at a desk or driving; take frequent breaks and adjust the car seat and headrest for maximum support.

Strategies for Action

An important step in taking action is assessing your current status. The Healthy Back Tests consist of eight pass or fail items that will give you an idea of the areas in which you might need improvement. The Healthy Back Tests are described in *Lab Resource Materials*. You will take these tests in Lab 11A. Experts have identified behaviors associated with potential future back and neck problems. A questionnaire is also provided for assessing these risk factors.

Adopting and maintaining good posture promotes good back health. Lab 11B includes a posture test to help you evaluate your posture. Identify possible postural problems and take appropriate corrective action to reduce stress and strain on your back and neck.

Specific exercises are sometimes needed to prevent or help rehabilitate postural, neck, and back problems. Exercises included in previous concepts were presented with health-related fitness in mind. The exercises included in this concept are not so different. They are either flexibility or strength/muscle endurance exercises for specific muscle groups; however, each is selected specifically to help correct a postural problem or to remove the cause of neck and back pain. To that extent, these exercises may be classified as therapeutic. The same exercises may be called preventive because they can be used to prevent postural or spine problems. People who have back and neck pain should seek the advice of a physician to make certain that it is safe for them to perform the exercises.

The exercises in Tables 4 to 10 are not necessarily intended for all people. Rather, use your results on the Healthy Back Tests and the posture test to determine the exercises that are most appropriate for you. Table 3 (pages 242–248) provides information on "Questionable Exercises and Safe Alternatives."

To facilitate the use of these exercises for back or postural problems, the most effective exercises for various maladies are organized in Tables 4 to 10. Lab 11C is designed to help you choose specific exercises related to test items in Lab 11A.

Keep records of progress to maintain a back care program. Lab 11C provides an activity logging sheet for keeping records of your progress as you regularly perform exercises to build and maintain good back and neck fitness.

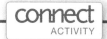

Web Resources

American Physical Therapy Association **www.apta.org**

American Spine Center **www.americanback.com**

Back and Body Care **www.backandbodycare.com**

Back Pain (Medline Plus-NIH) **www.nlm.nih.gov/ medlineplus/backpain.html**

Guide to Clinical Preventive Services **www .thecommunityguide.org/about/guide.html**

Low Back Pain (American Academy of Orthopaedic Surgeons) **http://orthoinfo.aaos.org/topic .cfm?topic=A00311**

Low Back Pain Fact Sheet (NIH) **www.ninds.nih.gov/ disorders/backpain/detail_backpain.htm**

MedX **www.medxonline.com**

National Osteoporosis Foundation **www.nof.org**

National Safety Council **www.nsc.org**

National Strength and Conditioning Association **www.nsca-cc.org**

Suggested Readings

Bird, M., et al. 2011. The long-term benefits of a multi-component exercise intervention to balance and mobility in healthy older adults. *Archives of Gerontology and Geriatrics* 52(2):211–216.

Brumitt, J. 2010. *Core Assessment and Training.* Champaign, IL: Human Kinetics.

Chang, Y., et al. 2010. Physical activity and cognition in older adults: The potential of Tai Chi Chuan. *Journal of Aging and Physical Activity* 18:451–472.

Ellingson, L. D., L. H. Colbert, and D. B. Cook. 2012. Physical activity is related to pain sensitivity in healthy women. *Medicine and Science in Sports and Exercise* 44(7):1401–1406.

Freburger, J. K., et al. 2009. The rising prevalence of chronic low back pain. *Archives of Internal Medicine* 169(3):251–258.

Jahnke, R., et al. 2010. A comprehensive review of health benefits of Qigong and Tai Chi. *American Journal of Health Promotion* 24(6):e1–e25.

Kiesel, K., Plisky, P., and R. Butler. 2011. Functional movement test scores improve following a standardized off-season intervention program in professional football players. *Scandinavian Journal of Medicine and Science in Sports* 21(2):287–292.

Martin, R. A., et al. 2008. Expenditures and health status among adults with back and neck problems. *Journal of the American Medical Association* 299(6):656–664.

Nelson, A., and J. Kokkonen. 2007. *Stretching Anatomy.* Champaign, IL: Human Kinetics.

O'Connor, F. G., et al. 2011. Functional movement screening: Predicting injuries in officer candidates. *Medicine and Science in Sports and Exercise* 43(12):2224–2230.

Rahman, S., et al. 2010. The association between obesity and low back pain: A meta-analysis. *American Journal of Epidemiology* 171(2):135–154.

Ratliff, J., A. Hilibrand, and A. R. Vaccaro. 2008. Spine-related expenditures and self-reported health status. *Journal of the American Medical Association* 299(22):2627.

Reid, Kieran F., and Roger A. Fielding. 2012. Skeletal muscle power: A critical determinant of physical functioning in older adults. *Exercise & Sport Sciences* 40(1):4–12.

Sanders, M. E. 2009. Off the floor exercises for back health. *ACSM's Health and Fitness Journal* 13(6):33–35.

Sherman, K. J., et al. 2011. A randomized trial comparing yoga, stretching, and a self-care book for chronic low back pain. *Archives of Internal Medicine* 171(22):2019–2026.

Tilbrook, H. E., et al. 2011. Yoga for chronic low back pain: A randomized trial. *Annals of Internal Medicine* 155(9):569–578.

Healthy People 2020

The objectives listed below are societal goals designed to help all Americans improve their health between now and the year 2020. They were selected because they relate to the content of this concept.

- Attain high-quality, longer lives free of preventable injury.
- Reduce activity limitations due to chronic back pain.
- Reduce joint pain in adults who have doctor-diagnosed arthritis.
- Reduce proportion of adults with arthritis limitations.
- Reduce prevalence of osteoporosis and hip fractures.
- Reduce sports and recreation injuries.
- Increase access to employee-based exercise facilities and programs.

A national goal is to increase the proportion of people who have activity limitations due to chronic back pain and recreational injuries. This concept provided information about the effects of questionable exercises, poor posture, and poor body mechanics on back and neck problems. It also described how functional fitness and core strength can help promote better posture and improve functional fitness. Do you think the overall prevalence of back and neck problems are caused by a lack of awareness of good posture/body mechanics, poor fitness, and core strength, or a combination?

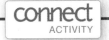

Table 3

Table 3 Questionable Exercises and Safer Alternatives

1. Questionable Exercise: The Swan

This exercise hyperextends the lower back and stretches the abdominals. The abdominals are too long and weak in most people and should not be lengthened further. Extension can be harmful to the back, potentially causing nerve impingement and facet joint compression. Other exercises in which this occurs include: cobras, backbends, straight-leg lifts, straight-leg sit-ups, prone-back lifts, donkey kicks, fire hydrants, backward trunk circling, weight lifting with the back arched, and landing from a jump with the back arched.

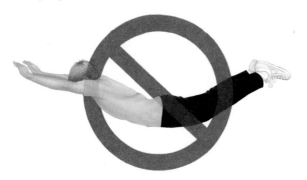

Safer Alternative Exercise: Back Extension

Lie prone over a roll of blankets or pillows and extend the back to a neutral or horizontal position.

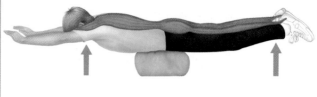

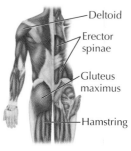

- Deltoid
- Erector spinae
- Gluteus maximus
- Hamstring

2. Questionable Exercise: Back-Arching Abdominal Stretch

This exercise can stretch the hip flexors, quadriceps, and shoulder flexors (such as the pectorals), but it also stretches the abdominals, which is not desired. Because of the armpull, it can potentially hyperflex the knee joint and strain neck musculature.

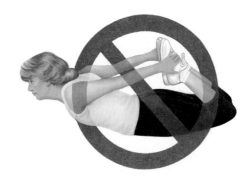

Note: All safer alternative exercises should be held 15 to 30 seconds unless otherwise indicated.

Safer Alternative Exercise: Wand Exercise

This exercise stretches the front of the shoulders and chest. Sit with wand grasped at ends. Raise wand overhead. Be certain that the head does not slide forward. Keep the chin tucked and neck straight. Bring wand down behind shoulder blades. Keep spine erect. Hold. Press forward on the wand simultaneously by pushing with the hands. Relax; then try to move the hands lower, sliding the wand down the back. Hold again. Hands may be moved closer together to increase stretch on

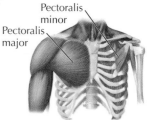

- Pectoralis minor
- Pectoralis major

chest muscles. If this is an easy exercise for you, try straightening the elbows and bringing the wand to waist level in back of you.

3. Questionable Exercise: Seated Forward Arm Circles with Palms Down

This exercise (arms straight out to the sides) may cause pinching of the rotator cuff and biceps tendons between the bony structures of the shoulder joint and/or irritate the bursa in the shoulder. The tendency is to emphasize the use of the stronger chest muscles (pectorals) to perform the motion rather than emphasizing the weaker upper back muscles.

Safer Alternative Exercise: Seated Backward Arm Circles with Palms Up

Sit, turn palms up, pull in chin, and contract abdominals. Circle arms backward.

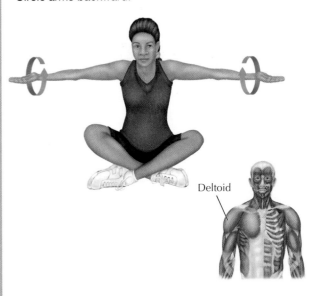

Deltoid

4. Questionable Exercise: Double-Leg Lift

This exercise is usually used with the intent of strengthening the abdominals, when in fact it is primarily a hip flexor (iliopsoas) strengthening exercise. Most people have overdeveloped the hip flexors and do not need to further strengthen those muscles because this may cause forward pelvic tilt. Even if the abdominals are strong enough to contract isometrically to prevent hyperextension of the lower back, the exercise produces excess stress on the discs.

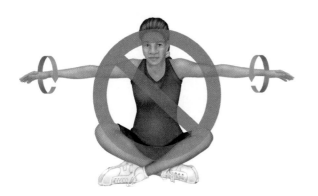

Safer Alternative Exercise: Reverse Curl

This exercise strengthens the lower abdominals. Lie on your back on the floor and bring your knees in toward the chest. Place the arms at the sides for support. For movement, pull the knees toward the head, raising the hips off the floor. Do not let knees go past the shoulders. Return to starting position and repeat.

Rectus abdominis

Table 3

Table 3 Questionable Exercises and Safer Alternatives

5. Questionable Exercise: The Windmill

This exercise involves simultaneous rotation and flexion (or extension) of the lower back, which is contraindicated. Because of the orientation of the facet joints in the lumbar spine, these movements violate normal joint mechanics, placing tremendous torsional stress on the joint capsule and discs.

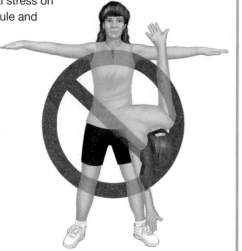

Safer Alternative Exercise: Back-Saver Toe Touch

Sit on the floor. Extend leg and bend the other knee, placing the foot flat on the floor. Bend at the hips and reach forward with both hands. Grasp one foot, ankle, or calf depending upon the distance you can reach. Pull forward with your arms and bend forward. Slight bend in the knee is acceptable. Hold. Repeat with the opposite leg.

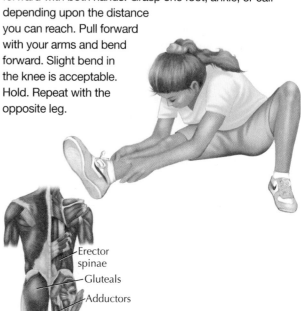

- Erector spinae
- Gluteals
- Adductors

6. Questionable Exercise: Neck Circling

This exercise and other exercises that require neck hyperextension (e.g., neck bridging) can pinch arteries and nerves in the neck and at the base of the skull, cause wear and tear to small joints of the spine, and produce dizziness or myofascial trigger points. In people with degenerated discs, it can cause dizziness, numbness, or even precipitate strokes. It also aggravates arthritis and degenerated discs.

Safer Alternative Exercise: Head Clock

This exercise relaxes the muscle of the neck. Assume a good posture (seated with legs crossed or in a chair), and imagine that your neck is a clock face with the chin at the center. Flex the neck and point the chin at 6:00, hold, lift the chin; repeat pointing chin to 4:00, to 8:00, to 3:00 and finally to 9:00. Return to center position with chin up after each movement.

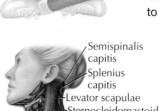

- Semispinalis capitis
- Splenius capitis
- Levator scapulae
- Sternocleidomastoid
- Scalenes
- Trapezius

7. Questionable Exercise: Shoulder Stand Bicycle

This exercise and the yoga positions called the plough and the plough shear (not shown) force the neck and upper back to hyperflex. It has been estimated that 80 percent of the population has forward head and kyphosis (humpback) with accompanying weak muscles. This exercise is especially dangerous for these people. Neck hyperflexion results in excessive stretch on the ligaments and nerves. It can also aggravate preexisting arthritic conditions. If the purpose for these exercises is to reduce gravitational effects on the circulatory system or internal organs, lie on a tilt board with the feet elevated. If the purpose is to warm up the muscles in the legs, slow jog in place. If the purpose is to stretch the lower back, try the leg hug exercise.

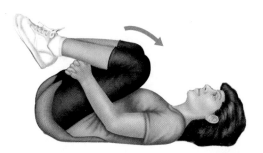

Safer Alternative Exercise: Leg Hug

Lie on your back with the knees bent at about 90 degrees. Bring your knees to the chest and wrap the arms around the back of the thighs. Pull knees to chest and hold.

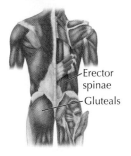

Erector spinae
Gluteals

8. Questionable Exercise: Straight-Leg and Bent-Knee Sit-Ups

There are several valid criticisms of the sit-up exercise. Straight-leg sit-ups can displace the fifth lumbar vertebra, causing back problems. A bent-knee sit-up creates less shearing force on the spine, but some recent studies have shown it produces greater compression on the lumbar discs than the straight-leg sit-up. Placing the hands behind the neck or head during the sit-up or during a crunch results in hyperflexion of the neck.

Safer Alternative Exercise: Crunch

Lie on your back with the knees bent more than 90 degrees. Curl up until the shoulder blades lift off the floor, then roll down to starting position and repeat. There are several safe arm positions. The easiest is with the arms extended straight in front of the body. Alternatives are with the arms crossed over the chest or the palms or fist held beside the ears.

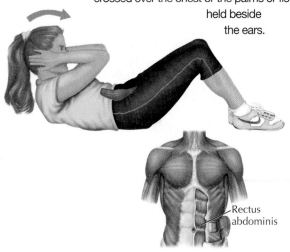

Rectus abdominis

Table 3 Questionable Exercises and Safer Alternatives

Table 3

9. Questionable Exercise: Standing Toe Touches or Double-Leg Toe Touches

These exercises—especially when done ballistically—can produce degenerative changes at the vertebrae of the lower back. They also stretch the ligaments and joint capsule of the knee. Bending the back while the legs are straight may cause back strain, particularly if the movement is done ballistically. If performed only on rare occasions as a test, the chance of injury is less than if incorporated into a regular exercise program. Safer stretches of the lower back include the leg hug, the single knee-to-chest, the back-saver hamstring stretch, and the back-saver toe touch.

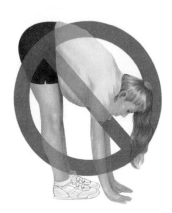

Safer Alternative Exercise: Back-Saver Hamstring Stretch

This exercise stretches the hamstring and lower back muscles. Sit with one leg extended and one knee bent, foot turned outward and close to the buttocks. Clasp hands behind back. Bend forward from the hips, keeping the low back as straight as possible. Allow bent knee to move laterally so trunk can move forward. Stretch and hold. Repeat with the other leg.

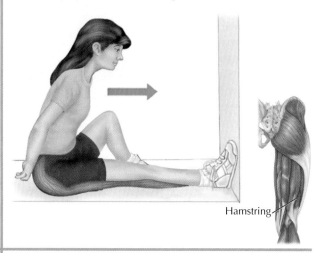

Hamstring

10. Questionable Exercise: Bar Stretch

This type of stretch may be harmful. Some experts have found that when the extended leg is raised 90 degrees or more and the trunk is bent over the leg, it may lead to **sciatica** and **piriformis syndrome,** especially in the person who has limited flexibility.

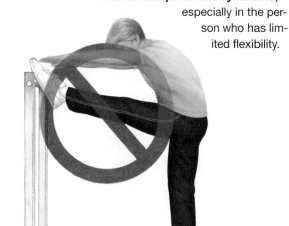

Safer Alternative Exercise: One-Leg Stretch

This exercise stretches the hamstring muscles. Stand with one foot on a bench, keeping both legs straight. Hinge forward from the hips keeping shoulders back and chest up. Bend forward until a pull is felt on the back side of the thigh. Hold. Repeat.

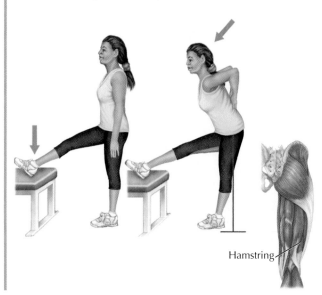

Hamstring

11. Questionable Exercise: Shin and Quadriceps Stretch

This exercise causes hyperflexion of the knee. When the knee is hyperflexed more than 120 degrees and/or rotated outward by an external **torque,** the ligaments and joint capsule are stretched, and damage to the cartilage may occur. Note: one of the quadriceps, the rectus femoris, is not stretched if the trunk is allowed to bend forward because it crosses the hip as well as the knee joint. If the exercise is used to stretch the quadriceps, substitute the hip and thigh stretch. For most people it is not necessary to stretch the shin muscles, since they are often elongated and weak; however, if you need to stretch the shin muscles to relieve muscle soreness, try the shin stretch.

Safer Alternative Exercise: Hip and Thigh Stretch

Kneel so that the front leg is bent at 90 degrees (front knee directly above the front ankle). The knee of the back leg should touch the floor well behind the front foot. Press the pelvis forward and downward. Hold. Repeat with the opposite leg forward. Do not bend the front knee more than 90 degrees.

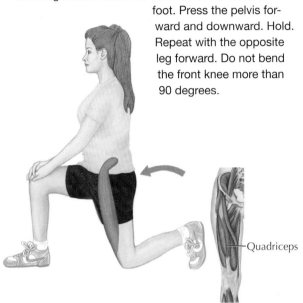

Quadriceps

12. Questionable Exercise: The Hero

Like the shin and quadriceps stretch, this exercise causes hyperflexion of the knee. It also causes torque on the hyperflexed knee. For these reasons the ligaments and joint capsule are stretched and the cartilage may be damaged. For most people it is not necessary to stretch the shin muscles since they are often elongated and weak; however, if you need to stretch the shin muscles, use the shin stretch. If this exercise is used to stretch the quadriceps, substitute the hip and thigh stretch.

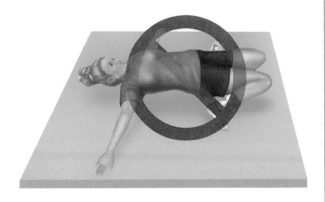

Safer Alternative Exercise: Shin Stretch

Kneel on your knees, turn to right and press down on right ankle with right hand. Hold. Keep hips thrust forward to avoid hyperflexing the knees. Do not sit on the heels. Repeat on the left side.

Tibialis anterior

Extensor digitorum longus

Extensor hallucis longus

Sciatica Pain along the sciatic nerve in the buttock and leg.

Piriformis Syndrome Muscle spasm and nerve entrapment in the pyriformis muscle of the buttocks region, causing pain in the buttock and referred pain down the leg (sciatica).

Torque A twisting or rotating force.

Table 3 Questionable Exercises and Safer Alternatives

Table 3

13. Questionable Exercise: Deep Squatting Exercises

This exercise, with or without weights, places the knee joint in hyperflexion, tends to "wedge it open," stretching the ligaments, irritating the synovial membrane, and possibly damaging the cartilage. The joint has even greater stress when the lower leg and foot are not in straight alignment with the knee. If you are performing squats to strengthen the knee and hip extensors, try substituting the alternate leg kneel or half-squat with free weight or leg presses on a resistance machine.

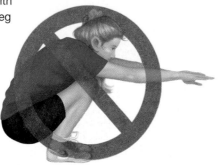

Safer Alternative Exercise: Half Squat

This exercise develops the muscles of the thighs and buttocks. Stand upright with feet shoulder width apart. Squat slowly by moving hips backwards, then bending knees. Keep shins vertical. Bend knees 45–90 degrees. Repeat.

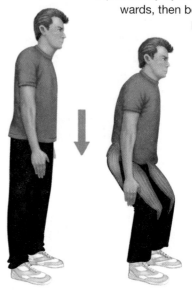

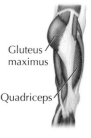

Gluteus maximus

Quadriceps

14. Questionable Exercise: Knee Pull-Down

This exercise can result in hyperflexion of the knee. The arms or hands placed on top of the shin places undue stress on the knee joint.

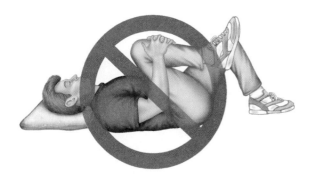

Safer Alternative Exercise: Single Knee-to-Chest

Lie down with both knees bent, draw one knee to the chest by pulling on the thigh with the hands, then extend the knee and point the foot toward the ceiling. Hold. Pull to chest again and return to starting position. Repeat with other leg.

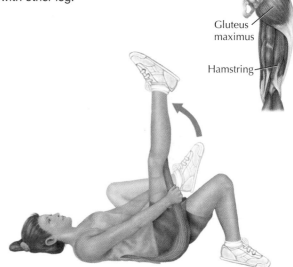

Gluteus maximus

Hamstring

Stretching Exercises for the Hip Flexors and Hamstrings Table 4

Table 4

When performed on a regular basis, these exercises will help maintain neutral spine posture and improve the flexibility of the hip flexor and hip extensor musculature. (Tightness of these muscles can, respectively, contribute to a forward or backward pelvic tilt due to their attachments to the pelvis.) Hold stretches for 15 to 30 seconds.

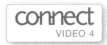

1. Back-Saver Hamstring Stretch

This exercise stretches the hamstrings and calf muscles. Sit on the floor with the feet against the wall or an immovable object. Bend left knee and bring foot close to buttocks. Clasp hands behind back. Bend forward from hips, keeping lower back as straight as possible. Let bent knee rotate outward so trunk can move forward keeping back flat. Hold and repeat on each leg.

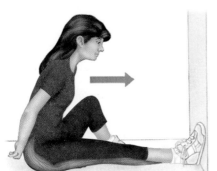

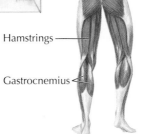

Hamstrings —

Gastrocnemius ◄—

3. Hip and Low Back Stretch

This exercise stretches the hip flexors of one leg and the gluteals and lumbar muscles of the opposite leg. Lie on your back. Draw one knee up to the chest and pull thigh toward chest with the hands; then slowly return to the original position. Repeat with other knee. Do not grasp knee— grasp thigh. If a partner or a weight stabilizes the extended leg, the hip flexor muscles on that leg will be stretched.

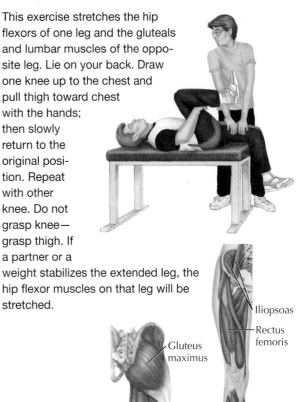

Iliopsoas

Rectus femoris

Gluteus maximus

2. Single Knee-to-Chest

This exercise stretches the lower back, gluteals, and hamstring muscles. Lie on your back with knees bent. Use hands on back of thigh to draw one knee to the chest. Hold. Then extend the knee and point the foot toward the ceiling. Hold. Return to the starting position without arching your back. Repeat with other leg.

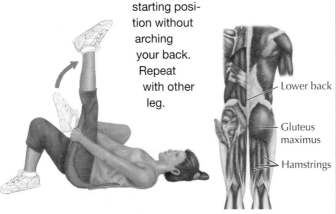

— Lower back

— Gluteus maximus

► Hamstrings

4. Hip and Thigh Stretch

This exercise stretches the hip flexor muscles and helps prevent or correct forward pelvic tilt, lumbar lordosis, and backache. Place right knee directly above right ankle and stretch left leg backward so knee touches floor. If necessary, place hands on floor for balance. Press pelvis forward and downward. Hold. Repeat on opposite side. Caution: Do not bend front knee more than 90 degrees.

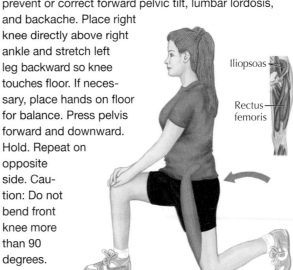

Iliopsoas

Rectus femoris

Table 5

Table 5 Core Stabilization Exercises

These exercises help train the abdominal and buttock muscles to provide postural stability by maintaining the pelvis in a neutral position during activity. They help prevent or correct lumbar lordosis, abdominal ptosis (see Table 1), and backache. Hold exercises for 15 to 30 seconds.

1. Abdominal Hollowing on Hands and Knees

Begin on hands and knees with lower back in a neutral position, stomach muscles relaxed and sag-

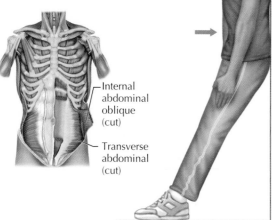

ging and eyes looking at the floor. Hands should be aligned directly below shoulders and knees directly below hips. The action is to pull the belly button "in and up," drawing it toward the spine. If performed correctly, the muscles below the umbilicus will flatten, rather than bulge. Recruitment of the transverse abdominus may be facilitated by coughing and then holding the muscle contraction. The exercise is held for 10–30 seconds. Breathe normally throughout the contraction. Repeat 10 times.

Internal abdominal oblique (cut)
Transverse abdominal (cut)

2. Abdominal Hollowing in Wall Support

Begin standing with feet 6 inches from the wall and back gently resting against the surface. Maintain a neutral spine. Contract the muscles below the belly button by pulling the abdominal wall "in and up." The pelvic floor may be contracted at the same time by pulling it "up and in" in a gripping motion. Breathe throughout the contraction. Hold 10–30 seconds. Repeat 10 times.

Internal abdominal oblique (cut)

Transverse abdominal (cut)

3. Horizontal Side Support

Begin in side lying position with the body resting on the forearm. Slowly lift the pelvis until the body forms a straight line from foot to shoulder. Hold 10–30 seconds. Repeat 8–12 times.

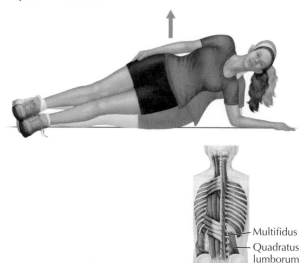

Multifidus
Quadratus lumborum

4. Head Nod

Lie flat on the back without a pillow. Gently nod the head in a "yes" motion. Motion should result in the tightening of muscles deep in the front of the neck. Place two fingers over the sides of the neck to monitor for the undesirable substitution of stronger muscles in this region.

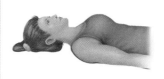

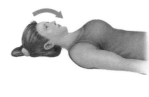

Hold 10–30 seconds (or as long as can be maintained without substitution). Repeat 10 times. Progress this exercise by first nodding "yes" and then lifting the head ¼ inch to ½ inch off the surface.

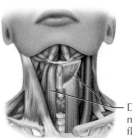

Deep neck flexors

Exercises for Muscle Fitness of the Abdominals Table 6

These exercises are designed to increase the strength of the abdominal muscles. Strong abdominal muscles are important for maintaining a neutral pelvis, maintaining good posture, and preventing backache associated with lordosis.

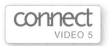

Table 6

1. Reverse Curl

Lie on your back. Bend the knees and bring knees in toward the chest. Place arms at sides for balance and support. Pull the knees toward the chest, raising the hips off the floor. Do not let the knees go past the shoulders. Return to the starting position. Repeat.

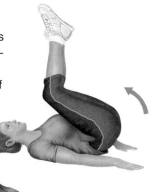

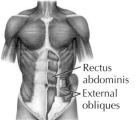

Rectus abdominis
External obliques

3. Crunch with Twist (on Bench)

Lie on your back with your feet on a bench, knees bent at 90 degrees. Arms may be extended or on shoulders or hands on ears (the most difficult). Same as crunch except twist the upper trunk so the right shoulder is higher than the left.

Reach toward the left knee with the right elbow. Hold. Return and repeat to the opposite side. (This exercise is not recommended for people with lower back pain due to the combined motions of flexion and rotation.)

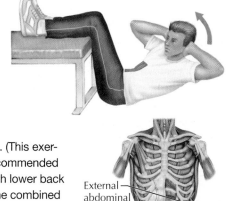

External abdominal oblique (cut)
Internal abdominal oblique

2. Crunch (Curl-Up)

Lie on your back with your knees bent and palms on ears. If desired, legs may rest on bench to increase difficulty. For less resistance, place hands at side of body. For more resistance, move hands higher. Curl up until shoulder blades leave floor, then roll down to the starting position. Repeat. Variation: extend the arms or cross the arms over your chest.

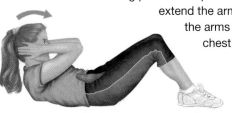

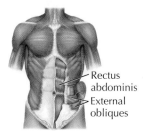

Rectus abdominis
External obliques

4. Sitting Tucks

Sit on floor with feet raised, arms extended for balance. Alternately bend and extend legs without letting your back or feet touch floor. (This is an advanced exercise and is not recommended for people who have back pain.)

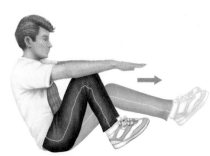

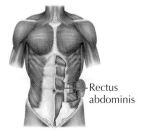

Rectus abdominis

Table 7

Table 7 Stretching and Strengthening Exercises for the Muscles of the Neck

These exercises are designed to increase strength in the neck muscles and to improve neck range of motion. They are helpful in preventing and resolving symptoms of neck pain and for relieving trigger points. Hold stretches for 15–30 seconds.

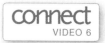

1. Neck Rotation Exercise

This PNF exercise strengthens and stretches the neck rotators. It should always be done with the head and neck in axial extension (good alignment). It is particularly useful for relieving trigger point pain and stiffness. Place palm of left hand against left cheek. Point fingers toward ear and point elbow forward. Turn head and neck to the left; contract while gently resisting with left hand. Contract neck muscle for 6 seconds. Relax and turn head to right as far as possible; hold stretch. Repeat four times; repeat on opposite side.

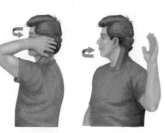
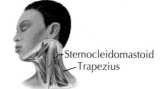

Sternocleidomastoid
Trapezius

2. Isometric Neck Exercises

This exercise strengthens the neck muscles. Sit and place one or both hands on the head as shown. Assume good head and neck posture by tucking the chin, flattening the neck, and pushing the crown of the head up (axial extension). Apply resistance (a) sideward, (b) backward, and (c) forward. Contract the neck muscles to prevent the head and neck from moving. Hold contraction for 6 seconds. Repeat each exercise up to six times. Note: for neck muscles, it is probably best to use a little less than a maximal contraction, especially in the presence of arthritis, degenerated discs, or injury.

Neck flexors

Neck rotator and extensors

3. Chin Tuck

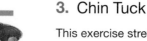

This exercise stretches the muscles at the base of the skull and reduces headache symptoms. Place hands together at the base of the head. Tuck in the chin and gently press head backward into your hands, while looking straight ahead. Hold.

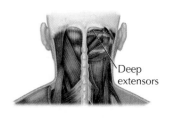

Deep extensors

4. Upper Trapezius Stretch

This exercise stretches the upper trapezius muscle and relieves neck pain and headache. To stretch the right upper trapezius, place left hand on top of head, right hand behind back. Gently turn head toward left underarm and tilt chin toward chest. Increase stretch by gently drawing head forward with left hand. Hold. Repeat to opposite side.

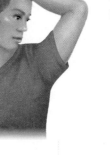

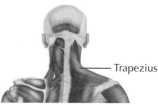

Trapezius

Table 8

Exercises for Trunk Mobility Table 8

These exercises are designed to increase the strength and mobility of the muscles that move the trunk. They are especially helpful for people with chronic back pain. Hold stretches for 15 to 30 seconds.

connect VIDEO 7

1. Upper Trunk Lift

Lie on a table, bench, or special-purpose bench designed for trunk lifts with the upper half of the body hanging over the edge. Have a partner stabilize the feet and legs while the trunk is raised parallel to the floor; then lower the trunk to the starting position. Lift smoothly, one segment of the back at a time. Place hands behind neck or on ears. Do not raise past the horizontal or arch the back or neck.

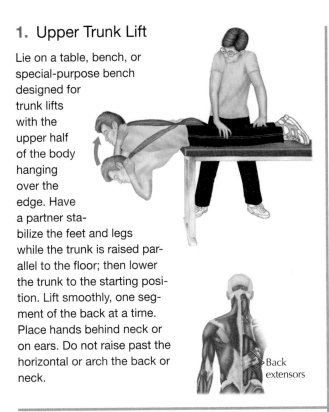

Back extensors

3. Side Bend

This exercise stretches the trunk lateral flexors. Stand with feet shoulder-width apart. Stretch left arm overhead to right. Bend to right at waist, reaching as far to right as possible with left arm; reach as far as possible to the left with right arm. Hold. Do not let trunk rotate or lower back arch. Repeat on opposite side. Note: this exercise is more effective if a weight is held down at the side in the hand opposite the side being stretched. More stretch will occur if the hip on the stretched side is dropped and most of the weight is borne by the opposite foot.

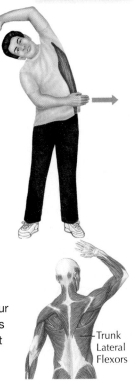

Trunk Lateral Flexors

2. Trunk Lift

This exercise develops the muscles of the upper back and corrects round shoulders. Lie face down with hands clasped behind the neck. Pull the shoulder blades together, raising the elbows off the floor. Slowly raise the head and chest off the floor by arching the upper back. Return to the starting position. Repeat. For less resistance, hands may be placed under thighs. Caution: Do not arch the lower back or neck. Lift only until the sternum (breastbone) clears the floor. Variations: arms down at sides (easiest), hands by head, hands extended (hardest).

Trunk extensors

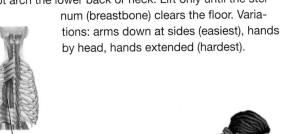

4. Supine Trunk Twist

This exercise increases the flexibility of the spine and stretches the rotator muscles. Lie on your back with your arms extended at shoulder level. Place left foot on right knee cap. Twist the lower body by lowering left knee to touch floor on right. Turn head to left. Keep shoulders and arms on floor. Hold.

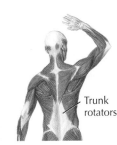

Trunk rotators

Table 8

Table 8 Exercises for Trunk Mobility

5. Lower Trunk Lift

This exercise develops low back and hip strength. Lie on your stomach on a bench or table with legs hanging over the edge. Have a partner stabilize the upper back or grasp the edges of the table with hands. Raise the legs parallel to the floor and lower them. Do not raise past the horizontal or arch the back. Suggested progression: (1) Begin by alternating legs; (2) when you can do 25 reps, add ankle weights; (3) when you can do 25 reps, lift both legs simultaneously (no weights).

Erector spinae

Gluteus maximus

6. Press-Up (McKenzie Extension Exercise)

This exercise increases flexibility of the lumbar spine and restores normal lordotic curve, especially for people with a flat lumbar spine. Lie on your stomach with hands under the face. Slowly press up to a rest position on forearms. Keep pelvis on floor. Relax and hold 10 seconds. Perform 5–10 repetitions. Do several times a day. Progress to gradually straightening the elbows while keeping the pubic bone on the floor. Caution: do not perform if you have lordosis or if you feel any pain or discomfort in the back or legs. Note: a prone press-up will feel good as a stretch after doing abdominal strength or endurance exercises. This relaxed lordotic position can be performed while standing. Place the hands in the small of the back and gently arch the back and hold. This should feel good after sitting for a long period with the back flat.

Stretching and Strengthening Exercises for Round Shoulders

Table 9

These exercises are designed to stretch the muscles of the chest and strengthen the muscles that keep the shoulders pulled back in good alignment (scapular adduction).

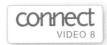

Table 9

1. Arm Lift

This exercise strengthens the scapular adductors. Lie on stomach with arms in reverse-T. Rest forehead on floor. Maintain the arm position and contract the muscles between the shoulder blades, lifting the arms as high as possible without raising head and trunk. Hold. Relax and repeat. Note: if the arms are first pressed against the floor before lifting, this becomes a PNF exercise and range of motion may be greater. Variation: this more advanced exercise is performed in the same way except the arms are extended overhead.

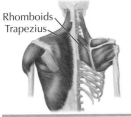

Rhomboids
Trapezius

2. Seated Rowing

This exercise strengthens the scapular adductors (rhomboid and trapezius). Sit facing pulley, feet braced and knees slightly bent. Grasp bar, palms down with hands shoulder-width apart. Pull bar to chest, keeping elbows high, and return.

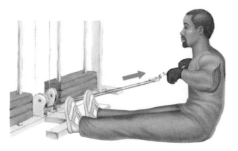

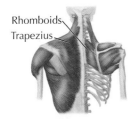

Rhomboids
Trapezius

3. Wand Exercise

This exercise stretches the muscles on the front of the shoulder joint. Sit with wand grasped at ends. Raise wand overhead. Be certain that the head does not slide forward into a "poke neck" position. Keep the chin tucked and neck straight. Bring wand down behind shoulder blades. Keep spine erect; hold. Hands may be moved closer together to increase stretch on chest muscles.

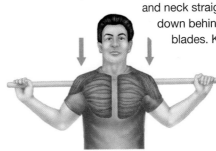

Pectoralis major

4. Pectoral Stretch

This exercise stretches the chest muscle (pectorals).

1. Stand erect in doorway with arms raised 45 degrees, elbows bent, and hands grasping door jambs, feet in front stride position. Press out on door frame, contracting the arms maximally for 3 seconds. Relax and shift weight forward on legs. Lean into doorway, so muscles on front of shoulder joint and chest are stretched. Hold.
2. Repeat with arms raised 90 degrees.
3. Repeat with arms raised 135 degrees.

(This exercise is not recommended for people with shoulder instability. Discontinue if it causes numbness in the arms or hands.)

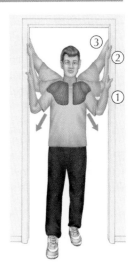

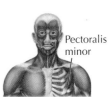

Pectoralis minor

Table 10

Table 10 Lumbar Stabilization Exercises with Stability Balls

These exercises are designed to help improve the ability of the back to stabilize and support the trunk. The physioballs provide a useful way to learn to balance the body in these positions.

1. Balancing

Contract abdominal muscles. Straighten one knee and raise opposite arm over head. Alternate sides. To increase difficulty, position ball farther from your body. Variation: slowly walk ball forward or backward with legs. Be careful not to arch back.

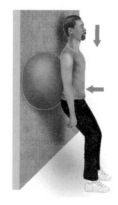

3. Wall Support

Stand against a wall with ball supporting low back. Contract abdominal muscles. Slowly bend knees 45 to 90 degrees and hold 5 seconds. Straighten knees and repeat. Raise both arms over head to increase difficulty.

2. Marching

Sit up straight with hips and knees bent 90 degrees. Contract abdominal muscles. Slowly raise one heel off the ground and opposite arm over head. Alternate sides. To increase difficulty, slowly raise one foot 2 inches from floor, alternating sides.

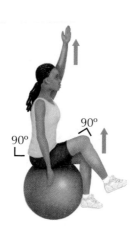

4. Stomach Roll

Lie prone over ball with abdominal region supported. Lower back and neck should be in neutral position with hands supported on floor directly under shoulders. Raise one leg off the floor while maintaining balance and a neutral spine. Alternate sides. To increase difficulty, raise one leg and opposite arm.

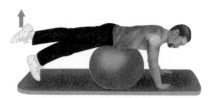

Lab Resource Materials: Healthy Back Tests

Chart 1 Healthy Back Tests

Physicians and therapists use these tests, among others, to make differential diagnoses of back problems. You and your partner can use them to determine if you have muscle tightness that may put you at risk for back problems. Discontinue any of these tests if they produce pain, numbness, or tingling sensations in the back, hips, or legs. Experiencing any of these sensations may be an indication that you have a low back problem that requires diagnosis by your physician. Partners should use *great caution* in applying force. Be gentle and listen to your partner's feedback.

FLEXIBILITY

Test 1—Straight-Leg Lift

Lie on your back with hands behind your neck. The partner on your left should stabilize your right leg by placing his or her right hand on your knee. With the left hand, your partner should grasp your left ankle and raise your left leg as near to a right angle as possible. In this position (as shown in the diagram), your lower back should be in contact with the floor. Your right leg should remain straight and on the floor throughout the test.

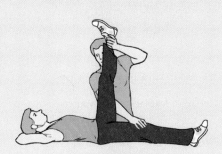

If your left leg bends at the knee, this indicates short hamstring muscles. If your back arches and/or your right leg does not remain flat on the floor this indicates short lumbar muscles or hip flexor muscles. To pass the test, each leg should be able to reach approximately 90 degress without the knee or back bending. (Both sides must pass in order to pass the test.)

Test 2—Thomas Test

Lie on your back on a table or bench with your right leg extended beyond the edge of the table (approximately one-third of your thigh off the table). Bring your left knee to your chest and pull your thigh down tightly with your hands. Lower your right leg. Your lower back should remain flat against the table, as shown in the diagram. To pass the test, your right thigh should be at table level or lower.

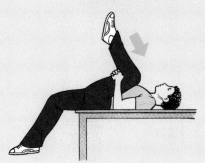

Test 3—Ober Test

Lie on your left side with your left leg flexed 90 degrees at the hip and 90 degrees at the knee. A partner should place your right hip in slight extension and right knee with just a slight bend (~20 degrees flexion). Your partner stabilizes your pelvis with the left hand to prevent movement. Your partner then allows the weight of the top leg to lower the leg to the floor. To pass the test your knee or upper leg should be able to touch the table.

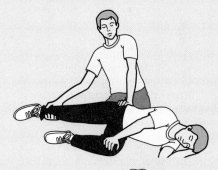

CORE TRUNK ENDURANCE TESTS

Test 4—Leg Drop Test*

Lie on your back on a table or on the floor with both legs extended overhead. Flatten your low back against the table or floor by tightening your abdominals. Slowly lower your legs while keeping your back flat.

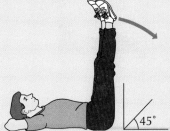

If your back arches before you reach a 45-degree angle, your abdominal muscles are too weak and you fail the test. A partner should be ready to support your legs if needed to prevent your lower back from arching or strain to the back muscles.

*The Leg Drop Test is suitable as a diagnostic test when performed one time. It is not a good exercise to be performed regularly by most people. If it causes pain, stop the test.

Chart 1 Healthy Back Tests *(Continued)*

Test 5—Isometric Abdominal Test. Lie supine with hips bent 45 degrees, feet flat on the floor and arms by the side. Draw a line 4 1/2 inches beyond fingertips. Tuck chin and curl trunk forward, touching line with fingers. To pass, hold for 30 seconds.

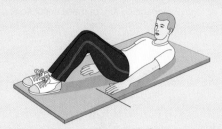

Test 6—Isometric Extensor Test. Lie on a table with upper half of the body hanging over the edge and arms crossed in front of chest. Have a partner stabilize your feet and legs. Raise your trunk smoothly until your back is in a horizontal position parallel to the floor. Do not arch the back. To pass the test hold this position for 30 seconds.

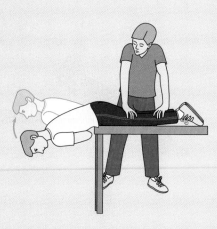

Test 7—Prone Bridge. Support yourself on the floor by resting on forearms and balls of feet, body extended and back straight. Elbows are placed directly underneath shoulders. Look straight down toward hands. Do not arch the back. To pass the test hold this position for 30 seconds.

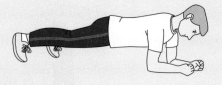

Test 8—Quadruped Stabilization. Begin on hands and knees. Place hands directly below shoulders and knees directly below hips. Draw abdominals in. Extend one arm and opposite leg to a horizontal position. Do not allow back to arch or body to sway. To pass, hold position for 30 seconds.

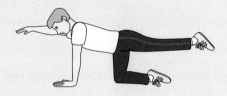

Test 9—Right Lateral Bridge. Lie on your right side with legs extended. Raise pelvis off the floor until trunk is straight and body weight is supported on arm and feet. Do not roll forward or backward. Do not arch back. Hold this position for 30 seconds.

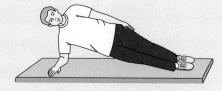

Test 10—Left Lateral Bridge. Lie on your left side with legs extended. Raise pelvis off the floor until trunk is straight and body weight is supported on arm and feet. Do not roll forward or backward or arch back. To pass the test, hold this position for 30 seconds.

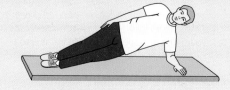

Chart 2 Healthy Back Test Ratings

Classification	Number of Tests Passed
Excellent	8–10
Very good	7
Good	6
Fair	5
Poor	1–4

Lab 11A The Healthy Back Tests and Back/Neck Questionnaire

Name   **Section**   **Date**

Purpose: To self-assess your potential for back problems using the Healthy Back Tests and the back/neck questionnaire

Procedures

1. Answer the questions in the following back/neck questionnaire. Count your points for nonmodifiable factors, modifiable factors, and total score, and record these scores in the Results section. Use Chart 1 to determine your rating for all three scores and record them in the Results section.
2. With a partner, administer the Healthy Back Tests to each other (see *Lab Resource Materials*). Determine your rating using Chart 2. Record your score and rating in the Results section. If you did not pass a test, list the muscles you should develop to improve on that test.
3. Complete the Conclusions and Implications section.

Risk-Factor Questionnaire for Back and Neck Problems

Directions: Place an X in the appropriate circle after each question. Add the scores for each of the circles you checked to determine your modifiable risk, nonmodifiable risk, and total risk scores.

Nonmodifiable

1. Do you have a family history of osteoporosis, arthritis, rheumatism, or other joint disease?   (0) No   (X) Yes

2. What is your age?   (X) <40   (1) 40–50   (2) 51–60   (3) 61+

3. Did you participate extensively in these sports when you were young: gymnastics, football, weight lifting, skiing, ballet, javelin, or shot put?   (0) No   (1) Some   (X) Extensive

4. How many previous back or neck problems have you had?   (0) None   (1) 1   (2) 2   (X) 3+

Modifiable

5. Does your daily routine involve heavy lifting?   (X) No   (1) Some   (3) A lot

6. Does your daily routine require you to stand for long periods?   (0) No   (X) Some   (3) A lot

7. Do you have a high level of job-related stress?   (0) No   (X) Some   (3) A lot

8. Do you sit for long periods of time (computer operator, typist, or similar job)?   (0) No   (X) Some   (3) A lot

9. Does your daily routine require doing repetitive movements or holding objects (e.g., baby, briefcase, sales suitcase) for long periods of time?   (0) No   (X) Some   (3) A lot

10. Does your daily routine require you to stand or sit with poor posture (e.g., sitting in a low car seat, reaching overhead with head tilted back)?   (0) No   (X) Some   (3) A lot

11. What is your score on the Healthy Back Tests?   (0) 6–7   (X) 5   (3) 4   (5) 0–3

12. What is your score on the posture test in Lab 11B?   (0) 0–2   (X) 3–4   (3) 5–7   (5) 8+

Results

Tests	Pass	Fail	If you failed, what exercise should you do?
1. Straight-leg lift	⊗	○	
2. Thomas test	⊗	○	
3. Ober test	⊗	○	
4. Leg drop test	⊗	○	
5. Isometric abdominal test	⊗	○	
6. Isometric extensor test	⊗	○	
7. Prone bridge	⊗	○	
8. Quadruped stabilization	⊗	○	
9. Right lateral bridge	⊗	○	
10. Left lateral bridge	⊗	○	

Total ☐

Chart 1 Back/Neck Questionnaire Ratings

Rating	Modifiable Score	Nonmodifiable Score	Total Score
Very high risk	7+	12+	19+
High risk	5–6	8–11	13–17
Average risk	3–4	4–7	7–11
Low risk	0–2	0–3	0–5

Chart 2 Healthy Back Tests Ratings

Classification	Number of Tests Passed
Excellent	8–10
Very good	7
Good	6
Fair	5
Poor	1–4

Back/Neck Questionnaire

Score ☐ 1.6 ☐ Rating high risk

Back Tests

Score ☐ 10 ☐ Rating Excellent

Conclusions and Implications: In several sentences, discuss your need to do exercises for care of the back and neck. Include in your discussion whether you think your muscles are fit enough to prevent problems, the areas in which you are most likely to experience problems, and steps you might take to prevent future problems. Use your test results to answer.

I have a history of things that would cause back problems. I need to stretch, work out, work on my posture, and just be more aware of back issues.

Lab 11B Evaluating Posture

Name _Jason Herm___

Section

Date

Purpose: To learn to recognize postural deviations and thus become more posture conscious and to determine your postural limitations in order to institute a preventive or corrective program

Procedures

1. Wear as little clothing as possible (bathing suits are recommended) and remove shoes and socks.
2. Work in groups of two or three, with one person acting as the subject while partners serve as examiners; then alternate roles.
   a. Stand by a vertical plumb line.
   b. Using Chart 1 and Figure 1, check any deviations and indicate their severity using the following point scale (0 = none, 1 = slight, 2 = moderate, and 3 = severe).
   c. Total the score and determine your posture rating from the Posture Rating Scale (Chart 2).
3. If time permits, perform back and posture exercises (see Lab 11C).
4. Complete the Conclusions and Implications section.

Results

Record your posture score: **4**

Record your posture rating from the Posture Rating Scale in Chart 2: 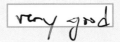 *very good*

Chart 1 Posture Evaluation

Side View	Points
Forward head	0
Rounded shoulders	2
Excessive lordosis (lumbar)	0
Abdominal ptosis	1
Hyperextended knees	1
Total scores	4

Chart 2 Posture Rating Scale

Classification	Total Score
Excellent	0–3
Very good	4–6
Good	7–9
Fair	10–12
Poor	12 or more

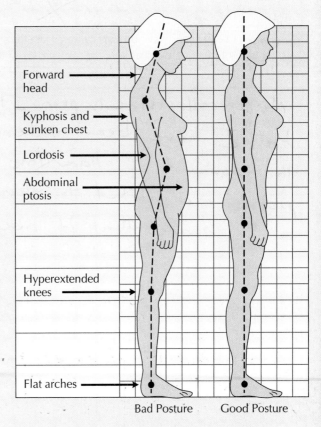

Figure 1 ▶ Comparison of bad and good posture.

Conclusions and Implications

Were you aware of the deviations that were found?   Yes ⊗   No ◯

1. List the deviations that were moderate or severe (use several complete sentences).

○ Shoulders were not rounded.
○ hunched over at times
○ Abdominal pushed in at times

My shoulders were not rounded and should be more pulled back. My abs were also slouched forward a bit and caused me to be hunched over.

2. In several sentences, describe your current posture status. Include in this discussion your overall assessment of your current posture, whether you think you will need special exercises in the future, and the reasons your posture rating is good or not so good.

My overall posture is poor. It used to be much worse but I have been made aware and have worked to improve it. I have done more exercises to correct posture and worked to think about my posture more to be aware that it needs constant correction.

Lab 11C Planning and Logging Exercises:
Care of the Back and Neck

Name: Jason Herrin

Section: _____ Date: _____

Purpose: To select several exercises for the back and neck that meet your personal needs and to self-monitor progress for one of these

Procedures

1. On Chart 1, check the tests from the Healthy Back Tests that you did *not* pass. Select at least one exercise from the group associated with those items. In addition, select several more exercises (a total of 8 to 10) that you think will best meet your personal needs. If you passed all of the items, select 8 to 10 exercises that you think will best prevent future back and neck problems. Check the exercises you plan to perform in Chart 1.
2. Perform each of the exercises you select 3 days in 1 week.
3. Keep a 1-week log of your actual participation using the last three columns in Chart 1. If possible, keep the log with you during the day. Place a check by each of the exercises you perform for each day, including ones that you didn't originally plan. If you cannot keep the log with you, fill in the log at the end of the day. If you choose to keep a log for more than 1 week, make extra copies of the log before you begin.
4. Answer the question in the Results section.

Chart 1 Back and Neck Exercise Plan

Check the tests you failed.	✓	Write in a selected exercise for each test that you can plan to perform this week. [The core tests (5–10) may be used as strengthening exercises]. Check the dates you performed the exercises.	Day 1 Date:	Day 2 Date:	Day 3 Date:
1. Straight-leg lift					
2. Thomas test					
3. Ober test					
4. Leg drop test		leg lifts	3/21	3/23	3/25
5. Isometric abdominal test		sit ups			
6. Isometric extensor test		Reverse situps			
7. Prone bridge		Pushup to plank			
8. Quadruped stabilization		Donkey kicks			
9. Right lateral bridge		Pelvis raises			
10. Left lateral bridge					

Results

Did you do 8 to 10 exercises at least 3 days in the week? Yes 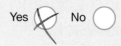 No ◯

Conclusions and Interpretations

1. Do you feel that you will use back and neck exercises as part of your regular lifetime physical activity plan, either now or in the future? Use several sentences to explain your answer.

> I need to do these exercises more than others because of my history of back problems and my high risk. I plan on continuing to work on my posture and reducing back problem risk through exercise and stretching

2. Discuss the exercises you did. What exercises would you continue to do, and which ones would you change? Use several sentences to explain your answer.

> I mainly did core exercises like leg lifts and sit ups. Doing reverse sit ups help because they balance the abdominals. I need to work on both front and back of my core.

Performance Benefits of Physical Activity

LEARNING OBJECTIVES

After completing the study of this concept, you will be able to:

▶ Describe characteristics of high-level performance and the training necessary for high-level performance.

▶ Identify the unique training considerations for endurance, speed, strength, muscular endurance, power, functional fitness, and flexibility.

▶ Explain how principles of periodization are used to optimize training effectiveness.

▶ Describe types of ergogenic aids and how they may or may not work to improve performance.

▶ Evaluate your personal skill-related fitness.

▶ Identify and self-assess overtraining symptoms.

Specialized forms of training are needed to optimize adaptations to exercise and performance in sports.

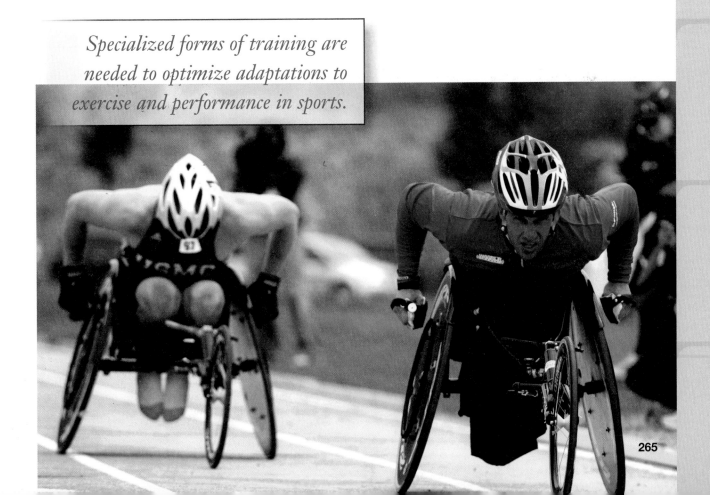

Sports and competitive athletics provide opportunities for individuals to explore the limits of their ability and to challenge themselves in competition. Some individuals enjoy challenges associated with competitive aerobic activities, such as running, cycling, swimming, and triathlons. Others enjoy the challenges associated with competitive resistance training activities, such as powerlifting and bodybuilding. High-level performance is also a requirement for some types of work, such as fire safety, military service, and police work.

In this concept, specific attention is devoted to the methods used to train for high-level performance. The amount of effort and training required to excel in sports, competitive athletics, or work requiring high-level performance is greater than the amount needed for good health and wellness. Because adaptations to exercise are specific to the type of activity that is performed, training should be matched to the specific needs of a given activity. Several types of training are discussed in detail, including endurance and speed training, specialized forms of resistance training, and other advanced training techniques, such as plyometrics, ballistic stretching, and functional balance training. Strategies for maximizing skill-related fitness and planning effective programs are also presented.

A full understanding of performance training requires a working knowledge of exercise physiology, an area of exercise science devoted to understanding how the body responds and adapts to exercise. This concept provides a basic introduction to these principles and some practical guidelines for individuals interested in athletic performance.

High-Level Performance and Training Characteristics

High-level performance requires health-related and skill-related fitness and the specific motor skills necessary for the performance. Improving performance requires more specific training than the type needed to improve health. **Training** (regular physical activity) builds health-related fitness which enhances both health and high-level performance (see Figure 1). High-performance levels are not necessary for all people, only those who need exceptional performances. A distance runner needs exceptional cardiovascular fitness and muscular endurance, a lineman in football needs exceptional strength, and a gymnast needs exceptional flexibility.

Exceptional performance also requires high-level skill-related physical fitness and good physical and motor skills. It is important to understand that skill-related fitness and skills are not the same thing. Skill-related fit-

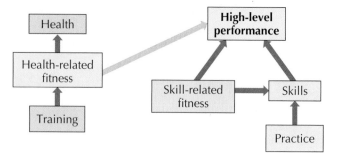

Figure 1 ▶ Factors influencing high-level performance.

components are abilities that help you learn skills faster and better, thus the arrow in Figure 1 from skill-related fitness to skills. Skills, on the other hand, are things such as throwing, kicking, catching, and hitting a ball. Practice enhances skills. Practicing the specific skills of a sport or a job is more productive to performance enhancement than more general drills associated with changing skill-related fitness.

Success in endurance sports requires a high aerobic capacity. Distance runners, cyclists, and swimmers must be able to perform activity for long periods of time without stopping. These types of performers need high levels of cardiovascular fitness, defined as aerobic capacity. In aerobic exercise, adequate oxygen is available to allow the body to rebuild the high-energy fuel the muscles need to sustain performance. Aerobic exercise increases aerobic capacity (cardiovascular fitness) by enhancing the body's ability to supply oxygen to the muscles as well as their ability to use it. Slow-twitch muscle fibers are most suited for aerobic exercise, and these fibers adapt most to aerobic training. Activities and events that require sustained, high-intensity, aerobic exercise place special demands on the slow-twitch fibers and require a high level of aerobic capacity (see Concept 7).

Many types of high-level performance require anaerobic capacity. While all athletes benefit from aerobic fitness, success in many sports is determined more by speed, strength, and power. The sprinting, jumping, and powerful movements needed in most competitive sports are good examples. Strength competitions and sprint events in running, bicycling, and swimming also require short bursts of high-intensity activity. These activities use more energy than can be provided with aerobic metabolism. Anaerobic processes (i.e., processes that do not require oxygen) provide the additional energy needs, but a by-product of these processes (**lactic acid**) eventually causes the muscles to fatigue.

When you do **anaerobic exercise,** the body cannot supply enough oxygen to sustain performance. So the body uses a high-energy fuel that the body has stored.

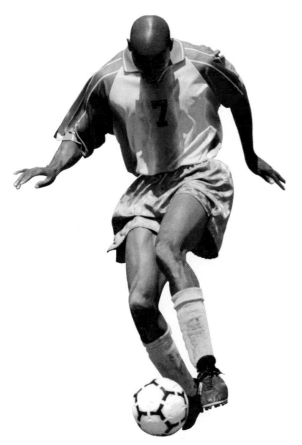

Performance in most sports requires good levels of fitness (health-related and skill-related) as well as practice to improve skills.

a combination of aerobic and anaerobic capacity, so it is important to conduct training that is most specific to the needs of a given activity.

Genetics can influence a person's potential for high-level performance. Each person inherits a unique genetic profile, which may predispose him or her to success in different sports and activities. A higher percentage of slow-twitch muscle fibers allow a person to adapt most effectively to aerobic exercise, while a higher percentage of fast-twitch muscle fibers enhance adaptations from and performance in anaerobic exercise. Heredity also influences the dimensions of skill-related fitness, such as balance, coordination, and reaction time, that enhance development of motor skills. The most successful performers are those who inherit good potential for health- and skill-related fitness, who train to improve their health-related fitness, and who do extensive practice to improve the skills associated with the specific activity in which they hope to excel.

Training for Endurance and Speed

Specific forms of training are needed to optimize endurance performance and speed. Speed and endurance are at opposite ends of the performance continuum. Speed events in running are as short as 100 meters, while endurance events, such as a marathon, last 26 miles. Middle-distance events, such as the mile run, fall between these extremes and present unique challenges, since it is important for athletes to have both speed and endurance. While these examples all involve running, the types of training needed for these events are very different.

When the high-energy fuel is used up, you cannot continue to perform. After the exercise you keep breathing fast and the heart continues to beat fast for a while, because the body needs to take in extra oxygen to rebuild the stores of the high-energy fuel used in anaerobic exercise. This is sometimes called **oxygen debt**. The body "borrows" oxygen that it cannot provide when it is using high-energy fuel during anaerobic exercise and then "pays back the debt" by supplying extra oxygen after the anaerobic exercise. Your body also breaks down lactic acid during the recovery period after anaerobic exercise. In some ways "borrowing" oxygen during anaerobic exercise, and paying back the oxygen debt later, is like using a credit card to borrow money that is paid back later.

Athletes involved in anaerobic activities typically perform specialized forms of anaerobic exercise to help improve their bodies' ability to produce energy anaerobically and to tolerate higher levels of lactic acid. Using the credit card analogy, this is equivalent to the increases in available credit that are provided to customers who demonstrate they can pay their credit card bills. Fast-twitch muscle fibers are used primarily during intense anaerobic activity, and these fibers are more likely to adapt and respond to anaerobic exercise. Most sports require

---

Anaerobic Exercise *Anaerobic* means "in the absence of oxygen." Anaerobic exercise is performed at an intensity so great that the body's demand for oxygen exceeds its ability to supply it.

Training Physical activity performed by people interested in high-level performance—e.g., athletes, people in specialized jobs.

Lactic Acid Substance that results from the process of supplying energy during anaerobic exercise; a cause of muscle fatigue.

Oxygen Debt The oxygen consumed following anaerobic exercise that is used to rebuild the supply of high-energy fuel.

A common feature in advanced training programs is the need to continually challenge the body. Involvement in regular physical activity will lead to increases in cardiovascular fitness in most people, but improvements are harder to achieve once a good level of fitness has been attained (the principle of diminishing returns). To maximize performance, it is necessary to perform more specific types of workouts that provide a greater challenge (overload) to the cardiovascular system. Serious athletes may exercise 6 or 7 days a week, but easier workouts are generally done after harder and more intense workouts. The hard workouts are generally very specific and are designed to challenge the body in different ways. Supplemental training to improve technique and efficiency are also used to enhance performance.

Long-slow distance training is important for endurance performance. Extended periods of aerobic exercise are needed to achieve high-level endurance performance. Athletes generally refer to this type of training as **long-slow distance (LSD) training**. Emphasis is placed on the overall duration or length of the exercise session rather than on speed. The reason for this is that specific adaptations take place within the muscles when used for long periods of time. These adaptations improve the muscles' ability to take up and use the oxygen in the bloodstream. Adaptations within the muscle cell also improve the body's ability to produce energy from fat stores. Long-slow distance training involves performances longer than the event for which you are performing but at a slower pace. For example, a mile runner will regularly perform 6- to 7-mile runs (at 50 to 60 percent of racing pace) to improve aerobic conditioning, even though the event is much shorter. A marathoner may perform runs of 20 miles or more to achieve even higher levels of endurance. Although this 20-mile distance is shorter than the marathon race distance, research suggests that ample adaptations occur from this volume of exercise. Excess mileage in this case may just wear the body down. Long-slow distance training should be performed once every 1 to 2 weeks, and a rest day is recommended on the subsequent day to allow the body to recover fully.

Improved anaerobic capacity can contribute to performance in aerobic activities. Many physical activities commonly considered to be aerobic—such as tennis, basketball, and racquetball—have an anaerobic component. These activities require periodic vigorous bursts of exercise. Regular anaerobic training will help you resist fatigue in these activities. Even participants in activities such as long-distance running can benefit from anaerobic training, especially if performance times or winning races is important. A fast start, a sprint past an opponent, and a kick at the end are typically anaerobic.

Interval training can be effective in building both aerobic and anaerobic capacity. High-level performance requires high-level training. **Interval training** is an advanced training technique that helps athletes optimize the effectiveness of their training. The premise behind interval training is that by providing periodic rest you can increase the overall intensity of the exercise session and provide a greater stimulus to the body. Interval training can be performed in different ways to achieve different training goals (see Table 1). It can be done at lower intensities to improve the aerobic metabolism or at extremely high intensities to enhance the anaerobic capacity. Interval training can also be done using a series of shorter intervals that are strung together after short rest. Alternately, intervals can also be done using longer and more sustained bouts. The purpose of the training session should dictate the intensity, duration, and rest intervals. A highly fit person may use shorter rests and repeat the interval session multiple times in a given workout. Descriptions of the primary types are summarized at right.

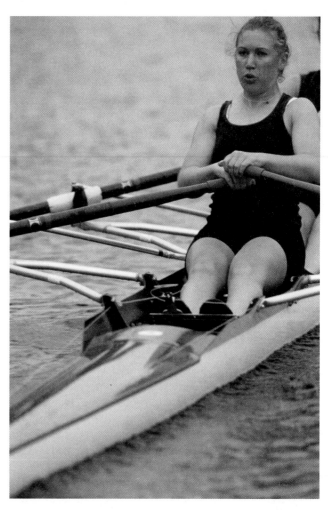

Interval training can be adapted for performers in a variety of activities.

Table 1 ▶ Work and Rest Bouts for Different Types of Interval-Training Workouts

Type of Interval	Short-Length Intervals			Long-Length Intervals		
	Intensity	Duration	Frequency	Intensity	Duration	Frequency
Aerobic Intervals	50–70%	2–3 minutes	Perform 7–8 with rest	50–60%	15–20 minutes	Perform full bout
(50–70% MaxHR)		10–15 seconds rest	Repeat after 3–4 minutes (recovery)			Repeat after 3–4 minutes (recovery)
Aerobic/Anaerobic Intervals	75–85%	1–2 minutes	Perform 5–6 with rest	70–75%	6–8 minutes	Perform full bout
(70–90% MaxHR)		30–60 seconds rest	Repeat after 5–6 minutes (recovery)			Repeat after 5–6 minutes (recovery)
Anaerobic Intervals	90–95%	10–15 seconds	Perform 3–4 with rest	85–90%	30–60 seconds	Perform 10–12 intervals with rest
(85–95% MaxHR)		15–120 seconds rest	Repeat after 7–8 minutes (recovery)		60–240 seconds rest	Repeat after 7–8 minutes (recovery)

- *Aerobic intervals improve the efficiency of the aerobic metabolism.* The goal of aerobic intervals is to provide a sustained challenge to the cardiovascular system. The intensity should be challenging (but manageable) since the goal is to train the aerobic system to function efficiently over an extended period of time. In general, the pace would be similar to (or slightly slower) than the pace used for a 30- to 40-minute continuous event (about 50 to 70 percent of max heart rate). The body adapts to the pace and becomes better at providing oxygen to the muscles and clearing lactic acid that accumulates during the bout. Aerobic interval training can be done using a series of short 2- to 3-minute intervals (with short 10- to 15-second rests). Alternately, it can be done as a pace workout using a longer continuous bout lasting 15 to 20 minutes. Advanced athletes may repeat the workout after a short recovery period to further enhance the training stimulus.

- *Aerobic/anaerobic intervals help to improve maximal aerobic capacity.* To improve aerobic capacity ($\dot{V}O_2$ max). it is necessary to push the body to perform near your aerobic capacity for an extended period of time (4 to 6 minutes is a good target). A person's aerobic capacity is reached at intensities above the anaerobic threshold, so this requires a fairly high intensity (typically about 70 to 85 percent maximum heart rate). For runners, a series of repeated mile runs at a faster than normal training pace provides a good challenge to the aerobic system. However, a series of quarter-mile repeats can also achieve the same goal as long as the total time at a high intensity is similar. In this case, the rest intervals for the set must be short enough to allow only partial recovery between intervals. The adaptations here are based on sustaining a high intensity for the 4- to

6-minute period so full recovery is desirable between sets. Similar workouts can be devised for other sports.

- *Anaerobic intervals improve the function of anaerobic energy processes.* This is typically accomplished with a series of high-intensity bouts of activity at 85 to 95 percent of maximum heart rate. In response to this training, the body improves its ability to produce energy anaerobically and to tolerate anaerobic by-products such as lactic acid. A series of 4 to 5 short bouts of activity that are 10 to 15 seconds long at maximum speed provide a good stimulus (e.g., 100-yard dash). Work-to-rest ratios may range from 1:1 to 1:10 depending on the individual's fitness and the goal of the training. Longer intervals (30 to 60 seconds) at a slightly slower speed (85 to 90 percent of maximum heart rate) with more extended rest breaks (60 to 240 seconds) can also be effective.

Recently, there has been considerable interest in a specific interval-training regimen referred to as *high intensity interval training* or *HIIT*. The workouts generally involve repeated 60-second bouts of high intensity exercise (90 percent maximum) followed by 60 seconds of rest. These

Long-Slow Distance (LSD) Training Training technique used by marathon runners and other endurance performers that emphasizes slow, sustained exercise rather than speed.

Interval Training A training technique often used for high-level aerobic and anaerobic training; uses repeated bouts of activity followed by rest to maximize the quality of the workout.

In the News

High Intensity Interval Training (HIIT)

Interval training has been used by athletes for many years to optimize the effectiveness of their training. Recently, several highly publicized articles reported on the benefits of interval training for weight loss, general conditioning, and metabolic/cardiovascular health. Popularized with the acronym HIIT (high intensity interval training), it represents a fairly standard interval-training regimen (60-second bouts followed by 60-seconds of rest). The novelty is that researchers have reported benefits for clinical populations. Advocates highlight the fact that a HIIT workout can be done in shorter periods of time than a more traditional cardiovascular exercise and therefore may improve adherence. While this may be true, it is not clear if HIIT can be recommended to all segments of the population or whether people would burn out from the emphasis on high-intensity exercise.

Would you be inclined to adopt HIIT in your workouts or would this type of training make exercise more like work and detract from your enjoyment of exercise?

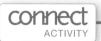

workouts are consistent with standard interval-training techniques but they have been popularized since they provide a good training dose in a short period of time. A typical HIIT workout consisting of 10 intervals can provide significant cardiovascular and health benefits in a short period of time (approximately 20 minutes with the associated rest breaks). Research suggests that this regimen can be done safely by non-athletes but additional research is needed to verify the utility for the general population (see In the News for details).

Principles of interval training can be adapted for different activities. The principles of interval training can be integrated into workouts in less structured ways. Runners sometimes use *fartlek* training to break up their workouts. A fartlek training run incorporates bursts of higher-intensity running followed by recovery periods of lower intensity. The difference from interval training is that the intermittent bursts in fartlek training are dictated by the nature of the terrain or the feelings of the moment. The term is from a Swedish word meaning "speed play," because the unstructured nature is more relaxed than structured interval training.

Many competitive sports involve alternating bursts of high-intensity activity followed by periods of recovery. Basketball, for example, involves intermittent sprints and jumps interspersed with periods of short recovery. Similarly, tennis involves bursts of activity separated by short recovery periods between points. To prepare for success in sports, it is important for athletes to incorporate intermittent interval-type training into their conditioning. Simulated games that require repeated sprints up and down the basketball court are a form of interval training specific to basketball players. Tennis players can incorporate a variety of forward and lateral movements into a high-intensity agility drill to improve conditioning for tennis.

Training for Strength and Muscular Endurance

Specific progressive resistance training programs are needed to achieve high-level muscular performance. A basic progressive resistance program for overall good health might involve performing a single exercise for each major muscle group two or three times a week. This level of training provides a regular stimulus to maintain healthy levels of muscular strength and endurance. However, many people challenge themselves to achieve higher levels of muscular performance. Olympic weight-lifting competitors use free weights and compete in two exercises: the snatch and the clean and jerk. Powerlifting competitors use free weights and compete in three lifts: the bench press, squat, and dead lift. Bodybuilding competitors use several forms of resistance training and are judged on muscular hypertrophy (large muscles) and **definition of muscle.** Performers in these activities and athletes in strength-related sports need to use more advanced training methods to reach their full potential. The essential goal in high-level training is to provide the optimal stimulus, so that the muscles adapt in the desired way. Because the goals are clearly different for athletes interested in strength/power, muscular hypertrophy, or muscular endurance, it is important to follow appropriate programs. The essential aspects of these different training programs are described in the sections that follow. The basic concepts are summarized in Figure 2.

Performers training for high-level strength should use multiple sets with heavier weights. The best stimulus for strength gains is repeated lifts with very heavy loads. Guidelines for intermediate lifters call for multiple sets of 6 to 12 reps performed using 70 to

Strength/power

	Low	Medium	High
Load			
Reps			
Sets			
Volume			
Rest			

Hypertrophy/size

	Low	Medium	High
Load			
Reps			
Sets			
Volume			
Rest			

Muscular endurance

	Low	Medium	High
Load			
Reps			
Sets			
Volume			
Rest			

Figure 2 ▶ Differences in training stimulus for different resistance training programs.

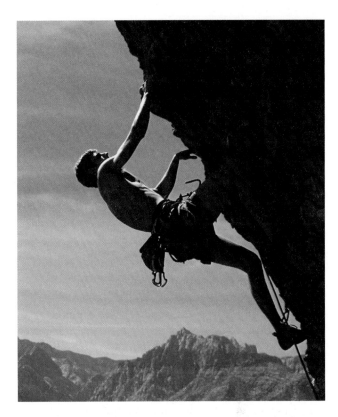

Good muscular endurance (and strength) are needed for performance in rock climbing.

80 percent of 1RM values. The load and intensity guidelines are higher for advanced lifters (1 to 12 reps performed using 70 to 100 percent 1RM) because they may need to use a higher overload to get continued improvements. Rest intervals must be long (2 to 3 minutes) for high-intensity strength training to allow full recovery of the muscles between sets.

Multiple joint exercises, such as the bench press, have been found to be more effective in strength enhancement, since they allow a greater load to be lifted. The sequencing of exercises within a workout is also an important consideration for strength development. When training all major muscle groups in a workout, large muscle groups should be done before small muscle groups, and multiple-joint exercises should be done before single-joint ones.

Performers training for muscular endurance should emphasize many repetitions with lighter weights. Completing multiple sets of 10 to 25 repetitions is required to build endurance. Short rest periods of 1 to 2 minutes are recommended for high-repetition sets, and periods of less than 1 minute should be used for lower-repetition sets. This challenges the muscles to perform repeatedly and with little or no rest. Variation in the order in which exercises are performed is also recommended to vary the stimulus. Intermediate lifters should aim for two to four times per week, but advanced lifters may perform up to six sessions per week if appropriate variation in muscle groups is used between workouts.

Performers training for bulk and definition often use extra reps and/or sets. Bodybuilders are more interested in definition and hypertrophy than in absolute strength. Gaining both size and definition requires a balance between strength and muscle endurance training. Most bodybuilders use 3 to 7 sets of 10 to 15 repetitions, rather than the 3 sets of 3 to 8 repetitions recommended for most weight lifters. Sometimes definition is difficult to obtain because it is obscured by fat. It should be noted that people with the largest looking muscles are not always the strongest.

Definition of Muscle The detailed external appearance of a muscle.

Training for cardiovascular fitness along with strength training can limit adaptations. The body adapts to the type of training that is performed. If too much endurance training is performed, the body tries to adapt to the needs of aerobic activity, and this makes it more difficult to gain muscle mass or achieve maximal increases in strength. The effect would only be an issue for competitive strength or power athletes and should not deter people from getting the important health benefits associated with moderate amounts of aerobic activity. Regular aerobic activity is considered essential for bodybuilders to help them reduce unwanted body fat.

Training for Power

Power is a combination of strength and speed, and it is both health-related and skill-related. Most experts classify power as a skill-related component of fitness because it depends partially on speed. However, power also depends on strength and can be classified as a health-related component. Thus, power falls somewhere between the two distinct groups.

Some experts consider power to be the most functional mode in which all human motion occurs. Power is exceptionally important in sport activities such as hitting a baseball, blocking in football, putting the shot, and throwing the discus. Power is also essential for good vertical jumping—a movement critical for basketball and many other sports. While power is emphasized in sports training, it is also now viewed as an important attribute for successful aging. A typical progressive resistance exercise program will build sufficient power for normal activities of daily living; however, people interested in high-level performance should consider using additional exercises that specifically develop power.

The stronger person is not necessarily the more powerful. Power is the amount of work per unit of time. To increase power, you must do more work in the same time or the same work in less time. If you extend your knee and move a 100-pound weight through a 90-degree arc in 1 second, you have twice as much power as a person who needs 2 seconds to complete the same movement. Power requires both strength and speed. Increasing one without the other limits power. Some power athletes (for example, football players) might benefit by achieving less strength and more speed.

The principle of specificity applies to power development. If you need power for an activity in which you are required to move heavy weights, then you need to develop *strength-related power* by working against heavy resistance at slower speeds. If you need to

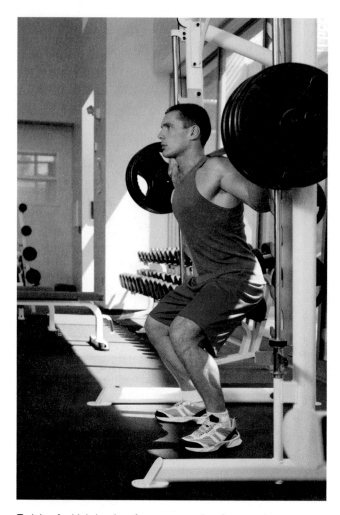

Training for high-level performance requires focus and determination.

move light objects at great speed, such as in throwing a ball, you need to develop *speed-related power* by training at high speeds with relatively low resistance. There must be trade-offs between speed and power because the heavier the resistance, the slower the movement. Training adaptations are also specific to the type of training performed. Power exercises done at high speeds will help enhance muscular endurance, whereas power exercises that use heavy resistance at lower speeds will increase strength.

Performers who need explosive power to perform their events should use training that closely resembles those events. Jumpers, for example, should jump as a part of their training programs in order to learn correct timing and mechanics. If they use machines, it is better to use the leg press than a knee extension machine because the press more nearly resembles the leg action of the jump.

The performer's program should use similar speed, force, angle, and range of motion as the activity. However,

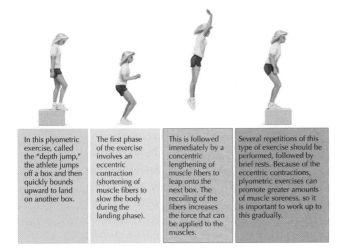

In this plyometric exercise, called the "depth jump," the athlete jumps off a box and then quickly bounds upward to land on another box.

The first phase of the exercise involves an eccentric contraction (shortening of muscle fibers to slow the body during the landing phase).

This is followed immediately by a concentric lengthening of muscle fibers to leap onto the next box. The recoiling of the fibers increases the force that can be applied to the muscles.

Several repetitions of this type of exercise should be performed, followed by brief rests. Because of the eccentric contractions, plyometric exercises can promote greater amounts of muscle soreness, so it is important to work up to this gradually.

Figure 3 ▶ Plyometric exercise—a technique for developing power

if a performer is unable to do the specific skill because of weather or injury or is seeking variety, then plyometrics, isokinetics, and weight training (especially with free weights or pulleys if simulating a sport skill) are effective means of developing power.

Power training can be done with weight equipment, but care is needed to ensure safety and efficacy. Resistance training can be performed to optimize power development, but these movements are not recommended for beginning lifters. Studies have shown that heavy resistance training can actually decrease power unless training also includes some explosive movements. Guidelines from the ACSM recommend heavy loading (85 to 100 percent of 1RM) to increase the force component of the power equation and light to moderate loading (30 to 60 percent of 1RM) performed at an explosive velocity to enhance the speed component of power. The guidelines recommend that a multiple-set power program (3 to 6 sets) be integrated within an overall strength training program. Exercises for power are most effectively done with free weights or pulleys to simulate sport-related movements more effectively. Isokinetic devices, such as isokinetic swim benches, may also be useful for enhancing sport-specific power.

Plyometrics may be useful in training for tasks or events requiring power. Plyometrics is an advanced training technique used by many athletes. It takes advantage of a quick prestretch prior to a movement to increase power. By repeatedly doing these movements in training, athletes can provide a greater stimulus to their muscles and improve their body's ability to perform power movements. Track and field athletes may do a hopping drill

Table 2 ▶ Safety Guidelines for Plyometrics

- Plyometrics for growing teens should begin moderately and progress slowly, compared with plyometrics for adults.
- Progression should be gradual to avoid extreme muscle soreness.
- Adequate strength should be developed prior to plyometric training. (As a general rule, you should be able to do a half-squat with one-and-a-half times your body weight.)
- Get a physician's approval prior to doing plyometrics if you have a history of injuries or if you are recovering from injury to the body part being trained.
- The landing surface should be semiresilient, dry, and unobstructed.
- Shoes should have good lateral stability, be cushioned with an arch support, and have a nonslip sole.
- Obstacles used for jumping-over should be padded.
- The training should be preceded by a general and specific warm-up.
- The training sequence should. . .
  - precede all other workouts (while you are fresh);
  - include at least one spotter;
  - be done no more than twice per week, with 48 hours' rest between bouts;
  - last no more than 30 minutes;
  - include 3 or 4 drills (for beginners), with 2 or 3 sets per drill, 10–15 reps per set, and 1–2 minutes' rest between sets.

Source: Adapted from Brittenham.

for 30 to 100 meters or alternate jumping from a box to the floor and back to the box (called depth jumping, drop jumping, or bounce loading). As the body lands, some of the major leg muscles lengthen in an eccentric contraction, then follow immediately with a strong concentric contraction as the legs push off for the next jump or stride. The prestretch of the muscle during landing adds an elastic recoil that provides extra force to the push-off (see Figure 3).

Plyometrics are used to apply the specificity principle to training for certain skills. Because eccentric exercise tends to result in more muscular soreness, proceed slowly with this type of training. It is also important to have good flexibility before beginning a plyometrics program. Table 2 lists safety guidelines for plyometrics.

Plyometrics A training technique used to develop explosive power. It involves the use of concentric-isotonic contractions performed after a prestretch or an eccentric contraction of a muscle.

Training for Functional Fitness and Flexibility

Functional fitness training builds motor skills such as balance, coordination, gait, and agility as well as strength and flexibility. Functional fitness training (also called neuromotor training) refers to specific efforts to improve the integration of the body's motor (muscle) system with the neural (sensory) system. This integration can improve the body's ability to perform real-life activities such as bending, squatting, lunging, kicking, climbing, reaching, or lifting. Functional fitness training is characterized by smooth movements that mimic functional motions of the limbs and trunk—the synchronized recruitment of multiple muscle groups to create motion in all three cardinal planes and movements that require both concentric (shortening) and eccentric (lengthening) muscle action. Exercises and movements of functional training generally target the major muscle groups of the body including the chest, arms, shoulders, trunk, back, hip, and legs since these groups are involved in typical functional movements of the body.

Functional fitness training can be conducted in a variety of ways but athletes often use task-specific or sports-specific training regimens such as squatting, tossing a ball against a rebounder, performing carioca, or running through agility ladders. Resistance needed for building strength comes from the weight of the moving body part(s) or the movement of devices such as kettlebells, medicine balls, or elastic cords. These devices are swung, tossed, caught, stretched, or pulled to provide added resistance to the workout. Recent ACSM guidelines specifically recognize the importance of neuromotor training exercises for the general population. The guidelines recommend that individuals participate in functional fitness activities 20 to 30 minutes/day at least two to three times per week. The ideal dosage (intensity, repetitions, and sets) have not been determined but would likely depend upon the type of functional fitness exercise being performed.

Functional balance training is a specific type of functional fitness training that can promote better body control. Functional balance training involves the execution of skilled movements that improve **proprioception** and promote balance. The unique aspect of the movements is that they typically require movement and stabilization force production at the same time. In other words, one part of the body is in motion while another is stabilized. These actions essentially train the body's many somatic sensory organs to respond and adjust to different postures and positions—thereby improving balance. Functional balance training is frequently performed with exercise balls, balance boards, or BOSU trainers (see Concept 9). It is important to start slowly with easy movements and work up to more challenging positions and movements. This type of training is not recommended for people who have had recent orthopedic injuries, who have degenerative joint disease, or individuals with knee instability.

Dynamic stretching provides some advantages for athletes preparing for competition. While static stretching is often recommended for general applications, athletes often need to perform more active (dynamic) stretching to prepare for activity. More dynamic forms of stretching (including ballistic stretching) are considered appropriate for high-level performers because many of the motions of the activities in which they perform require dynamic movements. Although ballistic stretching movements have an associated risk, athletes are trained to tolerate them, and the risk is not as significant. The ballistic movements also better prepare an athlete for the dynamic nature of activities during competition.

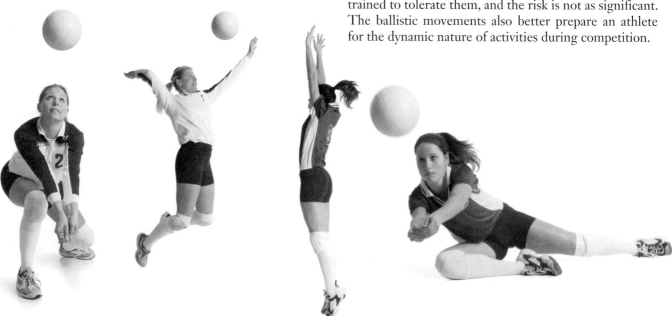

Sports-specific training and warm-up help prepare athletes for the unique demands of their sport.

Table 3 ▶ Skill-Related Requirements of Sports and Other Activities

Activity	Balance	Coordination	Reaction Time	Agility	Power	Speed
Archery	***	****	*	*	*	*
Backpacking	**	**	*	**	**	*
Badminton	**	****	***	***	**	***
Baseball/softball	***	****	****	***	****	***
Basketball	***	****	****	****	****	***
Bicycling	****	**	**	*	**	**
Bowling	***	****	*	**	**	**
Canoeing	***	***	**	*	***	*
Circuit training	**	**	*	**	***	**
Dance, aerobic	**	****	**	***	**	*
Dance, ballet	****	****	**	****	***	*
Dance, disco	**	***	**	****	*	**
Dance, modern	****	****	**	****	***	*
Dance, social	**	***	**	***	*	**
Fencing	***	****	****	***	***	****
Fitness calisthenics	**	**	*	***	**	*
Football	***	***	****	****	****	****
Golf (walking)	**	****	*	**	***	*
Gymnastics	****	****	***	****	****	**
Handball	**	****	***	****	***	***
Hiking	**	**	*	**	**	*
Horseback riding	***	***	**	***	*	*
Interval training	**	**	*	*	*	**
Jogging	**	**	*	*	*	*
Judo	***	****	****	****	****	****
Karate	***	****	****	****	****	****
Mountain climbing	****	****	**	***	***	*
Pool/billiards	**	***	*	**	**	*
Racquetball	**	****	***	****	**	***
Rope jumping	**	***	**	***	**	*
Rowing, crew	**	****	*	***	****	**
Sailing	***	***	***	***	**	*
Skating	****	***	**	***	**	***
Skiing, cross-country	**	****	*	***	****	**
Skiing, downhill	****	****	***	****	***	*
Soccer	**	****	***	****	****	***
Surfing	****	****	***	****	***	*
Swimming (laps)	**	***	*	***	**	*
Table tennis	**	***	***	**	**	**
Tennis	**	****	***	***	***	***
Volleyball	**	****	***	***	**	**
Walking	**	**	*	*	*	*
Waterskiing	***	***	*	***	**	*
Weight training	**	**	*	*	**	*

* = minimal needed; **** = a lot needed.

Dynamic stretching may provide other advantages for athletes. Static stretching may impair performance if done right before a competition. The reason for this is that the neuromuscular system somewhat fights the stretch with an inhibitory response. The muscles become less responsive and stay weakened for up to 30 minutes after stretching and this is certainly not beneficial for performance. Dynamic forms of stretching that stretch muscles while moving avoid this problem. Dynamic stretching is thought to enhance performance since muscles receive more of a stimulation response rather than an inhibition. Examples of ballistic stretches for sport-related activities include practice swings with a baseball bat, a golf club, or a tennis racquet. In each case, start by swinging backward and forward rhythmically and continuously. Gradually increase the speed and vigor of the swing until it approaches the speed used in the actual movement.

Training for High-Level Performance: Skill-Related Fitness and Skill

Good skill-related fitness is needed for success in many sports. As described in Concept 1, there are six primary components of skill-related fitness (agility, coordination, balance, reaction time, speed, and power). Having these attributes can make it easier to learn the necessary skills for many competitive sports. Balance and reaction time are critical for hitting a baseball, considered by many to be the toughest skill in sports. Similarly, agility and coordination may help one master advanced dribbling skills for sports such as basketball or soccer. Because skill-related fitness can enhance performance in sports, it is often called **motor fitness** or **sports fitness**. Table 3 summarizes the general skill-related fitness requirements of 44 sport activities. In Lab 12A, you will evaluate your skill-related fitness and learn what activities you are most suited for.

Good skills are needed for success in sports and other competitive activities. Skill-related fitness helps you learn skills, but possessing the specific skills of an activity is probably more important. As noted in Concept 8, skill is not the same as skill-related fitness. Skill refers to the ability to perform specific tasks. Sports examples include throwing, kicking, striking (as in hitting a baseball), and jumping. There are thousands of skills specific to different

Proprioception Awareness of body movements and orientation of the body in space; often used synonymously with *kinesthesis*.

Motor Fitness (Sports Fitness) Skill-related physical fitness.

sports and other competitive activities. A person with good skill-related fitness may learn skills easier and ultimately be able to achieve a higher level of skills than other people, but with practice anyone can learn skills. High-level performers typically must practice more often than recreational athletes and typically require more coaching on the specific skills of their chosen activity. Feedback is especially important to high-level performance and skill improvement-but not all feedback is effective. Studies show that feedback provided after successful performances (i.e. good feedback) reinforces good skill patterns while feedback provided after poor performances (i.e. bad feedback) is less effective. Feedback from coaches, peers, or video analyses can help to improve skill learning and performance if it is provided and utilized appropriately.

Fitness and skills interact to influence high-level performance. You may possess ability in one area and not in another. For this reason, general motor ability probably does not really exist, and individuals do not have one general capacity for performing. Rather, the ability to play games or sports is determined by combined abilities in each of the separate skill-related components. However, some performers will probably be above average in many areas. Following are key points about skill-related fitness.

- *Exceptional performers tend to be outstanding in more than one component of skill-related fitness.* Though people possess skill-related fitness in varying degrees, great athletes are likely to be above average in most, if not all, aspects.
- *Excellence in one skill-related fitness component may compensate for a lack in another.* Each individual possesses a specific level of each skill-related fitness aspect. The performer should learn his or her other strengths and weaknesses in order to produce optimal performances. For example, a tennis player may use good coordination to compensate for lack of speed.
- *Excellence in skill-related fitness may compensate for a lack of health-related fitness when playing sports and games.* As you grow older, health-related fitness potential declines more rapidly than many components of skill-related fitness. You may use superior skill-related fitness to compensate. For example, a baseball pitcher who lacks the power to dominate hitters may rely on a pitch such as a knuckle ball, which depends more on coordination than on power.

Guidelines for High-Performance Training

The quality of training is clearly more important than the quantity. A characteristic of high-performance training is the need to continually challenge the body (overload principle). Involvement in regular physical activity will lead to improvements in fitness for most people, but they are harder to achieve once a good level of fitness has been attained (the principle of diminishing returns). It takes considerably more training to improve fitness than it does to maintain fitness.

To maximize performance, perform more specific types of workouts that provide a greater challenge to the body. Serious athletes may exercise 6 or 7 days a week, but easier workouts are generally done after harder and more intense workouts. The hard workouts are generally very specific and are designed to challenge the body in different ways. The easier workouts provide time to recover while building other dimensions of fitness. Quality is clearly more important than quantity.

Overtraining is a common problem among athletes. Most Americans suffer from hypokinetic conditions resulting from too little activity. Athletes, on the other hand, often push themselves too hard and do not allow adequate time for rest, making them susceptible to a variety of hyperkinetic conditions, such as *overload syndrome*. This condition is characterized by fatigue, irritability, and sleep problems, as well as an increased risk for injuries. Performance can decline sharply in an overtrained status, causing athletes to train even harder and become even more overtrained. Athletes should pay close attention to possible symptoms of overtraining and back off their training if they notice increased fatigue, lethargy, or unexpected decreases in their performance. Lab 12B helps you identify some symptoms of overtraining.

A slightly elevated morning heart rate (four or five beats more than normal values) is a useful physical indicator of overtraining. The body has had to work too hard to recover from the exercise and isn't in its normal resting mode. To use this indicator, regularly monitor your resting heart rate before getting out of bed in the morning. Another indicator that is increasingly used by elite endurance athletes is compressed or reduced "heart rate variability." A lower beat-to-beat variability indicates fatigue or overtraining, since it reflects sympathetic dominance over the normally dominant parasympathetic system that exists during more rested states. Newer heart rate monitors provide an indicator of heart rate variability.

Rest and a history of regular exercise are both important for reducing the risks for overuse injuries. Adequate rest helps the body recover from the stress of vigorous training—it promotes the physiological adaptations that improve performance and reduces the likelihood of developing overuse injuries.

A history of regular exercise is also important for reducing risks for injury. Research conducted by the military has determined that recruits with a history of regular exercise were less likely to get injured during basic training than recruits without this experience. This suggests that regular exercise can build up the strength and integrity of bones and joints and reduce the risk for injury. While experienced athletes may have less risk for injuries, they often push themselves too hard and succumb to other conditions. An increased number of cases of rhabdomyolysis (breakdown of muscle fibers) have been reported among athletes, presumably because they were asked (or wanted) to push too hard in training (see Thomas, Suggested Readings). Listening to your body and getting rest are important for decreasing risk of overtraining.

Periodization of training may help prevent overtraining. When training for a single performance or perhaps several competitive events, such as games or matches during a sport season, you must plan carefully to reach peak performance at the right time and to avoid overtraining and injuries. **Periodization** is a modern concept of manipulating repetition, resistance, and exercise selection so there are periodic peaks and valleys during the training program. The peaks are needed to challenge the body, and the valleys allow the body to recover and adapt fully.

A training program is usually divided into a series of cycles that allow the intensity and volume to change in a systematic way. A hypothetical periodization cycle is depicted in Figure 4. Note that the overall training program (1 macrocycle) is made up of three mesocycles that are each made up of three microcycles. Note that the intensity increases gradually in each microcycle to provide a progressive training stimulus. Also note that the volume increases somewhat in opposition to the intensity with volume actually decreasing at the higher-intensity phases. The overall training stimulus increases throughout the mesocycle. Rest is a critical point of an effective periodization program as the body needs time to recover from (and adapt to) the challenging training stimulus. The intensity and volume drop to lower levels at the start of each

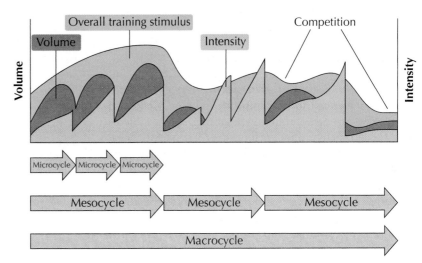

Figure 4 ▶ Conceptual pattern of cycles within a periodized training program.

microcycle with larger drops after each mesocycle. Periodization training is usually focused on preparing a person for a competition and, as the competition gets closer, the athlete typically begins a **tapering** plan to ensure a full recovery prior to the event. The tapering plan typically involves reductions in both intensity and volume of training to help facilitate recovery. Following a periodization plan helps an athlete optimize the effectiveness of training while also decreasing the risk of overtraining.

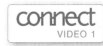

Athletes should be aware of various psychological disorders related to overtraining. Compulsive physical activity, often referred to as activity neurosis or exercise addiction, can be considered a hyperkinetic condition. People with activity neurosis become irrationally concerned about their exercise regimen. They may exercise more than once a day, rarely take a day off, or feel the need to exercise even when ill or injured. One condition related to body neurosis is an obsession with having an attractive body. Among females, it is usually associated with an extreme desire to be thin, whereas among males it is more often associated with an extreme desire to be muscular. This excessive desire to be fit or thin can negatively affect other aspects of life, threaten personal relationships, and cause extreme stress. Anorexia nervosa, an eating disorder associated with an excessive drive to be thin, has frequently been associated with compulsive exercise.

HELP **Health is available to Everyone for a Lifetime, and it's Personal**

Energy drinks are increasingly popular among young people. Improved athletic performance, better attention span, and staying awake to study are just a few of the reasons given for using them, but most users are not aware of how much caffeine they are truly consuming. Recent studies suggest that high consumption of energy drinks is a risky behavior and it is associated with other risky health behaviors.

What factors contribute to the popularity of these drinks among college students?

connect ACTIVITY

Periodization A planned sequence of training designed to optimize adaptations and minimize overtraining.

Tapering A reduction in training volume and intensity prior to competition to elicit peak performance.

Performance Trends and Ergogenic Aids

Many athletes look to ergogenic aids as an additional way to improve performance. Athletes are always looking for a competitive edge. In addition to pursuing rigorous training programs, many athletes look for alternative ways to improve their performance. Substances, strategies, and treatments designed to improve physical performance beyond the effects of normal training are collectively referred to as **ergogenic aids.** People interested in improving their appearance (including those with body neurosis) also abuse products they think will enhance their appearance. Ergogenic aids can be classified as mechanical, psychological, and physiological. Each category will be discussed in the subsequent sections.

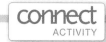

Mechanical ergogenics may improve efficiency and performance. Mechanical ergogenic aids consist of equipment or devices that aid performance. Examples include oversized tennis racquets, more flexible poles for pole vaulting, spring-loaded ice skates (klap skates), lycra body suits for reducing drag in swimming and running, and carbon fiber bike frames to increase stiffness and force transmission. While mechanical ergogenic aids may help maximize performance, the advantages are probably noticeable only for highly elite athletes. For example, a recreational athlete may not play any better with an expensive tennis racquet or new golf clubs. Expert players, on the other hand, can appreciate subtle differences in equipment and may benefit. Athletes, however, should continue to focus on improving fitness and practicing skills, since these will have bigger impacts on performance.

Psychological ergogenics can often improve concentration, improve motivation, and reduce anxiety during competitive activities. Many competitive activities require extreme levels of concentration, motivation, and focus. Athletes who maintain a mental edge during an event are at a clear advantage over athletes who cannot. Competitive anxiety can impair performance, and psychological ergogenics can help reduce anxiety before and during an event. Psychological ergogenics include mental imagery, hypnosis, modeling performance, and establishing skill routines, to name but a few.

Physiological ergogenics are designed to improve performance by enhancing biochemical and physiological processes in the body. Physiological ergogenics are primarily nutritional supplements thought to have a positive effect on various metabolic processes. Because the supplement industry is largely unregulated, many products are developed and marketed with little

TECHNOLOGY UPDATE

Performance Technology

Technological advancements in sports equipment have contributed to record-setting performances and improved performance. Specific applications of nano-technology have resulted in equipment that is lighter, yet stronger, including: lighter golf clubs for faster swing speed; golf balls with high precision for a more even spin and truer flight path; lighter and stronger tennis rackets for higher serve speed; tennis balls that keep bounce longer because of a nano-composite barrier that prevents leaks; high-tech ski wax that allows faster skiing; and lighter bicycles for greater speed and more efficient performance. Advances in clothing technology have also improved performance. High-tech swimsuits used by top swimmers reduce drag and improve speed. Made of a customized, water-repellent fabric (a combination of spandex and nylon yarn), the suit feels almost slippery to the touch. It weighs 70 percent less than other swimsuits and retains almost no water.

Do the advances in technology improve sports or does it detract from competition and give some people an unfair advantage?

or no research to document their effects. Producers of these products prey on an athlete's lack of knowledge and concern over performance.

Products with little or no evidence of benefits also have questionable safety. For example, protein supplements are unregulated products for which evidence of effectiveness is lacking. Many strength athletes continue to believe that extra protein in the diet can contribute to strength and muscle mass gains, despite the fact that this has been clearly refuted in the scientific literature. The aggressive marketing and propaganda in many muscle-related fitness publications convince many people to buy and try unproven supplements. Do not be swayed by ads and unsubstantiated claims.

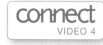

Physiological ergogenics with established performance benefits are described below. Concept 23 presents strategies for detecting quackery.

- *Fluid replacement beverages and energy bars.* Fluid replacement beverages, such as Gatorade, Exceed, and Powerade, contain carbohydrates needed for

Ergogenic Aids Substances, strategies, and treatments intended to improve performance in sports or competitive athletics.

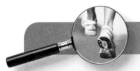

A CLOSER LOOK

Improved Education about Supplement Risks

The use of illegal (and legal), performance enhancing drugs and supplements continues to be a problem in competitive sports. The United States Anti-Doping Agency has launched a new website called "Supplement 411" to educate athletes about the risks and problems associated with use of various supplements. The site features the stories of prominent athletes who were disqualified from competition after illegal substances (originating from supplements) were found in their urine. The site also provides detailed information about the risks associated with various supplements.

Do you think this innovative (personalized) effort to educate athletes about supplements will have positive effects? Why or why not?

connect
ACTIVITY

endurance exercise. People exercising for more than an hour can benefit from these supplements, and research shows that they can replace fluid lost in sweat at the same or a faster rate than water. Energy bars (e.g., Power Bars and Clif Bars), energy gels (e.g., GU), or energy chews (e.g., Clif Shot Blocks) also provide valuable energy for extended endurance exercise. Consumers should be wary of other "energy" products that tout energy without calories. These are simply stimulants or caffeine products.

- *Creatine.* As described in Concept 9, creatine is a nutrient involved in the production of energy during intense exercise. The body produces it naturally from foods containing protein, but some athletes take creatine supplements (usually a powder dissolved in a liquid) to increase the amounts available in the muscle. The idea behind supplementation is that additional creatine intake enhances energy production and therefore increases the body's ability to maintain force and delay fatigue. Some studies have shown improvements in performance and anaerobic capacity, but recent reviews indicate that the supplement may be effective only for athletes who are already well trained. Products containing creatine do not work by themselves; instead, they only help athletes maximize their training or performance during an event. Effects are not evident unless training is performed while taking the supplements.

connect
VIDEO 5

Strategies for Action

Select activities that match your abilities. People differ in many factors, including skills and abilities that influence sports and athletic performance. You may be well suited to some sports but not to others. Behavioral scientists have also determined that perceptions of competence are important predictors of long-term exercise adherence. To give yourself the best chance of being successful in sports (and exercise involvement), choose activities that are well matched to your abilities. Lab 12A provides an assessment for evaluating your levels of skill-related physical fitness. Use Table 3 on page 275 to determine the sports and activities that best match your individual abilities.

The assessments in Lab 12A are but a few of the many tests that can be done for each of the skill-related fitness parts. If you have a personal desire to train for a specific sport or activity, but do not have a fitness profile that predicts success, do not be discouraged. Lab 12A will help you find an activity that you will enjoy and in which you have a good chance of success.

Take time to plan and record your training sessions. Coaches handle these tasks for many competitive athletes, but recreational athletes typically have to plan their own program. Although you can contract with a personal trainer to help you, adequate planning can be done by applying the principles described in this book. The key is to write a workout plan and keep careful records to monitor how your training program is progressing.

Get adequate rest and listen to your body. Many athletes make the mistake of training too hard and don't include enough time for rest. Without rest, the body does not have sufficient time to make the needed adaptations, and overtraining syndrome can result. Lab 12B helps you learn how to monitor for signs of overtraining.

connect
ACTIVITY

Web Resources

Gatorade Sports Science Institute **www.gssiweb.com**

National Athletic Trainers Association **www.nata.org**

National Collegiate Athletic Association **www.ncaa.org**

National Strength and Conditioning Association
www.nsca-cc.org

Promote Performance Newsletter (free) **www
.performancemattersinc.com/newsletters**

Special Olympics International **www.specialolympics.org**

Sports Injuries (Medline Plus-NIH) **www.nlm.nih
.gov/medlineplus/sportsinjuries.html**

Sports Injuries (NIAMSD) **www.niams.nih.gov/Health_Info/
sports_injuries/**

United States Anti-Doping Agency **www.usada.org/
supplement411**

United States Olympic Committee **www.teamusa.org**

Women's Sports Foundation **www
.womenssportsfoundation.org**

Suggested Readings

Bompa, T., and G. G. Haff. 2009. *Periodization.* 5th ed. Champaign, IL: Human Kinetics.

Brotherhood, J. R. 2008. Heat stress and strain in exercise and sport. *Journal of Science and Medicine in Sport* 11(1):3–5.

Faigenbaum, A. D. 2009. Overtraining in young athletes: How much is too much? *ACSM's Health and Fitness Journal* 13(4):8–13.

Gibala, M. J. 2010. A practical model of low-volume high-intensity interval training induces mitochondrial biogenesis in human skeletal muscle: Potential mechanisms. *Journal of Physiology* 588:1011–1022.

Gibala, M. J. 2012. Active voice: Is high-intensity interval training a time-efficient exercise strategy to promote health? *Sports Medicine Bulletin,* February 28.

Henschke, N., and Lin, C. C. Lin. 2011. Stretching before or after exercise does not reduce delayed-onset muscle soreness. *British Journal of Sports Medicine* 45:1249–1250.

Hibbs, A. E., et al. (2008). Optimizing performance by improving core stability and core strength. *Sports Medicine* 38(12):995–1008.

Kay, A. D., and A. J. Blazevich. 2011. Effect of acute static stretch on maximal muscle performance: A systematic review. *Medicine and Science in Sports and Exercise* 44(1):154–164.

Khan, K. M. et al. 2012. Sport and exercise as contributors to the health of nations. *Lancet* 380(9836):59–64.

Kovacs, M. 2009. *Dynamic Stretching: The Revolutionary New Warm-up Method to Improve Power, Performance and Range of Motion.* Berkeley, CA: Ulysses Press.

Lederman E. 2010. The myth of core stability. *Journal of Bodywork and Movement Therapies* 14(1):84–98.

Little, J. P., et al. 2011. Low-volume high-intensity interval training reduces hyperglycemia and increases muscle mitochondria capacity in patients with type 2 diabetes. *Journal of Applied Physiology* 111(6):1554–1660.

McHugh, M. P., and C. H. Cosgrave. 2010. To stretch or not to stretch: The role of stretching in injury prevention and performance. *Scandinavian Journal of Medicine and Science in Sports* 20:169–181.

Noakes, T. D. 2008. Heat stress in sport—Fact or fiction. *Journal of Science and Medicine in Sport* 11(1):3–5.

Ratamess, N. 2012. *ACSM's Foundations of Strength Training and Conditioning.* Philadelphia: Lippincott, Williams & Wilkins.

Thomas, D. Q., et al. 2012. Exertional rhabdomyolysis: What is it and why should we care? *Journal of Physical Education, Recreation and Dance* 83(1):46–49.

Healthy People 2020

The objectives listed below are societal goals designed to help all Americans improve their health between now and the year 2020. They were selected because they relate to the content of this concept.

- Reduce sports and recreation injuries.
- Reduce injuries from overexertion.
- Increase the proportion of adults who meet guidelines for aerobic and muscle fitness activity.
- Reduce steroid use by adolescents.
- Reduce percentage of adults who do no leisure-time activity.
- Reduce adverse events from medical products.

A national goal is to reduce use of steroids and illegal sports supplements by adolescents. While the media has focused on the use of steroids in professional sports, the bigger concern is the use of steroids and supplements by adolescents and young adults that are attracted by the allure of professional sports. Considering the established risks of steroids, does it surprise you that steroid use is a problem in mainstream society?

Lab Resource Materials: Skill-Related Physical Fitness

Important Note: Because skill-related physical fitness does not relate to good health, the rating charts used in this section differ from those used for health-related fitness. The rating charts that follow can be used to compare your scores with those of other people. You *do not* need exceptional scores on skill-related fitness to be able to enjoy sports and other types of physical activity; however, it is necessary for high-level performance. After the age of 30, you should adjust ratings by 1 percent per year.

Evaluating Skill-Related Physical Fitness

I. Evaluating Agility: The Illinois Agility Run

An agility course using four chairs 10 feet apart and a 30-foot running area will be set up as depicted in this illustration. The test is performed as follows:

1. Lie prone with your hands by your shoulders and your head at the starting line. On the signal to begin, get on your feet and run the course as fast as possible.
2. Your score is the time required to complete the course.

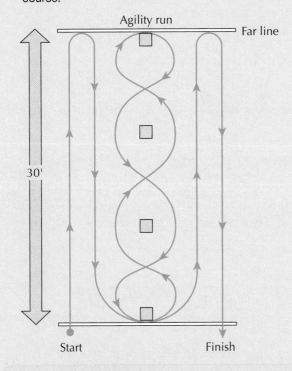

II. Evaluating Balance: The Bass Test of Dynamic Balance

Eleven circles (9½ inches) are drawn on the floor as shown in the illustration. The test is performed as follows:

1. Stand on the right foot in circle X. *Leap* forward to circle 1, then circle 2 through 10, alternating feet with each leap.
2. The feet must leave the floor on each leap and the heel may not touch. Only the ball of the foot and toes may land on the floor.
3. Remain in each circle for 5 seconds before leaping to the next circle. (A count of 5 will be made for you aloud.)
4. Practice trials are allowed.
5. The score is 50, plus the number of seconds taken to complete the test, minus the number of errors.
6. For every error, deduct 3 points each. Errors include touching the heel, moving the supporting foot, touching outside a circle, and touching any body part other than the supporting foot to the floor.

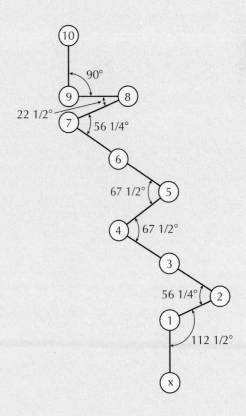

Chart 1 Agility Rating Scale

Classification	Men	Women
Excellent	15.8 or faster	17.4 or faster
Very good	16.7–15.9	18.6–17.5
Good	18.6–16.8	22.3–18.7
Fair	18.8–18.7	23.4–22.4
Poor	18.9 or slower	23.5 or slower

Source: Adams et al.

Chart 2 Balance Rating Scale

Rating	Score
Excellent	90–100
Very good	80–89
Good	70–79
Fair	60–69
Poor	50–59

Chart 3 Coordination Rating Scale

Classification	Men	Women
Excellent	14–15	13–15
Very good	11–13	10–12
Good	5–10	4–9
Fair	3–4	2–3
Poor	0–2	0–1

III. Evaluating Coordination: The Stick Test of Coordination

The stick test of coordination requires you to juggle three wooden sticks. The sticks are used to perform a one-half flip and a full flip, as shown in the illustrations.

1. *One-half flip.* Hold two 24-inch (½ inch in diameter) dowel rods, one in each hand. Support a third rod of the same size across the other two. Toss the supported rod in the air, so that it makes a half turn. Catch the thrown rod with the two held rods.
2. *Full flip.* Perform the preceding task, letting the supported rod turn a full flip.

The test is performed as follows:

1. Practice the half-flip and full flip several times before taking the test.
2. When you are ready, attempt a half-flip five times. Score 1 point for each successful attempt.
3. When you are ready, attempt the full flip five times. Score 2 points for each successful attempt.

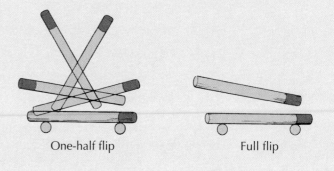

One-half flip   Full flip

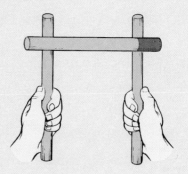

Hand position

IV. Evaluating Power: The Vertical Jump Test

The test is performed as follows:

1. Hold a piece of chalk so its end is even with your fingertips.
2. Stand with both feet on the floor and your side to the wall and reach and mark as high as possible.
3. Jump upward with both feet as high as possible. Swing arms upward and make a chalk mark on a 5′ × 1′ wall chart marked off in half-inch horizontal lines placed 6 feet from the floor.
4. Measure the distance between the reaching height and the jumping height.
5. Your score is the best of three jumps.

Chart 4 Power Rating Scale

Classification	Men	Women
Excellent	25½″ or more	23½″ or more
Very good	21″–25″	19″–23″
Good	16 ½″–20½″	14½″–18½″
Fair	12½″–16″	10½″–14″
Poor	12″ or less	10″ or less

Metric conversions for this chart appear in Appendix A.

V. Evaluating Reaction Time: The Stick Drop Test

To perform the stick drop test of reaction time, you will need a yardstick, a table, a chair, and a partner to help with the test. To perform the test, follow this procedure:

1. Sit in the chair next to the table so that your elbow and lower arm rest on the table comfortably. The heel of your hand should rest on the table so that only your fingers and thumb extend beyond the edge of the table.
2. Your partner holds a yardstick at the top, allowing it to dangle between your thumb and fingers.
3. The yardstick should be held so that the 24-inch mark is even with your thumb and index finger. No part of your hand should touch the yardstick.
4. Without warning, your partner will drop the stick, and you will catch it with your thumb and index finger.
5. Your score is the number of inches read on the yardstick just above the thumb and index finger after you catch the yardstick.
6. Try the test three times. Your partner should be careful not to drop the stick at predictable time intervals, so that you cannot guess when it will be dropped. It is important that you react only to the dropping of the stick.
7. Use the middle of your three scores (for example: if your scores are 21, 18, and 19, your middle score is 19). The higher your score, the faster your reaction time.

Chart 5 Reaction Time Rating Scale

Classification	Score
Excellent	More than 21″
Very good	19″–21″
Good	16″–18¾″
Fair	13″–15¾″
Poor	Below 13″

Metric conversions for this chart appear in Appendix A.

VI. Evaluating Speed: 3-Second Run

To perform the running test of speed, it will be necessary to have a specially marked running course, a stopwatch, a whistle, and a partner to help you with the test. To perform the test, follow this procedure:

1. Mark a running course on a hard surface so that there is a starting line and a series of nine additional lines, each 2 yards apart, the first marked at a distance 10 yards from the starting line.

2. From a distance 1 or 2 yards behind the starting line, begin to run as fast as you can. As you cross the starting line, your partner starts a stopwatch.

3. Run as fast as you can until you hear the whistle, which your partner will blow exactly 3 seconds after the stopwatch is started. Your partner marks your location at the time the whistle was blown.

4. Your score is the distance you covered in 3 seconds. You may practice the test and take more than one trial if time allows. Use the better of your distances on the last two trials as your score.

Chart 6 Speed Rating Scale

Classification	Men	Women
Excellent	24–26 yards	22–26 yards
Very good	22–23 yards	20–21 yards
Good	18–21 yards	16–19 yards
Fair	16–17 yards	14–15 yards
Poor	Less than 16 yards	Less than 14 yards

Metric conversions for this chart appear in Appendix A.

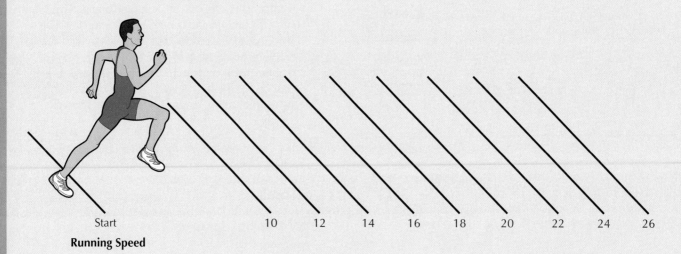

Start   10   12   14   16   18   20   22   24   26

Running Speed

Lab 12A Evaluating Skill-Related Physical Fitness

Name	Section	Date

Purpose: To help you evaluate your own skill-related fitness, including agility, balance, coordination, power, speed, and reaction time; this information may be of value in helping you decide which sports match your skill-related fitness abilities

Procedures

1. Read the direction for each of the skill-related fitness tests presented in *Lab Resource Materials.*
2. Take as many of the tests as possible, given the time and equipment available.
3. Be sure to warm up before and to cool down after the tests.
4. It is all right to practice the tests before trying them. However, you should decide ahead of time which trial you will use to test your skill-related fitness.
5. After completing the tests, write your scores in the appropriate places in the Results section.
6. Determine your rating for each of the tests from the rating charts in *Lab Resource Materials.*

Results

Place a check in the circle for each of the tests you completed.

Agility (Illinois run) ◯

Balance (Bass test) ◯

Coordination (stick test) ◯

Power (vertical jump) ◯

Reaction time (stick drop test) ◯

Speed (3-second run) ◯

Record your score and rating in the following spaces.

	Score	Rating	
Agility			(Chart 1)
Balance			(Chart 2)
Coordination			(Chart 3)
Power			(Chart 4)
Reaction time			(Chart 5)
Speed			(Chart 6)

Conclusions and Implications: In two or three paragraphs, discuss the results of your skill-related fitness tests. Comment on the areas in which you did well or did not do well, the meaning of these findings, and the implications of the results, with specific reference to the activities you will perform in the future.

Lab 12B Identifying Symptoms of Overtraining

Name	Section	Date

Purpose: To help you identify the symptoms of overtraining

Procedures

1. Answer the questions concerning overtraining syndrome in the Results section. If you are in training, rate yourself; if not, evaluate a person you know who is in training. As an alternative, you may evaluate a person who was formerly in training (and who experienced symptoms) or evaluate yourself when you were in training (if you trained for performance in the past).
2. Use Chart 1 (below) to rate the person (yourself or another person) who is (or was) in training.
3. Use Chart 2 (page 288) to identify some strategies you can try to treat or prevent overtraining syndrome.
4. Answer the questions in the Conclusions and Implications section.

Results

Answer "Yes" (place a check in the circle) to any of the questions relating to overtraining symptoms you (or the person you are evaluating) experienced.

○ 1. Has performance decreased dramatically in the last week or two?

○ 2. Is there evidence of depression?

○ 3. Is there evidence of atypical anger?

○ 4. Is there evidence of atypical anxiety?

○ 5. Is there evidence of general fatigue that is not typical?

○ 6. Is there general lack of vigor or loss of energy?

○ 7. Have sleeping patterns changed (inability to sleep well)?

○ 8. Is there evidence of heaviness of the arms and/or legs?

○ 9. Is there evidence of loss of appetite?

○ 10. Is there a lack of interest in training?

Chart 1 Ratings for Overtraining Syndrome

Number of "Yes" Answers	Rating
9–10	Overtraining syndrome is very likely present. Seek help.
6–8	Person is at risk for overtraining syndrome if it is not already present. Seek help to prevent additional symptoms.
3–5	Some signs of overtraining syndrome are present. Consider methods of preventing further symptoms.
0–2	Overtraining syndrome is not present, but attention should be paid to the few symptoms that do exist.

Conclusions and Implications

Chart 2 lists some of the strategies that may help eliminate or prevent overtraining syndrome. Check the strategies that you think would be (or would have been) most useful to the person you evaluated.

Chart 2 Strategies for Treating or Preventing Overtraining Syndrome

○ 1. Consider a break from training.

○ 2. Taper the program to help reduce symptoms.

○ 3. Seek help to redesign the training program.

○ 4. Alter your diet.

○ 5. Evaluate other stressors that may be producing symptoms.

○ 6. Reset performance goals.

○ 7. Talk to someone about problems.

○ 8. Have a medical checkup to be sure there is no medical problem.

○ 9. If you have a coach, consider a talk with him or her.

○ 10. Add fluids to help prevent performance problems from dehydration.

Discuss overtraining syndrome in general. Elaborate on one or two of the strategies in Chart 2 that you think would be (or would have been) most effective in treating or preventing overtraining syndrome for the person you evaluated.

Body Composition

LEARNING OBJECTIVES

After completing the study of this concept, you will be able to:

▶ Understand and interpret body composition measures.

▶ Describe common methods of assessing body composition.

▶ List health risks associated with overfatness.

▶ List health risks associated with excessively low body fatness.

▶ Identify and describe the origins of body fatness.

▶ Explain the relationship between physical activity and body composition and apply the FIT formula for achieving and maintaining a healthy body composition.

▶ Evaluate your body composition using several self-assessments and identify personal needs, set goals, and create a plan for achieving and maintaining a healthy body composition.

▶ Self-assess your daily energy expenditure.

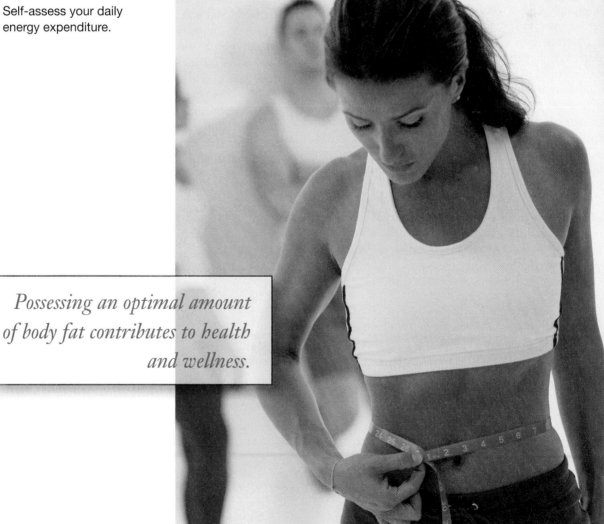

Possessing an optimal amount of body fat contributes to health and wellness.

The topic of overweight and obesity is in the news almost on a daily basis. Reports describe the health effects of obesity, the social and environmental factors that contribute to obesity, and the overall impact that it has on society. Ironically, in a society in which being thin or lean is almost obsessively valued, the incidence of overweight and obesity continues to increase. The most recent statistics indicate that approximately 17 percent of youth and 66 percent of adults are overweight or obese in the United States. Surveys indicate that only 52 percent believe they are overweight. About one-third of American adults are classified as obese, but only 12 percent classify themselves in this category. A decade ago, no state had an obesity rate higher than 25 percent. Recent statistics indicate that no state has a rate lower than 20 percent, and 36 have obesity rates higher than 25 percent, with Mississippi having the highest rate (34 percent) and Colorado the lowest (21 percent).

The health implications of this obesity epidemic are hard to quantify and predict, but it is clear that obesity has become one of our greatest public health challenges. Health-care dollars spent annually on medical conditions associated with obesity have been estimated at over $147 billion. It is estimated that by the year 2018 the cost will be $334 billion, accounting for 21 percent of health-care spending. Currently the yearly cost of medical care for the obese exceeds the cost for a normal-weight person by $2,460. When absenteeism from work is considered, the differences in health-care costs are even greater. Collectively, the obesity epidemic has placed a tremendous burden on our economy as well as on our health-care system. The problem is not unique to the United States, since similar trends are evident in almost all developed countries.

This concept describes issues associated with overweight and obesity as well as the health risks associated with being too lean. Developing a healthy body image and avoiding disordered patterns of eating are critical for optimal health and wellness.

Understanding and Interpreting Body Composition Measures

Body composition is considered a component of health-related fitness but can also be considered a component of metabolic fitness. Body composition is generally considered to be a health-related component of physical fitness. However, body composition is unlike the other parts of health-related physical fitness in that it is not a performance measure. Cardiovascular fitness, strength, muscular endurance, and flexibility can be assessed using movement or performance, such as running, lifting, or stretching. Body composition requires no movement or performance. This is one reason some experts prefer to consider body composition as a component of metabolic fitness. Whether you consider body composition to be a part of health-related or metabolic fitness, it is an important health-related factor.

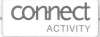

connect
VIDEO 1

Standards have been established for healthy levels of body fatness. Fat has important functions in the body, and it is distributed naturally into different tissues and storage depots. The indicator of **percent body fat** is typically used to reflect the overall fat content of the body. This indicator takes into account differences in body size and allows recommendations to be made for healthy levels of body fatness.

A certain minimal amount of fat is needed to allow the body to function. This level of **essential fat** is necessary for temperature regulation, shock absorption, and the regulation of essential body nutrients, including vitamins A, D, E, and K. The exact amount of fat considered essential to normal body functioning has been debated, but most experts agree that males should possess no less than 5 percent and females no less than 10 percent. For females, an exceptionally low body fat percentage (**underfat**) is of special concern, particularly when associated with overtraining, low calorie intake, competitive

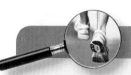

A CLOSER LOOK

Let's Move!

The childhood obesity epidemic is one of the biggest public health challenges facing our country. A number of national campaigns have been created to mobilize action and create change. These initiatives use a variety of social media to generate interest and momentum. The Let's Move! campaign addresses childhood obesity by adopting a broad community approach that enlists a variety of partners (community leaders, physicians, teachers, and parents) to help create healthier environments. The goal is to solve the epidemic of childhood obesity within a generation.

What changes in society would be needed to reach this goal?

connect
ACTIVITY

	Too low	Borderline	Good fitness	Marginal	At risk	
Male	5 or less	6–9	10–20	21–25	26+	Body fatness (percent body fat)
Female	10 or less	11–16	17–28	29–35	36+	

	Too low	Borderline	Good fitness	Overweight*	Obesity*	
Male	12 or less	13–16	17–25	26–30	30+	Body mass Index (kg/m²)
Female	12 or less	13–16	17–25	26–30	30+	

Figure 1 ▶ Health-related standards for body fatness (percent body fat) and body mass index.

*Note: Based on international standards used for BMI classification.

stress, and poor diet. **Amenorrhea** may occur, placing the woman at risk for bone loss (osteoporosis) and other health problems. A body fat level below 10 percent is one of the criteria often used by clinicians for diagnosing eating disorders, such as anorexia nervosa.

Figure 1 shows the health-related standards for body composition (percent body fat) for both males and females. Because individuals differ in their response to low fatness, a borderline range is provided above the essential fat (too low) zone. Values in this zone are not necessarily considered to be healthy, but some individuals may seek to have lower body fat levels to enhance performance in certain sports. These levels can be acceptable for nonperformers if they can be maintained on a healthy diet and without overtraining. If symptoms such as amenorrhea, bone loss, and frequent injury occur, then levels of body fatness should be reconsidered, as should training techniques and eating patterns. For many people in training, maintaining performance levels of body fatness is temporary; thus, the risk for long-term health problems is diminished.

Fat that is stored above essential fat levels is classified as **nonessential fat.** Just as percent body fat should not drop too low, it should not get too high. The healthy range for body fatness in males is between 10 and 20 percent, while the healthy range for women is between 17 and 28 percent. These levels are associated with good metabolic fitness, good health, and wellness. The marginal zone includes levels that are above the healthy fitness zone but not quite into the range used to reflect **obesity.** The term *obesity* often carries negative connotations and stereotypes, but it is important to understand that it is a clinical term that simply means excessively high body fat. Lab 13A provides opportunities for you to assess your level of body fatness.

Health standards have been established for the Body Mass Index. The **Body Mass Index (BMI)** is a commonly used indicator of **overweight** and obesity in our

society but is often misunderstood. The measure of BMI is basically an indicator of your weight relative to your height. It does not provide an indicator of body fatness, although BMI values tend to correlate with body fatness in most people. Because of this association, it is widely used in clinical settings and as a general indicator of body composition.

Because BMI is a frequently used measure, you should know how to calculate and interpret your BMI and your "healthy weight range." Mathematically, BMI is calculated with the following formula: BMI = weight (kg)/ (height [m] × height [m]). Instructions for calculating BMI, including the nonmetric formula and rating charts, are provided in the *Lab Resource Materials* (page 311). There are also many BMI calculators on the Internet that make it easy to calculate.

Percent Body Fat The percentage of total body weight that is composed of fat.

Essential Fat The minimum amount of fat in the body necessary to maintain healthful living.

Underfat Too little of the body weight composed of fat.

Amenorrhea Absent or infrequent menstruation.

Nonessential Fat Extra fat or fat reserves stored in the body.

Obesity A clinical term for a condition characterized by an excessive amount of body fat (or extremely high BMI).

Body Mass Index (BMI) A measure of body composition using a height-weight formula. High BMI values have been related to increased disease risk.

Overweight A clinical term that implies higher than normal levels of body fat and potential risk for development of obesity.

The accepted international standards for defining overweight and obesity are the same for both men and women. BMI values over 25 are used to define overweight, and values over 30 are used to define obesity. Figure 1 provides additional information concerning BMI standards.

While the use of BMI is widely accepted, it does have limitations. Individuals who do regular physical activity and who possess considerable muscle mass may show up as overweight using the BMI. This is because muscle weighs more than fat, but height and weight measurements do not detect differences in muscle and fat in the body.

Assessing body weight too frequently can result in making false assumptions about body composition changes. People vary in body weight from day to day and even hour to hour, based solely on their level of hydration. Short-term changes in weight are often due to water loss or gain, yet many people erroneously attribute the weight changes to their diet, a pill they have taken, or the exercise they recently performed. There is some evidence that monitoring weight daily can help normal-weight people from gaining weight. For people trying to lose weight, monitoring weight less frequently—once a week, for example—is more useful than taking daily or multiple daily measures. When you do weigh yourself, weigh at the same time of day, preferably early in the morning, because it reduces the chances that your weight variation will be a result of body water changes. Of course, it is best to use body composition assessments in addition to those based on body weight. These are described in the next section.

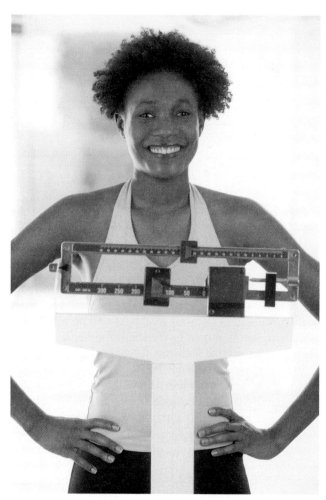

Monitoring weight can be helpful, but measures of body fatness provide a better indication of body composition.

Methods Used to Assess Body Composition

Methods of body composition vary in accuracy and practicality. A number of techniques have been developed to assess body composition. They vary in terms of practicality and accuracy, so it is important to understand the limitations of each method. Even established techniques have potential for error. The most common methods are summarized below.

connect
VIDEO 2

Dual-energy absorptiometry (DXA) has emerged as the accepted "gold standard" measure of body composition. The DXA technique uses the attenuation of two energy sources to estimate the density of the body. A specific advantage of DXA is that it can provide whole-body measurements of body fatness as well as amounts stored in different parts of the body. An additional advantage is that it provides estimates of bone density. For the procedure, the person lies on a table and the machine scans up along

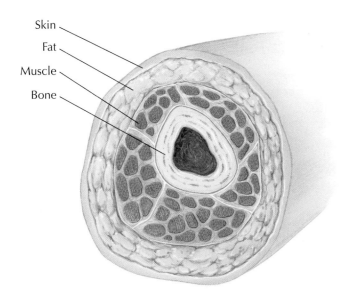

Figure 2 ▶ Location of body fat.

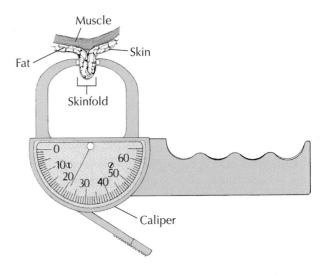

Figure 3 ▶ Measuring skinfold thickness with calipers.

the body. While some radiation exposure is necessary with the procedure, it is quite minimal compared with X-ray and other diagnostic scans. Because the machine is quite expensive, this procedure is found only in medical centers and well-equipped research laboratories. The DXA (also called DEXA) procedure provides scientists with a highly accurate measure of body composition for research and a criterion measure that has been used to validate other, more practical measures of body composition.

Underwater weighing and Bod Pod are two highly accurate methods. Underwater weighing is another excellent method of assessing body fatness. Before the development of DXA it was considered to be the "gold standard" method of assessment. In this technique, a person is weighed in air and underwater, and the difference in weight is used to assess the levels of body fatness. People with a lot of muscle, bone, and other lean tissue sink like a rock in water because muscle and other lean tissue are dense. Fat is less dense, so people with more fat tend to float in a water environment. A limitation of this method is that participants must exhale all their air while submerged in order to obtain an accurate reading. Additional error from the estimations of residual lung volumes also tends to reduce the accuracy of this approach.

A device called the Bod Pod uses the same principles as underwater weighing, but relies on air displacement to assess body composition. Evidence suggests that it provides an acceptable alternative to underwater weighing and is particularly useful for special populations (obese older people and the physically challenged).

Skinfold measurements are a practical method of assessing body fatness. About one-half of the body's fat is located around the various body organs and in the muscles. The other half of the body's fat is located just under the skin, or in skinfolds. A skinfold (Figure 2) is two thicknesses of skin and the amount of fat that lies just under the skin. By measuring skinfold thicknesses of various sites around the body, it is possible to estimate total body fatness (Figure 3). Skinfold measurements are often used because they are relatively easy to do. They are not nearly as costly as underwater weighing and other methods that require expensive equipment. Research-quality skinfold calipers cost more than $100, but consumer models are available for $10 to $20.

In general, the more skinfolds measured, the more accurate the fatness estimate. However, measurements with two or three skinfolds have been shown to be reasonably accurate and can be done in a relatively short period. Two skinfold techniques are used in Lab 13A. You are encouraged to try both. With adequate training, most people can learn to use calipers to get a good estimate of fatness.

Bioelectric impedance analysis has become a practical alternative for body fatness assessment. Bioelectric impedance analysis (BIA) ranks quite favorably for accuracy and has overall rankings similar to those of skinfold measurement techniques. The test can be performed quickly and is more effective for people high in body fatness (a limitation of skinfolds). The technique is based on measuring resistance to current flow. Electrodes are placed on the body and low doses of current are passed through the skin. Because muscle has greater water content than fat, it is a better conductor and has less resistance to current. The overall amount of resistance and body size are used to predict body fatness. The results depend heavily on hydration status, so do not test after exercising or immediately after eating or drinking. Accuracy is also affected by the quality of the equipment. Portable BIA scales are available that allow you to simply stand on metal plates to get an estimate of body fatness. These devices are easier to use but are less accurate than those that use electrodes for both upper and lower body.

Infrared sensors are sometimes used to assess body fatness. Near-infrared interactance machines use the absorption of light to estimate body fatness. The technique was originally developed to measure the fat content of meats. Commercially available units for humans have not been shown to be effective for estimating body fat, and at least one company has faced sanctions from the government for selling an unapproved product. For this reason, this type of device is not recommended.

Health Risks Associated with Overfatness

Obesity contributes directly and indirectly to a number of major health problems. The presence of excess body fat impairs the function of most systems of the body (e.g., the cardiovascular system, the pulmonary system, the skeletal system, the reproductive system, and the metabolic system). It also increases risks for a variety of diseases, including a variety of cancers. The American Heart Association classifies obesity as a primary risk factor, along with high blood pressure and high blood lipids (both associated with overweight and obesity). When all the evidence is considered, it is clear that overweight is associated with many health problems and obesity places a person at special risk (see Figure 4).

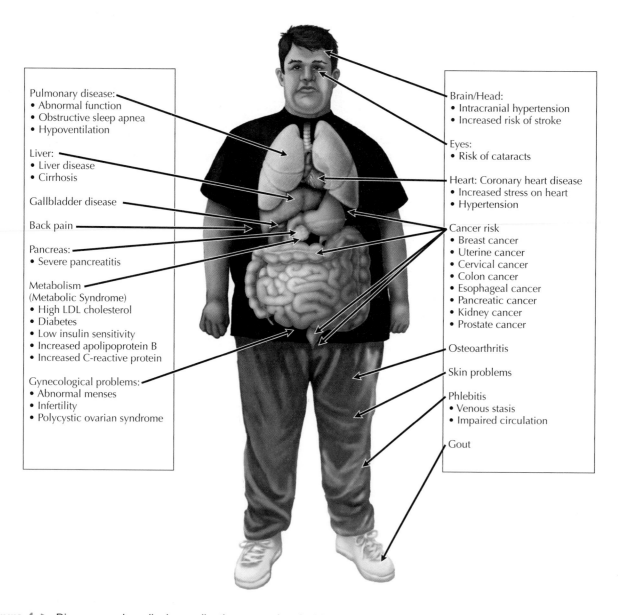

Pulmonary disease:
• Abnormal function
• Obstructive sleep apnea
• Hypoventilation

Liver:
• Liver disease
• Cirrhosis

Gallbladder disease

Back pain

Pancreas:
• Severe pancreatitis

Metabolism
(Metabolic Syndrome)
• High LDL cholesterol
• Diabetes
• Low insulin sensitivity
• Increased apolipoprotein B
• Increased C-reactive protein

Gynecological problems:
• Abnormal menses
• Infertility
• Polycystic ovarian syndrome

Brain/Head:
• Intracranial hypertension
• Increased risk of stroke

Eyes:
• Risk of cataracts

Heart: Coronary heart disease
• Increased stress on heart
• Hypertension

Cancer risk
• Breast cancer
• Uterine cancer
• Cervical cancer
• Colon cancer
• Esophageal cancer
• Pancreatic cancer
• Kidney cancer
• Prostate cancer

Osteoarthritis

Skin problems

Phlebitis
• Venous stasis
• Impaired circulation

Gout

Figure 4 ▶ Diseases and medical complications associated with obesity.

Studies indicate that overweight and obesity and associated unhealthy lifestyles (e.g., sedentary living and unhealthy eating) are the second leading actual cause of death. One study indicates that obesity and smoking are equal in their overall burden on the health-care system. Smoking has decreased 18.5 percent in the past two decades, while obesity rates increased by 85 percent. If current trends continue, obesity and overweight will soon surpass smoking as the number one cause of early death.

Obesity contributes to early death. In addition to the higher incidence of certain diseases and health problems, people who are moderately overfat have a 40 percent higher than normal risk of shortening their lifespan. More severe obesity results in a 70 percent higher than normal death rate. A study of nearly one million adults suggests that obesity can cut 8 to 10 years from life expectancy. Another recent study indicates that extreme obesity shortens life by 12 years.

Statistics indicate that underweight people also have a higher than normal risk for premature death. Though adequate evidence shows extreme leanness (e.g., anorexia nervosa) can be life threatening, underweight people may have lost weight because of a medical condition such as cancer. It appears that the medical problems are often the reason for low body weight rather than low body weight being the source of the medical problem. Most experts agree that people who are free from disease and who have lower than average amounts of body fat have a lower than average risk for premature death.

Physical fitness provides protection from the health risks of obesity. A general assumption in our society is that if you are thin, you are probably fit and healthy and if you are overweight, you are unfit and unhealthy. A series of studies from the Aerobic Center Longitudinal Study (a large cohort study of patients from the Cooper Clinic in Dallas, Texas) has demonstrated that the health risks associated with overweight are greatly reduced by regular physical activity and reasonable levels of cardiovascular

fitness (see Figure 5). In fact, the findings consistently show that active people who have a high BMI are at less risk than inactive people with normal BMI levels. Even high levels of body fatness may not be especially likely to increase disease risk if a person has good metabolic fitness as indicated by healthy blood fat levels, normal blood pressure, and normal blood sugar levels. It is when several of these factors are present at the same time that risk levels increase dramatically. For this reason, it is important to consider your cardiovascular and metabolic fitness levels before drawing conclusions about the effects of high body weight or high body fat levels on health and wellness. This information also points out the importance of periodically assessing your cardiovascular and metabolic fitness levels.

Excessive abdominal fat and excessive fat of the upper body can increase the risk for various diseases. The location of body fat can influence the health risks associated with obesity. Fat in the upper part of the body is sometimes referred to as "Northern Hemisphere" fat, and a body type high in this type of fat is called the "apple" shape (see Figure 6). Upper-body fat is also referred to as android fat because it is more characteristic of men than women. Postmenopausal women typically have a higher amount of upper body fat than premenopausal women. Lower body fat, such as in the hips and upper legs, is sometimes referred to as "Southern Hemisphere" fat. This body type is called the "pear"

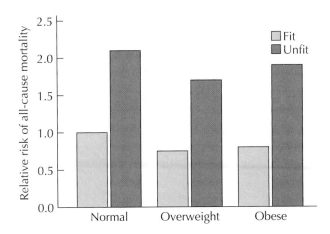

Figure 5 ► Risks of fatness vs. fitness.
Source: Lee, C. D., et al.

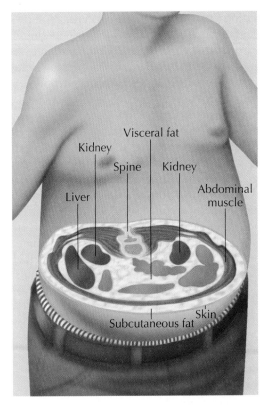

Figure 6 ► Visceral, or abdominal, fat is associated with increased disease risk.

shape. Lower-body fat is also referred to as gynoid fat because it is more characteristic of women than men.

Body fat located in the core of the body is referred to as central fat or visceral fat. Visceral fat is located in the abdominal cavity (see Figure 6), as opposed to subcutaneous fat, which is located just under the skin. Though subcutaneous fat (skinfold measures) can be used to estimate body fatness, it is not a good indicator of central fatness. Your waist size is a useful indicator of visceral fat distribution. It can be used alone, in combination with BMI, in combination with your gender and height, and/or in combination with hip size (waist-to-hip ratio) to determine health risk (see *Lab Resource Materials*). Visceral fat is considered more harmful than other forms and is associated with high blood fat levels as well as other metabolic problems. It is also associated with high incidence of heart attack, stroke, chest pain, breast cancer, and early death.

Part of the benefit of aerobic activity for health appears to be its ability to promote the preferential loss of abdominal body fat. Several recent studies have shown that higher levels of activity and/or higher cardiorespiratory fitness are associated with lower levels of abdominal body fatness independent of body mass index. In other words, if one person who is fit and active has the same height and weight as a less active person, he or she will likely have a lower amount of abdominal fat. These studies provide a clear understanding of how fitness may protect against the health risks of obesity and improve overall health.

Health effects of obesity may be mediated by circulating "adipokines." Research has recently shown that the fat cell is not only a storage depot, but also an active protein-secreting organ. The biomolecules secreted by adipose tissue are known as adipokines or adipocytokines. A number of adipokines have been identified, including adiponectin, visfatin, resistin, and leptin. Each has an important role, but adiponectin appears to play a particularly important role in energy balance, insulin resistance, and atherosclerosis. Studies show that adiponectin has an anti-atherosclerotic effect while also reducing platelet aggregation, which can contribute to formation of blood clots. In contrast, adiponectin deficiency appears to lead to metabolic dysfunction, insulin resistance, fatty liver disease, and also to a wide array of cancers. Current evidence supports that aerobic exercise, alone or combined with hypocaloric diet, improves symptoms of the metabolic syndrome, possibly by altering levels of adipokines.

Health Risks Associated with Excessively Low Body Fatness

Excessive desire to be thin or low in body weight can result in health problems. In Western society, the near obsession with thinness has been, at least in part, responsible for eating disorders. Eating disorders, or altered eating habits, involve extreme restriction of food intake and/or regurgitation of food to avoid digestion. The most common disorders are anorexia nervosa, binge-eating, bulimia, and anorexia athletica. All of these disorders are most common among highly achievement-oriented girls and young women, although they affect virtually all segments of the population. Patterns of "disordered eating" are not the same as clinically diagnosed eating disorders. People who adopt disordered eating, however, tend to have a greater chance of developing an eating disorder. It is interesting to note that in 1974 the percentage of underweight Americans was 3.6. Today half that percentage (1.8) of Americans is classified as underweight.

Anorexia nervosa is the most severe eating disorder. If untreated, it is life threatening. Anorexics restrict food intake so severely that their bodies become emaciated. Among the many characteristics of anorexia nervosa are fear of maturity and inaccurate body image. The anorexic starves himself or herself and may exercise compulsively or use laxatives to prevent the digestion of food in an attempt to attain excessive leanness. The anorexic's self-image is one of being too fat, even when the person is too lean for good health. Assessing body fatness using procedures such as skinfolds and observation of the eating habits may help identify people with anorexia. Among anorexic girls and women, development of an adult figure is often feared. People with this disorder must obtain medical and psychological help immediately, as the consequences are severe. About 25 percent of those with anorexia do compulsive exercise in an attempt to stay lean. Anorexia is a very serious medical condition that deserves more discussion than can be provided in this book.

Binge-eating is the most common eating disorder in the United States. According to the American Psychiatric Association, you are a binge-eater if you meet these three criteria: (1) eat larger amounts of food than most people eat in a short time; (2) feel out of control while bingeing at least once a week for three months; and (3) do three or more behaviors, such as feeling depressed about your binges, eating alone to avoid embarrassment about amounts eaten, eating large amounts when not hungry, eating more rapidly than normal, or continuing to eat when you feel full. While binge-eating can be a serious disorder, it can be treated effectively. One study showed that 64 percent of binge-eaters who received therapy and reading material were binge free after only one year.

Bulimia is a common eating disorder characterized by bingeing and purging. Disordered eating patterns become habitual for many people with bulimia.

A bulimic might binge after a relatively long period of dieting and consume excessive amounts of junk foods containing empty calories. After a binge, the bulimic purges the food by forced regurgitation or the use of laxatives. Another form of bulimia is bingeing on one day and starving on the next. The consequences of bulimia include serious mental, gastrointestinal, and dental problems. Bulimics may or may not be anorexic. It may not be possible to use measures of body fatness to identify bulimia, as the bulimic may be lean, normal, or excessively fat.

Anorexia athletica is a more recently identified eating disorder that appears to be related to participation in sports and activities emphasizing body leanness. Studies show that participants in sports such as gymnastics, wrestling, and bodybuilding and activities such as ballet and cheerleading are most likely to develop anorexia athletica. This disorder has many of the symptoms of anorexia nervosa, but not of the same severity. In some cases, anorexia athletica leads to anorexia nervosa.

Female athlete triad is an increasingly common condition among female athletes. The triad refers to the presence of three related and linked symptoms that affect some women athletes (eating disorders/low energy availability, amenorrhea, and decreased bone mineral density). The conditions are linked because low body fat levels lead to the amenorrhea. The alterations in menstrual cycles lead to low levels of estrogen which subsequently lead to the reduced bone density and risk for osteoporosis.

The female athlete triad is one of the more challenging conditions to treat because it often goes undetected. Once identified or diagnosed, it is hard to change because the three components of the triad are thought to be linked pathophysiologically. The athlete is very serious about performance and has likely developed altered eating patterns to control body weight. Efforts to bring about change often result in resistance, since the compulsion to be thin and perform well overrides other concerns, such as eating well, moderating exercise, and having a normal menstrual cycle. The ACSM recommends regular screening exams to identify those with the triad and rule changes in women's sports to "discourage unhealthy weight loss practices." Nutrition counseling is recommended for those with the triad, and psychotherapy is recommended for athletes with eating disorders.

Many female athletes train extensively and have relatively low body fat levels but experience none of the symptoms of the triad. Eating well, training properly, using stress-management techniques, and monitoring health symptoms are the keys to their success.

Muscle dysmorphia is an emerging problem among male athletes. Muscle dysmorphia is a body dysmorphic disorder in which a male becomes preoccupied with the idea that his body is not sufficiently lean and/or muscular. Athletes with this condition may be more inclined to use performance-enhancing drugs, to exercise while sick, or to have an eating disorder. Additional risks include depression and social isolation.

Fear of obesity and purging disorder are other identified conditions. Fear of obesity is most common among achievement-oriented teenagers who impose a self-restriction on caloric intake because they fear obesity. Consequences include stunting of growth, delayed puberty, delayed sexual development, and decreased physical attractiveness. Purging disorder, a condition that results in purging similar to bulimia, but without the bingeing, has recently been identified. People with these conditions should seek assistance.

The Origin of Fatness

Obesity is a multifactorial disease that is influenced by both genetics and the environment. The evidence documenting a genetic component to human obesity is quite compelling. There is clear clustering of obesity within families, and studies have documented high concordance of body composition in identical twins. Studies of adopted children have also demonstrated that there is an association between the BMI of adoptees and the biologic parents, but not with the adoptee parents. Despite the clear evidence, the role of genetic factors is still not well understood. Genetic mapping studies suggest that a number of genes may work in combination to influence susceptibility to obesity. These *susceptibility genes* may not lead directly to obesity but may predispose a person to overweight or obesity if exposed to certain environmental conditions.

Thus, the prevailing model guiding obesity research is that complex genetic and environmental variables interact to increase potential risks for obesity. Genetic factors, by themselves, cannot account for the increases in obesity because the gene pool does not change that rapidly. Recent research has shown that lack of sleep can increase risk for overweight (particularly in youth). Excessive screen time (TV and computer use) and sitting time increase risk of obesity. Future research will allow genetic factors to be integrated with behavioral and environmental data so that the combined effects can be better understood.

connect
VIDEO 3

Body weight is regulated and maintained through complex regulatory processes. Some scholars have suggested that the human body type, or **somatotype,**

In the News

Lack of Sleep Is Associated with Overweight

Most people know that sleep is important for good health, but it also may contribute to maintaining a healthy weight. A number of studies have demonstrated inverse associations between sleep and overweight but it has proven difficult to understand the biological mechanisms. Recent studies suggest that sleep loss may impose demands on the metabolism that trigger hormonal and behavior adaptations that increase food intake and conservation of energy.

Scientists speculate that this response may have evolved as a way for primitive man to conserve energy during periods with limited food availability but it is problematic in modern society with food abundance. The findings point out how different lifestyles can interact to influence weight status and wellness.

How do these findings about sleep influence your views about health and wellness?

is inherited. Clearly, some people have more difficulty than others controlling fatness, and this may be because of their somatotype and genetic predisposition. Regulatory processes appear to balance energy intake and energy expenditure so that body weight stays near a biologically determined **set-point.** The regulation is helpful for maintaining body weight but can be frustrating for people trying to lose weight. If a person slowly tries to cut calories, the body perceives an energy imbalance and initiates processes to protect the current body weight. The body can accommodate to a new, higher set-point if weight gain takes place over time, but there is greater resistance to adopting a lower set-point. Many people lose weight, only to see the weight come back months later. One of the reasons exercise is so critical for weight maintenance is that it may help in resetting this set-point.

In recent years, the mechanisms involved in the regulation of the biological set-point have become better understood. The current view is that there are complex feedback loops among fatty tissues, the brain, and endocrine glands, such as the pancreas and the thyroid. The compound leptin plays a crucial role in altering appetite and in speeding up or slowing down the metabolism. Leptin levels rise during times of energy excess in order to suppress appetite and fall when energy levels are low to stimulate appetite. Resistance to leptin has been hypothesized as a possible contributor to obesity. A number of other compounds also appear to be involved in the complex processes regulating energy balance. Problems with the thyroid gland can lead to impairments in metabolic regulation, but these do not contribute to overfatness in most people.

Fatness early in life leads to adult fatness. Although there are exceptions, individuals who are overweight or obese as children are more likely to be overweight or obese as adults. One explanation for this is that overfatness in children causes the body to produce more fat cells. Research has even suggested that the neonatal environment that the child is exposed to during development may also influence future risks for obesity. It appears that hormones and lipids circulating in the maternal blood can interact with genetic factors to establish metabolic conditions that contribute to overfatness. While these factors influence body composition, it is still possible to improve body composition by adopting healthy lifestyles.

Maintaining healthy levels of body fat is an important objective for children and adults. It was previously thought that only adult obesity was related to health problems, but it is now apparent that teens who are overfat are at a greater risk for heart problems and cancer than leaner peers. Obese children have been found to have symptoms of "adult-onset diabetes," and obese children have a higher than normal risk of premature death, indicating that the effects of obesity can impair health, even for young people. Concerns about the current and future implications of childhood obesity have made it one of the greatest public health concerns facing our country. A variety of national organizations have targeted obesity prevention as a top priority. (See information on the Let's Move! campaign on page 290.) The momentum generated from these campaigns is encouraging, but it must translate into progressive policies and programming to create such a change.

Changes in basal metabolic rate can be the cause of obesity. Your **basal metabolic rate (BMR)** is the largest component of total daily energy expenditure. BMR is typically expressed in the number of **calories** needed to maintain your body functions under resting conditions. When resting, your body expends calories because your heart is pumping and other body organs are working. Processing the food you eat also expends calories. People with more lean tissue have a higher BMR

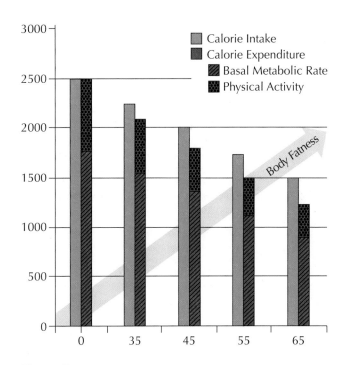

Figure 7 ▶ Creeping obesity.

than those with less lean tissue and greater amounts of body fat. People that are physically active will also have a higher BMR on days they exercise, contributing to long-term weight control.

BMR is highest during the growing years. The amount of food eaten increases to support this increased energy expenditure. When a person reaches full growth, the BMR is determined primarily by the amount of muscle mass a person has. Regular physical activity throughout life helps keep the muscle mass higher, resulting in a higher BMR. Evidence suggests that regular exercise can contribute in other ways to increased BMR. For example, BMR can stay elevated for up to 10 hours following a bout of vigorous physical activity. The higher BMR helps burn extra calories during the day.

"Creeping obesity" is a problem as you grow older. With age, people tend to become less active, causing declines in BMR. Caloric intake does seem to decrease somewhat with age, but the decrease does not adequately compensate for the decreases in BMR and activity levels. For this reason, body fat increases gradually with age for the typical person (see Figure 7). This increase in fatness over time is commonly referred to as "creeping obesity" because the increase in fatness is gradual. For a typical person, creeping obesity can result in a gain of 1/2 to 1 pound per year. People who stay active can keep muscle mass high and delay changes in BMR. For those who are not active, it is suggested that caloric intake decrease by 3 percent each decade after 25 so that by age 65 caloric intake is at least 10 percent less than it was at age 25. The decrease in caloric intake for active people need not be as great.

The Relationship between Physical Activity and Body Composition

A combination of regular physical activity and dietary restriction is the most effective means of losing body fat. Studies indicate that regular physical activity combined with dietary restriction is the most effective method of losing fat. **Diet** alone can contribute to weight loss, but much of this loss is actually lean tissue. When physical activity and diet are both used in a

Somatotype A term that refers to a person's body type. One researcher (Sheldon) suggested that there are three basic body types: ectomorph (linear), mesomorph (muscular), and endomorph (round).

Set-point A theoretical concept that describes the way the body protects current weight and resists change.

Basal Metabolic Rate (BMR) Energy expenditure in a basic, or rested, state.

Calories Units of energy supplied by food; the quantity of heat necessary to raise the temperature of a kilogram of water 1°C (actually, a kilocalorie, but usually called a calorie for weight control purposes).

Diet The usual food and drink for a person or an animal.

Table 1 ▶ Threshold of Training and Target Zones for Body Fat Reduction

	Threshold of Training*		Target Zones*	
	Physical Activity	Diet	Physical Activity	Diet
Frequency	• To be effective, activity must be regular, preferably daily, though fat can be lost over the long term with almost any frequency that results in increased caloric expenditure.	• Reduce caloric intake consistently and daily. To restrict calories only on certain days is not best, though fat can be lost over a period of time by reducing caloric intake at any time.	• Daily moderate activity is recommended. For people who do regular vigorous activity, 3 to 6 days per week may be best.	• It is best to diet consistently and daily.
Intensity	• To lose 1 pound of fat, you must expend 3,500 calories more than you normally expend.	• To lose 1 pound of fat, you must eat 3,500 calories fewer than you normally eat.	• Slow, low-intensity aerobic exercise that results in no more than 1 to 2 pounds of fat loss per week is best.	• Modest caloric restriction resulting in no more than 1 to 2 pounds of fat loss per week is best.
Time	• To be effective, exercise must be sustained long enough to expend a considerable number of calories. At least 15 minutes per exercise bout are necessary to result in consistent fat loss.	• Eating moderate meals is best. Do not skip meals.	• Exercise durations similar to those for achieving aerobic cardiovascular fitness seem best. Exercise of 30 to 60 minutes in duration is recommended.	• Eating moderate meals is best. Skipping meals or fasting is not most effective.

Note: A gram of fat is 9 calories; thus, a pound is equal to 4,086 calories (9 cal/g × 454 g/pound). However, fat in the body is 10 percent water and contains some protein and minerals that reduce the effective caloric equivalent to 3,500 calories (the accepted standard).

*It is best to combine exercise and diet to achieve the 3,500-calorie imbalance necessary to lose a pound of fat. Using both exercise and diet in the target zone is most effective.

weight loss program, the same amount of weight may be lost but more of it is from fat. This is obviously beneficial for appearance and for participation in physical activity, but it can also help maintain resting metabolic rate at a higher level. This can contribute to further weight loss or facilitate weight maintenance. For optimal results, all weight loss programs should combine a lower caloric intake with a good physical exercise program. Table 1 presents thresholds of training and target zones for body fat reduction, including information for both physical activity and diet. A general guideline is to try to lose no more than 1 to 2 pounds a week. Because a pound of fat contains 3,500 calories (see note in Table 1), this requires a caloric deficit of approximately 500 calories per day. Individuals interested in maintaining body composition should aim for **caloric balance.** Individuals who want to increase lean body mass need to increase caloric intake while carefully increasing the intensity and duration of their physical activity (mainly muscular activity).

connect
VIDEO 4

Physical activity can help expend extra energy needed to promote weight loss. The ACSM and national activity guidelines recommend a minimum of 30 minutes of moderate to vigorous activity a day or 150 minutes per week (see Table 1) but acknowledge that this may not be enough for some people. More time is often needed either to maintain weight over time or to

lose weight. The ACSM guidelines suggest that it may be necessary to work progressively up to 200 to 300 minutes a week to expend enough calories to lose weight. One study found that women who maintained weight across the lifespan average approximately 60 minutes of activity per day. Calories expended in various activities are presented in Table 2.

Energy balance principles apply for both weight maintenance and weight gain. Table 1 focuses on weight loss because overweight and obesity are prevalent in our society and many adults are currently dieting (approximately 33 percent), while another one-third are taking other steps to lose weight. For normal-weight people, maintenance is important, and balancing energy intake with energy expenditure is the key. There is little doubt that preventing overweight in the first place will help people avoid the more difficult task of losing weight. For those interested in weight gain, extra calorie intake is required, following the sound eating practices described in Concepts 14 and 15. Resistance training is also recommended because it builds muscle mass.

Caloric Balance Consuming calories in amounts equal to the number of calories expended.

Table 2 ▶ Calories Expended per Hour in Various Physical Activities (Performed at a Recreational Level)*

Activity	Calories Used per Hour				
	100 lb. (46 kg)	120 lb. (55 kg)	150 lb. (68 kg)	180 lb. (82 kg)	200 lb. (91 kg)
Archery	180	204	240	276	300
Backpacking (40-lb. pack)	307	348	410	472	513
Badminton	255	289	340	391	425
Baseball	210	238	280	322	350
Basketball (half-court)	225	255	300	345	375
Bicycling (< 10 mph)	182	218	273	327	364
Bowling	136	164	205	245	273
Canoeing	227	273	341	409	455
Circuit training	247	280	330	380	413
Dance, aerobics	315	357	420	483	525
Dance, ballet (choreographed)	240	300	360	432	480
Dance, modern (choreographed)	240	300	360	432	480
Dance, social	205	245	307	368	409
Fencing	225	255	300	345	375
Fitness calisthenics	232	263	310	357	388
Football	225	255	300	345	375
Golf (walking)	250	300	375	450	500
Gymnastics	232	263	310	357	388
Handball	450	510	600	690	750
Hiking	225	255	300	345	375
Horseback riding	182	218	273	327	364
Interval training	487	552	650	748	833
Jogging (5 1/2 mph)	487	552	650	748	833
Judo/karate	232	263	310	357	388
Mountain climbing	450	510	600	690	750
Pool/billiards	97	110	130	150	163
Racquetball/paddleball	450	510	600	690	750
Rope jumping (continuous)	525	595	700	805	875
Rowing, crew	615	697	820	943	1025
Running (10 mph)	625	765	900	1035	1125
Sailing (pleasure)	135	153	180	207	225
Skating, ice	262	297	350	403	438
Skating, roller/inline	262	297	350	403	438
Skiing, cross-country	318	382	477	573	636
Skiing, downhill	450	510	600	690	750
Soccer	405	459	540	621	775
Softball (fast-pitch)	210	238	280	322	350
Softball (slow-pitch)	217	246	290	334	363
Surfing	416	467	550	633	684
Swimming (fast laps)	420	530	630	768	846
Swimming (slow laps)	273	327	409	491	545
Table tennis	182	218	273	327	364
Tennis	315	357	420	483	525
Volleyball	262	297	350	403	483
Walking	173	207	259	311	346
Waterskiing	306	390	468	564	636
Weight training	352	399	470	541	558

*Locate your weight to determine the calories expended per hour in each of the activities shown in the table based on recreational involvement. More vigorous activity, as occurs in competitive athletics, may result in greater caloric expenditures.

Source: Corbin and Lindsey.

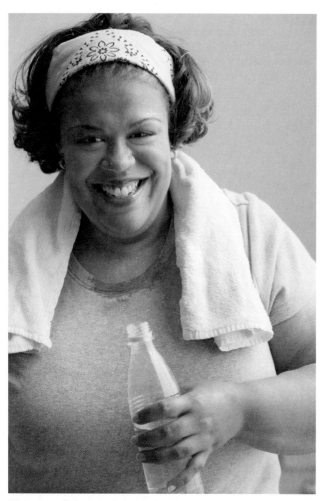

Water contains zero calories and is an excellent alternative to sugary drinks that are high in calorie content.

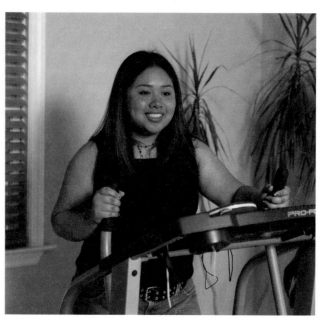

Physical activity can help in regulating body fatness.

Whether you are trying to maintain, gain, or lose weight, know how many calories you consume in food and expend in the activities you perform. Appendix C provides estimates of calories in some common foods. The MyPlate (Food-A-Pedia)

website included in the Web Resources for this concept provides a comprehensive list of calories in foods.

Strength training can be effective in maintaining a desirable body composition. Performing exercises from the strength and muscular endurance level of the physical activity pyramid can be effective in maintaining desirable body fat levels. People who do strength training increase their muscle mass (lean body mass). This extra muscle mass expends extra calories at rest, resulting in a higher metabolic rate. Also, people with more muscle mass expend more calories when doing physical activity.

connect
VIDEO 5

Strategies for Action

Doing several self-assessments can help you make informed decisions about body composition. In Labs 13A and 13B, you will take various body composition self-assessments. It is important that you take all of the measurements and consider all of the information before making final decisions about your body composition. Each self-assessment technique has strengths and weaknesses to be aware of when you make personal decisions. The importance you place on

one particular measure may be different from the importance another person places on that measure; you are a unique individual and should use information that is more relevant for you personally.

Self-assessment results for body composition are personal and confidential. There are steps that can be taken to assure confidentiality. When performing the self-assessments, be aware of the following:

1. If doing a self-assessment around other people makes you self-conscious, do the measurement in private. If the measurement requires the assistance of another person, choose a person you trust and feel comfortable with.

2. Estimates of body composition from even the best techniques may be off by as much as 2 to 3 percent. The values should be interpreted only as estimates.

3. The formulas used to determine body fatness from skinfolds and other procedures are based on typical body types. Measurement will be larger for the very lean and for people with higher than normal levels of fat.

4. Some measurements, such as the thigh skinfold, are hard to take on some people. This is one reason two different skinfold procedures are presented.

5. Self-assessments require skill. With practice, you can become skillful in making measurements. Your first few attempts will, no doubt, lack accuracy.

6. Use the same measuring device each time you measure (scale, calipers, measuring tape, etc.). This assures that any measurement error is constant and allows you to track your progress over time.

7. Once you have tried all of the self-assessments in Lab 13A, choose the ones you want to continue to do and use the same measurement techniques each time. Consider assessing your body composition with some of the other techniques described in the concept.

Estimate your BMR to determine the number of calories you expend each day. In Lab 13C, you can estimate your BMR, giving you an idea of how much energy you expend when you are resting. Use this information together with the information about the energy you expend in activities to help you balance the calories you consume with the calories you expend each day.

Log your daily activities to determine the number of calories you expend each day in these activities. In Lab 13C, you will also log the activities you perform in a day. Then determine your energy expenditure in these activities. Combine this information with the information about your basal metabolism to determine your total daily energy expenditure.

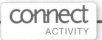

connect
ACTIVITY

Web Resources

Centers for Disease Control and Prevention BMI Information **www.cdc.gov/nccdphp/dnpa/bmi/adult_BMI/about_adult_BMI.htm**

Centers for Disease Control and Prevention Growth Chart Information **www.cdc.gov/growthcharts**

FDA Consumer **www.fda.gov/fdac**

Let's Move! Campaign **www.letsmove.gov**

MyPlate **www.choosemyplate.gov**

MyPlate Food-A-Pedia **www.choosemyplate.gov/SuperTracker/foodapedia.aspx**

MyPlate Food Tracker **www.choosemyplate.gov/SuperTracker/foodtracker.aspx**

National Heart Lung and Blood Institute (BMI Calculator) **www.nhlbisupport.com/bmi**

Nutriwatch (nutrition facts and fallacies) **www.nutriwatch.org**

Partnership for Healthy Weight Management **www.ftc.gov/bcp/edu/pubs/consumer/health/hea05.pdf**

Shape Up America **www.shapeup.org**

STOP Obesity Alliance **www.stopobesityalliance.org**

Surgeon General's Call to Reduce Overweight and Obesity **www.surgeongeneral.gov/library/calls/obesity/index.html**

"We Can" Program **www.nhlbi.nih.gov/health/public/heart/obesity/wecan/index.htm**

Suggested Readings

ACSM. 2010. *ACSM's Resource Manual for Guidelines for Exercise Testing and Prescription.* 6th ed. Philadelphia: Lippincott, Williams & Wilkins, Chapter 10.

Ball, S., P. Swan, and T. Altena. 2006. Skinfold assessment: Accuracy and application. *Measurement in Physical Education and Exercise Science* 10(4):255–264.

Chan, R. S., and J. Woo. 2010. Prevention of overweight and obesity: How effective is the current public health approach. *International Journal of Environmental Research on Public Health* 7(3):765–783.

Christakis, N. A., and J. H. Fowler. 2007. The spread of obesity in a large social network over 32 years. *New England Journal of Medicine* 375(4):370–379.

Cohen, D. A., et al. 2010. Not enough fruit and vegetables or too many cookies, candies, salty snacks, and soft drinks? *Public Health Reports* 125(1):88–95.

Eisenmann, et al. 2008. Combined influence of physical activity and television viewing on the risk of overweight in US youth. *International Journal of Obesity* 32(4):613–618.

Finkelstein, E. A. 2010. Individual and aggregate years of life lost associated with overweight and obesity. *Obesity* 18(2):333–339.

Flegal, K. M., and B. I. Graubard. 2009. Estimates of excess deaths associated with body mass index and other anthropometric variables. *American Journal of Clinical Nutrition* 89(4):1213–1219.

Flegal, K. M., et al. 2010. Prevalence and trends in obesity among U.S. adults, 1999–2008. *Journal of the American Medical Association* 303(3):235–241.

Hardy, L. L., et al. 2010. Screen time and metabolic risk factors among adolescents. *Archives of Pediatric and Adolescent Medicine* 164(7):643–649.

Herman, K. M., et al. 2009. Tracking of obesity and physical activity from childhood to adulthood: The Physical Activity

Longitudinal Study. *International Journal of Pediatric Obesity* 4(4):281–288.

Herman, K. M., et al. 2012. Physical activity, body mass index, and health-related quality of life in Canadian adults. *Medicine and Science in Sports and Exercise* 44(4):625–636.

John, J., et al. 2010. Recent economic findings on childhood obesity: Cost-of-illness and cost-effectiveness of interventions. *Current Opinions in Clinical Nutrition and Metabolic Care* 13(3):305–313.

Keel, P. K., et al., 2007. Clinical features and psychological response to a test meal in purging disorder and bulimia nervosa. *Archives of General Psychiatry* 64:1058–1066.

Kuk, J. L., et al. 2006. Visceral fat is an independent predictor of all-cause mortality in men. *Obesity Research* 14:336–341.

Kwon, S., et al. 2011. Effects of adiposity on physical activity in childhood: Iowa bone development study. *Medicine & Science in Sports & Exercise* 4(3):443–448.

Li, S., and R. J. Loos. 2008. Progress in the genetics of common obesity: Size matters. *Current Opinions in Lipidology* 19(2):113–121.

Liou, Y. M., et al. 2010. Obesity among adolescents: Sedentary leisure time and sleeping as determinants. *Journal of Advances in Nursing* 66(6):1246–1256.

Lynch, F. L., et al. 2010. Cognitive behavioral guided self-help for the treatment of recurrent binge eating. *Journal of Consulting and Clinical Psychology* 78(3):312–321.

Lynch, F. L., et al. 2010. Cost-effectiveness of guided self-help treatment for recurrent binge eating. *Journal of Consulting and Clinical Psychology* 78(3):322–333.

Maine, M., B. H. McGilley, and D. Bunnell (Eds.). 2010. *Treatment of Eating Disorders: Bridging the Research-Practice Gap.* London: Academic Press.

Ogden, C. L., et al. 2012. Prevalence of obesity and trends in body mass index among US children and adolescents, 1999–2010. *JAMA* 307(5):483–490.

Penev, P. D. 2012. Update on energy homeostasis and insufficient sleep. *Journal of Clinical Endocrinology and Metabolism.* March.

Perusse, L., et al. 2005. The human obesity gene map: The 2004 update. *Obesity Research* 13(3):381–490.

Phillips, K. A., et al. 2010. Body dysmorphic disorder: Some key issues for DSM-V. *Depression and Anxiety* 27(6):573–591.

Prospective Studies Collaboration. 2009. Body-mass index and cause-specific mortality in 900,000 adults: Collaborative analyses of 57 prospective studies. *Lancet* 373(9669):1083–1096.

Ruiz, J. R., et al. 2010. Attenuation of the effect of the FTO rs9939609 polymorphism on total and central body fat by physical activity in adolescents: The HELENA Study. *Archives of Pediatric and Adolescent Medicine* 164(4):328–333.

Shehzad, A., et al. 2012. Adiponectin: Regulation of its production and its role in human diseases. *Hormones* 11(1):8–20.

Stewart, S. 2009. Forecasting the effects of obesity and smoking on U.S. life expectancy. *New England Journal of Medicine* 361(23):2252–2260.

Surgeon General's Vision for a Healthy and Fit Nation. 2010 (fact sheet). Available at **www.surgeongeneral.gov.**

Vella-Zarb, R. A., and F. J. Elgar. 2009. The 'freshman 5': A meta-analysis of weight gain in the freshman year of college. *Journal of American College Health* 58(2):161–166.

Wang, Y., et al. 2008. Will all Americans become overweight or obese? Estimating the progression and cost of the U.S. obesity epidemic. *Obesity* 16(10):2323–2330.

Westcott, W. 2009. ACSM strength training guidelines: Role in body composition and health enhancement. *ACSM's Health and Fitness Journal* 13(4):14–22.

Yates, T., et al. 2012. Self-reported sitting time and markers of inflammation, insulin resistance, and adiposity. *American Journal of Preventive Medicine* 42(1):1–7.

Healthy People 2020

The objectives listed below are societal goals designed to help all Americans improve their health between now and the year 2020. They were selected because they relate to the content of this concept.

- Increase proportion of adults with healthy weight.
- Reduce childhood overweight and obesity.
- Reduce disorder eating among adolescents.
- Increase proportion of adults with high LDL who control weight and get activity.
- Reduce percentage of adults who do no leisure-time activity.
- Increase work sites that offer nutrition and weight management classes and counseling.

- Increase physician counseling on nutrition and weight management.
- Increase BMI measurement by primary doctors.
- Increase policies that give retail food outlets incentives for foods that meet dietary guidelines.

A national goal is to increase the proportion of adults with a healthy weight. More than twice as many adults are overweight or obese than youth. However, studies show that overweight youth are more likely to become overweight adults. Is it important to focus on obesity prevention at all ages or should more concentrated efforts be focused specifically on children to help prevent problems in the future? What changes would you implement first to help reverse the obesity epidemic in society?

Lab Resource Materials: Evaluating Body Fat

General Information about Skinfold Measurements

It is important to use a consistent procedure for "drawing up" or "pinching up" a skinfold and making the measurement with the calipers. The following procedures should be used for each skinfold site.

1. Lay the calipers down on a nearby table. Use the thumbs and index fingers of both hands to draw up a skinfold, or layer of skin and fat. The fingers and thumbs of the two hands should be about 1 inch apart, or 1/2 inch on each side of the location where the measurement is to be made.

2. The skinfolds are normally drawn up in a vertical line rather than a horizontal line. However, if the skin naturally aligns itself less than vertical, the measurement should be done on the natural line of the skinfold, rather than on the vertical.

3. Do not pinch the skinfold too hard. Draw it up so that your thumbs and fingers are not compressing the skinfold.

4. Once the skinfold is drawn up, let go with your right hand and pick up the calipers. Open the jaws of the calipers and place them over the location of the skinfold to be measured and 1/2 inch from your left index finger and thumb. Allow the tips, or jaw faces, of the calipers to close on the skinfold at a level about where the skin would be normally.

5. Let the reading on the calipers settle for 2 or 3 seconds; then note the thickness of the skinfold in millimeters.

6. Three measurements should be taken at each location. Use the middle of the three values to determine your measurement. For example, if you had values of 10, 11, and 9, your measurement for that location would be 10. If the three measures vary by more than 3 millimeters from the lowest to the highest, you may want to take additional measurements.

Skinfold Measurement Methods

You will be exposed to two methods of using skinfolds. The first method (FITNESSGRAM) uses the same sites for men and women. It was originally developed for use with schoolchildren but has since been modified for adults. The second method (Jackson-Pollock) is the most widely used method. It uses different sites for men and women and considers your age in estimating your body fat percentage. You are encouraged to try both methods.

Calculating Fatness from Skinfolds (FITNESSGRAM Method)

1. Sum the three skinfolds (triceps, abdominal, and calf) for men and women. Use horizontal abdominal measure.

2. Use the skinfold sum and the appropriate column (men or women) to determine your percent fat using Chart 1. Locate your sum of skinfold in the left column at the top of the chart. Your estimated body fat percentage is located where the values intersect.

3. Use the Standards for Body Fatness (Chart 2) to determine your fatness rating.

FITNESSGRAM Locations (Men and Women)

Triceps

Make a mark on the back of the right arm, one-half the distance between the tip of the shoulder and the tip of the elbow. Make the measurement at this location.

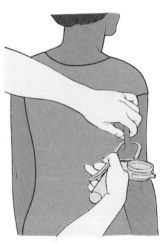

Abdominal

Make a mark on the skin approximately 1 inch to the right of the navel. Unlike the Jackson-Pollock method (done vertically), make a horizontal measurement.

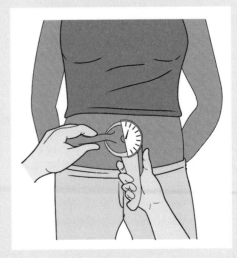

305

FITNESSGRAM Locations *(continued)*

Calf skinfold

Make a mark on the inside of the calf of the right leg at the level of the largest calf size (girth). Place the foot on a chair or other elevation so that the knee is kept at approximately 90 degrees. Make a vertical measurement at the mark.

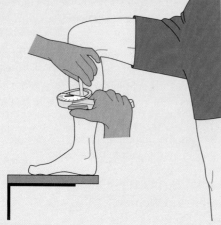

Self-Measured Triceps Skinfold

This measurement is made on the left arm so that the calipers can easily be read. Hold the arm straight at shoulder height. Make a fist with the thumb faced upward. Place the fist against a wall. With the right hand, place the calipers over the skinfold as it "hangs freely" on the back of the tricep (halfway from the tip of the shoulder to the elbow).

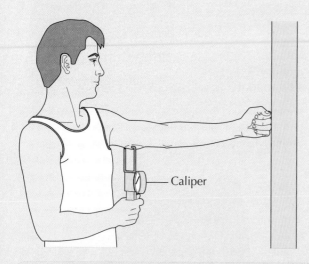

Caliper

Chart 1 Percent Fat for Sum of Triceps, Abdominal, and Calf Skinfolds (Fitnessgram)

Men		Women	
Sum of Skinfolds	Percent Fat	Sum of Skinfolds	Percent Fat
8–10	3.2	23–25	16.8
11–13	4.1	26–28	17.7
14–46	5.0	29–31	18.5
17–19	6.0	32–34	19.4
20–22	6.0	35–37	20.2
23–25	7.8	38–40	21.0
26–28	8.7	41–43	21.9
29–31	9.7	44–46	22.7
32–34	10.6	47–49	23.5
35–37	11.5	50–52	24.4
38–40	12.5	53–55	25.2
41–43	13.4	56–58	26.1
44–46	14.3	59–61	26.9
47–49	15.2	62–64	27.7
50–52	16.2	65–67	28.6
53–55	17.1	68–70	29.4
56–58	18.0	71–73	30.2
59–61	18.9	74–76	31.1
62–64	19.9	77–79	31.9
65–67	20.8	80–82	32.7
68–70	21.7	83–85	33.6
71–73	22.6	86–88	34.4
74–76	23.6	89–91	35.5
77–79	24.5	92–94	36.1
80–82	25.4	95–97	36.9
83–85	26.4	98–100	37.8
86–88	27.3	101–103	38.6
89–91	28.2	104–106	39.4
92–94	29.1	107–109	40.3
95–97	30.1	110–112	41.1
98–100	31.0	113–115	42.0
101–103	31.9	116–118	42.8
104–106	32.8	119–121	43.6
107–109	33.8	122–124	44.5
110–112	34.7	125–127	45.3
113–115	35.6	128–130	46.1
116–118	36.6	131–133	47.0
119–121	37.5	134–136	47.8
122–124	38.4	137–139	48.7
125–127	39.3	140–142	49.5

Chart 2 Standards for Body Fatness (Percent Body Fat)

	Too Low	Borderline	(Healthy) Good Fitness	Marginal	(At Risk) Overfat
	Below Essential Fat Levels	Unhealthy for Many People	Optimal for Good Health	Associated with Some Health Problems	Unhealthy
Males	No less than 5%	6–9%	10–20%	21–25%	>25%
Females	No less than 10%	11–16%	17–28%	29–35%	>35%

Calculating Fatness from Skinfolds (Jackson-Pollock Method)

1. Sum three skinfolds (tricep, iliac crest, and thigh for women; chest, abdominal [vertical], and thigh for men).

2. Use the skinfold sum and your age to determine your percent fat using Chart 3 for women and Chart 4 for men. Locate your sum of skinfold in the left column and your age at the top of the chart. Your estimated body fat percentage is located where the values intersect.

3. Use the Standards for Body Fatness (Chart 2) to determine your fatness rating.

Jackson-Pollock Locations (Women)

Triceps

Same as FITNESSGRAM (see page 305).

Iliac crest

Make a mark at the top front of the iliac crest. This skinfold is taken diagonally because of the natural line of the skin.

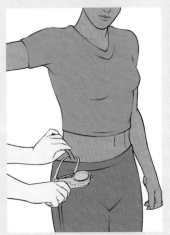

Thigh

Make a mark on the front of the thigh midway between the hip and the knee. Make the measurement vertically at this location.

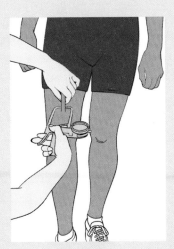

Jackson-Pollock Locations (Men)

Chest

Make a mark above and to the right of the right nipple (one-half the distance from the midline of the side and the nipple). The measurement at this location is often done on the diagonal because of the natural line of the skin.

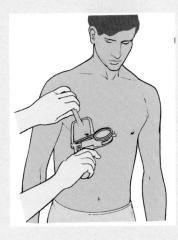

Abdominal

Make a mark on the skin approximately 1 inch to the right of the navel. Make a vertical measure for the Jackson-Pollock method and horizontally for the FITNESSGRAM method.

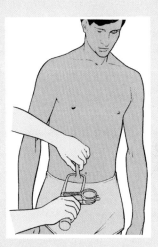

Thigh

Same as for women.

Note: Research has identified other methods that can also be used to calculate body fatness using skinfold measurements. See below.

- Ball, S., Altena, T., and P. Swan. 2004. Accuracy of anthropometry compared to dual energy x-ray absorptiometry: A new generalizable equation for men. *European Journal of Clinical Nutrition* 58:1525–1531.

- Ball, S., Swan, P., and R. Desimone. 2004. Comparison of anthropometry compared to dual energy x-ray absorptiometry: A new generalizable equation for women. *Research Quarterly for Exercise and Sports* 75:248–258.

Chart 3 Percent Fat for Women (Jackson-Pollock: Sum of Triceps, Iliac Crest, and Thigh Skinfolds)

Sum of Skinfolds (mm)	Age to the Last Year								
	22 and Under	23 to 27	28 to 32	33 to 37	38 to 42	43 to 47	48 to 52	53 to 57	Over 57
23–25	9.7	9.9	10.2	10.4	10.7	10.9	11.2	11.4	11.7
26–28	11.0	11.2	11.5	11.7	12.0	12.3	12.5	12.7	13.0
29–31	12.3	12.5	12.8	13.0	13.3	13.5	13.8	14.0	14.3
32–34	13.6	13.8	14.0	14.3	14.5	14.8	15.0	15.3	15.5
35–37	14.8	15.0	15.3	15.5	15.8	16.0	16.3	16.5	16.8
38–40	16.0	16.3	16.5	16.7	17.0	17.2	17.5	17.7	18.0
41–43	17.2	17.4	17.7	17.9	18.2	18.4	18.7	18.9	19.2
44–46	18.3	18.6	18.8	19.1	19.3	19.6	19.8	20.1	20.3
47–49	19.5	19.7	20.0	20.2	20.5	20.7	21.0	21.2	21.5
50–52	20.6	20.8	21.1	21.3	21.6	21.8	22.1	22.3	22.6
53–55	21.7	21.9	22.1	22.4	22.6	22.9	23.1	23.4	23.6
56–58	22.7	23.0	23.2	23.4	23.7	23.9	24.2	24.4	24.7
59–61	23.7	24.0	24.2	24.5	24.7	25.0	25.2	25.5	25.7
62–64	24.7	25.0	25.2	25.5	25.7	26.0	26.2	26.4	26.7
65–67	25.7	25.9	26.2	26.4	26.7	26.9	27.2	27.4	27.7
68–70	26.6	26.9	27.1	27.4	27.6	27.9	28.1	28.4	28.6
71–73	27.5	27.8	28.0	28.3	28.5	28.8	28.0	29.3	29.5
74–76	28.4	28.7	28.9	29.2	29.4	29.7	29.9	30.2	30.4
77–79	29.3	29.5	29.8	30.0	30.3	30.5	30.8	31.0	31.3
80–82	30.1	30.4	30.6	30.9	31.1	31.4	31.6	31.9	32.1
83–85	30.9	31.2	31.4	31.7	31.9	32.2	32.4	32.7	32.9
86–88	31.7	32.0	32.2	32.5	32.7	32.9	33.2	33.4	33.7
89–91	32.5	32.7	33.0	33.2	33.5	33.7	33.9	34.2	34.4
92–94	33.2	33.4	33.7	33.9	34.2	34.4	34.7	34.9	35.2
95–97	33.9	34.1	34.4	34.6	34.9	35.1	35.4	35.6	35.9
98–100	34.6	34.8	35.21	35.3	35.5	35.8	36.0	36.3	36.5
101–103	35.3	35.4	35.7	35.9	36.2	36.4	36.7	36.9	37.2
104–106	35.8	36.1	36.3	36.6	36.8	37.1	37.3	37.5	37.8
107–109	36.4	36.7	36.9	37.1	37.4	37.6	37.9	38.1	38.4
110–112	37.0	37.2	37.5	37.7	38.0	38.2	38.5	38.7	38.9
113–115	37.5	37.8	38.0	38.2	38.5	38.7	39.0	39.2	39.5
116–118	38.0	38.3	38.5	38.8	39.0	39.3	39.5	39.7	40.0
119–121	38.5	38.7	39.0	39.2	39.5	39.7	40.0	40.2	40.5
122–124	39.0	39.2	39.4	39.7	39.9	40.2	40.4	40.7	40.9
125–127	39.4	39.6	39.9	40.1	40.4	40.6	40.9	41.1	41.4
128–130	39.8	40.0	40.3	40.5	40.8	41.0	41.3	41.5	41.8

Source: Baumgartner and Jackson.

Note: Percent fat calculated by the formula by Siri. Percent fat = $[(4.95/BD) - 4.5] \times 100$, where BD = body density.

Chart 4 Percent Fat for Men (Jackson-Pollock: Sum of Thigh, Chest, and Abdominal Skinfolds)

Sum of Skinfolds (mm)	Age to the Last Year								
	22 and Under	23 to 27	28 to 32	33 to 37	38 to 42	43 to 47	48 to 52	53 to 57	Over 57
8–10	1.3	1.8	2.3	2.9	3.4	3.9	4.5	5.0	5.5
11–13	2.2	2.8	3.3	3.9	4.4	4.9	5.5	6.0	6.5
14–16	3.2	3.8	4.3	4.8	5.4	5.9	6.4	7.0	7.5
17–19	4.2	4.7	5.3	5.8	6.3	6.9	7.4	8.0	8.5
20–22	5.1	5.7	6.2	6.8	7.3	7.9	8.4	8.9	9.5
23–25	6.1	6.6	7.2	7.7	8.3	8.8	9.4	9.9	10.5
26–28	7.0	7.6	8.1	8.7	9.2	9.8	10.3	10.9	11.4
29–31	8.0	8.5	9.1	9.6	10.2	10.7	11.3	11.8	12.4
32–34	8.9	9.4	10.0	10.5	11.1	11.6	12.2	12.8	13.3
35–37	9.8	10.4	10.9	11.5	12.0	12.6	13.1	13.7	14.3
38–40	10.7	11.3	11.8	12.4	12.9	13.5	14.1	14.6	15.2
41–43	11.6	12.2	12.7	13.3	13.8	14.4	15.0	15.5	16.1
44–46	12.5	13.1	13.6	14.2	14.7	15.3	15.9	16.4	17.0
47–49	13.4	13.9	14.5	15.1	15.6	16.2	16.8	17.3	17.9
50–52	14.3	14.8	15.4	15.9	16.5	17.1	17.6	18.1	18.8
53–55	15.1	15.7	16.2	16.8	17.4	17.9	18.5	18.2	19.7
56–58	16.0	16.5	17.1	17.7	18.2	18.8	19.4	20.0	20.5
59–61	16.9	17.4	17.9	18.5	19.1	19.7	20.2	20.8	21.4
62–64	17.6	18.2	18.8	19.4	19.9	20.5	21.1	21.7	22.2
65–67	18.5	19.0	19.6	20.2	20.8	21.3	21.9	22.5	23.1
68–70	19.3	19.9	20.4	21.0	21.6	22.2	22.7	23.3	23.9
71–73	20.1	20.7	21.2	21.8	22.4	23.0	23.6	24.1	24.7
74–76	20.9	21.5	22.0	22.6	23.2	23.8	24.4	25.0	25.5
77–79	21.7	22.2	22.8	23.4	24.0	24.6	25.2	25.8	26.3
80–82	22.4	23.0	23.6	24.2	24.8	25.4	25.9	26.5	27.1
83–85	23.2	23.8	24.4	25.0	25.5	26.1	26.7	27.3	27.9
86–88	24.0	24.5	25.1	25.5	26.3	26.9	27.5	28.1	28.7
89–91	24.7	25.3	25.9	25.7	27.1	27.6	28.2	28.8	29.4
92–94	25.4	26.0	26.6	27.2	27.8	28.4	29.0	29.6	30.2
95–97	26.1	26.7	27.3	27.9	28.5	29.1	29.7	30.3	30.9
98–100	26.9	27.4	28.0	28.6	29.2	29.8	30.4	31.0	31.6
101–103	27.5	28.1	28.7	29.3	29.9	30.5	31.1	31.7	32.3
104–106	28.2	28.8	29.4	30.0	30.6	31.2	31.8	32.4	33.0
107–109	28.9	29.5	30.1	30.7	31.3	31.9	32.5	33.1	33.7
110–112	29.6	30.2	30.8	31.4	32.0	32.6	33.2	33.8	34.4
113–115	30.2	30.8	31.4	32.0	32.6	33.2	33.8	34.5	35.1
116–118	30.9	31.5	32.1	32.7	33.3	33.9	34.5	35.1	35.7
119–121	31.5	32.1	32.7	33.3	33.9	34.5	35.1	35.7	36.4
122–124	32.1	32.7	33.3	33.9	34.5	35.1	35.8	36.4	37.0
125–127	32.7	33.3	33.9	34.5	35.1	35.8	36.4	37.0	37.6

Source: Baumgartner and Jackson.

Note: Percent fat calculated by the formula by Siri. Percent fat = $[(4.95/BD) - 4.5] \times 100$, where BD = body density.

Calculating Fatness from Self-Measured Skinfolds

1. Use either the Jackson-Pollock or Fitnessgram method, but make the measures on yourself rather than have a partner do the measures. When doing the triceps measure, use the self-measurement technique for men and women. (See page 306.)
2. Calculate fatness using the methods described previously.

Height-Weight Measurements

1. *Height*—Measure your height in inches or centimeters. Take the measurement without shoes, but add 2.5 centimeters or 1 inch to measurements, as the charts include heel height.

2. *Weight*—Measure your weight in pounds or kilograms without clothes. Add 3 pounds or 1.4 kilograms because the charts include the weight of clothes. If weight must be taken with clothes on, wear indoor clothing that weighs 3 pounds, or 1.4 kilograms.

3. Determine your frame size using the elbow breadth. The measurement is most accurate when done with a broad-based sliding caliper. However, it can be done using skinfold calipers or can be estimated with a metric ruler. The right arm is measured when it is elevated with the elbow bent at 90 degrees and the upper arm horizontal. The back of the hand should face the person making the measurement. Using the calipers, measure the distance between the epicondyles of the humerus (inside and outside bony points of the elbow). Measure to the nearest millimeter (1/10 centimeter). If a caliper is not available, place the thumb and the index finger of the left hand on the epicondyles of the humerus and measure the distance between the fingers with a metric ruler. Use your height and elbow breadth in centimeters to determine your frame size (Chart 5); you need not repeat this procedure each time you use a height and weight chart.

4. Use Chart 6 to determine your healthy weight range. The new healthy weight range charts do not account for frame size. However, you may want to consider frame size when determining a personal weight within the healthy weight range. People with a larger frame size typically can carry more weight within the range than can those with a smaller frame size.

Chart 5 Frame Size Determined from Elbow Breadth (mm)

Height	Elbow Breadth (mm)		
	Small Frame	Medium Frame	Large Frame
Males			
5'2 1/2" or less	<64	64–72	>72
5'3"–5'6 ½"	<67	67–74	>74
5'7"–5'10 ½"	<69	69–76	>76
5'11"–6'2 ½"	<71	71–78	>78
6'3" or more	<74	74–81	>81
Females			
4'10 ½" or less	<56	56–64	>64
4'11"–5'2 ½"	<58	58–65	>65
5'3"–5'6 ½"	<59	59–66	>66
5'7"–5'10 ½"	<61	61–68	>69
5'11" or more	<62	62–69	>69

Source: Metropolitan Life Insurance Company.

Height is given including 1-inch heels.

Chart 6 Healthy Weight Ranges for Adult Women and Men

Height			Height		
Feet	Inches	Pounds	Feet	Inches	Pounds
4	10	91–119	5	9	129–169
4	11	94–124	5	10	132–174
5	0	97–128	5	11	136–179
5	1	101–132	6	0	140–184
5	2	104–137	6	1	144–189
5	3	107–141	6	2	148–195
5	4	111–146	6	3	152–200
5	5	114–150	6	4	156–205
5	6	118–155	6	5	160–211
5	7	121–160	6	6	164–216
5	8	125–164			

Source: U.S. Department of Agriculture and Department of Health and Human Services.

Chart 7 Body Mass Index (BMI)

Height	100	105	110	115	120	125	130	135	140	145	150	155	160	165	170	175	180	185	190	195	200	205	210	215	220	225	230	235	240	245	250
5'0"	20	21	21	22	23	24	25	26	27	28	29	30	31	32	33	34	35	36	37	38	39	40	41	42	43	44	45	46	47	48	49
5'1"	19	20	21	22	23	24	25	26	26	27	28	29	30	31	32	33	34	35	36	37	38	39	40	41	42	43	43	44	45	46	47
5'2"	18	19	20	21	22	23	24	25	26	27	27	28	29	30	31	32	33	34	35	36	37	37	38	39	40	41	42	43	44	45	46
5'3"	18	19	19	20	21	22	23	24	25	26	27	27	28	29	30	31	32	33	34	35	35	36	37	38	39	40	41	42	43	43	44
5'4"	17	18	19	20	21	21	22	23	24	25	26	27	27	28	29	30	31	32	33	33	34	35	36	37	38	39	39	40	41	42	43
5'5"	17	17	18	19	20	21	22	22	23	24	25	26	27	27	28	29	30	31	32	32	33	34	35	36	37	37	38	39	40	41	42
5'6"	16	17	18	19	19	20	21	22	23	23	24	25	26	27	27	28	29	30	31	31	32	33	34	35	36	36	37	38	39	40	40
5'7"	16	16	17	18	19	20	20	21	22	23	23	24	25	26	27	27	28	29	30	31	31	32	33	34	34	35	36	37	37	38	39
5'8"	15	16	17	17	18	19	20	21	21	22	23	24	24	25	26	27	27	28	29	30	30	31	32	33	33	34	35	36	36	37	38
5'9"	15	16	16	17	18	18	19	20	21	21	22	23	24	24	25	26	27	27	28	29	29	30	31	32	32	33	34	35	35	36	37
5'10"	14	15	16	17	17	18	19	19	20	21	22	22	23	24	24	25	26	27	27	28	29	29	30	31	31	32	33	34	34	35	36
5'11"	14	15	15	16	17	17	18	19	20	20	21	22	22	23	24	24	25	26	26	27	28	29	29	30	31	31	32	33	33	34	35
6'0"	14	14	15	16	16	17	18	18	19	20	20	21	22	22	23	24	24	25	26	26	27	28	28	29	30	31	31	32	33	33	34
6'1"	13	14	15	15	16	16	17	18	18	19	20	20	21	22	22	23	24	24	25	26	26	27	28	28	29	30	30	31	32	32	33
6'2"	13	13	14	15	15	16	17	17	18	19	19	20	21	21	22	22	23	24	24	25	26	26	27	28	28	29	30	30	31	31	32
6'3"	12	13	14	14	15	16	16	17	17	18	19	19	20	21	21	22	22	23	24	24	25	26	26	27	27	28	29	29	30	31	31
6'4"	12	13	13	14	15	15	16	16	17	18	18	19	19	20	21	21	22	23	23	24	24	25	26	26	27	27	28	29	29	30	30

Weight

☐ Low   ☐ Normal (good fitness zone)   ☐ Overweight   ☐ Obese

Body Mass Index (BMI)

Use the steps listed below or use Chart 7 to calculate your BMI.

1. Divide your weight in pounds by 2.2 to determine your weight in kilograms.

2. Multiply your height in inches by 0.0254 to determine your height in meters.

3. Square your height in meters (multiply your height in meters by your height in meters).

4. Divide your weight in kilograms from step 1 by your height in meters squared from step 3.

5. If you use these steps to determine your BMI, use the Rating Scale for Body Mass Index (Chart 8) to obtain a rating for your BMI.

Chart 8 Rating Scale for Body Mass Index (BMI)

Classification	BMI
Obese (high risk)	Over 30
Overweight	25–30
Normal (good fitness zone)	17–24.9
Low	Less than 17

Note: An excessively low BMI is not desirable. Low BMI values can indicate eating disorders and other health problems.

Formula

$$BMI = \frac{\text{weight in kilograms (kg)}}{(\text{height in meters}) \times (\text{height in meters})}$$

$$BMI = \frac{\text{weight in pounds (lb)}}{(\text{height in inches}) \times (\text{height in inches})} \times 703$$

Determining the Waist-to-Hip Circumference Ratio

The waist-to-hip circumference ratio is recommended as the best available index for determining risk for disease associated with fat and weight distribution. Disease and death risk are associated with abdominal and upper body fatness. When a person has high fatness and a high waist-to-hip ratio, additional risks exist. The following steps should be taken in making measurements and calculating the waist-to-hip ratio.

1. Both measurements should be done with a nonelastic tape. Make the measurements while standing with the feet together and the arms at the sides, elevated only high enough to allow the measurements. Be sure the tape is horizontal and around the entire circumference. Record scores to the nearest millimeter or 1/16th of an inch. Use the same units of measure for both circumferences (millimeters or 1/16th of an inch). The tape should be pulled snugly but not to the point of causing an indentation in the skin.

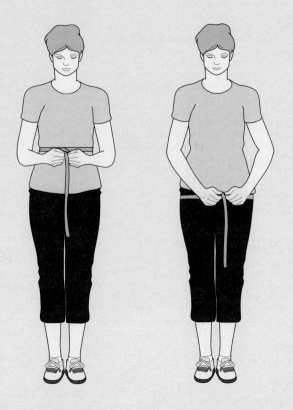

2. Waist measurement—Measure at the natural waist (smallest waist circumference). If no natural waist exists, the measurement should be made at the level of the umbilicus. Measure at the end of a normal inhale.

3. *Hip measurement*—Measure at the maximum circumference of the buttocks. It is recommended that you wear thin-layered clothing (such as a swimming suit or underwear) that will not add significantly to the measurement.

4. Divide the hip measurement into the waist measurement or use the waist-to-hip nomogram (Chart 9) to determine your waist-to-hip ratio.

5. Use the Waist-to-Hip Ratio Rating Scale (Chart 10) to determine your rating for the waist-to-hip ratio.

Chart 9 Waist-to-Hip Ratio Nomogram

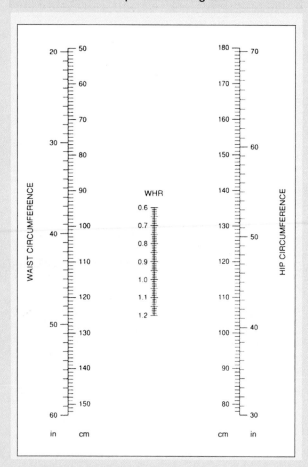

Note: Using a partner or mirror will aid you in keeping the tape horizontal.

Determining Disease Risk Based on BMI and Waist Circumference

Use Chart 11 to determine a BMI and Waist Circumference Rating. In the first column of Chart 11, locate your BMI. Locate your Waist Circumference in either column 2 or 3 depending on your age. Your rating is located at the point where the appropriate rows and columns intersect.

Chart 11 BMI and Waist Circumference Rating Scale

	Waist Circumference (in.)	
BMI	**Men 40 or less Women 34.5 or less**	**Men above 40 Women above 34.5**
Less than 18.5	Normal	Normal
18.5–24.9	Normal	Normal
25.0–29.9	Increased risk	High risk
30.0–34.9	High risk	Very high risk
35.0–39.9	Very high risk	Very high risk
40 or more	Extremely high risk	Extremely high risk

Source: Adapted from ACSM.

Chart 10 Waist-to-Hip Ratio Rating Scale

Classification	Men	Women
High risk	>1.0	>0.85
Moderately high risk	0.90–1.0	0.80–0.85
Lower risk	<0.90	<0.80

Lab 13A Evaluating Body Composition: Skinfold Measures

Name Jason Hernin

Section

Date

Purpose: To estimate body fatness using two skinfold procedures; to compare measures made by an expert, by a partner, and by self-measurements; to learn the strengths and weaknesses of each technique; and to use the results to establish personal standards for evaluating body composition

General Procedures: Follow the specific procedures for the two self-assessment techniques. If possible, have one set of measurements made by an expert (instructor) for each of the two techniques. Next, work with a partner you trust. Have the partner make measurements at each site for both techniques. Finally, make self-measurements for each of the sites. If you are just learning a measurement technique, it is important to practice the skills of making the measurement. If you do measurements over time, use the same instrument (if possible) each time you measure. If your measurements vary widely, take more than one set until you get more consistent results.

If you have had an underwater weighing, a bioelectric impedance measurement, a near-infrared interactance measure, or some other body fatness measurement done recently, record your results below.

Measurement Technique	% Body Fat	Rating
1. Tri, Ab, Calf	a 11.5	36
2. chest	12.8	31

Skinfold Measurements (Jackson-Pollock Method)

Procedures for Jackson-Pollock Method

1. Read the directions for the Jackson-Pollock method measurements in *Lab Resource Materials*.
2. If possible, observe a demonstration of the proper procedures for measuring skinfolds at each of the different locations before doing partner or self-measurements.
3. Make expert, partner, and self-measurements (see *Lab Resource Materials*). When doing the self-measure of the triceps, use the self-measurement technique described in *Lab Resource Materials* (women only).
4. Record each of the measurements in the Results section.
5. Calculate your body fatness from skinfolds by summing the appropriate skinfold values (chest, thigh, and abdominal for men; triceps, iliac crest, and thigh for women). Using your age and the sum of the appropriate skinfolds, determine your body fatness using Charts 3 and 4 in *Lab Resource Materials*.
6. Rate your fatness using Chart 2 in *Lab Resource Materials*.

Results for Jackson-Pollock Method

Skinfolds by an Expert (If Possible)	Skinfolds by Partner	Self-Measurements
Male	*Male*	*Male*
Chest	Chest 4	Chest 4
Thigh	Thigh 10	Thigh 10
Abdominal	Abdominal 22	Abdominal 2 3
Sum	Sum 36	Sum 37
% body fat	% body fat 10.9	% body fat 10.9
Rating	Rating Good	Rating Good
Female	*Female*	*Female*
Triceps	Triceps	Triceps
Iliac crest	Iliac crest	Iliac crest
Thigh	Thigh	Thigh
Sum	Sum	Sum
% body fat	% body fat	% body fat
Rating	Rating	Rating

Make a check by the statements that are true about your measurements.

☐ The person doing measurements has experience with these three skinfold measurements.

☑ Self-measurements were practiced until measurements became consistent.

☑ Results of several trials for each measure are consistent (do not vary more than 2–3 mm).

☑ You are not exceptionally low or exceptionally high in body fat.

The more checks you have, the more likely your measurements are accurate.

Skinfold Measurements (FITNESSGRAM Method)

Procedures for FITNESSGRAM Method

1. Read the directions for the FITNESSGRAM measurements in *Lab Resource Materials.*
2. Use the procedures as for the FITNESSGRAM method using the triceps, abdominal, and calf sites described in *Lab Resource Materials.* When doing the self-measure of the triceps, use the self-measurement technique shown earlier.
3. Calculate your body fatness from skinfolds by summing the appropriate skinfold values (same for both men and women). Using the sum of the appropriate skinfolds, determine your body fatness using Chart 1 in *Lab Resource Materials.*
4. Rate your fatness using Chart 2 in *Lab Resource Materials.*

Results for FITNESSGRAM Method

Skinfolds by an Expert (If Possible)	Skinfolds by Partner	Self-Measurements
Triceps	Triceps: 6	Triceps: 5
Abdominal: 20	Abdominal: 23	Abdominal: 22
Calf	Calf: 8	Calf: 9
Sum	Sum: 37	Sum: 36
% body fat	% body fat: 11.5	% body fat: 11.5
Rating	Rating: good	Rating: good

Make a check by the statements that are true about your measurements.

[ ] The person doing measurements has experience with these three skinfold measurements.

[✓] Self-measurements were practiced until measurements became consistent.

[✓] Results of several trials for each measure are consistent (do not vary more than 2 to 3 mm).

[✓] You are not exceptionally low or exceptionally high in body fat.

The more checks you have, the more likely your measurements are accurate.

Conclusions and Implications

In the space provided below, discuss your current body composition based on the two skinfold procedures and any other measures of body fatness you did. Note any discrepancies in the measurements and discuss which of the measurements you think provide the most useful information. To what extent do you think you need to alter your level of body fatness?

Overall my body fatness levels are good but not great. I have more fat around my abs than other areas of my body. I need to be more consistent in my exercise to reduce belly fat. Also, my diet could be much better.

Lab 13B Evaluating Body Composition: Height, Weight, and Circumference Measures

Name _____   **Section** _____   **Date** _____

Purpose: To assess body composition using a variety of procedures, to learn the strengths and weaknesses of each technique, and to use the results to establish personal standards for evaluating body composition

General Procedures: Follow the specific procedures for the three self-assessment techniques. If possible, work with a partner you trust to help with measurements that you have difficulty making yourself. If you are just learning a measurement technique, it is important to practice the skills of making the measurement. If you do measurements over time, use the same instrument (if possible) each time you measure. If your measurements vary widely, take more than one set until you get more consistent results. If possible, have an expert make measurements on you using these procedures.

Height and Weight Measurements

Procedures

1. Read the directions for height and weight measurements in *Lab Resource Materials*.
2. Determine your healthy weight range using Chart 6 in *Lab Resource Materials*. You may want to use your elbow breadth (Chart 5). People with a smaller frame size should typically weigh less than those with a larger frame size within the healthy weight range. You may need the assistance of a partner to make the elbow breadth measurement.
3. Record your scores in the Results section.

Results

Weight [ ]   Healthy weight range [ ]

Height [ ]

Make a check by the statements that are true about your measurements.

[✓] You are confident in the accuracy of the scale you used.

[✓] You are confident that the height technique is accurate.

The more checks you have, the more likely your measurements are accurate.
If you are a very active person with a high amount of muscle, use this method with caution.

Body Mass Index

Procedures

1. Use the height and weight measures from above.
2. Determine your BMI score by using Chart 7 or the directions in *Lab Resource Materials*. Determine your rating using Chart 8.
3. Record your score and rating in the Results section.

Results

Body mass index [25]   Rating [ ]

If you are a very active person with a high amount of muscle, use this method with caution.

Waist-to-Hip Ratio

Procedures

1. Measure your waist and hip circumferences using the procedures in *Lab Resource Materials*.
2. Divide your hip circumference into your waist circumference, or use Chart 9 in *Lab Resource Materials* to calculate your waist-to-hip ratio.
3. Determine your rating using Chart 10 in *Lab Resource Materials*.
4. Record your scores in the Results section.

Results

Waist circumference 32   Hip circumference 32   Waist-to-hip ratio 1:1   Rating moderate

Make a check by the statements that are true about you.

- [ ] I am a male 5′9″ or less and have a waist girth of 34 inches or more.
- [ ] I am a male 5′10″ to 6′4″ and have a waist girth of 36 inches or more.
- [ ] I am a male 6′5″ or more and have a waist girth of 38 inches or more.
- [ ] I am a female 5′2″ or less and have a waist girth of 29 inches or more.
- [ ] I am a female 5′3″ to 5′10″ and have a waist girth of 31 inches or more.
- [ ] I am a female 5′11″ or more and have a waist girth of 33 inches or more.

If you checked one of the boxes above, the waist-to-hip ratio is especially relevant for you.

BMI and Waist Circumference Rating

Procedures

1. Locate your BMI and Waist Circumference from previous Results sections in this Lab.
2. Use these values to calculate your BMI and Waist Circumference Rating using Chart 11. Record the rating in the Results section.

Results

BMI and Waist Circumference Rating  high

Conclusions and Implications

In the space below, discuss your results for the height, weight, and circumference procedures. Note any discrepancies in the measurements. Indicate the strengths and weaknesses of the various methods. Which of the measures do you think provided you with the most useful information? If you also did the skinfold measures (Lab 13A), discuss your body composition based on all the information you have collected (skinfolds and height, weight, and circumference measures).

Overall I have a high risk rating. I need to reduce my waist fat. I don't think the height-weight ratio is accurate because if you lift weights you could be heavy but have low body fat.

Lab 13C Determining Your Daily Energy Expenditure

Name	Section	Date

Purpose: To learn how many calories you expend in a day

Procedures

1. Estimate your basal metabolism using step 1 in the Results section in this Lab. First determine the number of minutes you sleep.
2. Monitor your activity expenditure for 1 day using Chart 1 (page 321). Record the number of 5-, 15-, and 30-minute blocks of time you perform each of the different types of physical activities (e.g., if an activity lasted 20 minutes, you would use one 15-minute block and one 5-minute block). Be sure to distinguish between moderate (Mod) and vigorous (Vig) intensity in your logging. If you perform an activity that is not listed, specify the activity on the line labeled "Other" and estimate if it is moderate or vigorous. You may want to keep copies of Chart 1 for future use. One extra copy is provided on page 322.
3. Sum the total number of minutes of moderate and vigorous activity. Determine your calories expended during moderate and vigorous activity using steps 2 and 3.
4. Determine your nonactive minutes using step 4. This is all time that is not spent sleeping or being active.
5. Determine your calories expended in nonactive minutes using step 5.
6. Determine your calories expended in a day using step 6.

Results

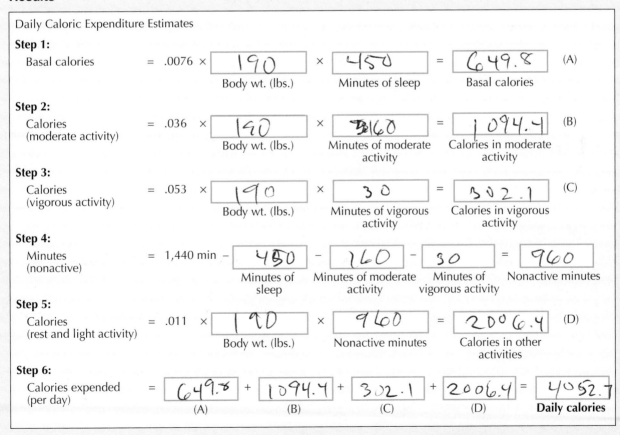

Daily Caloric Expenditure Estimates

Step 1:
Basal calories = .0076 × [190] Body wt. (lbs.) × [450] Minutes of sleep = [649.8] Basal calories (A)

Step 2:
Calories (moderate activity) = .036 × [190] Body wt. (lbs.) × [3160] Minutes of moderate activity = [1,094.4] Calories in moderate activity (B)

Step 3:
Calories (vigorous activity) = .053 × [190] Body wt. (lbs.) × [30] Minutes of vigorous activity = [302.1] Calories in vigorous activity (C)

Step 4:
Minutes (nonactive) = 1,440 min − [450] Minutes of sleep − [160] Minutes of moderate activity − [30] Minutes of vigorous activity = [960] Nonactive minutes

Step 5:
Calories (rest and light activity) = .011 × [190] Body wt. (lbs.) × [960] Nonactive minutes = [2006.4] Calories in other activities (D)

Step 6:
Calories expended (per day) = [649.8] (A) + [1094.4] (B) + [302.1] (C) + [2006.4] (D) = [4052.7] **Daily calories**

Answer the following questions about your daily caloric expenditure estimate.

Yes **No**

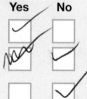

☑ ☐ Were the activities you performed similar to what you normally perform each day?

☐ ☑ Do you think your daily estimated caloric expenditure is an accurate estimate?

☐ ☑ Do you think you expend the correct number of calories in a typical day to maintain the body composition (body fat level) that is desirable for you?

Conclusions and Interpretations: In several paragraphs, discuss your daily caloric expenditure. Comment on your answers to the preceding questions. In addition, comment on whether you think you should modify your daily caloric expenditure for any reason.

I think the caloric numbers were a little higher then actual. If these numbers were accurate I would be burning more calories and be much more lean. I should reduce my caloric intake however.

Chart 1 Daily Activity Log

Day of Monitoring:

Physical Activity Category	5 Minutes	15 Minutes	30 Minutes	Minutes
Lifestyle Activity	1 2 3 4 5 6	1 2 3 4 5 6	1 2 3	
Dancing (general) — Mod			X	30
Gardening — Mod		X		15
Home repair/maintenance — Mod				30
Occupation — Mod			X	
Walking/hiking — Mod	XXXXXX	XXXXXX		120
Other: — Mod				
Aerobic Activity	1 2 3 4 5 6	1 2 3 4 5 6	1 2 3	
Aerobic dance (low-impact) — Mod / Vig				
Aerobic machines (rowing, stair, ski) — Mod / Vig				
Bicycling — Mod / Vig				
Running — Mod / Vig		X X X	X X	105
Skating (roller/ice) — Mod / Vig				
Swimming (laps) — Mod / Vig				
Other: — Mod / Vig				
Sport/Recreation Activity	1 2 3 4 5 6	1 2 3 4 5 6	1 2 3	
Basketball — Mod / Vig				
Bowling/billiards — Mod				
Golf — Mod				
Martial arts (judo, karate) — Mod / Vig				
Racquetball/tennis — Mod / Vig				
Soccer/hockey — Mod / Vig				
Softball/baseball — Mod				
Volleyball — Mod / Vig				
Other: — Mod	X X X	XX		45
Flexibility Activity	1 2 3 4 5 6	1 2 3 4 5 6	1 2 3	
Stretching — Mod	XX X X			20
Other: — Mod				
Strengthening Activity	1 2 3 4 5 6	1 2 3 4 5 6	1 2 3	
Calisthenics (push-ups/sit-ups) — Mod				
Resistance exercise — Mod				
Other: — Mod			X X	40

Minutes of moderate activity	425
Minutes of vigorous activity	0
Total minutes of activity	425

Chart 1 Daily Activity Log

Day of Monitoring:

Physical Activity Category		5 Minutes 1 2 3 4 5 6	15 Minutes 1 2 3 4 5 6	30 Minutes 1 2 3	Minutes
Lifestyle Activity		1 2 3 4 5 6	1 2 3 4 5 6	1 2 3	
Dancing (general)	Mod				
Gardening	Mod			X	3 0
Home repair/maintenance	Mod				3 0
Occupation	Mod				
Walking/hiking	Mod		XXX XX	X	105
Other:	Mod				
Aerobic Activity		1 2 3 4 5 6	1 2 3 4 5 6	1 2 3	
Aerobic dance (low-impact)	Mod				
	Vig				
Aerobic machines	Mod				
(rowing, stair, ski)	Vig				
Bicycling	Mod				
	Vig				
Running	Mod			X X	60
	Vig			X	30
Skating (roller/ice)	Mod				
	Vig				
Swimming (laps)	Mod				
	Vig				
Other:	Mod				
	Vig		XX X X		60
Sport/Recreation Activity		1 2 3 4 5 6	1 2 3 4 5 6	1 2 3	
Basketball	Mod			X	30
	Vig			X	30
Bowling/billiards	Mod	X		X	30
Golf	Mod				
Martial arts (judo, karate)	Mod				
	Vig				
Racquetball/tennis	Mod				
	Vig				
Soccer/hockey	Mod				
	Vig				
Softball/baseball	Mod				
Volleyball	Mod				
	Vig				
Other:	Mod				
Flexibility Activity		1 2 3 4 5 6	1 2 3 4 5 6	1 2 3	
Stretching	Mod	XX	XX		40
Other:	Mod				
Strengthening Activity		1 2 3 4 5 6	1 2 3 4 5 6	1 2 3	
Calisthenics (push-ups/sit-ups)	Mod		X X X		45
Resistance exercise	Mod				
Other:	Mod				

Minutes of moderate activity	460
Minutes of vigorous activity	3 d
Total minutes of activity	490

Nutrition

LEARNING OBJECTIVES

After completing the study of this concept, you will be able to:

▶ Apply basic guidelines for healthy eating.

▶ List and apply dietary recommendations for carbohydrates, fats, proteins, vitamins, minerals, and water.

▶ Interpret and use food labels to make healthy decisions.

▶ Describe and incorporate sound eating practices.

▶ Describe and apply nutrition guidelines for active people and those interested in performance (e.g., sports).

▶ Analyze your diet to determine nutrient quality.

▶ Compare nutritional quality of various foods.

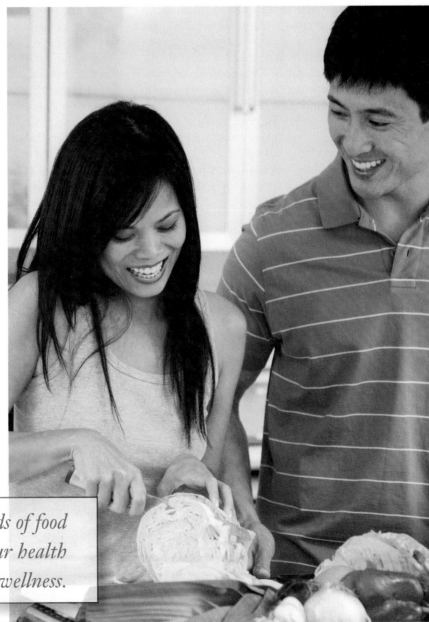

The amount and kinds of food you eat affect your health and wellness.

The importance of good nutrition for optimal health is well established. Eating patterns have been related to four of the seven leading causes of death, and poor nutrition increases the risks for numerous diseases, including heart disease, obesity, stroke, diabetes, hypertension, osteoporosis, and many cancers (e.g., colon, prostate, mouth, throat, lung, and stomach). The American Cancer Society estimates that 35 percent of cancer risks are related to nutritional factors. In addition to helping avoid these health risks, proper nutrition can enhance the quality of life by improving appearance and increasing the ability to carry out work and leisure-time activity without fatigue.

Most people believe that nutrition is important but still find it difficult to maintain a healthy diet. One reason for this is that foods are usually developed, marketed, and advertised for convenience and taste rather than for health or nutritional quality. Another reason is that many individuals have misconceptions about what constitutes a healthy diet. Some of these misconceptions are propagated by commercial interests and so-called experts with less than impressive credentials. Other misconceptions are created by the confusing, and often contradictory, news reports about new nutrition research. In spite of the fact that nutrition is an advanced science, many questions remain unanswered. This concept reviews important national guidelines and recommendations for healthy eating. The significance of essential dietary nutrients is also described along with strategies for adopting and maintaining a healthy diet.

Guidelines for Healthy Eating

National dietary guidelines provide a sound plan for good nutrition. The U.S. Department of Agriculture (USDA) and the Department of Health and Human Services (DHHS) publishes a definitive report called the *Dietary Guidelines for Americans* to help consumers make healthier food choices. Federal law requires that these guidelines be updated every 5 years to incorporate new research findings. The most recent USDA nutrition guidelines were published in 2010. Many other countries release similar sets of guidelines specific to their population (e.g., Health Canada's *Food Guide*).

The MyPlate model conveys a variety of key nutrition principles. The U.S. Dietary Guidelines are developed largely to help promote education about healthy eating. Many of the key elements of the guidelines are summarized in the MyPlate model (see Figure 1) which replaces the previous MyPyramid model as the primary symbol or icon of the program. The four colored areas represent the different food groups (fruits, grains, vegetables, and proteins) and a glass represents the dairy food group (including solid dairy products). The pyramid included the same categories, but the plate helps a person visualize the recommended allocations in a typical meal. Fruits and vegetables are emphasized in the MyPlate model (representing half of the plate) because they are high in nutrients and fiber and low in calories. The MyPlate model also emphasizes healthy food choices in each category. For example, they recommend low-fat dairy choices (e.g., shifting to skim milk) and making half of your grains "whole" (i.e., whole grains). Key principles highlighted in the MyPlate model are summarized to the left of Figure 1. Like the pyramid, the MyPlate image is widely promoted and displayed to help remind consumers about the key principles of good nutrition. There are a number of other resources available to help consumers apply these principles and guidelines at the MyPlate website (www.choosemyplate.gov).

National dietary guidelines provide suggestions for healthy eating. The current version of the national Dietary Guidelines for Americans emphasizes a "total diet" approach, which is defined as the "combination of foods and beverages that provide energy and nutrients, and constitute an individual's complete dietary intake, on average,

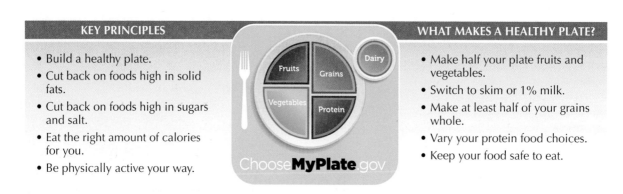

Figure 1 ▶ MyPlate presents a combination of nutrition guidelines and healthy food choices.

Source: Adapted from the USDA 2010, www.choosemyplate.gov

over time." The information at the right of Figure 1 tells how to "build a plate" to meet the "total diet" goal. The report further describes other key components of a nutrient-dense total diet:

- *Eat the right amount of calories for you.* Effective weight control requires balancing energy intake with energy expenditure. The new guidelines encourage Americans to achieve their recommended nutrient intakes by consuming foods within a total diet that meets, but does not exceed, energy needs. This should be done using personal information such as age, gender, current body weight, and current physical activity levels. Studies indicate that Americans underestimate the number of calories they eat and only about 9 percent regularly keep track of the calories in the foods they eat.

- *Consume nutrient-dense foods.* Americans consume less than 20 percent of the recommended intakes for whole grains, less than 60 percent for vegetables, less than 50 percent for fruits, and less than 60 percent for milk and milk products. Consuming nutrient-dense foods improves the overall quality of the diet. Examples of nutrient-dense foods include vegetables, fruits, high-fiber whole grains, fat-free or lowfat milk and milk products, seafood, lean meat and poultry, eggs, soy products, nuts, seeds, and oils.

- *Reduce solid fats and added sugars (SoFAS).* Evidence indicates that solid fats and added sugars (SoFAS) contribute about 35 percent of total calories, leading to excessive intake of saturated fat and cholesterol and insufficient intake of dietary fiber and other nutrients. The guidelines recommend reducing consumption of SoFAS as an important diet strategy.

- *Reduce sodium intake.* Excessive sodium in the diet can increase blood pressure and lead to health problems.

- *Be physically active your way.* The USDA nutrition guidelines also emphasize the importance of daily physical activity (60 minutes each day) in energy balance. Most Americans overestimate the number of calories that they expend in activity.

Specific Dietary Reference Intakes (DRI) provide a target zone for healthy eating. About 45 to 50 nutrients in food are believed to be essential for the body's growth, maintenance, and repair. These are classified into six categories: carbohydrates (and fiber), fats, proteins, vitamins, minerals, and water. The first three provide energy, which is measured in calories. Specific dietary recommendations for each of the six nutrients are presented later in this concept.

In the United States, guidelines specifying the nutrient requirements for good health are developed by the Food and Nutrition Board of the National Academy of Science's Institute of Medicine. **Recommended Dietary**

Allowance (RDA) historically was used to set recommendations for nutrients, but the complexity of dietary interactions prompted the board to develop a more comprehensive and functional set of dietary intake recommendations. These broader guidelines, referred to as **Dietary Reference Intake (DRI)**, include RDA values when adequate scientific information is available and estimated **Adequate Intake (AI)** values when sufficient data aren't available to establish a firm RDA. The DRI values also include **Tolerable Upper Intake Level (UL),** which reflects the highest level of daily intake a person can consume without adverse effects on health (see Table 1). The guidelines make it clear that although too little of a nutrient can be harmful to health, so can too much. The distinctions are similar to the concept of the target zone used to prescribe exercise levels. The Recommended Dietary Allowance (RDA) or Adequate Intake (AI) values are analogous to the threshold levels (minimal amount needed to meet guidelines), while the Upper Limit values represent amounts that should not be exceeded.

A unique aspect of the DRI values is that they are categorized by function and classification in order to facilitate awareness of the different roles that nutrients play in the diet. Specific guidelines have been developed for B-complex vitamins; vitamins C and E; bone-building nutrients, such as calcium and vitamin D; micronutrients, such as iron and zinc; and the class of macronutrients that includes carbohydrates, fats, proteins, and fiber. Table 1 includes the DRI values (including the UL values) for most of these nutrients.

Nutrition recommendations are flexible, but also highly individualized. A unique aspect of the nutrition guidelines is that they highlight a variety of dietary patterns. The established DASH-style and Mediterranean-style dietary patterns were cited as examples of healthy diets because they have been well-supported in the scientific literature. The guidelines also referenced traditional Asian dietary patterns and vegetarian diets as

Recommended Dietary Allowance (RDA) Dietary guideline that specifies the amount of a nutrient needed for almost all of the healthy individuals in a specific age and gender group.

Dietary Reference Intake (DRI) Appropriate amounts of nutrients in the diet (AI, RDA, and UL).

Adequate Intake (AI) Dietary guideline established experimentally to estimate nutrient needs when sufficient data are not available to establish an RDA value.

Tolerable Upper Intake Level (UL) Maximum level of a daily nutrient that will not pose a risk of adverse health effects for most people.

Table 1 ▶ Dietary Reference Intake (DRI), Recommended Dietary Allowance (RDA), and Tolerable Upper Intake Level (UL) for Major Nutrients

	DRI/RDA			
	Males	**Females**	**UL**	**Function**
Energy and Macronutrients				
Carbohydrates (45–65%)	130 g	130 g	ND	Energy (only source of energy for the brain)
Fat (20–35%)	ND	ND	ND	Energy, vitamin carrier
Protein (10–35%)	.8 g/kg	.8 g/kg	ND	Growth and maturation, tissue formation
Fiber (g/day)	38 g/day*	25 g/day*	ND	Digestion, blood profiles
B-Complex Vitamins				
Thiamin (mg/day)	1.2	1.1	ND	Co-enzyme for carbohydrates and amino acid metabolism
Riboflavin (mg/day)	1.3	1.1	ND	Co-enzyme for metabolic reactions
Niacin (mg/day)	16	14	35	Co-enzyme for metabolic reactions
Vitamin B-6 (mg/day)	1.3	1.3	100	Co-enzyme for amino acid and glycogen reactions
Folate (µg/day)	400	400	1,000	Metabolism of amino acids
Vitamin B-12 (µg/day)	2.4	2.4	ND	Co-enzyme for nucleic acid metabolism
Pantothenic acid (mg/day)	5*	5*	ND	Co-enzyme for fat metabolism
Biotin (µg/day)	30*	30*	ND	Synthesis of fat, glycogen, and amino acids
Choline (mg/day)	550*	425*	3,500	Precursor to acetylcholine
Antioxidants and Related Nutrients				
Vitamin C (mg/day)	90	75	2,000	Co-factor for reactions, antioxidant
Vitamin E (mg/day)	15	15	1,000	Undetermined, mainly antioxidant
Selenium (µg/day)	55	55	400	Defense against oxidative stress
Bone-Building Nutrients				
Calcium (mg/day)	1,000*	1,000*	2,500	Muscle contraction, nerve transmission
Phosphorus (mg/day)	700	700	3,000	Maintenance of pH, storage of energy
Magnesium (mg/day)	400–420	310–320	350	Co-factor for enzyme reactions
Vitamin D (µg/day)	5*	5*	50	Maintenance of calcium and phosphorus levels
Fluoride (mg/day)	4*	3*	10	Stimulation of new bone formation
Micronutrients and Other Trace Elements				
Vitamin K (µg/day)	120*	90*	ND	Blood clotting and bone metabolism
Vitamin A (µg/day)	900	700	3,000	Vision, immune function
Iron (mg/day)	8	18	45	Component of hemoglobin
Zinc (mg/day)	11	8	40	Component of enzymes and proteins

Note: These values reflect the dietary needs generally for adults aged 19–50 years. Specific guidelines for other age groups are available from the Food and Nutrition Board of the National Academy of Sciences (www.iom.edu). Values labeled with an asterisk (*) are based on Adequate Intake (AI) values rather than the RDA values; ND = not determined.

examples of ways to achieve dietary goals. The new guidelines emphasize that a healthful total diet is not a rigid prescription but rather a flexible approach to eating that can be adjusted for a variety of individual tastes and preferences. The flexibility for individual eating patterns is also reflected in the wide ranges provided for various DRI categories. The recommended DRI values for carbohydrates range from 45 to 65 percent. The DRI values for protein range from 10 to 35 percent, while the DRI values for fat range from 20 to 35 percent. These ranges are much broader than recommendations from the USDA in previous versions of the dietary guidelines. According to the Institute of Medicine (IOM), this broader range was established to "help people make healthy and more realistic choices based on their own food preferences." Figure 2 illustrates the recommended DRI distributions for carbohydrates, fats, and proteins.

The quantity of nutrients recommended varies with age and other considerations; for example, young children need more calcium than adults and pregnant women, and postmenopausal women need more calcium than other women. Accordingly, DRIs, including RDAs, have been established for several age/gender groups. In this book, the values are appropriate for most adult men and women. The USDA has a website that calculates personally determined DRI values. You can enter data such as your gender, age, height, weight, and activity level, and the calculator determines your DRI values. (Search "USDA DRI calculator" on the Internet.)

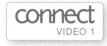

Dietary Recommendations for Carbohydrates

Complex carbohydrates should be the principal source of calories in the diet. Carbohydrates have gotten a bad rap in recent years due to the hype associated with low-carbohydrate diets. Carbohydrates have been unfairly implicated as a cause of obesity. The suggestion that they cause insulin to be released and that insulin, in turn, causes the body to take up and store excess energy as fat is overly simplistic and doesn't take into account differences in types of carbohydrates. Simple sugars (such as sucrose, glucose, and fructose) found in candy and soda lead to quick increases in blood sugar and tend to promote fat deposition. Complex carbohydrates (e.g., bread, pasta, rice), on the other hand, are broken down more slowly and do not cause the same effect on blood sugar. They contribute valuable nutrients and fiber in the diet and should constitute the bulk of a person's diet. Lumping simple and complex carbohydrates together is not appropriate, since they are processed differently and have different nutrient values.

A number of low-carb diet books have used an index known as the glycemic index (GI) as the basis for determining if foods are appropriate in the diet. Foods with a high GI value produce rapid increases in blood sugar, while foods with a low GI value produce slower increases. While this seems to be a logical way to categorize carbohydrates, it is misleading, since it doesn't account for the amount of carbohydrates in different servings of a food. A more appropriate indicator of the effect of foods on blood sugar levels is called the glycemic load. Carrots, for example, are known to have a very high GI value, but the overall glycemic load is quite low. The carbohydrates from most fruits and vegetables exhibit similar properties.

Despite the intuitive and logical appeal of this classification system, neither the glycemic index nor glycemic load have been consistently associated with body weight. Evidence also indicates no difference on weight loss between high glycemic index and low glycemic index diets. There is some evidence linking glycemic load to a higher risk for diabetes but no associations with cancer risk.

Additional research is needed, but excess sugar consumption appears to be problematic only if caloric intake is larger than caloric expenditure. Carbohydrates are the body's preferred form of energy for physical activity, and the body is well equipped for processing extra carbohydrates. Athletes and other active individuals typically have no difficulty burning off extra energy from carbohydrates. Sugar consumption, among people with an adequate diet, is also not associated with major chronic diseases.

Reducing dietary sugar can help reduce risk of obesity and heart disease. Although sugar consumption has not been viewed as harmful, people who consume high amounts of sugar also tend to consume excess calories. The new dietary guidelines clearly recommend decreasing consumption of added sugars to reduce risk of excess calorie consumption and weight gain. The American Heart Association also endorsed this position in a

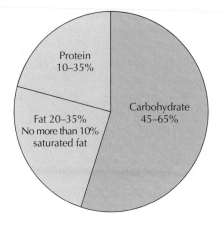

Figure 2 ▶ Dietary Reference Intake values.

scientific statement entitled "Dietary Sugars Intake and Cardiovascular Health."

The document notes that excessive consumption of sugars (sugars added to foods and drinks) contributes to overconsumption of discretionary calories. Among Americans, the current average daily sugars consumption is 355 calories per day (22.2 teaspoons) as opposed to 279 calories in 1970. Soft drinks and sugar-sweetened beverages are the primary sources of added sugars in the American diet. The AHA's scientific statement recommends no more than 100 calories of added sugars for most women and not more than 150 calories for most men. A typical 12-ounce sweetened soft drink contains 150 calories, mostly sugar. Reducing consumption of sugar-sweetened beverages is a simple, but important, diet modification.

Increasing consumption of dietary fiber is important for overall good nutrition and health. Diets high in complex carbohydrates and **fiber** are associated with a low incidence of coronary heart disease, stroke, and some forms of cancer. Long-term studies indicate that high-fiber diets may also be associated with a lower risk for diabetes mellitus, diverticulosis, hypertension, and gallstone formation. It is not known whether these health benefits are directly attributable to high dietary fiber or other effects associated with the ingestion of vegetables, fruits, and cereals.

A position statement from the American Dietetics Association summarizes the health benefits and importance of fiber in a healthy diet. It indicates that high-fiber diets provide bulk, are more satiating, and are linked to lower body weights. It also points out that a fiber-rich diet often has a lower fat content, is larger in volume, and is richer in micronutrients, all of which have beneficial health effects. Evidence for health benefits has become strong enough that the FDA has stated that specific beneficial health claims can be made for specific dietary fibers. The National Cholesterol Education Program also recommends dietary fiber as part of overall strategies for treating high cholesterol in adults.

In the past, clear distinctions were made between soluble fiber and insoluble fiber because they appeared to provide separate effects. Soluble fiber (typically found in fruits and oat bran) was more frequently associated with improving blood lipid profiles, while insoluble fiber (typically found in grains) was mainly thought to help speed up digestion and reduce risks for colon and rectal cancer. Difficulties in measuring these compounds in typical mixed diets led a National Academy of Sciences panel to recommend eliminating distinctions between soluble and insoluble fibers and instead to use a broader definition of fiber.

Currently, few Americans consume the recommended amounts of dietary fiber. The average intake of dietary fiber is about 15 g/day, which is much lower than the recommended 25 to 35 g/day. Foods in the typical American diet contain little, if any, dietary fiber, and servings of commonly consumed grains, fruits, and vegetables contain only 1 to 3 g of dietary fiber. Therefore, individuals have to look for ways to ensure that they get sufficient fiber in their diet. Manufacturers are allowed to declare a food as a "good source of fiber" if it contains 10 percent of the recommended amount (2.5 g/serving) and an "excellent source of fiber" if it contains 20 percent of the recommended amount (5 g/serving). Because fiber has known health benefits, the new dietary guidelines encourage consumers to select foods high in dietary fiber, such as whole-grain breads and cereals, legumes, vegetables, and fruit, whenever possible.

Fruits and vegetables are essential for good health. Fruits and vegetables are a valuable source of dietary fiber, are packed with vitamins and minerals, and contain many additional phytochemicals, which may have beneficial effects on health. The International Agency of Research on Cancer (IARC), an affiliate of the World Health Organization, did a comprehensive review on the links between dietary intake of fruits and vegetables and cancer. It concluded that both human studies and animal experimental studies "indicate that a higher intake of fruits and vegetables is associated with a lower risk of various types of cancer." The clearest evidence of a cancer-protective effect from eating more fruits is for stomach,

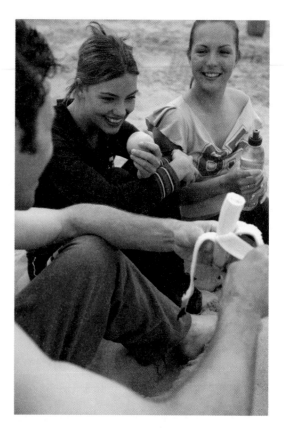

Plan ahead for healthy, low-fat snacks when on the run.

lung, and esophageal cancers. A higher intake of vegetables is also associated with reduced risks for cancers of the esophagus and colon-rectum. This evidence—plus the evidence of the beneficial effects of fruits and vegetables on other major diseases, such as heart disease—indicates that individuals should strive to increase their intake of these foods. Reports from the 2010 Dietary Guidelines Advisory Committee indicate that beneficial effects on health appear to be linked to a minimum of five servings of fruits and vegetables per day. Additional benefits were noted at even higher consumption levels. These findings contributed to the increased emphasis being placed on a plant-based diet in the new dietary guidelines.

Follow the recommendations to assure healthy amounts of carbohydrates in the diet. The following list summarizes key strategies to achieve dietary guidelines for carbohydrate content in the diet:

- Consume a variety of fiber-rich fruits and vegetables.
- Select whole-grain foods when possible.
- Choose and prepare foods and beverages with little added sugars or caloric sweeteners.

Dietary Recommendations for Fat

Fat is an essential nutrient and an important energy source. Humans need some fat in their diet because fats are carriers of vitamins A, D, E, and K. They are a source of essential linoleic acid, they make food taste better, and they provide a concentrated form of calories, which serve as a vital source of energy during moderate to vigorous exercise. Fats have more than twice the calories per gram as carbohydrates.

There are several types of dietary fat. **Saturated fats** come primarily from animal sources, such as red meat, dairy products, and eggs, but they are also found in some vegetable sources, such as coconut and palm oils. There are two basic types of **unsaturated fats**: polyunsaturated and monounsaturated. Polyunsaturated fats are derived principally from vegetable sources, such as safflower, cottonseed, soybean, sunflower, and corn oils (omega-6 fats), and cold-water fish sources, such as salmon and mackerel (omega-3 fats). Monounsaturated fats are derived primarily from vegetable sources, including olive, peanut, and canola oil.

Saturated fat is associated with an increased risk for disease, but polyunsaturated and monounsaturated fats can be beneficial. Excessive total fat in the diet (particularly saturated fat) is associated with atherosclerotic cardiovascular diseases and breast, prostate, and

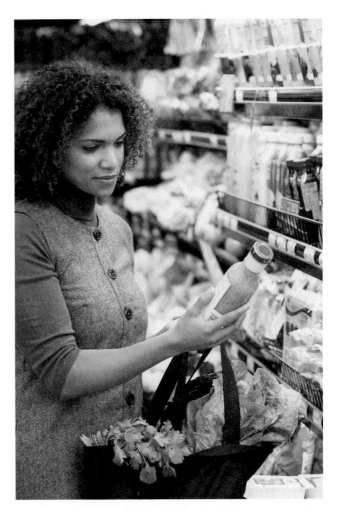

Being an informed and educated consumer can help you make healthier food choices.

colon cancer, as well as obesity. Excess saturated fat in the diet contributes to increased cholesterol and increased low-density lipoprotein (LDL) cholesterol in the blood. For this reason, no more than 10 percent of your total calories should come from saturated fats.

Unsaturated fats are generally considered to be less likely to contribute to cardiovascular disease, cancer, and obesity than saturated fats. Polyunsaturated fats can

Fiber Indigestible bulk in foods that can be either soluble or insoluble in body fluids.

Saturated Fats Dietary fats that are usually solid at room temperature and come primarily from animal sources.

Unsaturated Fats Monounsaturated or polyunsaturated fats that are usually liquid at room temperature and come primarily from vegetable sources.

reduce total cholesterol and LDL cholesterol, but they also decrease levels of high-density lipoprotein (HDL) cholesterol. Omega-3 fatty acids (a special type of polyunsaturated fat found in cold-water fish) have received a lot of attention due to their potential benefits in reducing the risk of cardiovascular disease. A plant source of omega-3 fatty acids (alpha-linolenic acid) found in walnuts, flaxseed, and canola oil may have similar benefits.

Monounsaturated fats have been shown to decrease total cholesterol and LDL cholesterol without an accompanying decrease in the desirable HDL cholesterol. Past dietary guidelines recommended a diet low in saturated fat and cholesterol but moderate in total fat, making it clear that excess saturated fat is the main concern and that some fat is necessary in the diet. Fat should account for 20 to 35 percent of calories in the diet, with no more than 10 percent of total calories from saturated fat. The remaining fat should come from plant-based sources, especially monounsaturated fats.

Trans fats and hydrogenated vegetable oils should be minimized in the diet. For decades, the public has been cautioned to avoid saturated fats and foods with excessive cholesterol. Many people switched from using butter to margarine because margarine is made from vegetable oils that are unsaturated and contain no cholesterol. The hydrogenation process used to convert oils into solids, however, is known to produce **trans fats,** which are just as harmful as saturated fats, if not more so. Trans fats are known to cause increases in LDL cholesterol and have been shown to contribute to the buildup of atherosclerotic plaque. Because of these effects, it is important to try to minimize consumption of trans fats in your diet.

The FDA requires trans fat content to be listed on the nutrition facts labels so that consumers can be more aware of foods high in this fat. The requirement to post trans fat content on food labels has prompted companies to look for ways to remove excess trans fats from products. Lay's uses cottonseed oil instead of sunflower oil to help eliminate trans fats from Fritos, Tostitos, and Cheetos. A number of margarines are also available with little or no trans fat (e.g., Smart Balance). These changes and the increased awareness about trans fat appear to have had a positive effect. The CDC reports that levels of trans fat have declined in the population by over 58 percent. These findings provide an effective example of how food policy (e.g., labeling) has prompted positive changes in food quality and food access. The Dietary Guidelines continue to recommend that consumers keep trans fat consumption as low as possible by limiting solid fats and foods that contain synthetic sources of trans fats. Foods that have trace amounts of trans fat (i.e., those containing less than .5 g of trans fat per serving) may still be listed as having no trans fat. Therefore, you should also look for foods that contain little or no hydrogenated vegetable oil.

Fat substitutes and neutraceuticals in food products may reduce fat consumption and lower cholesterol. Olestra is a synthetic fat substitute that passes through the gastrointestinal system without being digested. Thus, foods prepared with Olestra have fewer calories. For example, a chocolate chip cookie prepared in a normal way would have 138 calories, but an Olestra cookie would have 63. Some consumer groups warn that the promotion of Olestra-containing products may make individuals more likely to snack on less energy-dense snack foods. They also express concern that Olestra inhibits absorption of many naturally occurring antioxidants that have been shown to have many beneficial effects on health. Early warnings were required on the product because of fear that it caused gastric problems. These warnings were removed by the FDA soon after Olestra was introduced.

Several other new products offer potential to modify the amount and effect of dietary fat in our diets. The first is a naturally occurring compound included in several margarines (Benecol and Take Control). The active ingredient in this compound (sitostanol ester) comes from pine trees and has been shown to reduce total and LDL cholesterol in the blood. Several clinical trials have confirmed that these margarines are both safe and effective in lowering cholesterol levels. The products must be used regularly to be effective and may be useful only in individuals who have high levels of cholesterol. Food products that contain these medically beneficial compounds are often referred to as *neutraceuticals*, or *functional foods*, because they are a combination of pharmaceuticals and food.

Follow the recommendations to assure healthy amounts of fat in the diet. The 2010 Dietary Guidelines Advisory Committee emphasized that significant health benefits can be achieved by making several changes in consumption of dietary fats and cholesterol.

- Limit saturated fatty acid intake to less than 10 percent of total calories, with continued gradual reductions down to 7 percent. Substitute food sources of mono- or polyunsaturated fatty acids.

- Limit dietary cholesterol to less than 300 mg per day (200 mg per day for persons with or at high risk for cardiovascular disease or Type II diabetes).

- Avoid trans fatty acids from processed foods (except the small amounts that occur naturally from ruminant sources in animals).

- Limit cholesterol-raising fats (saturated fats exclusive of stearic acid and trans fatty acids) to less than 5 to 7 percent of energy.

- Consume two servings of seafood per week to provide healthy

connect
VIDEO 3

amounts of omega-3 fatty acids from marine sources (e.g., docosahexaenoic acid [DHA] and eicosapentaenoic acid [EPA]).

Dietary Recommendations for Proteins

Protein is the basic building block for the body, but dietary protein constitutes a relatively small amount of daily caloric intake. Proteins are often referred to as the building blocks of the body because all body cells are made of protein. More than 100 proteins are formed from 20 different **amino acids.** Eleven of these amino acids can be synthesized from other nutrients, but 9 **essential amino acids** must be obtained directly from the diet. One way to identify amino acids is the -*ine* at the end of their name. For example, arginine and lysine are two of the amino acids. Only 3 of the 20 amino acids do not have the -*ine* suffix. They are aspartic acid, glutamic acid, and tryptophan.

Certain foods, called complete proteins, contain all of the essential amino acids, along with most of the others. Examples are meat, dairy products, and fish. Incomplete proteins contain some, but not all, of the essential amino acids. Examples include beans, nuts, and rice.

Protein should account for at least 10 percent of daily calorie consumption, which can be met easily with complete (animal) or incomplete (vegetable) sources of protein. A person consuming a typical 2,000-calorie diet should consume approximately 200 calories from protein. Protein provides 4 calories per gram, so minimum daily protein needs are as low as 50 grams per day. Figure 3 shows the relative protein content of various foods.

To provide more flexibility, dietary guidelines indicate that protein can account for as much as 35 percent of calorie intake. Experts, however, agree that there are no known benefits and some possible risks associated with consuming excess protein, particularly animal protein. High-protein diets are damaging to the kidneys, as the body must process a lot of extra nitrogen. Excessive protein intake can also lead to urinary calcium loss, which can weaken bones and lead to osteoporosis.

People who eat a variety of foods, including meat, dairy, eggs, and plants rich in protein, virtually always consume more protein than the body needs. Because of the negative consequences associated with excess intake, dietary supplements containing extra protein are not recommended for the general population.

Vegetarian diets provide sufficient protein and may offer health benefits. Vegetarian diets provide ample sources of protein as long as a variety of protein-rich food sources are included in the diet. According to the American Dietetics Association, well-planned vegetarian diets "are appropriate for all stages of the life cycle, including during pregnancy, and lactation," and can "satisfy the nutrient needs of infants, children, and adolescents." You can get enough protein as long as the variety and amounts of foods consumed are adequate. **Vegans** must supplement the diet with vitamin B-12 because the only source of this vitamin is food from animal sources. **Lacto-ovo vegetarians** do not have the same concerns because vitamin B-12 can be obtained in dairy products.

There is an increased recognition of the importance of whole grains, fruits, and vegetables in the diet, but vegetarian diets based primarily on plants are still uncommon. A Harris poll estimates that approximately 3 percent of Americans are vegetarian (.5 percent vegan). However, an additional 10 percent of the population indicates they

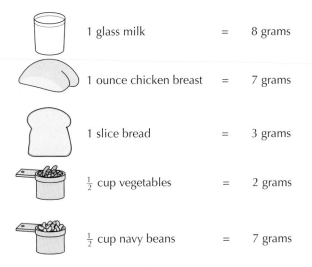

1 glass milk	=	8 grams
1 ounce chicken breast	=	7 grams
1 slice bread	=	3 grams
½ cup vegetables	=	2 grams
½ cup navy beans	=	7 grams

Figure 3 ▶ Protein content of various foods.
Source: Williams, M.

Trans Fats Fats that result when hydrogen is added to liquid oil to make it more solid. Hydrogenation transforms unsaturated fats so that they take on the characteristics of saturated fats, as is the case for margarine and shortening.

Amino Acids The 20 basic building blocks of the body that make up proteins.

Essential Amino Acids The nine basic amino acids that the human body cannot produce and that must be obtained from food sources.

Vegans Strict vegetarians, who exclude not only all forms of meat from the diet but also dairy products and eggs.

Lacto-Ovo Vegetarians Vegetarians who include dairy and eggs in the diet.

follow a vegetarian-inclined diet. Research has widely supported the health benefits associated with vegetarian diets and trends suggest that it is growing in popularity.

An increasing array of soy foods are available to provide alternative sources of protein. Soybeans and soy-based foods are a high-quality source of protein. They may also have beneficial effects on blood pressure and cholesterol levels, possibly contributing to reductions in risk for coronary heart disease. Soy-based foods contain compounds called isoflavones, a phytoestrogen that contributes to bone health, immune function, and maintenance of menopausal health in women. A variety of soy-based food products are commercially available as alternatives to traditional meat foods. Common options include tofu, tempeh, soy milk, or textured vegetable (soy) protein. Grocery stores carry a variety of other meatless products based on soy (e.g., veggie burgers). Soy foods that contain at least 6.25 grams per serving can be labeled with FDA-approved health claims.

Follow the recommendations to assure healthy amounts of protein in the diet. The following list summarizes some key dietary recommendations for protein:

- Of the three major nutrients that provide energy, protein should account for the smallest percentage of total calories consumed (10 to 35 percent).
- Protein in the diet should meet the RDA of 0.8 gram per kilogram (2.2 pounds) of a person's weight (about 54 grams for a 150-pound person).
- People on low-calorie diets need to consume a higher percentage of protein in the diet. In contrast, people consuming a lot of calories need a lower percentage.
- Vegetarians must eat a combination of foods to assure an adequate intake of essential amino acids. Vegans should supplement their diet with vitamin B-12.
- Excess protein can be harmful to the kidneys. Protein in the diet should not exceed twice the RDA (1.6 grams per kilogram of body weight).
- Dietary supplements of protein, such as tablets and powders, are not recommended.

Dietary Recommendations for Vitamins

Adequate vitamin intake is necessary for good health and wellness, but excessive vitamin intake is not necessary and can be harmful. Vitamins serve a variety of functions within the body. For example, they serve as co-enzymes for metabolism of different nutrients, contribute to the regulation of energy stores, and assist in immune function. Some vitamins (e.g.,

B-complex vitamins and vitamin C) are water soluble and are excreted in urine. These vitamins must be consumed on a daily basis. Other vitamins, such as A, D, E, and K, are fat soluble. These vitamins are stored over time, so daily doses of these vitamins are not necessary. Excess consumption of fat-soluble vitamins can actually build to toxic levels and harm cell function and health. The specific DRI values (minimal amounts) for some of the more important vitamins are shown in Table 1, along with the Tolerable Upper Intake Levels (maximum amounts).

Some vitamins act as antioxidants, but health benefits may depend on other compounds in foods. Carotenoid-rich foods, such as carrots and sweet potatoes, contain high amounts of vitamin A and high amounts of beta-carotene. Diets high in vitamin C (e.g., citrus fruits) and vitamin E (e.g., green leafy vegetables) are also associated with reduced risk of cancer. Vitamin E has also been associated with reduced risk of heart disease.

Vitamins A, C, and E (as well as beta-carotene) act as **antioxidants** within the body. Antioxidants are substances that are thought to inactivate free radicals (molecules

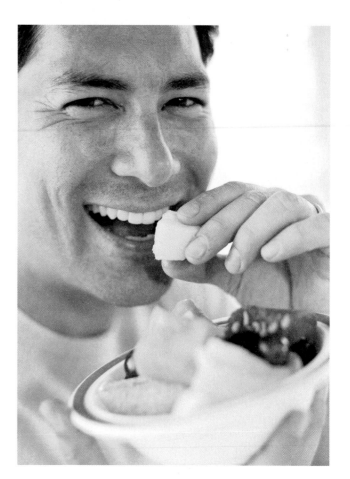

Fruits and vegetables contain vitamins as well as health-promoting phytochemicals.

that can cause cell damage and health problems). For this reason, health benefits have been attributed to anti-oxidant properties. However, several large-scale studies have shown no benefit (and possible risks) from taking beta-carotene supplements. Another study of over 20,000 people failed to find health benefits associated with consumption of a daily mixture of vitamin E, vitamin C, and beta-carotene. These results were difficult for scientists to interpret, but it is now known that there may be other beneficial substances in foods that contribute health benefits.

As mentioned earlier, the designation of "*functional foods*" has been coined to refer to foods or dietary components that may provide a health benefit beyond basic nutrition. Fruits and vegetables, for example, are loaded with a variety of powerful phytochemicals that have been shown to have potential health benefits (see Table 2). The relative importance to health of each compound is difficult to determine because the compounds may act synergistically with each other (and with antioxidant vitamins) to promote positive outcomes.

Other examples of functional foods include the beneficial types of fiber and beta glucan in whole grains, the isoflavones in soy products, the omega-3 fatty acids in cold-water fish, and the probiotic yeasts and bacteria in yogurts and other cultured dairy products. Most vitamins and minerals are also classified as functional foods, since they have functions beyond their primary role in basic nutrition. The examples listed here and in Table 2 should not be viewed as "magic bullets," since research is still accumulating on these compounds. In general, diets containing a lot of fruits and vegetables and whole grains (as recommended in MyPlate) will provide adequate intake of vitamins and other healthy food components.

Fortification of foods has been used to ensure adequate vitamin intake in the population. National policy requires many foods to be fortified. For example, milk is fortified with vitamin D, low-fat milk with vitamins A and D, and margarine with vitamin A. These foods were selected because they are common food sources for growing children. Many common grain products are fortified with folic acid because low folic acid levels increase the risk for birth defects in babies. Fortification is considered essential, since more than half of all women do not consume adequate amounts of folic acid during the first months of gestation (before most women even realize they are pregnant). Research clearly demonstrates the value of fortification. One study showed that neural tube defects are 19 percent less likely today than in 1996 (prior to fortification). Though other factors may have contributed to this decline, the study supports the benefits of fortification for improving nutritional intakes.

Table 2 ▶ Examples of Functional Foods and Potential Benefits

Carotenoids	Potential Benefits
Beta-carotene: found in carrots, pumpkin, sweet potato, cantaloupe	May bolster cellular antioxidant defenses
Lutein, zeaxanthin: found in kale, collards, spinach, corn, eggs, citrus	May contribute to healthy vision
Lycopene: Found in tomatoes, watermelon, red/pink grapefruit	May contribute to prostate health

Flavonoids	Potential Benefits
Anthocyanins: found in berries, cherries, red grapes *Flavanones:* found in citrus foods *Flavonols:* found in onions, apples, tea, broccoli	May bolster antioxidant defenses; maintain brain function and heart health

Isothiocyanates	Potential Benefits
Proanthocyanidins: found in cranberries, cocoa, apples, strawberries, grapes, peanuts	May contribute to maintenance of urinary tract health and heart health
Sulforaphane: found in cauliflower, broccoli, brussels sprouts, cabbage, kale, horseradish	May enhance detoxification of undesirable compounds; bolsters cellular antioxidant defenses

Phenolic Acids	Potential Benefits
Caffeic/ferulic acids: found in apples, pears, citrus fruits, some vegetables, coffee	May bolster cellular antioxidant defenses; may contribute to maintenance of healthy vision

Sulfides/Thioles	Potential Benefits
Sulfides: found in garlic, onions, leeks, scallions *Dithiolthiones:* found in cruciferous vegetables	May enhance detoxification of undesirable compounds; may contribute to maintenance of heart health and healthy immune function

Taking a daily multiple vitamin supplement may be a good idea. Sometimes supplements are needed to meet specific nutrient requirements for specific groups. For example, older people may need a vitamin D supplement if they get little exposure to sunlight, and iron supplements

Antioxidants Vitamins that are thought to inactivate "activated oxygen molecules," sometimes called free radicals. Free radicals may cause cell damage that leads to diseases of various kinds. Antioxidants may inactivate the free radicals before they do their damage.

are often recommended for pregnant women. Vitamin supplements at or below the RDA are considered safe; however, excess doses of vitamins can cause health problems. For example, excessively high amounts of vitamin C are dangerous for the 10 percent of the population who inherit a gene related to health problems. Excessively high amounts of vitamin D are toxic, and mothers who take too much vitamin A risk birth defects in unborn children.

In the past some medical groups recommended a daily multivitamin to insure adequate daily intake. However, national dietary guidelines specifically note that "For the general, healthy population, there is no evidence to support a recommendation for the use of multivitamin/mineral supplements in the primary prevention of chronic disease." In spite of this recommendation, some people may choose to take a multivitamin/mineral supplement. (Guidelines are presented in Table 3.)

Follow the recommendations to assure healthy amounts of vitamins in the diet. Vitamins in the amounts equal to the RDAs should be included in the diet each day. The following guidelines will help you implement this recommendation:

• Eat a diet containing the recommended servings for carbohydrates, proteins, and fats.

• Consume extra servings of green and yellow vegetables, citrus and other fruits, and other nonanimal food sources high in fiber, vitamins, and minerals.

Table 3 ▶ Vitamin and Mineral Supplements

• Limit the use of supplements unless warranted because of a health problem or a specific lack of nutrients in the diet.

• If you decide supplementation is necessary, select a multivitamin/mineral supplement that contains micronutrients in amounts close to the recommended levels (e.g., "one-a-day"-type supplements).

• If your diet is deficient in a particular mineral (e.g., calcium or iron), it may be necessary to incorporate dietary sources or an additional mineral supplement as well, since most multivitamins do not contain the recommended daily amount of minerals.

• Choose supplements that provide between 50 and 100 percent of the AI or RDA, and avoid those that provide many times the recommended amount. The use of supplements that hype "megadoses" of vitamins and minerals can increase the risk for some unwanted nutrient interactions and possible toxic effects.

• Buy supplements from a reputable company and look for supplements that carry the U.S. Pharmocopoeia (USP) notation (www.usp.org).

Source: Manore.

• People with special needs should seek medical advice before selecting supplements and should inform medical personnel as to the amounts and content of all supplements (vitamin and other).

Dietary Recommendations for Minerals

Adequate mineral intake is necessary for good health and wellness, but excessive mineral intake is not necessary and can be harmful. Like vitamins, minerals have no calories and provide no energy for the body. They are important in regulating various bodily functions. Two particularly important minerals are calcium and iron. Calcium is important to bone, muscle, nerve, and blood development and function and has been associated with reduced risk for heart disease. Iron is necessary for the blood to carry adequate oxygen. Other important minerals are phosphorus, which builds teeth and bones; sodium, which regulates water in the body; zinc, which aids in the healing process; and potassium, which is necessary for proper muscle function.

RDAs are established to determine the amounts of each mineral necessary for healthy daily functioning. A sound diet provides all of the RDA for minerals. Evidence indicating that some segments of the population may be mineral-deficient has led to the establishment of health goals identifying a need to increase mineral intake for some people.

A National Institutes of Health (NIH) consensus statement indicates that a large percentage of Americans fail to get enough calcium in their diet and emphasizes the need for increased calcium—particularly for pregnant women, postmenopausal women, and people over 65, who need 1,500 mg/day, which is higher than previous RDA amounts. The NIH has indicated that a total intake of 2,000 mg/day of calcium is safe and that adequate vitamin D in the diet is necessary for optimal calcium absorption to take place. Though getting these amounts in a calcium-rich diet is best, calcium supplementation for those not eating properly seems wise. Many multivitamins do not contain enough calcium for some classes of people, so some may want to consider additional calcium. Check with your physician or a dietitian before you consider a supplement because individual needs vary.

Another concern is iron deficiency among very young children and women of childbearing age. Low iron levels may be a special problem for women taking birth control pills because the combination of low iron levels and birth control pills has been associated with depression and generalized fatigue. Eating the appropriate number of servings recommended in MyPlate provides all the minerals necessary for meeting the RDA for minerals.

Nutrition goals for the nation emphasize the importance of adequate servings of foods rich in calcium, such as green, leafy vegetables and milk products; adequate servings of foods rich in iron, such as beans, peas, spinach, and meat; and reduced salt in the diet.

Follow the recommendations to assure healthy amounts of minerals in the diet. The following list includes basic recommendations for mineral content in the diet:

- Minerals in amounts equal to the RDAs should be consumed in the diet each day.
- In general, a calcium dietary supplement is not recommended for the general population; however, supplements (up to 1,000 mg/day) may be appropriate for adults who do not eat well. For postmenopausal women, a calcium supplement is recommended (up to 1,500 mg/day for those who do not eat well). A supplement may also be appropriate for people who restrict calories, but RDA values should not be exceeded unless the person consults with a registered dietitian or a physician.

The following guidelines will help you implement these recommendations:

- A diet containing the food servings recommended for carbohydrates, proteins, and fats will more than meet the RDA standards.
- Extra servings of green and yellow vegetables, citrus and other fruits, and other nonanimal sources of foods high in fiber, vitamins, and minerals are recommended as a substitute for high-fat foods.

Reducing salt in the diet can reduce health risks. Salt is common in many processed food products and most Americans consume way too much. Since the 1970s, salt consumption has gone up 55 percent for men and 60 percent for women. Salt intake increases the risk for hypertension, which is a major risk factor for heart disease and stroke. Many people have assumed that salt consumption is not a problem if you are not hypertensive, but this is not the case. Recent studies have shown that sodium intake increases risks of stroke independent of the presence of hypertension. Therefore, reducing salt consumption is important for everyone.

Reducing salt consumption was emphasized as a key priority in the latest Dietary Guidelines. The amount of salt recommended in the diet was reduced from 2.5 grams, slightly less than one teaspoon per day, to 1.5 grams (about half a teaspoon) for both adults and children. This is because of the strong link between salt intake and high blood pressure. The guidelines note it will take time for most people to reduce salt intake, so it may be done gradually. Increased potassium in the diet is recommended because it helps reduce the effects of sodium on blood pressure.

A prominent report by the Institute of Medicine and the National Academy of Sciences indicates that reducing salt intake could prevent 100,000 deaths and save $18 billion in medical expenses. A principal recommendation in the report is to encourage manufacturers to reduce salt content in processed foods. Sodium content is also high in fast foods. A study of 17 fast-food chains showed that 85 percent of meals served had more than a full day's allotment of salt. While changes in food supply are important, taking responsibility for lowering salt in the diet is the best way for an individual to make change.

Dietary Recommendations for Water and Other Fluids

Water is a critical component of a healthy diet. Though water is not in the MyPlate food groups because it contains no calories, provides no energy, and provides no key nutrients, it is crucial to health and survival. Water is a major component of most of the foods you eat, and more than half of all body tissues are composed of it. Regular water intake maintains water balance and is critical to many bodily functions. Though a variety of fluid-replacement beverages are available for use during and following exercise, replacing water is the primary need.

Beverages other than water are a part of many diets, but some beverages can have an adverse effect on good health. Coffee, tea, soft drinks, and alcoholic beverages are often substituted for water. Too much caffeine consumption has been shown to cause symptoms such as irregular heartbeat in some people. Tea has not been shown to have similar effects, though this may be because tea drinkers typically consume less volume than coffee drinkers, and tea has less caffeine per cup than coffee. Many soft drinks also have caffeine, though drip coffee typically contains two to three times the caffeine of a typical cola drink.

Excessive consumption of alcoholic beverages can have negative health implications because the alcohol often replaces nutrients. Excessive alcohol consumption is associated with increased risk for heart disease, high blood pressure, stroke, and osteoporosis. Long-term excessive alcoholic beverage consumption leads to cirrhosis of the liver and to increased risk for hepatitis and cancer. Alcohol consumption during pregnancy can result in low birth weight, fetal alcoholism, and other damage to the fetus. While there are clear risks associated with excessive alcohol consumption, the dietary guidelines indicate that alcohol used in moderation can enhance enjoyment of meals and reduce risks for coronary heart disease.

Follow the recommendations to assure healthy amounts of water and other fluids in the diet. The following list includes basic recommendations for water and other fluids in the diet:

- In addition to foods containing water, the average adult needs about eight glasses (8 ounces each) of water every day. Active people and those who exercise in hot environments require additional water.

- Coffee, tea, and soft drinks should not be substituted for sources of key nutrients, such as low-fat milk, fruit juices, or foods rich in calcium.

- Limit daily servings of beverages containing caffeine to no more than three.

- Limit sugared soft drinks.

- If you are an adult and you choose to drink alcohol, do so in moderation. The dietary guidelines for Americans indicate that moderation means no more than one drink per day for women and no more than two drinks per day for men (one drink equals 12 ounces of regular beer, 5 ounces of wine [small glass], or one average-size cocktail [1.5 ounces of 80-proof alcohol]).

Making Well-Informed Food Choices

Well-informed consumers eat better. Most people underestimate the number of calories they consume daily and the caloric content of specific foods. Not surprisingly, people who are better informed about the content of their food are more likely to make wise food choices. Ways to get better food choice information include accurate food labels on packages and information about food content on menus or signs in restaurants.

The content of food labels changes from time to time depending on federal guidelines and policies. The most recent change is the requirement to post trans fat content on labels (see Figure 4). This action was prompted by the clear scientific evidence that trans fats are more likely to cause atherosclerosis and heart disease than are other types of fat. Trans fats are discussed in a later section.

Reading food labels helps you be more aware of what you are eating and make healthier choices in your daily eating. In particular, paying attention to the amounts of saturated fat, trans fat, and cholesterol posted on food labels helps you make heart-healthy food choices. When comparing similar food products, combine the grams (g) of saturated fat and trans fat and look for the lowest combined amount. The listing of % Daily Value (% DV) can also be useful. Foods low in saturated fat and cholesterol generally have % DV values less than 5 percent, while foods high in saturated fat and cholesterol have values greater than 20 percent.

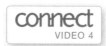

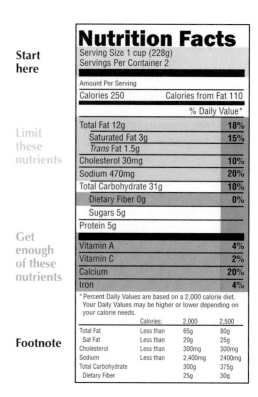

Figure 4 ▶ Sample food label for macaroni and cheese.
Source: U.S. Food and Drug Administration.

Supplemental food labels may not provide accurate information. Some manufacturers have used supplemental labels on foods to advertise healthy aspects of their products. An example is the "Smart Choice" designation created by a consortium of food manufacturers. The labels were placed prominently on the front of selected food packages to promote them as a healthy choice for good nutrition. While perhaps well-intentioned, the claims and designations were not approved by the FDA and could have swayed consumers to select the product. National nutrition groups criticized the name (Smart Choice) as well as the location and content of the labels. This action prompted the FDA to require manufacturers to cease using the potentially confusing labels. Care should be taken when considering claims on food packages.

Guides to food contents in restaurants can help consumers eat better. It is increasingly common for restaurants to post the calorie counts for the foods on their menu. Some restaurants also provide more detailed information about specific nutrients (e.g., protein, carbohydrate, salt, fiber). These changes have come about due, in part, to policy changes and USDA requirements; however, they also reflect an increased consumer demand for health and nutrition information. While some restaurants still emphasize gluttony and excess in advertisements and menus, there are many others that are positioning themselves to accommodate greater demand for healthier food choices. Posting the nutritional quality of foods allows restaurants to at least document that they have provided consumers with the information needed to make healthier choices.

Sound Eating Practices

Consistent eating patterns (with a daily breakfast) are important for good nutrition. Eating regular meals every day, including a good breakfast, is wise. Many studies have shown breakfast to be an important meal, in which one-fourth of the day's calories should be consumed. Skipping breakfast impairs performance because blood sugar levels drop in the long period between dinner the night before and lunch the following day. Eating every 4 to 6 hours is wise.

Moderation is a good general rule of nutrition. You do not have to permanently eliminate foods that you really enjoy, but some of your favorite foods may not be among the best choices. Enjoying special foods on occasion is part of moderation. The key is to limit food choices high in empty calories.

Portion sizes have increased in recent years. Cafeteria-style restaurants (and others) sometimes offer all you can eat meals, which encourage larger portions. Reducing portion size is very important when eating out and at home (see Concept 15 for more information).

Minimize your reliance on fast foods. Recent estimates suggest that 63 percent of Americans eat fast food one to three times a week and an additional 3 percent eat fast food three to five times a week. Unfortunately, many fast foods are poor nutritional choices. Hamburgers are usually high in fat, as are french fries (because they are usually cooked in saturated fat). Even chicken and fish are often high in fat and calories 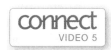 because they may be cooked in fat and covered with high-fat/high-calorie sauces. (Fast foods are also discussed in more detail in Concept 15.)

Healthy snacks can be an important part of good nutrition. For people who want to lose weight or maintain their current weight, small snacks of appropriate foods can help fool the appetite. For people wanting to gain weight, snacks provide additional calories. The calories consumed in snacks will probably necessitate limiting the calories from meals. The key is proper selection of the foods for snacking.

As with your total diet, the best snacks are nutritionally dense. Too many snacks are high in calories, fats, simple sugar, and salt. Even foods sold as "healthy snacks," such as granola bars, are often high in fat and simple sugar. Some common snacks, such as chips, pretzels, and even popcorn, may be high in salt and may be cooked in fat. Healthier snacks include ice milk (instead of ice cream), fresh fruits, vegetable sticks, popcorn not cooked in fat and with little or no salt, crackers, and nuts with little or no salt.

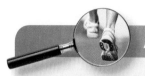

A CLOSER LOOK

MyPlate "SuperTracker" for Diet and Activity Monitoring

Self-monitoring is an important behavioral skill for adopting and maintaining healthy lifestyles. There are many cell phone apps and resources for monitoring your diet, but the web-based resources available through MyPlate provide a free, comprehensive set of tools (called Super-Tracker). An easy-to-use food database (Food-A-Pedia) allows you to enter the name of a specific food and get quick feedback concerning the food's content. A customized tool called the Food Tracker evaluates the nutrient quality of your diet and an accompanying Physical Activity Tracker evaluates activity levels compared to the U.S. Physical Activity Guidelines. An integrative tool (My Weight Manager) combines data on energy intake and expenditure to facilitate weight management. Companion tools let you set goals, use virtual coaches, and monitor progress over time. The comprehensive set of self-monitoring tools can assist consumers in adopting and maintaining a healthy and active lifestyle.

How would your diet stack up to the 2010 Dietary Guidelines? Would you benefit from tools designed to evaluate and track the quality of your diet over time?

connect
ACTIVITY

Minimize your consumption of overly processed foods and foods high in hydrogenated fat or saturated fat. Many foods available in grocery stores have been highly processed to enhance shelf life and convenience. In many cases, the processing of foods removes valuable nutrients and includes other additives that may compromise overall nutrition. Processing of grains, for example, typically removes the bran and germ layers, which contain fiber and valuable minerals. In regard to additives, there has been considerable attention on the possible negative effects of high fructose corn syrup, as well as the pervasive use of hydrogenated vegetable oils containing trans fatty acids. Table 4 compares food quality in each of the main food categories. To improve your diet, you should aim to choose foods in the "more desirable" category instead of those in the "less desirable" category.

Consider eating organic foods to reduce exposure to carcinogens. Consumers are often confused about what "organic" means. Organic food differs from conventionally produced food primarily in the way it is grown, handled, and processed. Organic food is produced without conventional pesticides and using natural fertilizers. Organic meat, poultry, eggs, and dairy products come from animals that are given no antibiotics or growth hormones. Organic foods are typically produced by farmers who emphasize the use of renewable resources and the conservation of soil and water. The benefits of organic farming production have led to initiatives to encourage farmers to adopt organic practices.

The U.S. Department of Agriculture (USDA) has recently established a new set of standards for foods labeled as "organic." The current labeling requires that a government-approved certifier inspect the farm where the food is grown or produced to ensure that the farmer is following all the rules necessary to meet USDA organic

Table 4 ▶ Comparing the Quality of Similar Food Products

Food Product	Less Desirable Option	More Desirable Option	Benefit of More Desirable Option in Nutrition Quality
Bread	White bread	Whole wheat bread	More fiber
Rice	White rice	Brown rice	More fiber
Juice	Sweetened juice	100% juice	More fiber and less fructose corn syrup
Fruit	Canned	Fresh	More vitamins, more fiber, less sugar
Vegetables	Canned	Fresh	More vitamins, less salt
Potatoes	French fries	Baked potato	Less saturated fat
Milk	2% milk	Skim milk	Less saturated fat
Meat	Ground beef (high fat)	Ground sirloin (low fat)	Less saturated fat
Oils	Vegetable oil	Canola oil	More monounsaturated fat
Snack food	Fried chips	Baked chips	Less fat/calorie content, less trans fat

In the News

Knowledge Doesn't Translate to Behavior

Nutrition remains a top priority for most Americans. A Harris poll found that awareness of key nutritional facts is high. At least three-quarters of all U.S. adults place importance on freshness (89 percent), fiber (81 percent), and whole grains (81 percent) when choosing foods. Consumers also carefully consider the fat content (80 percent), portion size (79 percent), calorie content (77 percent), and saturated fat (76 percent) when making food and beverage purchases. Over half of U.S. adults (57 percent) report monitoring or restricting consumption of some foods to improve their diet. Sugar and salt are the top two restricted items, with 34 percent and 32 percent restricting salt and sugar, respectively.

While awareness is high, it does not appear to translate into dietary change for most segments of the population. Fewer than half of Americans who rated sugar or salt as "important when managing their diet/weight" actually restrict their sugar (42 percent) or salt (47 percent) intake. Adherence to diet recommendations varies across the generations. Respondents over age 66 were the most likely to pay close attention to nutritional facts and translate their health consciousness into behavior. This was attributed to the greater need to follow a diet with specific restrictions. Overall, the results suggest that adherence to diet recommendations may be more driven by necessity than by knowledge.

Does your knowledge and awareness of nutrition directly impact your food choices?

---

standards. Companies that handle, process, or sell organic food must also be certified. The USDA does not imply that organically produced food is safer or more nutritious than conventionally produced food, but many health experts recommend organic foods to reduce exposure to pesticides and other chemicals and to help support more sustainable and environmentally friendly agricultural practices. Foods purchased at local farmer's markets may claim to be organic but may or may not meet FDA standards.

Nutrition and Physical Performance

Some basic dietary guidelines exist for active people. In general, the nutrition rules described in this concept apply to all people, whether active or sedentary, but some additional nutrition facts are important for exercisers and athletes. Because active people often expend calories in amounts considerably above normal, they need extra calories in their diet. To avoid excess fat and protein, complex carbohydrates should constitute as much as 70 percent of total caloric intake. A higher amount of protein is generally recommended for active individuals (1.2 grams per kg of body weight) because some protein is used as an energy source during exercise. Extra protein is obtained in the additional calories consumed. While the IOM range of 10 to 35 percent allows a "broader range" of choice, intake above 15 percent is not typically necessary.

Carbohydrate loading before exercise and carbohydrate replacement during exercise can enhance sustained aerobic performances. Athletes and vigorously active people must maintain a high level of readily available fuel, especially in the muscles. Consumption of complex carbohydrates is the best way to assure this.

Prior to an activity requiring an extended duration of physical performance (more than 1 hour in length, such as a marathon), **carbohydrate loading** can be useful. Carbohydrate loading is accomplished by resting 1 or 2 days before the event and eating a higher than normal amount of complex carbohydrates. This helps build up maximum levels of stored carbohydrate (**glycogen**) in the muscles and liver so it can be used during exercise. The key in carbohydrate loading is not to eat a lot but, rather, to eat a higher percentage of carbohydrates than normal.

Ingesting carbohydrate beverages during sustained exercise can also aid performance by preventing or forestalling muscle glycogen depletion. Fluid-replacement drinks containing 6 to 8 percent carbohydrates and no more than 6 to 8 percent sugar are very helpful in preventing dehydration and replacing energy stores. A number

Carbohydrate Loading The extra consumption of complex carbohydrates in the days prior to sustained performance.

Glycogen A source of energy stored in the muscles and liver necessary for sustained physical activity.

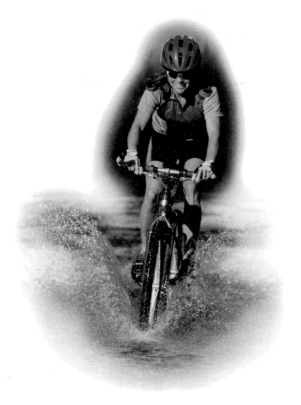

Good nutrition is essential for active people.

of companies also make concentrated carbohydrate gels that deliver carbohydrates (generally 80 percent complex, 20 percent simple) in a form the body can absorb quickly for energy. Examples are PowerGel and Gu. Energy bars, such as Powerbars and Clif bars, are also commonly eaten during or after exercise to enhance energy stores. The various carbohydrate supplements have been shown to be effective for exercise sessions lasting over an hour and are good for replacing glycogen stores after exercise. Consuming carbohydrates 15 to 30 minutes following exercise can aid in rapid replenishment of muscle glycogen, which may enhance future performance or training sessions.

These supplements have little benefit for shorter bouts of exercise. Because they contain considerable calories, they are not recommended for individuals primarily interested in weight control.

The timing may be more important than the makeup of a pre-event meal. If you are racing or doing high-level exercise early in the morning, eat a small meal prior to starting. Eat about 3 hours before competition or heavy exercise to allow time for digestion. Generally, athletes can select foods on the basis of experience, but easily digested carbohydrates are best. Generally, fat intake should be minimal because fat digests more slowly; proteins and high-cellulose foods should be kept to a moderate amount prior to prolonged events to avoid urinary and bowel excretion. Drinking 2 or 3 cups of liquid will ensure adequate hydration.

Consuming simple carbohydrates (sugar, candy) within an hour or two of an event is not recommended because it may cause an insulin response, resulting in weakness and fatigue, or it may cause stomach distress, cramps, or nausea.

Changes in the frequency and composition of meals are important to gain muscle mass. To increase muscle mass, the body requires a greater caloric intake. The challenge is to provide enough extra calories for the muscle without excess amounts going to fat. An increase of 500 to 1,000 calories a day will help most people gain muscle mass over time. Smaller, more frequent meals are best for weight gain, since they tend to keep the metabolic rate high. The majority of extra calories should come from complex carbohydrates. Breads, pasta, rice, and fruits such as bananas are good sources. Granola, nuts, juices (grape and cranberry), and milk also make good high-calorie, healthy snacks.

Diet supplements are not particularly effective unless used as part of a behaviorally based program. High-fat diets can result in weight gain but may not be best for good health, especially if they are high in saturated fat. If weight gain does not occur over a period of weeks and months with extra calorie consumption, individuals may need to seek medical assistance.

Strategies for Action

An analysis of your current diet is a good first step in making future decisions about what you eat. Many experts recommend keeping a log of what you eat over an extended period so you can determine the overall quality of your diet. In Lab 14A, you will have an opportunity to track your diet over several days. In addition to computing the amount of carbohydrates, fats, and proteins, you will also be able to monitor your consumption of fruits and vegetables. A number of online tools and personal software programs can make dietary calculations for you and provide a more comprehensive report of nutrient intake. Whether you use a Web-based tool or a paper and pencil log doesn't really matter—the key is to monitor and evaluate the quality of your diet.

Making small changes in diet patterns can have a big impact. Nutrition experts emphasize the importance of making small changes in your diet over time rather than trying to make comprehensive changes at one time. Try cutting back on sweets or soda. Simply adding a bit more fruit and vegetables to your diet can lead to major changes in overall diet quality. In Lab 14B, you will be given the opportunity to compare a "nutritious diet" to a "favorite diet." Analyzing two daily meal plans will help you get a more accurate picture as to whether foods you think are nutritious actually meet current healthy lifestyle goals.

Web Resources

American Dietetic Association **www.eatright.org**
Berkeley Nutrition Services **www.nutritionquest.com**
Center for Nutrition Policy and Promotion **www.usda
   .gov/cnpp**
Center for Science in the Public Interest **www.cspinet.org**
FDA Food Website **www.fda.gov/Food/default.htm**
Food and Drug Administration (FDA) **www.fda.gov**
Food Safety Database **www.foodsafety.gov**
Institute of Medicine **www.iom.edu**
Institute of Medicine—Food and Nutrition **www.iom
   .edu/Global/Topics/Food-Nutrition.aspx**
International Food Information Council Foundation
   www.ific.org
MyPlate **www.choosemyplate.gov**
MyPlate Food-A-Pedia **www.choosemyplate
   .gov/SuperTracker/foodapedia.aspx**
MyPlate SuperTracker **www.choosemyplate
   .gov/SuperTracker/foodtracker.aspx**
National Nutrition Summit Database **www.nlm.nih
   .gov/pubs/cbm/nutritionsummit.html**
Nutrition.gov **www.nutrition.gov**
Office of Dietary Supplements **http://ods.od.nih.gov**
Rudd Center for Food Policy and Obesity (Yale University)
   www.yaleruddcenter.org
U.S. Department of Agriculture (USDA) **www.usda.gov**
USDA Food and Nutrition Information Center **www
   .nal.usda.gov/fnic**
USDA MyFoodapedia (calorie calculator) **http://fnic
   .nal.usda.gov/dietary-guidance/interactive-tools/
   calculators-and-counters**

Suggested Readings

Dunford, M. 2010. *Fundamentals of Sport and Exercise Nutrition.* Champaign, IL: Human Kinetics.

Finkelstein, E. A., and L. Zuckerman. 2008. *The Fattening of America.* Hoboken, NJ: John Wiley and Sons.

Gardener, H., et al. 2012. Mediterranean diet and white matter hyperintensity volume in the Northern Manhattan Study. *Archives of Neurology* 69(2):251–256.

Institute of Medicine, Food and Nutrition Board. 2010. *Strategies to Reduce Sodium Intake in the United States.* Washington, DC: National Academies Press.

Johnson, R. K., et al. 2009. Dietary sugars intake and cardiovascular health: A scientific statement from the American Heart Association. *Circulation* 120(11):1011–1020.

Kessler, D. 2009. *The End of Overeating: Taking Control of the Insatiable American Appetite.* New York: Rodale Press.

Otten, J. J., Helwig, J. P., and L. D. Meyers (Eds.). 2006. *Dietary Referenced Intakes: The Essential Guide to Nutrient Requirements.* Washington, DC: Institute of Medicine, National Academy of Science Press.

Pan, A., et al. 2012. Red meat consumption and mortality: Results from 2 prospective cohort studies. *American Journal of Public Health* 100(2):312–318.

Roberto, C. A., et al. 2010. Evaluating the impact of menu labeling on food choices and intake. *American Journal of Public Health* 100(2):312–318.

Wardlaw, G. M. 2011. *Contemporary Nutrition.* New York: McGraw-Hill Higher Education.

Healthy People 2020

The objectives listed below are societal goals designed to help all Americans improve their health between now and the year 2020. They were selected because they relate to the content of this concept.

- Increase the contribution of fruits in the diet.
- Increase the variety and contribution of vegetables in the diet.
- Increase the contribution of whole grains in the diet.
- Reduce consumption of saturated fat in the diet.

- Reduce consumption of sodium.
- Increase consumption of calcium.
- Reduce iron deficiency.

A national goal is to increase fruit and vegetables in the diet. This is information children learn in elementary school, yet many Americans fail to meet the guideline that "half of the plate should be fruits and vegetables." What can be done to change the pattern of eating so that more people eat adequate fruits and vegetables?

connect
ACTIVITY

Lab 14A Nutrition Analysis

Name Jason Herrm

Section

Date

Purpose: To learn to keep a dietary log, to determine the nutritional quality of your diet, to determine your average daily caloric intake, and to determine necessary changes in eating habits

Procedures

1. Record your dietary intake for 2 days using the Daily Diet Record sheets (see pages 345–346). Record intake for 1 weekday and 1 weekend day. You may wish to make copies of the record sheet for future use.
2. Include the actual foods eaten and the amount (size of portion in teaspoons, tablespoons, cups, ounces, or other standard units of measurement). Be sure to include all drinks (coffee, tea, soft drinks, etc.). Include *all* foods eaten, including sauces, gravies, dressings, toppings, spreads, and so on. Determine your caloric consumption for each of the 2 days. Use the calorie guides at the **myplate.gov** website to assist in evaluating your diet.
3. List the number of servings from each food group by each food choice.
4. Estimate the proportion of complex carbohydrate, simple carbohydrate, protein, and fat in each meal and in snacks, as well as for the total day.
5. Answer the questions in Chart 1 on page 344, using information for a typical day based on the Daily Diet Record sheets. Score 1 point for each "yes" answer. Then use Chart 2 to rate your dietary habits (circle rating).
6. Complete the Conclusions and Implications sections

Results

Record the number of calories consumed for each of the 2 days.

Weekday [1080] calories   Weekend [ ] calories

Conclusions and Implications: In several sentences, discuss your diet as recorded in this lab. Explain any changes in your eating habits that may be necessary. Comment on whether the days you surveyed are typical of your normal diet.

Honestly for the assignment I ate fewer calories than I usually do. I think the reason is because I was more conscientous about my diet. Overall I have moderate eating habits. I could defmately improve

Chart 1 Dietary Habits Questionnaire

Yes **No**   **Answer questions based on a typical day (use your Daily Diet Records to help).**

○	Ø	1. Do you eat at least three healthy meals each day?
Ø	○	2. Do you eat a healthy breakfast?
Ø	○	3. Do you eat lunch regularly?
Ø	○	4. Does your diet contain 45 to 65 percent carbohydrates with a high concentration of fiber?*
○	Ø	5. Are less than one-fourth of the carbohydrates you eat simple carbohydrates?
Ø	○	6. Does your diet contain 10 to 35 percent protein?*
○	Ø	7. Does your diet contain 20 to 35 percent fat?*
○	Ø	8. Do you limit the amount of saturated fat in your diet (no more than 10 percent)?
Ø	○	9. Do you limit salt intake to acceptable amounts?
Ø	○	10. Do you get adequate amounts of vitamins in your diet without a supplement?
Ø	○	11. Do you typically eat 6 to 11 servings from the bread, cereal, rice, and pasta group of foods?
Ø	○	12. Do you typically eat 3 to 5 servings of vegetables?
Ø	○	13. Do you typically eat 2 to 4 servings of fruits?
○	Ø	14. Do you typically eat 2 to 3 servings from the milk, yogurt, and cheese group of foods?
Ø	○	15. Do you typically eat 2 to 3 servings from the meat, poultry, fish, beans, eggs, and nuts group of foods?
○	Ø	16. Do you drink adequate amounts of water?
Ø	○	17. Do you get adequate minerals in your diet without a supplement?
Ø	○	18. Do you limit your caffeine and alcohol consumption to acceptable levels?
Ø	○	19. Is your average caloric consumption reasonable for your body size and for the amount of calories you normally expend?

13	Total number of "yes" answers

*Based on USDA standards.

Chart 2 Dietary Habits Rating Scale

Score	Rating
18–19	Very good
15–17	Good
13–14	Marginal
12 or less	Poor

Daily Diet Record

Day 1

Breakfast Food	Amount (cups, tsp., etc.)	Calories	Bread/Cereal	Fruit/Veg.	Milk/Meat	Fat/Sweet	Estimated Meal Calories %
Smoothie	16 oz	220		3	1	1	
							10 % Protein
							0 % Fat
							45 % Complex carbohydrate
							45 % Simple carbohydrate
							100% Total
Meal Total	✕						

Lunch Food	Amount (cups, tsp., etc.)	Calories	Bread/Cereal	Fruit/Veg.	Milk/Meat	Fat/Sweet	Estimated Meal Calories %
Bagel	1	259	2				
Cream Cheese	1 tbls					1	
Cranberry Chicken Salad	2 C	526		3			3 % Protein
							30 % Fat
							60 % Complex carbohydrate
							7 % Simple carbohydrate
							100% Total
Meal Total	✕						

Dinner Food	Amount (cups, tsp., etc.)	Calories	Bread/Cereal	Fruit/Veg.	Milk/Meat	Fat/Sweet	Estimated Meal Calories %
Club Sandwich	10 oz	500	2	1	2	1	
Almond milk	2.5 c	200		1			15 % Protein
							20 % Fat
							40 % Complex carbohydrate
							25 % Simple carbohydrate
							100% Total
Meal Total	✕						

Snack Food	Amount (cups, tsp., etc.)	Calories	Bread/Cereal	Fruit/Veg.	Milk/Meat	Fat/Sweet	Estimated Snack Calories %
Sweet Potato Fries	1 C	440	2			1	
Coconut Water	17 oz	120	1	1			% Protein
							15 % Fat
							60 % Complex carbohydrate
							25 % Simple carbohydrate
							100% Total
Meal Total	✕						

							Estimated Daily Total Calories %
Daily Totals	✕	2265	7	9	3	4	20 % Protein
		Calories	Servings	Servings	Servings	Servings	5 % Fat
							60 % Complex carbohydrate
							25 % Simple carbohydrate
							100% Total

Daily Diet Record

Day 2

Breakfast Food	Amount (cups, tsp., etc.)	Calories	Food Servings				Estimated Meal Calories %
			Bread/Cereal	Fruit/Veg.	Milk/Meat	Fat/Sweet	
Kale Smoothie	16 oz	265		3	1	1	
Bagel Sandwich	2 C	330	2		1	1	20 % Protein
							20 % Fat
							40 % Complex carbohydrate
							20 % Simple carbohydrate
							100% Total
Meal Total	✕						

Lunch Food	Amount (cups, tsp., etc.)	Calories	Food Servings				Estimated Meal Calories %
			Bread/Cereal	Fruit/Veg.	Milk/Meat	Fat/Sweet	
Chicken Wings	1.5 serving	330			2	1	
							% Protein
							% Fat
							% Complex carbohydrate
							% Simple carbohydrate
							100% Total
Meal Total	✕						

Dinner Food	Amount (cups, tsp., etc.)	Calories	Food Servings				Estimated Meal Calories %
			Bread/Cereal	Fruit/Veg.	Milk/Meat	Fat/Sweet	
Chef Salad	2 C	400		3	1	1	
							20 % Protein
							20 % Fat
							40 % Complex carbohydrate
							20 % Simple carbohydrate
							100% Total
Meal Total	✕						

Snack Food	Amount (cups, tsp., etc.)	Calories	Food Servings				Estimated Snack Calories %
			Bread/Cereal	Fruit/Veg.	Milk/Meat	Fat/Sweet	
Bagel/cream cheese	1.5 C	330	2			1	
Lemon Bar	3 oz	160	1	0.5		1	34 % Fat
							60 % Complex carbohydrate
							6 % Simple carbohydrate
							% Protein
							100% Total
Meal Total	✕						

							Estimated Daily Total Calories %
Daily Totals	✕	1815	5	6.5	5	6	10 % Protein
		Calories	Servings	Servings	Servings	Servings	10 % Fat
							60 % Complex carbohydrate
							20 % Simple carbohydrate
							100% Total

Lab 14B Selecting Nutritious Foods

Name **Section** **Date**

Purpose: To learn to select a nutritious diet, to determine the nutritive value of favorite foods, and to compare nutritious and favorite foods in terms of nutrient content

Procedures

1. Select a favorite breakfast, lunch, and dinner from the foods list in Appendix C. Include between-meal snacks with the nearest meal. If you cannot find foods you would normally choose, select those most similar to choices you might make.
2. Select a breakfast, lunch, and dinner from foods you feel would make the most nutritious meals. Include between-meal snacks with the nearest meal.
3. Record your "favorite foods" and "nutritious foods" on page 348. Record the calories for proteins, carbohydrates, and fats for each of the foods you choose.
4. Total each column for the "favorite" and the "nutritious" meals.
5. Determine the percentages of your total calories that are protein, carbohydrate, and fat by dividing each column total by the total number of calories consumed.
6. Comment on what you learned in the Conclusions and Implications section.

Results: Record your results below. Calculate percentage of calories from each source by dividing total calories into calories from each food source (protein, carbohydrates, or fat).

Food Selection Results

Source	Favorite Foods Calories	Favorite Foods % of Total Calories	Nutritious Foods Calories	Nutritious Foods % of Total Calories
Protein				
Carbohydrates				
Fat				
Total 100%		100%		100%

Conclusions and Implications: In several sentences, discuss the differences you found between your nutritious diet and your favorite diet. Discuss the quality of your nutritious diet as well as other things you learned from doing this lab.

"Favorite" versus "Nutritious" Food Choices for Three Daily Meals

Breakfast Favorite — Food Choices

Food	Cal.	Pro. Cal.	Car. Cal.	Fat Cal.
Totals				

Breakfast Nutritious — Food Choices

Food	Cal.	Pro. Cal.	Car. Cal.	Fat Cal.
Totals				

Lunch Favorite — Food Choices

Food	Cal.	Pro. Cal.	Car. Cal.	Fat Cal.
Totals				

Lunch Nutritious — Food Choices

Food	Cal.	Pro. Cal.	Car. Cal.	Fat Cal.
Totals				

Dinner Favorite — Food Choices

Food	Cal.	Pro. Cal.	Car. Cal.	Fat Cal.
Totals				
Daily Totals (Calories)				
Daily % of Total Calories				

Dinner Nutritious — Food Choices

Food	Cal.	Pro. Cal.	Car. Cal.	Fat Cal.
Totals				
Daily Totals (Calories)				
Daily % of Total Calories				

Managing Diet and Activity for Healthy Body Fatness

LEARNING OBJECTIVES

After completing the study of this concept, you will be able to:

▶ Explain the principles for weight control and the concept of energy balance.

▶ Identify the features of an obesogenic environment that influence our behavior.

▶ Outline guidelines for weight loss treatments.

▶ Describe and apply, when appropriate, guidelines for losing body fat.

▶ Utilize healthy shopping and eating strategies and guidelines.

▶ Evaluate fast-food options.

Various management strategies for eating and performing physical activity are useful in achieving and maintaining optimal body composition.

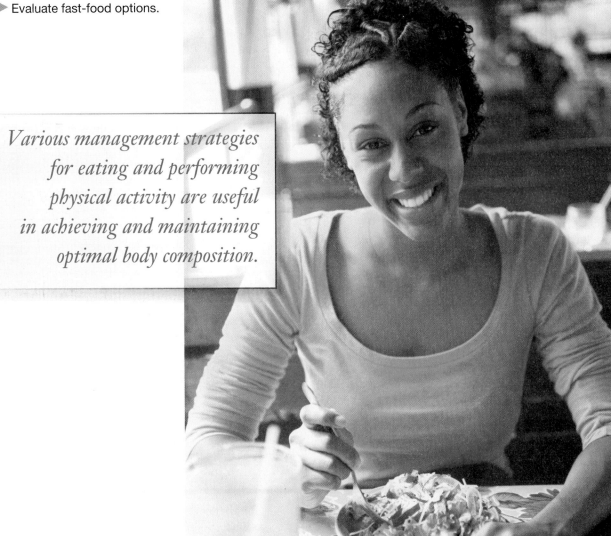

The fact that more than 67 percent of adult Americans are classified as overweight is clear evidence that weight control is a vexing problem for the majority of the population. Most recognize the importance of the problem and want to correct it. In fact, a recent national survey by the International Food Information Council (IFIC) reported that nearly two-thirds of Americans were either very concerned or somewhat concerned about their weight.

Too often, the focus is on appearance rather than health and on weight loss rather than fat loss. In attempts to lose weight, the dietary (energy intake) side of the energy balance equation is typically emphasized. However, the energy expenditure side of the equation is just as important, if not more so. Despite the documented benefits, few people trying to lose weight are physically active. A state-based survey determined that approximately one-half of individuals trying to lose weight do not engage in any physical activity, and only 15 percent report exercising regularly. The challenges many people experience with weight control may be an indirect reflection of the challenges people face in trying to be more active. Although being physically active cannot ensure you will become as thin as you desire, you may attain a body size that is appropriate for your genetics and body type.

The focus in this concept is on lifestyle patterns (both diet and physical activity) that will assist with losing body fat rather than weight. Guidelines for maintaining healthy body fat levels over time are also presented.

Factors Influencing Weight and Fat Control

Long-term weight control requires a balance between energy intake and energy expenditure. The relationships governing energy balance are very simple—the number of calories expended must match the number consumed. There may be subtle differences on a daily basis, but if intake exceeds expenditure over a period of time, a person will store the extra calories as body fat. The average person gains 1 pound of weight (i.e., fat) for every year over the age of 25. This may sound like a lot but it represents a calorie difference of only 10 kcal per day (approximately the calories found in a cracker or potato chip). This subtle difference shows the precise regulation of intake and expenditure that is normally in effect when a person maintains his or her body weight. The built-in regulation system is based on our appetite, which guides us when we might be running low on energy.

Figure 1 shows the hypothetical balance between energy intake and expenditure. Energy intake comes from the three major nutrients in our diet (carbohydrates, fats, and proteins) as well as from alcohol. Energy

expenditure can be divided into three major components as well. Basal metabolism accounts for the bulk of daily energy expenditure (60 percent to 75 percent) and this refers to the calories expended to maintain basic body functions while the body is at rest. A second category, called thermogenesis, captures the energy expended processing the food we eat (approximately 10 percent of total daily energy expenditure). The third and most variable component of energy expenditure rate is physical activity (typically accounting for 10 to 30 percent of total energy expenditure in most people). To maintain a healthy weight, a person's overall energy expenditure must offset energy intake. While it is difficult to monitor these directly, the body has built-in regulatory systems that help in weight regulation. Detailed coverage of these pathways is beyond the scope of the book, but the most important part of the system is your appetite because it helps prompt and influence eating.

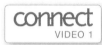

Physical activity contributes to energy balance in a number of ways. By maintaining an active lifestyle, you can burn off extra calories, keep your body's metabolism high, and prevent the decline in basal metabolic rate that typically occurs with aging (due to reduced muscle mass). All types of physical activity from the physical activity pyramid can be beneficial to weight control. Moderate physical activity (see Concept 6) is especially effective because people of all ages and abilities can perform it. It can be maintained for long periods of time and results in significant calorie expenditure. Long-term studies show that 60 or more minutes of moderate activity such as walking is very effective for long-term weight loss and maintenance.

Vigorous physical activity (see Concepts 7 and 8) can also be effective in maintaining or losing weight. For some people, especially older adults, vigorous activity may be more difficult to adhere to over a long time. However, for

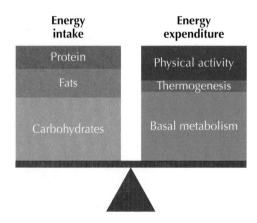

Figure 1 ▶ Components of energy intake must balance components of energy expenditure for weight maintenance.

those who stick with it, vigorous activity expends more calories in a shorter time, and for this reason, it can be a very good way to expend calories. Research shows that bouts of vigorous physical activity can lead to increases in basal metabolic rate that persist throughout the day. Therefore, vigorous activity can contribute to additional energy expenditure after the workout is done. There is now considerable evidence showing that muscle fitness exercise also contributes to maintaining a healthy body weight (see Concept 9). Muscle fitness exercise expends calories and increases muscle mass, leading to an increase in calories expended at rest. Flexibility exercises (see Concept 10) also expend calories, but are of lower intensity than other types of activities on the pyramid. They can still contribute to energy expenditure, however.

The accumulation of light physical activity can help burn extra calories. Most of the emphasis in this book has been on moderate and vigorous forms of physical activity. As described in Concept 6, "light" physical activity falls between rest and moderate physical activity on the energy expenditure continuum (1.5 to 3 METS). Research indicates that light activities may help reduce risks associated with excessive time spent being sedentary (e.g., sitting). The accumulation of light activity can also contribute to weight control by burning more calories. Researchers coined the term NEAT (non-exercise activity thermogenesis) to refer to the accumulation of activity from low-intensity movements throughout the day. Light activity may account for

as little as 15 percent of total daily energy expenditure in sedentary people and up to 50 percent in people with more active jobs and lifestyles. The weight maintenance benefits of light or NEAT activity are greatest when the activities replace sedentary activities such as sitting (e.g., TV watching and computer use). To further take advantage of NEAT, many people have started using active workstations that allow them to walk slowly on a treadmill or lightly pedal a bike while working at a computer.

Awareness and dietary restraint are needed to avoid excess caloric intake. In our modern society, it is very easy for people to meet their daily energy needs. In fact, considerable willpower is needed to keep energy intake at a manageable level. Having an extra cookie or brownie for a snack may sound like a good idea until you realize you would need to possibly walk between one and two miles to burn it off. Foods high in empty calories are easily available and are frequent selections of college students, who may be responsible for their food selection or preparation for the first time in their lives. Sugar, especially from soft drinks, and beer add calories. Learning to make healthy choices and showing some restraint with food intake are important skills for long-term weight control.

Many find it difficult to establish these patterns and develop unhealthy relationships with food, either restraining too much or using food as a source of comfort when feeling sad, anxious, or bored. The latter has been termed "emotional eating" since the consumption of food is directly tied to our emotions. The assumption has been that the food is consumed in response to emotional situations, but new research shows that consumption of some foods may actually have reciprocal effects on our emotions. One study showed that consumption of a high-fat snack helped people fend off negative emotions more effectively than a control snack. The biological connection between food and our brain may have had some evolutionary advantage in the past, but it can be problematic in our present society where food is abundant. While an occasional binge may not be a problem, emotional eating can escalate into a more compulsive habit that is hard to control. To avoid emotional eating, find other non-food-related methods to combat stress or help relax.

Confronting an Obesogenic Environment

An obesogenic environment makes it hard to maintain a healthy weight. Although traditional approaches to weight control have emphasized individual behaviors, public health leaders focus considerable

---

HELP **Health is available to Everyone for a Lifetime, and it's Personal**

A survey by the International Food Information Council reports that only 9 percent of people in the United States know the approximate number of calories they should eat in a day. About 9 percent report actually tracking their calories on a daily basis. Calorie requirements are unique to each person and are influenced by your gender, age, body size, and physical activity level. Typical ranges for a small sedentary woman may be 1,400 to 1,600 or 2,000 to 2,200 for a sedentary man. Our body has a natural ability to regulate intake (appetite) but people tend to disregard it or not pay attention to the cues. Some experts are concerned about the lack of awareness about calorie requirements. For example, if you knew your calorie requirement was 1,600 calories a day you may think twice about eating a burger and fries that contain 1,200 calories at one meal.

What steps can you take to make sure that you do not exceed recommended daily calorie requirements for your age, gender, and activity level?

connect ACTIVITY

energy on combating *"obesogenic environments"* that promote excessive eating and inactivity. For example, the 2010 Dietary Guidelines acknowledge that Americans have to make dietary choices *"within the context of an environment that promotes over-consumption of calories and discourages physical activity."* A variety of social-ecological models have been proposed to summarize and study these environments. A simplified model is depicted in Figure 2 to show the various sectors and settings that shape our environment and ultimately our behavior. The essence of the model is that we are continually confronted with environments that make it easy to consume large quantities of energy-dense food and limit our physical activity. On the energy-intake side, we have easy access to large quantities of low-cost, highly-palatable, high-calorie foods almost everywhere we go. The convenience and large portion sizes lead to increases in daily energy intake. On the energy expenditure side, we live in a world dominated by sedentary (computer-based) jobs and lifestyles dominated by automobiles and inactive recreation. These factors lead to reductions in daily energy expenditure. Small increases in energy intake combined with small decreases in energy expenditure lead to the storage of fat. While most people are aware of these general influences, they still find it hard to find ways to overcome them.

New public/private partnerships offer promise for promoting healthier environments. As shown in Figure 2, aspects of our environment are influenced by larger societal and economic forces. For example, it is unrealistic to expect changes in menu choices in a local fast-food restaurant since they receive their food from the corporate supply chain, which in turn receives ingredients

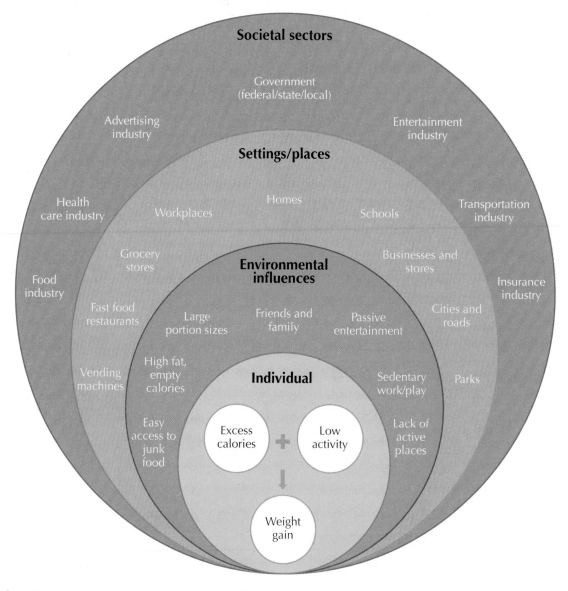

Figure 2 ▶ Social and environmental components of the obesogenic environment.

from other larger food conglomerates. To reverse the epidemic of obesity, a coordinated systemwide approach is needed. Changes in policy and the business supply chain offer the most promise since they can impact other aspects of the local environment. A number of large-scale public/private partnerships have shown potential for coordinated action. A few particularly prominent examples are highlighted below:

- *Healthy Weight Commitment Foundation* (www .healthyweightcommit.org). This large foundation is a consortium of grocery stores, food and beverage manufacturers, restaurants, sporting goods stores, insurance companies, and other health-related organizations that have joined forces to create healthier (less obesogenic) environments. This collaboration is unique because it is led by executives and CEOs of the various organizations. The group is committed to creating systematic changes in key segments of society in order to help reverse the obesity epidemic. The companies in the consortium may be in direct competition for consumer spending, yet here they are partnering together to help address a significant public health problem. For example, the food manufacturing companies in the group have pledged to work together to help reduce excess calorie consumption in their food products. They will do this by introducing lower-calorie options, changing recipes to lower the calorie content of current products, or by reducing portion sizes of existing single-serve products. The group has also launched several innovative social media tools and challenges to directly facilitate changes in society. One tool called Together Counts is designed to provide families with tools and resources to make (and track) healthy changes in their families. Another tool called Energy Balance 101 provides educational resources to teach principles of energy balance in schools.

- *Alliance for a Healthier Generation* (www.healthier generation.org). This nonprofit organization, formed as a partnership by the American Heart Association and the William J. Clinton Foundation, was established to specifically help to reverse the prevalence of childhood obesity. In 2006, the Alliance brokered agreements with beverage providers to limit portion sizes and reduce the number of beverage calories available to children during the school day. The agreement led to an 88 percent reduction in total beverage calories shipped to schools. A new agreement with leading food manufacturers, group purchasing organizations, and technology companies will enable America's schools to serve healthier meals at more affordable prices. Through the agreement, more than 30 million students across the country will have access to healthier school meals, including at least 14 million students who currently participate in the free and reduced lunch program. The Alliance also

established a new medically based partnership (Alliance Healthcare Initiative) that unites national medical associations, leading insurers, and employers to offer health benefits for the prevention, assessment, and treatment of childhood obesity. The agreement enables health-care providers to play a more active role in obesity treatment by making primary-care visits and visits to registered dietitians (RDs) a part of their health insurance benefits. The initiative will recruit additional health insurance companies and employers to participate so that more overweight American children have access to this care.

New public policies offer promise for promoting weight control. Public policy has a strong influence on behavior, because it has the potential to influence all segments of the population. Examples of recent public policy changes that have potential for helping reduce overweight are described below.

- *Posting food values in restaurants.* New legislation requires chain restaurants with 20 or more outlets to post calorie and other nutrition values for the foods they serve. The FDA has finalized guidelines for this legislation and new efforts will extend the labeling rules to vending machines. Posting food values has been shown to be effective in reducing calorie consumption in people eating at fast-food restaurants.

- *Restricting food commercials that target children.* The food industry adopted self-regulation on foods targeted for children, especially high-sugar, low-nutrient foods. Studies show that these self-regulations have made only small changes in advertising. Nutrition groups have proposed regulation requiring the food industry to advertise nutritious foods more often and to reduce advertising of non-nutritious foods during children's TV shows.

- *Ensuring healthy foods are available in school vending machines.* The USDA mandated that schools set formal policies for food service and vending machines. The requirements stipulate the latter must offer a balance of "healthy" and "unhealthy" food choices. Changes have also been made to limit soft drink consumption at schools.

- *Requiring more physical activity and physical education in schools.* Schools provide an infrastructure to help ensure that children get some regular physical activity each day. A national health goal is to increase the number of children who get daily physical education. Some states have imposed specific guidelines requiring schools to document that they are providing a certain amount of physical activity. Proposed federal legislation (Healthy Kids Outdoors Act) aims to increase children's access to outdoor recreational activities.

- *Promoting physical activity with incentives for participation.* Many companies provide employees with free access to employee-sponsored fitness centers or subsidies to use community fitness centers. Many also offer financial incentives for participation and flexible schedules for workouts during the day. Proposed changes in the Affordable Health Care Act would provide incentives for companies that adopt these types of measures.

- *Implementing policies and programs to promote active commuting.* Walk to school programs and Walking School Buses have become increasingly popular methods for promoting physical activity in youth. Different approaches are used for worksites but with the same goal of active commuting in mind. Buses and trains are often configured with bike racks. Many communities have also started investing in bike-share programs that allow individuals to check out a bike and drop it off at a different location. The systems are in widespread use in bicycle-friendly European countries and are slowly gaining momentum and visibility in the U.S.

- *Implementing empty calorie tax (also called fat tax).* Some public health experts have proposed a tax on foods low in nutritional density, such as sweetened soft drinks, candy, and fast food. Advocates of this type of tax propose that the proceeds go to campaigns to improve nutrition and increase activity levels.

Public support is strong for many of these policies. However, some people argue that policy changes such as a "fat tax" infringe on personal liberties. Nevertheless, changes in public policy have resulted in major reductions in smoking and smoking-related deaths over the past 20 years, and experts feel that similar policy changes can decrease obesity in America and reduce associated medical costs.

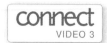

Guidelines for Losing Body Fat

Following appropriate weight loss guidelines is important for the best long-term results. There is considerable misinformation about diet and weight loss strategies, leading many people to use unsafe or ineffective weight loss supplements or to follow inappropriate exercise programs. Fat, weight, and body proportions are all factors that can be changed, but people often set goals that are impossible to achieve. Starting with small goals and aiming for reasonable rates of weight loss (1 to 2 pounds a week) are recommended. Setting unrealistic goals may result in eating disorders, failure to meet goals, or failure to maintain weight loss over time. Table 1 provides a summary of weight loss guidelines from the American College of Sports Medicine (ACSM).

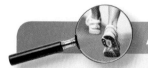

A CLOSER LOOK

Mindless Eating

In his book, *Mindless Eating*, Dr. Brian Wansink presents a somewhat different approach to eating. Based on his research, Dr. Wansink contends that subtle and almost imperceptible cues and prompts in our day contribute to a tendency to overeat ("*We overeat because of family and friends, packages and plates, names and numbers, labels and lights, colors and candles, shapes and smells, distractions and distances, cupboard and containers*"). His research on labels and containers led to the development of the 100-calorie snack packages. He also advocates for eating with smaller plates and drinking from taller glasses since it tricks our mind into thinking that we ate or drank more than we did. By better understanding cues that lead us to eat, we can set habits and environments that help us to eat less. According to Dr. Wansink, "The best diet is the one that you don't know that you are on."

Would this mental approach to weight control help you better regulate your weight?

Behavioral goals are more effective than outcome goals. Researchers have shown that setting only **outcome goals,** or goals that set a specific amount of weight or fat loss (or gain), can be discouraging. If a **behavioral goal** of eating a reasonable number of calories per day and expending a reasonable number of calories in exercise is met, outcome goals will be achieved. Most experts believe that behavioral goals work better than weight or fat loss goals, especially in the short term (see Concept 2 for tips about goal-setting principles and SMART goals).

A combination of physical activity and a healthy, low-calorie diet is the best approach for long-term weight control. The most effective diet for fat loss is a low-calorie diet that you can stick with over time. Reduced-calorie diets result in meaningful weight loss, regardless of the composition of the diet (e.g., carbohydrates, fats, proteins). Diets high in grains, fruits, and vegetables are generally recommended because they are typically low in calories and easy to maintain over time. Research also clearly indicates that regular exercise is crucial to long-term fat loss. Weight loss programs that do not include physical activity are likely to fail.

A major advantage of emphasizing both physical activity and dietary changes is that physical activity can help maintain basal metabolic rate and prevent the decline that occurs with calorie sparing. Studies have shown that programs that include both diet and physical activity promote greater loss of body fat than programs based solely

Table 1 ▶ Guidelines for Weight Loss Treatment

Questions about Weight Loss	Recommendations
Who should consider weight loss?	Individuals with a BMI of >25 or in the marginal or overfat zone *should consider* reducing their body weight—especially if it is accompanied by abdominal obesity. Individuals with a BMI of >30 *are encouraged to seek* weight loss treatment.
What types of goals should be established?	Overweight and obese individuals should target reducing their body weight by a minimum of 5 to 10 percent and should aim to maintain this long-term weight loss.
What about maintenance?	Individuals should strive for long-term weight maintenance and the prevention of weight regain over the long term, especially when weight loss is not desired or when attainment of ideal body weight is not achievable.
What should be targeted in a weight loss program?	Weight loss programs should target both eating and exercise behaviors, as sustained changes in both behaviors have been associated with significant long-term weight loss.
How should diet be changed?	Overweight and obese individuals should reduce their current intake by 500–1,000 kcal/day to achieve weight loss (<30% of calories from fat). Individualized levels of caloric intake should be established to prevent weight regain after initial loss.
How should activity be changed?	Overweight and obese individuals should progressively increase to a minimum of 150 minutes of moderate-intensity physical activity per week for health benefits. However, for long-term weight loss, the program should progress to higher amounts of activity (e.g., 200–300 minutes per week or >2,000 kcal/week).
What about resistance exercise?	Resistance exercise should supplement the endurance exercise program for individuals undertaking modest reductions in energy intake to lose weight.
What about using drugs for weight loss?	Pharmacotherapy (medicine/drugs) for weight loss should be used only by individuals with a BMI >30 or those with excessive body fatness. Weight loss medications should be used only in combination with a strong behavioral intervention that focuses on modifying eating and exercise behaviors.

Source: American College of Sports Medicine.

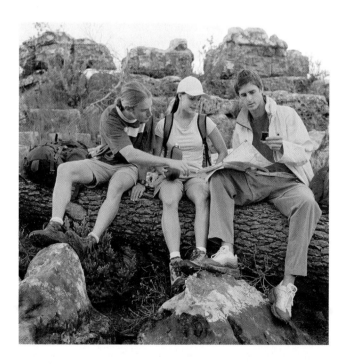

An active, healthy lifestyle is critical for long-term weight control.

on dietary changes. The total weight loss from the programs may be about the same, but a larger fraction of the weight comes from fat when physical activity is included. In contrast, programs based solely on diet result in greater loss of lean muscle tissue. A healthy diet and regular physical activity are the keys for long-term weight control. Small changes, such as eating a few hundred calories less per day or walking for 30 minutes every day, can make a big difference over time. The important point is to strive for permanent changes that can be maintained in a normal daily lifestyle.

Outcome Goal Statement of intent to achieve a specific test score or a specific standard associated with good health or wellness—for example, "I will lower my body fat level by 3 percent."

Behavioral Goal Statement of intent to perform a specific behavior (changing a lifestyle) for a specific period of time—for example, "I will reduce the calories in my diet by 200 a day for the next 4 weeks."

TECHNOLOGY UPDATE

Lifestyle Monitoring for Weight Control

The BodyMedia FIT system provides individuals with a comprehensive lifestyle monitoring tool to assist with weight control efforts. The advanced, multisensor, monitor (worn on the upper arm) tracks physical activity and energy expenditure while you go about your normal activities. Data can be displayed on a wrist display, linked to free smartphone apps, or uploaded to an online self-monitoring tool (Activity Manager). The online application makes it possible for users to record foods they eat in order to provide estimates of calorie intake, thereby aiding in energy balance (i.e., calories in minus calories out). The monitor and associated applications have been shown to facilitate weight loss in several controlled studies.

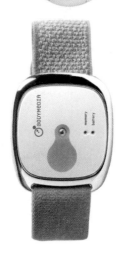

Motivation to lose weight may be enough for most people but a new partnership with a Web-based social media company (Earndit.com) allows users to earn financial rewards for their self-monitoring efforts. After registering through Earndit, you can associate your Bodymedia Fit monitor with your account. Earndit will then award points based upon the amount of activity you perform in a day. Similar to other social media tools (such as Groupon), the points are redeemable through associated vendors.

Would the extra motivation to monitor your activity help you maintain your weight loss goals?

connect
ACTIVITY

Small changes in eating patterns can be effective in fat loss. Experts suggest that we make over 200 food decisions in a given day. Making good food choices is generally easier at home than when eating at restaurants, work, or special occasions. Table 2 provides guidelines for making good selections when purchasing and preparing food at home as well as when you are away from home. Following are some specific steps you can take to improve your eating habits.

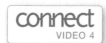

connect
VIDEO 4

- *Make small changes at first.* Small restrictions in caloric intake sustained over time are more effective than drastic short-term changers.

- *Eat breakfast every day.* Studies show that breakfast skipping is associated with an increased risk of obesity.

- *Consider eating smaller and more frequent meals in a day.* A common strategy in guided weight loss programs is to consume healthy, high protein snacks to help curb hunger and excess consumption at meals.

- *Eat less fat.* Research shows that reduction of fat in the diet results not only in fewer calories consumed (fats have more than twice the calories per gram as carbohydrates or proteins) but in greater body fat loss as well.

- *Restrict consumption of **empty calories**.* Foods that provide little nutrition often account for an excessive proportion of daily caloric intake. Examples of these foods are candy (often high in simple sugar) and potato chips (often fried in saturated fat).

- *Increase complex carbohydrates.* Foods high in fiber, such as fresh fruits and vegetables, contain few calories for their volume. They are nutritious and filling, and they are especially good foods for a fat loss program.

- *Learn the difference between craving and hunger.* Hunger is a physiological signal that helps promote an organism's drive to eat when energy supply gets low. A craving is simply a desire to eat something, often a food that is sweet or high in calories. When you feel the urge to eat, ask yourself, "Is this real hunger or a craving?"

- *Adopt a "mindful" approach to eating.* Most people consume food for enjoyment, but having a mindful approach to eating helps you learn to view food as sustenance or energy for healthy living. (See the Web Resources for more information on mindful eating.)

- *Use smaller plates and taller, thinner glasses for meals.* Research has shown that the size of serving dishes is related to the amount of food consumed. By using smaller plates and bowls and taller, thinner glasses you can help trick your mind into eating less.

- *Avoid negative self-talk.* One type of **negative self-talk** occurs when a person self-criticizes for not meeting a goal. For example, if you are determined not to eat more than one serving of food at a party but fail to meet this goal, you might say, "It's no use stopping now; I've already blown it." View this as a minor setback rather than a failure. A more appropriate response is **positive self-talk,** such as, "I'm not going to eat anything else tonight; I can do it."

Empty Calories   Calories in foods considered to have little or no nutritional value.

Negative Self-Talk   Self-defeating discussions with yourself focusing on your failures rather than your successes.

Positive Self-Talk   Telling yourself positive, encouraging things that help you succeed in accomplishing your goals.

Table 2 ▶ Guidelines for Healthy Shopping and Eating in a Variety of Settings

Guidelines for Shopping	• Shop from a list to avoid purchasing foods that contain empty calories and other foods that will tempt you to overeat. • Shop with a friend to avoid buying unneeded foods. For this technique to work, the other person must be sensitive to your goals. In some cases, a friend can have a bad, rather than a good, influence. • Shop on a full stomach to avoid the temptations of snacking on and buying junk food. • Check labels to avoid foods that are excessively high in fat or saturated fat.
Guidelines for How You Eat	• When you eat, do nothing else but eat. If you watch television, read, or do some other activity while you eat, you may be unaware of what you have eaten. • Eat slowly. Taste your food. Pause between bites. Chew slowly. Do not take the next bite until you have swallowed what you have in your mouth. Periodically take a longer pause. Be the last one finished eating. • Do not eat food you do not want. Some people do not want to waste food, so they clean their plate even when they feel full. • Follow an eating schedule. Eating at regular meal times can help you avoid snacking. Spacing meals equally throughout the day can help reduce appetite. • Leave the table after eating to avoid taking extra, unwanted bites and servings. • Eat meals of equal size. Some people try to restrict calories at one or two meals to save up for a big meal. • Eating several *small* meals helps you avoid hunger (fools the appetite), and this may help prevent overeating. • Avoid second servings. Limit your intake to one moderate serving. If second servings are taken, make them one-half the size of first servings. • Limit servings of salad dressings and condiments (e.g., catsup). These are often high in fat and sugar and can amount to greater caloric consumption than expected.
Guidelines for Controlling the Home Environment	• Store food out of sight. Avoid containers that allow you to see food. Limit the accessibility of foods that tempt you and foods with empty calories. Foods that are out of sight are out of mouth. • Do your eating in designated areas only, such as the kitchen and dining room, so you do not snack elsewhere. It is especially easy to eat too much while watching television. • If you snack, eat foods high in complex carbohydrates and low in fats, such as fresh fruits and carrot sticks. • Freeze leftovers so that it takes preparation to eat them, helping you avoid temptation.
Guidelines for Controlling the Work Environment	• Bring food from home rather than eating from vending machines or catering trucks. • Do not eat while working and take your lunch as a break. Do something active during breaks, such as taking a walk. • Avoid food provided by co-workers, such as snacks in work rooms, birthday cakes, or candy. • Have drinking water or low-calorie drinks available to substitute for snacks.
Guidelines for Eating on Special Occasions	• Practice ways to refuse food. Knowing exactly what to say will help you avoid being talked into eating something you do not want. • Eat before you go out, so you are not as hungry at parties and events. • Do not stand near food sources, and distract yourself if tempted to eat when you are not really hungry. • Limit servings of nonbasic parts of the meal, such as alcohol, soft drinks, appetizers, and desserts.
Guidelines for Eating at Restaurants	• Make healthy selections from the menu. Choose chicken without skin, fish, or lean cuts of meat. Grilled or broiled options are better than fried. Choose healthier options for dessert, as many decadent desserts can have more calories than the whole dinner. • Ask for the condiments (e.g., butter, mayonnaise, salad dressings) on the side, allowing you to determine how much to put on. • Do not feel compelled to eat everything on your plate. Many restaurants serve exceptionally large portions to try to please the customers. • Ask for a to-go box to divide big portions before eating. • Order à la carte rather than full meals to avoid multiple courses and servings. • Avoid supersizing your meals if eating at fast-food restaurants, as this can add unwanted calories. Opt for the child-sized meal if possible.

The support of family and friends can be of great importance in balancing caloric intake and caloric expenditure. Family and friends can help you adopt and maintain healthy eating practices and follow shopping guidelines (see Table 2). Sometimes, friends and family can "try too hard" to help. This can have the opposite effect if it is perceived as an attempt to control your behavior. Encouragement and support, rather than control of behavior, are the keys.

Group support can also be beneficial to many individuals attempting to change their behavior. Commercial

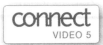

In the News

Diet Soft Drinks

Diet soft drinks are a popular, and seemingly healthy, choice for people concerned about excess calories. However, recent studies have reported that consumption of diet soft drinks may increase risk for Type 2 diabetes and cardiovascular disease. The most prominent findings have been from a 10-year longitudinal project called the Northern Manhattan Study. This study had a large sample of over 2,500 adults report on how much and what kind of soft drinks they drank. They followed participants for an average of 9 or more years and monitored risks for vascular events such as ischemic and hemorrhagic stroke. People who drank diet soft drinks every day had a 61 percent higher risk of vascular events than those who reported no soda drinking, even after controlling for a variety of demographic (e.g., age, gender, BMI) and lifestyle (smoking, alcohol, physical activity, calorie consumption) variables. The authors point out that diet soft drink drinkers should not be alarmed because the findings do not prove cause and effect. At present, there are no clear mechanisms that explain the findings, so additional work is clearly needed. The results, however, may lead some calorie-conscious consumers to rethink their beverage choices.

Do these results influence your thinking about the benefits and risks of diet soft drinks?

connect ACTIVITY

---

groups such as Overeaters Anonymous and Weight Watchers help those who need the support of peers in attaining and maintaining desirable fat levels for a lifetime. A number of new group-based lifestyle and fitness programs are available to provide social support for change (e.g., Kosama).

Facts about Fad Diets and Clinical Approaches to Weight Loss

Fad diets and extreme diets are not likely to be effective. Consumers are barraged with products and advertisements that claim easy weight loss solutions. Various fad diets capitalize on the consumer's concern about weight and a general lack of knowledge about diet and exercise. Fad diets often take some small fact about nutrition and claim they have uncovered some magic solution to weight loss that wasn't previously known. Consumers often believe the claims because they have a history of failing with past efforts to control their weight.

A common strategy in some fad diets is to restrict carbohydrates. Because water is required to store carbohydrates, reductions in carbohydrate intake leads to reductions in water storage—and weight. The person who restricts carbohydrates may see a reduction in "weight" (not fat!) and assume the diet worked when it didn't. Regardless of the approach, fad diets provide little hope since they typically can't

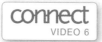
connect VIDEO 6

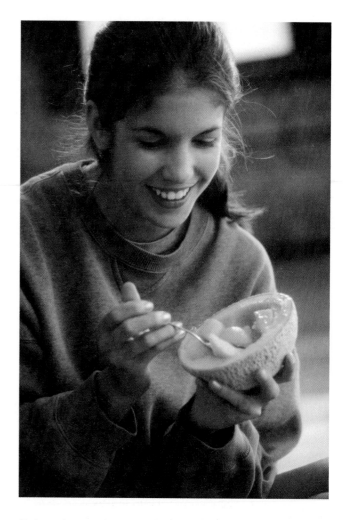

Fruits and vegetables are good snack choices to help reduce total calorie consumption and improve health.

be maintained over time. Constant losing and gaining, known as "yo-yo" dieting, is counterproductive and may lead to negative changes in the person's metabolism and unwanted shifts in sites of fat deposition.

Avoid diets that require severe caloric restriction and exercise programs that require exceptionally large caloric expenditure. These plans can be effective in fat loss over a short period but are seldom maintained for a lifetime. Studies show that extreme programs for weight control, designed to "take it off fast," result in long-term success rates of less than 5 percent. One reason extremely low calorie diets are ineffective is that they may promote "calorie sparing." When caloric intake is 800 to 1,000 or less, the body protects itself by reducing basal and resting metabolism levels (sparing calories). This results in less fat loss, even though the caloric intake is very low. When in doubt, avoid programs that promise fast and easy solutions, extreme diets that favor specific foods or eating patterns, and any product that makes unreasonable claims about easy ways to stimulate your metabolism or "melt away fat."

Artificial sweeteners and fat substitutes may help but do not provide a complete weight loss solution. Artificial sweeteners are frequently used in soft drinks and food to reduce the calorie content. Because they have few or no calories, these supplements were originally expected to help people with weight control. However, since they were introduced, the general public has not eaten fewer calories and more people are now overweight than before. People consuming these products end up consuming just as many calories per day as people consuming products with real sugar or sweeteners.

As described in Concept 14, a variety of artificial fat substitutes are now used to reduce fat content in foods. Potato chips and other fried foods cooked in these products as well as baked goods using these products have less fat and fewer calories. If you eat no more food than usual and substitute foods made with these products, you will consume fewer calories and less fat. Experts worry that consumers will not eat the same amount of foods with these fake fats but will feel they can eat more because the fake fats contain fewer calories and less fat.

A variety of appetite suppressants are available but all of them have limitations. Because long-term weight control is difficult, many individuals seek simple solutions from various nonprescription weight loss products. A common additive in dietary supplements has been the stimulant ephedra (or the herbal equivalent, Ma Huang). Many negative reactions and multiple deaths have been attributed to the use of ephedra, and this led the FDA to ban the sale and use of any products containing this compound. A concern among public health officials is that many products still do not accurately label the contents of their supplements. Manufacturers of supplements have recently started selling "ephedra-free" supplements that use other stimulants, but these have been shown to present similar health risks. Consumers should be wary of dietary supplements, due to the unregulated nature of the industry.

Four prescription drugs have been approved by the FDA to help patients curb appetite and lose weight. Sibutramine (Meridia) acts by inhibiting the reuptake of the neurotransmitters serotonin and noradrenaline, which regulate hunger. Orlistat (used in prescription Xenical and over-the-counter Alli) enhances weight loss by inhibiting the body's absorption of fat. Studies have confirmed that it can help patients lose more weight, but a limitation is that it also blocks the absorption of fat-soluble vitamins. Belviq, like Sibutramine, acts to inhibit the reuptake of neurotransmitters that regulate hunger. Qsymia (Qnexa), the most recently approved, suppresses appetite and increases feelings of fullness. All of the prescription medications are considered to be adjuncts to lifestyle modification and are designed for use with only obese patients or overweight adults with other comorbidities.

Products and procedures claiming to remove fat cells are not safe or effective. A procedure known as "lipodissolve" claims that it is possible to remove fat cells from the body with chemicals. A small amount of a chemical found in lecithin—a food ingredient derived from soybeans—is injected into fatty areas of the body, such as the buttocks or thighs. The fat absorbs the substance (phosphatidylcholine deoxycholate, or PCDC), resulting in an inflammation, followed by a hardening of the fat cells in the area. The fat cells are then allegedly eliminated from the body. The FDA has not approved the procedure, and the safety and effectiveness of the procedure has not been demonstrated by scientific evidence. However, there are reports of the procedure being marketed as a "quick fix" that "burns fat away with an injection." Companies promoting the injections have marketed them as a dietary supplement because the active ingredient (lecithin) has been approved for human consumption by mouth. However, because the PCDC is injected (rather than consumed by mouth), the FDA views the product as a drug and has ordered the manufacturer to stop marketing and distributing the product due to safety concerns. In addition to unproven effectiveness, the procedure can cause permanent scarring, skin deformation, and deep, painful knots under the skin where the lipodissolve treatments are given. This highlights why consumers should be wary of unproven procedures they see on the Internet.

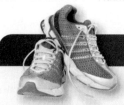

Strategies for Action

Knowing about guidelines for controlling body fat is not as important as following them. The guidelines in this concept work only if you use them. In Lab 15A, you will identify guidelines that may help you in the future.

Record keeping is important in meeting fat control goals and making moderation a part of your normal lifestyle. It is easy to fool yourself when determining the amount of food you have eaten or the amount of exercise you have done. Once fat control goals have been set, whether for weight loss, maintenance, or gain, keeping a diet log and an exercise log can help you monitor your behavior and maintain the lifestyle necessary to meet your goals. A log can also help you monitor changes in weight and body fat levels. But remember, avoid too much emphasis on short-term weight changes. Lab 15B will help you learn about the actual content of fast foods, so you can learn to make better choices when eating out.

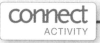

Web Resources

Academy of Nutrition and Dietetics **www.eatright.org**
Berkeley Nutrition Sciences **www.nutritionquest.com**
Center for Mindful Eating **www.tcme.org**
Mindless Eating **http://mindlesseating.org**
Nutrition Action Health Letter **www.cspinet.org/nah**
Nutriwatch (consumer website) **www.nutriwatch.org**
Office of Dietary Supplements **http://ods.od.nih.gov**
STOP Obesity Alliance **www.stopobesityalliance.org**
USDA Food and Nutrition Information Center **www.nal.usda.gov/fnic**

Suggested Readings

Burke, M. A., et al. 2010. From "Overweight" to "About Right": Evidence of a generational shift in body weight norms. *Obesity* 18(6):1226–1234.

Centers for Disease Control and Prevention. 2011. Beverage Consumption Among High School Students—United States, MMWR 60(23):778–780.

Chozen Bays, J. 2009. *Mindful Eating: A Guide to Rediscovering a Healthy and Joyful Relationship with Food.* Boston: Shambhala.

Harris, J. L., et al. 2009. Priming effects of television food advertising on eating behavior. *Health Psychology* 28(4): 404–413.

Katz, M. H., and R. Katz. 2010. Food surcharges and subsidies: Putting your money where your mouth is. *Archives of Internal Medicine* 170(5):405–406.

Kessler, D. 2009. *The End of Overeating: Taking Control of the Insatiable American Appetite.* New York: Rodale Press.

King, N. A., Horner, K., and A. P. Hills. 2012. Exercise, appetite and weight management: Understanding the compensatory responses in eating behavior and how they contribute to variability in exercise-induced weight loss. *British Journal of Sports Medicine* 46:315–322.

Lee, I., et al. 2010. Physical activity and weight gain prevention. *Journal of the American Medical Association* 303(12):1173–1179.

Lusk, A. C., et al. 2010. Bicycle riding, walking and weight gain in premenopausal women. *Archives of Internal Medicine* 170(12):1050–1056.

Lynch, F. L., et al. 2010. Cognitive behavioral guided self-help for the treatment of recurrent binge eating. *Journal of Consulting and Clinical Psychology* 78(3):312–321.

Lynch, F. L., et al. 2010. Cost-effectiveness of guided self-help treatment for recurrent binge eating. *Journal of Consulting and Clinical Psychology* 78(3):322–333.

Ogden, C. L., et al. 2012. Prevalence of obesity in the United States (2009–2010). NCHS data brief, no 82. Hyattsville, MD: National Center for Health Statistics.

Papalazarou, A., et al. 2010. Lifestyle intervention favorably affects weight loss and maintenance following obesity surgery. *Obesity* 18:1348–1353.

Shehzad, A., et al. 2012. Adiponectin: Regulation of its production and its role in human disease. *Hormones* 11(1):8–20.

Striegel-Moore, R., et al. 2010. Cognitive behavioral guided self-help for the treatment of recurrent binge eating. *Journal of Consulting and Clinical Psychology* 78(3):312–321.

Van Oudenhove, L., et al. 2011. Fatty acid-induced gut-brain signaling attenuates neural and behavioral effects of sad emotion in humans. *Journal of Clinical Investigation* 121(8):3094–3099.

Wansink, B. 2007. *Mindless Eating: Why We Eat More Than We Think.* New York: Bantam Books.

Wardlaw, G. M. 2011. *Contemporary Nutrition.* New York: McGraw-Hill Higher Education.

Westcott, W. 2009. ACSM strength training guidelines: Role in body composition and health enhancement. *ACSM's Health and Fitness Journal* 13(4):14–22.

Healthy People 2020

The objectives listed below are societal goals designed to help all Americans improve their health between now and the year 2020. They were selected because they relate to the content of this concept.

- Increase policies that give retail food outlets incentives for foods that meet dietary guidelines.

- Increase work sites that offer nutrition and weight management classes and counseling.

- Increase participation in employee wellness programs.

- Increase BMI measurement by primary care physicians.

- Increase physician counseling on nutrition and weight management.

- Reduce percentage of adults who do no leisure-time activity.

- Reduce consumption of calories from solid fats and added sugars.

- Decrease the consumption of sugar-sweetened beverages.

- Reduce consumption of saturated fat in the diet.

- Increase proportion of adults with healthy weight.

- Reduce childhood overweight and obesity.

A national goal is to reduce the consumption of sugar-sweetened beverages. A 12 oz. soft drink contains 10 teaspoons of sugar and has no other nutritional values. Substituting consumption of soft drinks with water, milk, or 100 percent fruit juice would improve overall nutrition quality and reduce calorie consumption. Do you agree with proposals that would tax soft drink consumption in order to reduce consumption and shift consumer choices to healthier beverages?

connect
ACTIVITY

Lab 15A Selecting Strategies for Managing Eating

Name: Jason Herron

Section: _____ Date: _____

Purpose: To learn to select strategies for managing eating to control body fatness

Procedures

1. Read the strategies listed in Chart 1.
2. Check the box beside 5 to 10 of the strategies that you think will be most useful for you.
3. Answer the questions in the Conclusions and Implications section.

Chart 1 Strategies for Managing Eating to Control Body Fatness

✔	Check 5 to 10 strategies that you might use in the future.
	Shopping Strategies
✔	Shop from a list.
	Shop with a friend.
✔	Shop on a full stomach.
✔	Check food labels.
	Consider foods that take some time to prepare.
	Methods of Eating
✔	When you eat, do nothing but eat. Don't watch television or read.
✔	Eat slowly.
✔	Do not eat food you do not want.
✔	Follow an eating schedule.
	Do your eating in designated areas, such as kitchen or dining room only.
	Leave the table after eating.
✔	Avoid second servings.
	Limit servings of condiments.
✔	Limit servings of nonbasics, such as dessert, breads, and soft drinks.
	Eat several meals of equal size rather than one big meal and two small ones.
	Eating in the Work Environment
✔	Bring your own food to work.
✔	Avoid snack machines.
	If you eat out, plan your meal ahead of time.
	Do not eat while working.
	Avoid sharing foods from co-workers, such as birthday cakes.
	Have activity breaks during the day.
✔	Have water available to substitute for soft drinks.
✔	Have low-calorie snacks to substitute for office snacks.

✔	Check 5 to 10 strategies that you might use in the future.
	Eating on Special Occasions
✔	Practice ways to refuse food.
✔	Avoid tempting situations.
	Eat before you go out.
	Don't stand near food sources.
	If you feel the urge to eat, find someone to talk to.
	Strategies for Eating Out
✔	Limit deep-fat fried foods.
	Ask for information about food content.
	Limit use of condiments.
	Choose low-fat foods (e.g., skim milk, low-fat yogurt).
✔	Choose chicken, fish, or lean meat.
	Order à la carte.
	Ask early for a to-go box and divide portions.
	If you eat desserts, avoid those with sauces or toppings.
	Eating at Home
	Keep busy at times when you are at risk of overeating.
	Store food out of sight.
	Avoid serving food to others between meals.
✔	If you snack, choose snacks with complex carbohydrates, such as carrot sticks or apple slices.
✔	Freeze leftovers to avoid the temptation of eating them between meals.

Conclusions and Implications

1. In several sentences, discuss your need to use strategies for effective eating. Do you need to use them? Why or why not?

My main strategyes is to track my eating. If I have a plan I am much more likely to eat well. When I plan my meals I don't stray from healthy food. I allow myself a cheat day to address cravings.

2. In several sentences, discuss the effectiveness of the strategies contained in Chart 1. Do you think they can be effective for people who have a problem controlling their body fatness?

I think the strategies listed are effective. The issue is discipline. People need to stick to whatever plan they have for themselves. Once self-control is developed these items are more effective

3. In several sentences, discuss the value of using behavioral goals versus outcome goals when planning for fat loss.

Behavioral goals are more important. The most important behavioral trait is self control. Outcome will come later if behavior is changed.

Lab 15B Evaluating Fast-Food Options

Name		Section	Date

Purpose: To learn about the energy and fat content of fast food and how to make better choices when eating at fast-food restaurants

Procedures

1. Select a fast-food restaurant and a typical meal that you might order. Then use an online food calculator to determine total calories, fat calories, saturated fat intake, and cholesterol for each food item.
2. Record the values in Chart 2.
3. Sum the totals for the meal in Chart 2.
4. Record recommended daily values by selecting an amount from Chart 1. The estimate should be based on your estimated needs for the day.
5. Compute the percentage of the daily recommended amounts that you consume in the meal by dividing recommended amounts (step 4) into meal totals (step 3). Record percent of recommended daily amounts in Chart 2.
6. Answer the questions in the Conclusions and Implications section.

Chart 1 Recommended Daily Amounts of Fat, Saturated Fat, Cholesterol, and Sodium

	2,000 kcal	3,000 kcal
Total fat	65 g	97.5 g
Saturated fat	20 g	30 g
Cholesterol	300 mg	450 mg
Sodium	2,400 mg	3,600 g

Results

Chart 2 Listing of Foods Selected for the Meal

Food Item	Total Calories	Total Fat (g)	Saturated Fat (g)	Cholesterol (mg)
1.				
2.				
3.				
4.				
5.				
6.				
Total for meal (sum up each column)				
Recommended daily amount (record your values from Chart 1)				
% of recommended daily amount (record your % of recommended)				

Consult an online fast food calculator to estimate calorie content of menu choices (see www.fastfoodnutrition.org).

Conclusions and Implications:

1. Describe how often you eat at fast-food restaurants and indicate whether you would like to reduce how much fast food you consume.

2. Were you surprised at the amount of fat, saturated fat, and cholesterol in the meal you selected?

3. What could you do differently at fast-food restaurants to reduce your intake of fat, saturated fat, and cholesterol?

Stress and Health

LEARNING OBJECTIVES

After completing the study of this concept, you will be able to:

▶ Identify major sources and types of stress.

▶ Explain the major bodily responses to stress.

▶ Describe the stages of the General Adaptation Syndrome.

▶ Identify common physical, emotional, and behavioral consequences of stress.

▶ Understand individual differences in both physiological reactivity and appraisals of stressful events.

▶ Describe personal characteristics that influence consequences of stress.

▶ Identify personal sources of stress and your approaches for dealing with stressful life events.

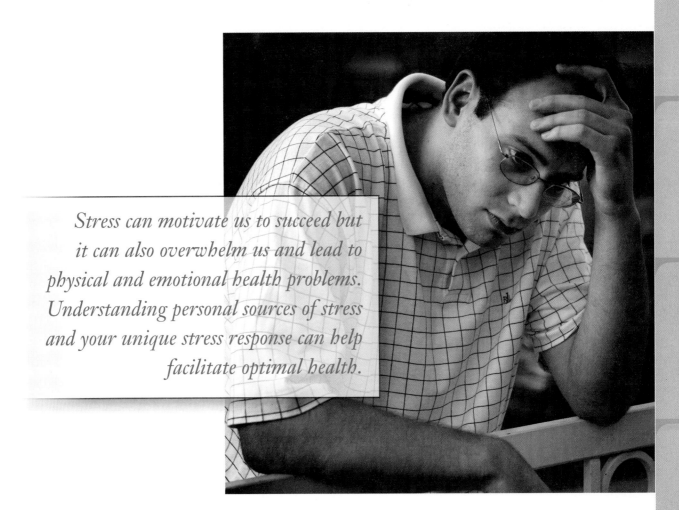

Stress can motivate us to succeed but it can also overwhelm us and lead to physical and emotional health problems. Understanding personal sources of stress and your unique stress response can help facilitate optimal health.

Stress affects everyone to some degree. In fact, approximately 75 percent of adults say they have experienced moderate to high levels of **stress** in the past month, and nearly half report that their level of stress has increased in the past year. **Stressors** come in many forms, and even positive life events can increase our stress levels.

At moderate levels, stress can motivate us to reach our goals and keep life interesting. However, when stressors are severe or chronic, our bodies may not be able to adapt successfully. Stress can compromise immune functioning, leading to a host of diseases of **adaptation.** In fact, stress has been linked to between 50 and 70 percent of all illnesses. Further, stress is associated with negative health behaviors, such as alcohol and other drug use, and to psychological problems, such as depression and anxiety. Although all humans have the same physiological system for responding to stress, stress reactivity varies across individuals. In addition, the way we think about or perceive stressful situations has a significant impact on how our bodies respond. Thus, there are large differences in individual responses to stress.

This concept reviews the causes and consequences of stress. First, the sources of stress (stressors), such as daily hassles and major life events, are described. Then the physiological responses to stress and the impact of these effects on physical and mental health are reviewed. Finally, individual differences in physiological and cognitive responses to stress and the implications of these individual differences for health and wellness are discussed.

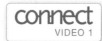

Sources of Stress

The first step in managing stress is to recognize the causes and to be aware of the symptoms. Identify the factors in your life that make you feel "stressed-out." Everything from minor irritations, such as traffic jams, to major life changes, such as births, deaths, or job loss, can be a stressor. A stress overload of too many demands on your time can make you feel that you are no longer in control. Recognizing the causes and effects of stress is important for learning how to manage it.

Stress has a variety of sources. There are many kinds of stressors. Environmental stressors include heat, noise, overcrowding, pollution, and second-hand smoke. Physiological stressors are such things as drugs, caffeine, tobacco, injury, infection or disease, and physical effort.

Emotional stressors are the most frequent and important stressors. Some people refer to these as *psychosocial stressors.* A national study of daily experiences indicated that more than 60 percent of all stressful experiences fall into a few areas (see Table 1).

Table 1 ▶ Ten Common Stressors in the Lives of College Students and Middle-Aged Adults	
College Students	**Middle-Aged Adults**
1. Troubling thoughts about the future	1. Concerns about weight
2. Not getting enough sleep	2. Health of a family member
3. Wasting time	3. Rising prices of common goods
4. Inconsiderate smokers	4. Home maintenance (interior)
5. Physical appearance	5. Too many things to do
6. Too many things to do	6. Misplacing or losing things
7. Misplacing or losing things	7. Yard work or outside home maintenance
8. Not enough time to do the things you need to do	8. Property, investments, or taxes
9. Concerns about meeting high standards	9. Crime
10. Being lonely	10. Physical appearance

Source: Kanner, et al.

Stressors vary in severity. Major stressors create major emotional turmoil or require tremendous amounts of adjustment. This category includes personal crises (e.g., major health problems or death in the family, divorce/separation, financial problems, legal problems) and job/school-related pressures or major age-related transitions (e.g., college, marriage, career, retirement). Daily hassles are generally viewed as shorter-term or less severe. This category includes events such as traffic problems, peer/work relations, time pressures, and family squabbles. In school, pressures such as grades, term papers, and oral presentations would likely fall into this category. Major stressors can alter daily patterns of stress and impair our ability to handle the minor stressors of life, while daily hassles can accumulate and create more significant problems. It is important to be aware of both types of stressors.

Negative, ambiguous, and uncontrollable events are usually the most stressful. Although stress can come from both positive and negative events, negative ones generally cause more distress because negative stressors usually have harsher consequences and little benefit. Positive stressors, on the other hand, usually have enough benefit to make them worthwhile. For example, the stress of starting a new job may be tremendous, but it is not as bad as the negative stress from losing a job.

Ambiguous stressors are harder to accept than more clearly defined problems. In most cases, if the cause of a stressor or problem can be identified, measures can be taken to improve the situation. For example, if you are stressed about a project at work or school, you can use specific strategies to complete the task on time. Stress brought on by a relationship with friends or co-workers, on the other hand, may be harder to understand. In some cases, it is not possible to determine the primary source or cause of the problem. These situations are more problematic because fewer clear-cut solutions exist. Another factor that makes events stressful is a lack of control. Because little can be done to change the situation, these events leave us feeling powerless.

Stress in Contemporary Society

Americans report high levels of stress. The American Psychological Association commissions an annual survey ("Stress in America") to monitor attitudes and perceptions of stress in the general public. The results from the most recent survey (2011) reveal a decline in overall ratings of stress, continuing a slow decline compared to peaks in 2007. However, more adults report that their stress is increasing instead of decreasing. In fact, over 44 percent reported that their stress increased over the past 5 years while only 27 percent reported a decrease. Money, work, and the economy were the three most commonly reported sources of stress, as they have been for the past 5 years. The most commonly reported physical symptoms of stress included irritability/anger, feeling nervous or anxious, and fatigue.

Although sources and consequences of stress are similar for men and women, and for younger and older Americans, the report highlights some important gender differences. Overall, women seem to be more aware of the potential negative impact of stress on health than men. With respect to age, older adults tend to report lower levels of stress and more successful efforts to manage their stress. (See A Closer Look on page 375 for more details.)

College presents unique challenges and stressors. For college students, schoolwork can be a full-time job, and those who have to work outside of school must handle the stresses of both jobs. Although the college years are often thought of as a break from the stresses of the real world, college life has its own stressors. Obvious sources of stress include taking exams, speaking in public, and becoming comfortable with talking to professors. Students are often living independently of family for the first time while negotiating new relationships—with

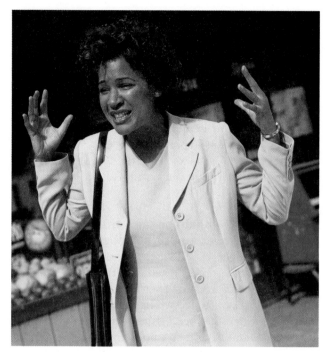
Daily hassles can contribute to stress.

roommates, dating partners, and so on. Young people entering college are also faced with a less structured environment and with the need to control their own schedules. Though this environment has a number of advantages, students are faced with a greater need to manage their stress effectively.

In addition to the traditional challenges of college, the new generation of students faces stressors that were not typical for college students in the past. According to the American Council on Education, only 40 percent of today's college students enroll full-time immediately after high school. More students now work, and many go back to school after spending time in the working world. More of today's college students are the first in their family to attend college. Perhaps as a result of some of these factors and the pressures that they create, rates of mental health problems among college students have

Stress The nonspecific response (generalized adaptation) of the body to any demand made on it in order to maintain physiological equilibrium. This positive or negative response results from emotions that are accompanied by biochemical and physiological changes directed at adaptation.

Stressors Things that place a greater than routine demand on the body or evoke a stress reaction.

Adaptation The body's efforts to restore normalcy.

increased dramatically in recent years (see Figure 1). In a 2011 survey of campus counseling center directors, 91 percent of respondents indicated that they believed that more students today have severe psychological problems. This impression is substantiated by the increasing percentage of students on psychiatric medications (9 percent in 1994 to 23 percent in 2011). Student surveys paint a similar picture. For example, a recent study found that 42 percent of students reported feeling "so depressed it was difficult to function" at some point during the past year.

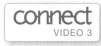

Some sources of stress are shared by entire communities, cultures, or societies. Although the stresses individuals experience are often unique to their particular circumstances, there are times when entire communities, cultures, or even countries have shared experiences of severe stress. The economic downturn in the United States has been a shared source of stress for everyone in this country. A poll developed by Gallup and Healthways to track the well-being of the U.S. population has documented the effects of shared stressors on well-being. The poll includes daily surveys of 1,000 Americans beginning in January 2008. As the economic downturn worsened in the latter half of 2008, dramatic decreases in well-being were observed, with low levels persisting through the early months of 2009. Although the economic crisis is far from over, Americans have shown themselves to be quite resilient. By June 2009, levels of well-being had returned to levels first assessed in January 2008, and levels have stayed relatively stable since that time.

Experiences of discrimination are a significant source of stress. In a 2009 meta-analysis of 134 previous studies, researchers found that higher levels of perceived discrimination were associated with both negative

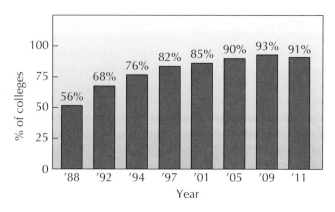

Figure 1 ▶ Colleges reporting increased psychological problems.
Source: R. Gallagher.

physical and psychological health outcomes. Perceived discrimination was also associated with more negative physiological and psychological stress responses, more negative health behaviors (e.g., smoking), and fewer positive health behaviors (e.g., exercise). With respect to physiological response, a recent study of Caucasian and African-American women found that higher levels of perceived discrimination were associated with higher levels of visceral fat, a known risk factor for cardiovascular disease. Regarding health risk behaviors, a recent study of college students found that students who reported more discrimination experiences had more negative moods, were more likely to drink as a way to cope with negative emotions, and were more likely to be heavy drinkers. These findings were consistent across a range of discrimination experiences (e.g., race/ethnicity, gender, weight, sexual orientation).

Reactions to Stress

All people have a general reaction to stress. In the early 1900s, Walter Cannon identified the fight-or-flight response to threat. According to his model, the body reacts to a threat by preparing either to fight or flee the situation. The body prepares for either option through the activation of the **sympathetic nervous system (SNS).** When the SNS is activated, epinephrine (adrenaline) and norepinephrine are released to focus attention on the task at hand. Heart rate and blood pressure increase to deliver oxygen to the muscles and essential organs, the eyes take in more light to increase visual acuity, and more sugar is released into the bloodstream to increase energy level. At the same time, nonessential functions like digestion and urine production are slowed. Figure 2 depicts some of the many physiological changes that occur during this process. Once the immediate threat has passed,

Health is available to Everyone for a Lifetime, and it's Personal

Once a year colleges all over the country participate in a National Stress Out Day where other college students and professionals provide pre-finals stress relief, educate about anxiety disorders, and help promote mental health awareness among college students. Between classes, finals, jobs, and family responsibilities, college students today have a lot on their plate.

Which types of stressors do you think have the most impact on college students?

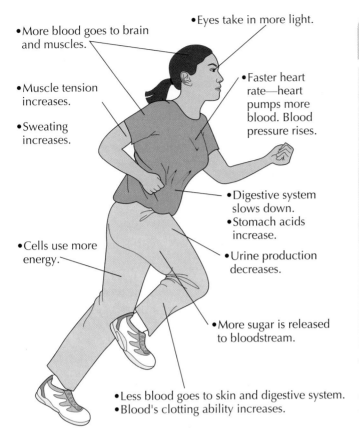

- More blood goes to brain and muscles.
- Eyes take in more light.
- Muscle tension increases.
- Sweating increases.
- Faster heart rate—heart pumps more blood. Blood pressure rises.
- Cells use more energy.
- Digestive system slows down.
- Stomach acids increase.
- Urine production decreases.
- More sugar is released to bloodstream.
- Less blood goes to skin and digestive system.
- Blood's clotting ability increases.

Figure 2 ▶ Physical symptoms of stress.

Table 2 ▶ The Three Stages in the General Adaptation Syndrome
Stage 1: Alarm Reaction   Any physical or mental trauma triggers an immediate set of reactions that combat the stress. Because the immune system is initially depressed, normal levels of resistance are lowered, making us more susceptible to infection and disease. If the stress is not severe or long-lasting, we bounce back and recover rapidly.
Stage 2: Resistance   Eventually, sometimes rather quickly, we adapt to stress, and we tend to become more resistant to illness and disease. The immune system works overtime during this period, keeping up with the demands placed on it.
Stage 3: Exhaustion   Because the body is not able to maintain homeostasis and the long-term resistance needed to combat stress, we invariably experience a drop in resistance level. No one experiences the same resistance and tolerance to stress, but everyone's immunity at some point collapses following prolonged stress reactions.

Source: H. Selye.

the **parasympathetic nervous system (PNS)** takes over in an attempt to restore the body to homeostasis and conserve resources. The PNS largely reverses the changes initiated by the SNS (e.g., slows heart rate and returns blood from the muscles and essential organs to the periphery).

Sometimes the fight-or-flight, or SNS, response is essential to survival, but when invoked inappropriately or excessively it may be more harmful than the effects of the original stressor. Hans Selye, another prominent scientist, was the first to recognize the potential negative consequences of this response. Selye suggested that this system could be invoked by mental as well as physical threats and that the short-term benefits might lead to long-term negative consequences. Based on these ideas, Selye described the general adaptation syndrome, which explains how the autonomic nervous system reacts to stressful situations and the conditions under which the system may break down (Table 2). The term *general* highlights the similarities in response to stressful situations across individuals. Selye's work led him to be referred to as the "father of stress."

Although chronic activation of the SNS is still believed to be important in the development of physical disease, other systems in the body are also involved. For example, the hypothalamic-pituitary-adrenal (HPA) axis is activated during stress, leading to the release of corticotropin-releasing hormone (CRH) and secondary activation of the pituitary gland. The pituitary releases a chemical called adrenocorticotropic hormone (ACTH), which ultimately causes the release of an active stress hormone called cortisol. With chronic exposure to stress, the HPA system can become dysregulated, and both over- and underactivation of the system are associated with risk for negative health outcomes.

Excessive stress reduces the effectiveness of the immune system. In addition to preparing the body for fight or flight, the stress-related activation of the SNS and the HPA axis slows down the functioning of the immune response. In the face of an immediate threat, mobilizing resources that will help in the moment is more important to the body than preventing or fighting infection. As

Sympathetic Nervous System (SNS) The component of the autonomic nervous system that responds to stressful situations by initiating the fight-or-flight response.

Parasympathetic Nervous System (PNS) The component of the autonomic nervous system that helps bring the body to a resting state following stressful experiences.

a result, if the stress response is chronically activated, high levels of adrenaline and cortisol continue to tell the body to mobilize resources at the expense of immune functioning. There are also normative developmental changes in the functioning of the HPA axis. Overall, HPA axis activity increases with age, and a recent study found that the HPA axis becomes more reactive to stress during adolescence. This increased reactivity may contribute to higher rates of negative outcomes during adolescence, including anxiety, depression, and substance use.

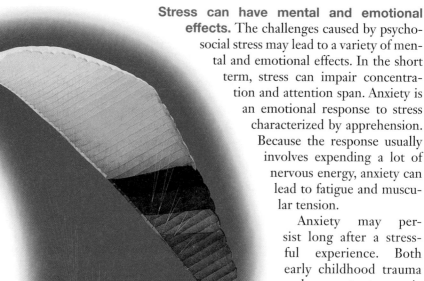

One person's stress is another's pleasure.

Stress Effects on Health and Wellness

Chronic or repetitive acute stress can lead to fatigue and can cause or exacerbate a variety of health problems. Some stress persists only as long as the stressor is present. For example, job-related stress caused by a challenging project generally subsides once that project is complete. In contrast, exposure to chronic stress or repeated exposure to acute stress may lead to a state of fatigue. Fatigue may result from lack of sleep, emotional strain, pain, disease, or a combination of these factors. Both **physiological fatigue** and **psychological fatigue** can result in a state of exhaustion, with resultant physical and mental health consequences. Chronic stress has been linked to health maladies that plague individuals on a daily basis, such as headaches, indigestion, insomnia, and the common cold. In fact, one study concluded that out-of-control stress is the leading preventable source of increased health-care cost in the workforce, roughly equivalent to the costs of the health problems related to smoking.

The effects of stress on health are not limited to minor physical complaints. Compelling evidence links psychological stress to a host of serious health problems, including cardiovascular disease, cancer, and HIV/AIDS. Stress may also increase the risk for upper respiratory tract infections, asthma, herpes, viral infections, autoimmune diseases, and slow wound healing. Reduced immune function due to negative emotions and stress appears to be a principal reason for these health problems. Stress may also increase the risk of early death. It is theorized that stress accelerates the aging process by causing a more rapid deterioration of chromosomes (changes in DNA proteins).

Stress can have mental and emotional effects. The challenges caused by psychosocial stress may lead to a variety of mental and emotional effects. In the short term, stress can impair concentration and attention span. Anxiety is an emotional response to stress characterized by apprehension. Because the response usually involves expending a lot of nervous energy, anxiety can lead to fatigue and muscular tension.

Anxiety may persist long after a stressful experience. Both early childhood trauma and recent traumatic experiences have been shown to alter functioning of the HPA axis, contributing to later risk for physical and mental health problems. In some cases, traumatic experiences lead to posttraumatic stress disorder (PTSD). Symptoms of PTSD include flashbacks of the traumatic event, avoidance of situations that remind the person of the event, emotional numbing, and increased level of arousal.

People who are excessively stressed are also more likely to be depressed than people who have optimal amounts of stress in their lives. Although drugs commonly prescribed to reduce depression can be effective in many cases, drugs do not get to the source of the life stressors that cause depression, and many have negative side effects.

Stress can alter both positive and negative health behaviors. In addition to direct effects on health, stress can contribute to negative health outcomes indirectly, through increased engagement in negative behaviors, such as smoking, alcohol use, and overeating. Stress may also decrease engagement in health-protective behaviors like exercise. During periods of increased stress, people may also get insufficient sleep and have sleep difficulties associated with the causes of stress. For example, an individual experiencing severe stress related to finances may pick up additional shifts at work, leaving less time for sleep. The person may also have difficulty sleeping due to worry associated with the financial situation. Unfortunately, reduced or disrupted sleep may exacerbate the problem. Studies have consistently found a link between sleep difficulties and stress-related physical and mental

In the News

Telehealth

Rates of mental health problems in the military are increasing dramatically as a consequence of combat stress associated with deployments in Iraq and Afghanistan. A 2010 study found that, even using the most stringent criteria, rates of depression ranged from 5 to 9 percent and rates of PTSD ranged from 6 to 11 percent. Given the large number of veterans currently in need of services and the perceived stigma associated with mental health problems, the Veterans Administration (VA) has embraced telehealth as an approach to providing mental health services to veterans in need. This includes use of videoconferencing, anonymous Internet-based treatment delivery, use of smartphone applications, and development of a new website dedicated to delivering wellness resources to veterans and their families (www.afterdeployment.org).

If you were in need of mental health services, would you favor these telehealth applications or would you rather visit with a real person?

connect ACTIVITY

---

health problems, including cardiovascular disease and depression, and a recent study found a strong link between stress and sleep disturbances among college students.

Eustress is an optimal amount of stress. We all need sufficient stress to motivate us to engage in activities that make our lives meaningful. Otherwise, we would be in a state of **hypostress,** which leads to apathy, boredom, and less than optimal health and wellness. An example of hypostress is a person working on an assembly line. Because the same task is repeated without variation, the level of stimulation is quite low and might lead to a state of boredom and job dissatisfaction. In fact, a certain level of stress, called **eustress,** is experienced positively. In contrast, **distress** is a level of stress that compromises performance and well-being. Each of us possesses a system that allows us to mobilize resources when necessary and seeks to find a homeostatic level of arousal (see Figure 3). Although we all have an optimal level of arousal, it varies considerably. What one person finds stressful another may find exhilarating. For example, riding a roller coaster is thrilling for some people, but stressful and unpleasant for others.

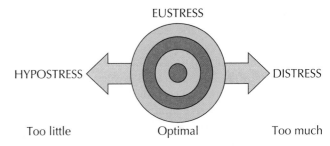

Figure 3 ▶ Stress target zone.

TECHNOLOGY UPDATE

Effect of Smartphones on Stress

A recent Gallup poll found that 78 percent of young adults (age 18 to 29) own smartphones. Although smartphones may facilitate organization and time-management, recent studies suggest that excessive use of smartphones may negatively impact well-being. According to one study, the more hours people spent on their smartphones, the higher their levels of stress. Interestingly, it was time spent on social networking rather than school- or work-related activities that produced the most stress. Many respondents said they spend too much time on their phones (58 percent) and on social networking (about 50 percent).

Are you adding stress to your life through your use of a mobile phone? How might you better manage your use of this technology?

connect ACTIVITY

Physiological Fatigue A deterioration in the capacity of the neuromuscular system as a result of physical overwork and strain; also referred to as true fatigue.

Psychological Fatigue A feeling of fatigue, usually caused by such things as lack of exercise, boredom, or mental stress, that results in a lack of energy and depression; also referred to as subjective or false fatigue.

Hypostress Insufficient levels of stress leading to boredom or apathy.

Eustress Positive stress, or stress that is mentally or physically stimulating.

Distress Negative stress, or stress that contributes to health problems.

Individual Differences in the Stress Response

Individuals respond differently to stress. Individuals exposed to high levels of stress are most at risk for negative health consequences. However, not everyone exposed to severe or chronic stress will experience negative outcomes. The events that occurred on September 11, 2001, provide a vivid example of the very different reactions that people have to the same or similar stressors. Everyone who witnessed these events, in person or on television, was profoundly impacted. At the same time, individual reactions varied dramatically. Most felt overwhelming sadness, many felt extreme anger, others felt hopeless or desperate, and yet others felt lost or confused. Undoubtedly, there were some who were simply too shocked to process their emotional experience at all. With time, most Americans began to experience a wave of additional emotions, such as hope and patriotism. Figure 4 depicts the role that stress appraisals play in mediating relations between stress and its emotional, physical, and behavioral consequences.

Reactions to stress depend on one's appraisal of both the event and the subsequent physiological response. Stressors by themselves generally do not cause problems unless they are perceived as stressful. As shown in Figure 4, two specific factors are thought to influence individual susceptibility to negative stress-related outcomes: stress appraisal and stress reactivity.

Stress appraisal refers to an individual's perceptions of a stressor and the person's resources for managing stressful situations. Appraisal usually involves consideration of the consequences of the situation (primary appraisal) and an evaluation of the resources available to cope with the situation (secondary appraisal). If one sees a stressor as a challenge that can be tackled, one is likely to respond in a more positive manner than if the stressor is viewed as an obstacle that cannot be overcome. Individual differences in appraisal are due to inherited predispositions as well as our unique histories of experiencing and attempting to cope with stress.

Individual appraisal of the body's response to a stressful event is also important. Stress reactivity refers to the extent to which the sympathetic nervous system, or fight-or-flight system, is activated by a stressor. The degree of activation influences how one will react emotionally and behaviorally, but some react more than others. For example, public speaking is a situation that leads to significant autonomic arousal for most people. Those who handle these situations well probably recognize that these sensations are normal and may even interpret them as excitement about the situations. In contrast, those who experience severe and sometimes debilitating anxiety are probably interpreting the same sensations as indicators of fear, panic, and loss of control. The combination of individual differences in stress reactivity and appraisals may lead to characteristic ways of responding to stress that either confer risk or protect against risk for physical and mental health problems. In fact, several different patterns of behavior (or personality styles) have been clearly identified.

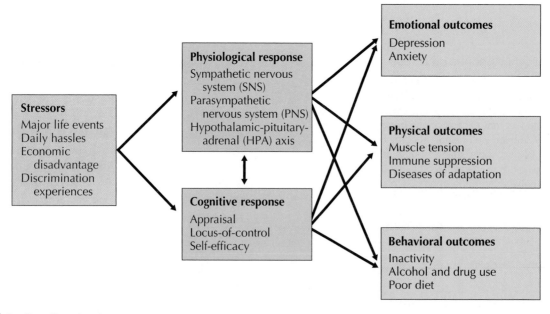

Figure 4 ▶ Reactions to stress.

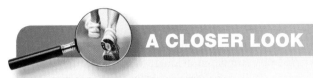

A CLOSER LOOK

Gender Differences in Stress

The recent "Stress in America" report from the American Psychological Association provides insights about patterns and trends in stress. Although sources and consequences of stress are similar for men and women, there are many key differences in how each gender reports and perceives stress. Women tend to report higher levels of stress than men, but they also appear to be following better stress management practices than men. The report suggests that men may be less concerned about managing stress and feel they are doing enough in this area. Women, in contrast, tend to place more emphasis on the need to manage stress, but feel they are not doing a good enough job of it.

Are you surprised that there are gender differences in ratings of stress?

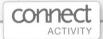

Type A and Type D personalities may increase risk for negative health outcomes. The best-known "personality" style associated with risk for negative health outcomes is the **Type A behavior pattern.** Several decades ago psychologists Friedman and Rosenman identified a subgroup of goal-oriented, or "driven," patients, whom they believed were at increased risk based on their pattern of behavior. These individuals demonstrated a sense of time urgency, were highly competitive, and tended to experience and express anger and hostility under conditions of stress. In contrast, individuals with the Type B behavior pattern were relatively easygoing and less reactive to stress. Although early research on Type A behavior demonstrated increased risk for heart disease, it now appears that certain aspects of the Type A behavior pattern pose greater risk than others. In particular, hostility and anger appear to be consistently associated with risk for cardiovascular disease. Although most studies have not found time urgency or competitiveness predictive of risk for cardiovascular disease, a recent study found that people who scored high on a measure of impatience were nearly twice as likely to have high blood pressure relative to individuals lower on this trait. At the same time, certain aspects of the Type A behavior pattern (other than hostility) may lead to higher levels of achievement and an increased sense of personal accomplishment. Although the Type A behavior pattern has often been referred to as Type A personality, it was not the intention of those who developed the concept to identify a "personality type."

In contrast, the more recently identified **Type D,** or "distressed," **behavior pattern** is associated with two well-defined personality characteristics based on personality theory. Individuals with Type D personality are characterized by high levels of "negative affectivity," or negative emotion, and "social inhibition," or the tendency not to express negative emotions in social interactions. The combination of these characteristics appears to constitute risk for cardiovascular disease and other negative health outcomes. Converging evidence from recent research on both Type A and Type D behaviors has led some to conclude that negative affectivity, in general, is a more important risk for negative health outcomes than any emotion in particular. In other words, anger and hostility (Type A), as well as anxiety and depressed mood (Type D), pose a health risk. Several other well-established personality traits, including neuroticism and novelty seeking, have also been linked to morbidity and mortality.

Several personality traits are associated with resilience in the face of stress. Resilience is not simply due to an absence of risk factors, but also to the presence of protective factors that lead to adaptive functioning. The experience of positive emotion is one well-established protective factor. Individuals who experience more positive emotion are more likely to adopt healthy lifestyles, and their physical responses to stress are more adaptive than those who experience less positive emotion. For example, patterns of cortisol response, heart rate, and blood pressure under stress are all more favorable among individuals who experience higher levels of positive emotion. Positive emotion may also be an effective coping mechanism for managing acute stress. Positive moods have been shown to undo some of the cardiovascular effects associated with negative emotions. Individuals who have more positive moods are also more socially integrated and report higher levels of social support, both characteristics associated with health benefits. **Optimism** is a trait associated with more positive emotional experiences and a more positive outlook on the future. Extensive research demonstrates that optimistic individuals have better physical and mental health outcomes than pessimistic individuals.

Type A Behavior Pattern Characterized by impatience, ambition, and aggression; Type A personalities may be more susceptible to the effects of stress but may also be more able to cope with stress.

Type D Behavior Pattern Characterized by high levels of negative emotion and the tendency to withhold expression of these emotions.

Resilience Positive outcomes in the face of stress or disadvantage.

Optimism The tendency to have a positive outlook on life or a belief that things will work out favorably.

An individual's **locus of control** can also have a significant impact on how he or she responds to a stressful situation. Research has consistently found that having an internal locus of control is associated with better health outcomes. People with an internal locus of control are more likely to take steps to address the problems that created the stress, rather than avoiding them. Those with an external locus of control tend to use passive methods for managing stress. In addition, an external locus of control is related to higher perceived levels of stress, lower job satisfaction, and poorer school achievement.

Although an internal locus of control generally promotes health, this is not always the case. This truth is apparent in depressed individuals with a pessimistic explanatory style. They believe that their failures are due to internal factors, squarely placing the control of these events within themselves. Even though they believe stressors are under their control, they don't believe in their ability to initiate change. Thus, for an internal locus of control to be beneficial to well-being, it must be combined with the belief that one is capable of making changes to prevent future problems. The belief in one's ability to reach a desired goal is often referred to as **self-efficacy.** Finally, studies have consistently shown health benefits of **conscientiousness,** the tendency to be organized, thoughtful, and goal directed. Highly conscientious individuals are at decreased risk for a range of negative outcomes, including asthma, stroke, depression, and panic attacks. It appears that conscientiousness contributes to better health outcomes both through

reduced engagement in health risk behaviors like alcohol use and through more adaptive responses to stressful experiences. For example, individuals higher in conscientiousness are more likely to exercise on days that they experience high levels of stress.

As noted earlier, individuals who possess characteristics that protect them from the negative health consequences of stress are said to be resilient. **Hardiness** is one constellation of characteristics associated with resilience. Hardy individuals are strongly committed to their goals, view difficult situations as challenges rather than stressors, and find ways to assume control over their problems.

Locus of Control The extent to which we believe the outcomes of events are under our control (internal locus) or outside our personal control (external locus).

Self-Efficacy The belief in one's ability to take action that will lead to the attainment of a goal.

Conscientiousness Associated with high levels of organization, thoughtfulness, and goal-directed activity.

Hardiness A collection of personality traits thought to make a person more resistant to stress.

Strategies for Action

Self-assessments of stressors in your life can be useful in managing stress. As discussed in the text, to effectively manage stress, you first must identify the sources of stress in your life. In Lab 16A you will have the opportunity to evaluate your stress levels using the Life Experience Survey.

Learning to appraise stressful events in a more positive way can help you respond to stress more effectively. Personality characteristics have been associated with reactions to stress. Although overall personality structure has proven somewhat resistant to change, it is certainly possible to change your appraisal of stressful events and thereby diminish the resulting emotional, physical, and behavioral outcomes. In Lab 16B you can assess your hardiness and locus of control, characteristics associated with appraising and coping effectively with stress.

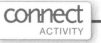

Web Resources

American Institute of Stress **www.stress.org**
APA Stress in America Press Room **www.apa.org/news/ press/index.aspx**
Gallup-Healthways Well-Being Index **www.well-beingindex.com**
National Center for Post Traumatic Stress Disorder **www.ptsd.va.gov**

National Mental Health Information Center **www.mentalhealth.samhsa.gov**
Ulifeline: The online behavioral support system for young adults **www.ulifeline.org**
U.S. Health and Human Services **www.womenshealth.gov/ publications/our-publications/fact-sheet/stress-your-health.cfm**

Suggested Readings

American College Counseling Association. 2011. *National Survey of Counseling Center Directors.* Alexandria, VA: The International Association of Counseling Services, Inc.

American Psychological Association. 2012. *Stress in America.* Washington, DC: American Psychological Association.

Greenberg, J. S. 2011. *Comprehensive Stress Management.* 12th ed. New York: McGraw-Hill.

Hatzenbuehler, M. L., Corbin, W. R., and K. Fromme. 2011. Discrimination and alcohol-related problems among college students: A prospective examination of mediating effects. *Drug and Alcohol Dependence* 115(3):213–220.

Lewis, T. T., et al. 2011. Self-reported experiences of discrimination and visceral fat in middle-aged African-American and Caucasian women. *American Journal of Epidemiology* 173(11):1223–1231.

Lund, H. G., et al. 2010. Sleep patterns and predictors of disturbed sleep in a large population of college students. *Journal of Adolescence Health* 46:124–132.

O'Connor, D. B., et al. 2009. Exploring the benefits of conscientiousness: An investigation of the role of daily stressors and health behaviors. *Annals of Behavioral Medicine* 37:184–196.

Pascoe, E. A., and L. S. Richman. 2009. Perceived discrimination and health: A meta-analytic review. *Psychological Bulletin* 135 (4):531–554.

Sloan, D. M., Marx, B. P., and T. M. Keane. 2011. Reducing the burden of mental illness in military veterans: Commentary on Kazdin and Blase. *Perspectives on Psychological Science* 6(5):503–506.

Steptoe, A., S. Dockray, and J. Wardle. 2009. Positive affect and psychobiological processes relevant to health. *Journal of Personality* 77:1747–1776.

Healthy People 2020

The objectives listed below are societal goals designed to help all Americans improve their health between now and the year 2020. They were selected because they relate to the content of this concept.

- Promote quality of life, healthy development, and healthy behaviors across all stages of life.
- Increase screening for and treatment of mental health problems.
- Reduce suicide and suicide attempts.
- Increase availability of work-site stress-reduction programs.

- Reduce rates of depression and disordered eating.
- Increase levels of social support among adults.
- Increase the proportion of primary care facilities that provide mental health treatment.

A national goal is to improve mental health through prevention and by ensuring access to appropriate, quality mental health services. What are some of the activities your school offers to address mental health issues (e.g., depression, anxiety)? Are adequate facilities available on your campus for students in need of mental health services?

Lab 16A Evaluating Your Stress Level

Name _____   Section _____   Date _____

Purpose: To evaluate your stress during the past year and determine its implications

Procedures

1. Complete the Life Experience Survey (page 380) based on your experiences during the past year. This survey lists a number of life events that may be distressful or eustressful. Read all of the items. If you did not experience an event, leave the box blank. In the box after each event that you did experience, write a number ranging from –3 to +3 using the scale described in the directions. Extra blanks are provided to write in positive or negative events not listed. Some items apply only to males or females. Items 48 to 56 are only for current college students.
2. Add all of the negative numbers and record your score (distress) in the Results section. Add the positive numbers and record your score (eustress) in the Results section. Use all of the events in the past year.
3. Find your scores on Chart 1 and record your ratings in the Results section.
4. Interpret the results by discussing the Conclusions and Implications in the space provided.

Results

Sum of negative scores [21] (distress)

Sum of positive scores [28] (eustress)

Rating on negative scores [May need counseling]

Rating on positive scores [Above]

Chart 1 Scale for Life Experiences and Stress

	Sum of Negative Scores (Distress)	Sum of Positive Scores (Eustress)
May need counseling	14+	
Above average	9–13	11+
Average	6–8	9–10
Below average	<6	<9

Scoring the Life Experience Survey

1. Add all of the negative scores to arrive at your own distress score (negative stress).
2. Add all of the positive scores to arrive at a eustress score (positive stress).

Conclusions and Implications: In several sentences, discuss your current stress rating and its implications.

> I currently have high stress levels. I am actually seeing a councelor to address stress levels. If I ignored my stress level it could lead to further negative outcomes.

Life Experience Survey

Directions: If you did not experience an event, leave the box next to the event empty. If you experienced an event, enter a number in the box based on how the event impacted your life. Use the following scale:

Extremely negative impact = –3
Moderately negative impact = –2
Somewhat negative impact = –1
Neither positive nor negative impact = 0
Somewhat positive impact = +1
Moderately positive impact = +2
Extremely positive impact = +3

1. Marriage — **3**
2. Detention in jail or comparable institution —
3. Death of spouse —
4. Major change in sleeping habits (much more or less sleep) — **–1**
5. Death of close family member:
   a. Mother —
   b. Father —
   c. Brother —
   d. Sister —
   e. Child —
   f. Grandmother —
   g. Grandfather — **–2**
   h. Other (specify) _____ —
6. Major change in eating habits (much more or much less food intake) — **–1**
7. Foreclosure on mortgage or loan —
8. Death of a close friend —
9. Outstanding personal achievement —
10. Minor law violation (traffic ticket, disturbing the peace, etc.) — **–1**
11. *Male:* Wife's/girlfriend's pregnancy — **3**
    Female: Pregnancy —
12. Changed work situation (different working conditions, working hours, etc.) — **2**
13. New job — **2**
14. Serious illness or injury of close family member:
    a. Father —
    b. Mother —
    c. Sister —
    d. Brother — **–1**
    e. Grandfather — **–1**
    f. Grandmother —
    g. Spouse —
    h. Child — **–1**
    i. Other (specify) _____ —
15. Sexual difficulties — **–2**
16. Trouble with employer (in danger of losing job, being suspended, demoted, etc.) — **–2**
17. Trouble with in-laws —
18. Major change in financial status (a lot better off or a lot worse off) — **1**
19. Major change in closeness of family members (decreased or increased closeness) — **–1**

20. Gaining a new family member (through birth, adoption, family member moving in, etc.) — **3**
21. Change of residence — **1**
22. Marital separation from mate (due to conflict) —
23. Major change in church activities (increased or decreased attendance) — **1**
24. Marital reconciliation with mate — **2**
25. Major change in number of arguments with spouse (a lot more or a lot fewer arguments) — **1**
26. *Married male:* Change in wife's work outside the home (beginning work, ceasing work, changing to a new job) — **2**
    Married female: Change in husband's work (loss of job, beginning new job, retirement, etc.) —
27. Major change in usual type and/or amount of recreation —
28. Borrowing more than $10,000 (buying a home, business, etc.) — **–1**
29. Borrowing less than $10,000 (buying car or TV, getting school loan, etc.) — **–1**
30. Being fired from job —
31. *Male:* Wife/girlfriend having abortion —
    Female: Having abortion —
32. Major personal illness or injury —
33. Major change in social activities, such as parties, movies, visiting (increased or decreased participation) — **–1**
34. Major change in living conditions of family (building new home, remodeling, deterioration of home or neighborhood, etc.) — **–2**
35. Divorce —
36. Serious injury or illness of close friend —
37. Retirement from work —
38. Son or daughter leaving home (due to marriage, college, etc.) —
39. Ending of formal schooling —
40. Separation from spouse (due to work, travel, etc.) —
41. Engagement — **2**
42. Breaking up with boyfriend/girlfriend — **–2**
43. Leaving home for the first time — **1**
44. Reconciliation with boyfriend/girlfriend — **2**

Other recent experiences that have had an impact on your life: list and rate.

45. LDS mission — **2**
46. _____ —
47. _____ —

For Students Only

48. Beginning new school experience at a higher academic level (college, graduate school, professional school, etc.) —
49. Changing to a new school at same academic level (undergraduate, graduate, etc.) —
50. Academic probation —
51. Being dismissed from dormitory or other residence —
52. Failing an important exam — **–1**
53. Changing a major —
54. Failing a course —
55. Dropping a course —
56. Joining a fraternity/sorority —

Source: **Sarason, Johnson, and Siegel.**

Lab 16B Evaluating Your Hardiness and Locus of Control

Name	Section	Date

Purpose: To evaluate your level of hardiness and locus of control and to help you identify the ways in which you appraise and respond to stressful situations

Procedures

1. Complete the Hardiness Questionnaire and the Locus of Control Questionnaire. Make an X over the circle that best describes what is true for you personally.
2. Compute the scale scores and record the values in the Results section.
3. Evaluate your scores using the Rating chart (Chart 1), and record your ratings in the Results section.
4. Interpret the results by answering the questions in the Conclusions and Implications section.

Hardiness Questionnaire

	Not True	Rarely True	Sometimes True	Often True	Score
1. I look forward to school and work on most days.	1	2	3	4	
2. Having too many choices in life makes me nervous.	4	3	2	1	
3. I know where my life is going and look forward to the future.	1	2	3	4	
4. I prefer not to get too involved in relationships.	4	3	2	1	
Commitment Score, Sum 1–4					
5. My efforts at school and work will pay off in the long run.	1	2	3	4	
6. I just have to trust my life to fate to be successful.	4	3	2	1	
7. I believe that I can make a difference in the world.	1	2	3	4	
8. Being successful in life takes more luck and good breaks than effort.	4	3	2	1	
Control Score, Sum 5–8					
9. I would be willing to work for less money if I could do something really challenging and interesting.	1	2	3	4	
10. I often get frustrated when my daily plans and schedule get altered.	4	3	2	1	
11. Experiencing new situations in life is important to me.	1	2	3	4	
12. I don't mind being bored.	4	3	2	1	
Challenge Score, Sum 9–12					

Locus of Control Questionnaire

					Score
13. Hard work usually pays off.	1	2	3	4	
14. Buying a lottery ticket is not worth the money.	1	2	3	4	
15. Even when I fail I keep trying.	1	2	3	4	
16. I am usually successful in what I do.	1	2	3	4	
17. I am in control of my own life.	1	2	3	4	
18. I make plans to be sure I am successful.	1	2	3	4	
19. I know where I stand with my friends.	1	2	3	4	
Locus of Control, Sum 13–19					

Results

Hardiness

Commitment score [ ]

Commitment rating [ ]

Control score [ ]

Control rating [ ]

Challenge score [ ]

Challenge rating [ ]

Hardiness score [ ]

Hardiness rating [ ]

Locus of Control

Locus of Control score [ ]

Locus of Control rating [ ]

Chart 1 Rating Chart

Rating	Individual Hardiness Scale Scores	Total Hardiness Score	Locus of Control Score
High	14–16	40–48	24–28
Moderate	10–13	30–39	12–23
Low	<10	<30	<12

Conclusions and Implications

1. In several sentences, discuss your commitment, control, and challenge ratings, as well as your overall hardiness rating. Are they what you expected? Do you think they are true indications of your hardiness? Explain.

2. In several sentences, discuss your locus of control rating. Is it what you expected (a high rating indicates an internal locus of control)? Do you think your rating is a realistic indicator of your locus of control? Explain.

Stress Management, Relaxation, and Time Management

LEARNING OBJECTIVES

After completing the study of this concept, you will be able to:

▶ Describe the stress-buffering effects of physical activity that contribute to positive psychological health.

▶ Identify behaviors that contribute to better sleep hygiene.

▶ Describe the benefits of recreation, leisure, and play to overall quality of life.

▶ Identify a variety of strategies for effective time management.

▶ Understand the unique benefits of cognitive-, emotion-, and problem-focused coping strategies.

▶ Describe the mental health benefits of mindfulness, spirituality, and emotional expression.

▶ Determine several relaxation techniques that can be used to effectively manage stress.

▶ Describe different types of social support and ways in which it facilitates effective stress management.

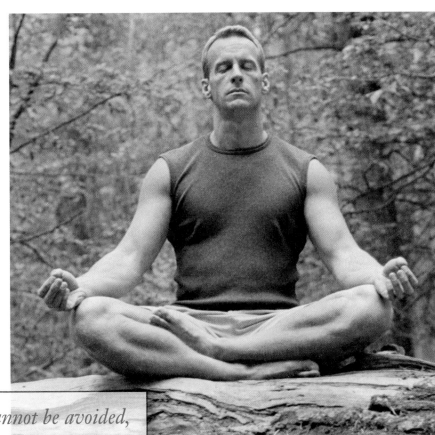

Although stress cannot be avoided, proper stress-management techniques can help reduce the impact of stress in your life.

As outlined in Concept 16, we all experience stress on a daily basis and must find ways to manage stress effectively. We can do many things to prevent excessive levels of stress, including exercising regularly, getting sufficient sleep, and allowing time for recreation. Effective time management is essential for balancing work and other activities. Despite our best efforts, stressful situations will occur, and we must find a way to deal with them. Later in this concept, three effective methods for managing stress are described.

Physical Activity and Stress Management

Regular activity and a healthy diet can help you adapt to stressful situations. An individual's capacity to adapt is not a static function but fluctuates as situations change. The better your overall health, the better you can withstand the rigors of tension without becoming susceptible to illness or other disorders. Physical activity is especially important because it conditions your body to function effectively under challenging physiological conditions.

Physical activity can provide relief from stress and aid muscle tension release. Physical activity has been found to be effective at relieving stress, particularly white-collar job stress. Studies show that regular exercise decreases the likelihood of developing stress disorders and reduces the intensity of the stress response. It also shortens the period of recovery from an emotional trauma. Its effect tends to be short-term, so exercise regularly for it to have a continuing effect. Whatever your choice of exercise, it is likely to be more effective as an antidote to stress if it is something you find enjoyable.

Regular physical activity reduces reactivity to stress. Physical activity is associated with a physiological response that is similar, in many ways, to the body's response to psychosocial stressors. Individuals who are physically fit have a reduced physiological response to exercise. Therefore, it makes sense that someone who is physically fit would also have a reduced response to psychosocial stressors. Research supports this hypothesis indicating that regular exercise reduces physiological reactivity to non-exercise stressors. For example, a recent study found that children's responses to stress are dampened by engagement in exercise. Compared to children who watched television before a stressor, those who exercised showed lower systolic and diastolic blood pressure and reduced heart rate reactivity. A recent study suggests that exercising after a stressor may also be an effective coping mechanism.

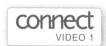

Physical activity has many other positive effects on mental health. Exercise can reduce anxiety, aid in recovery from depression, and assist in efforts to eliminate negative health behaviors, such as smoking. It also appears to buffer the effects of stress on cellular aging. Key findings related to mental health are summarized below.

- *Physical activity can reduce anxiety.* Evidence shows that physical activity leads to reductions in anxiety in non-clinical samples. One study found that exercise may also be effective in reducing anxiety among individuals with panic disorder. An aerobic exercise program led to reductions in panic symptoms relative to a control group. Although exercise was not as effective as medication, it may be a useful addition to other treatment methods for anxiety disorders.

- *Physical activity can reduce depression.* A randomized clinical trial compared antidepressant medication and aerobic exercise with a combined antidepressant and exercise condition in the treatment of major depressive disorder. The aerobic exercise group fared as well as the other two at the end of treatment. In addition, the patients who only exercised were less likely to have a remission to depression at a 6-month follow-up.

- *Physical activity can aid in health behavior change.* One study tested vigorous physical activity as an adjunct to a cognitive-behavioral smoking cessation program for women. Women who received the exercise intervention were able to sustain continuous abstinence from smoking for a longer period relative to those who did not receive the exercise intervention. Women in the exercise program also gained less weight during smoking cessation.

- *Physical activity buffers the negative impact of stress on cellular aging.* Stress can reduce the length of telomeres (protective ends of DNA strands), leading to more rapid cell aging. Recent studies suggest that regular physical activity can prevent stress-induced damage to DNA. One recent study found that sedentary individuals showed stress induced decreases in telomere length, whereas those who engaged in at least 75 minutes of weekly exercise demonstrated no relation between stress and telomere length.

Stress, Sleep, and Recreation

In order to adapt effectively to stressful situations, one must get adequate sleep. Although the number of hours needed varies, the average adult needs between 7 and 8 hours of sleep per night. Teenagers and young adults (those in their early 20s) may need slightly more sleep. Unfortunately, many do not get this extra amount of sleep. As noted in a later section, full-time college students get an average of 8.4 hours of sleep on weekday nights. However, more than one-fourth of college students average 7 or fewer hours of sleep on weekdays. Thus, a substantial number of students fail to get adequate sleep. With insufficient sleep, many people resort to caffeine to stay awake, leading to an endless cycle of deficient sleep and caffeine usage and compromised health and wellness. Table 1 presents guidelines for good sleep.

All work and no play can lead to poor mental and physical health. Between 1860 and 1990, the number of hours typically spent working in industrialized countries decreased relatively dramatically. While that trend has continued in most countries, work hours in the United States have increased considerably over the past two decades. A major reason for this increase is that more people now hold second jobs than in the past. Also, some jobs of modern society have increasing rather than decreasing time demands. For example, many medical doctors and other professionals work more hours than the 35 to 44 hours that most people work. Nearly three times as many married women with children work full-time now, as compared with 1960.

Table 1 ▶ Guidelines for Good Sleep

- Be aware of the effects of medications. Some medicines, such as weight loss pills and decongestants, contain caffeine or other ingredients that interfere with sleep.

- Avoid tobacco use. Nicotine is a stimulant and can interfere with sleep.

- Avoid excess alcohol use. Alcohol may make it easier to get to sleep but may be a reason you wake up at night and are unable to get back to sleep.

- You may exercise late in the day, but do not do vigorous activity right before bedtime.

- Sleep in a room that is cooler than normal.

- Avoid hard-to-digest foods late in the day, as well as fatty and spicy foods.

- Avoid large meals late in the day or right before bedtime. A light snack before bedtime should not be a problem for most people.

- Avoid too much liquid before bedtime.

- Avoid naps during the day.

- Go to bed and get up at the same time each day.

- Do not study, read, or engage in other activities in your bed. You want your brain to associate your bed with sleep, not with activity.

- If you are having difficulty falling asleep, do not stay in bed. Get up and find something to do until you begin to feel tired, and then go back to bed.

Experts have referred to young adults as the "overworked Americans" because they work several jobs and maintain dual roles (full-time employment coupled with normal family chores), or they work extended hours in demanding professional jobs. A Gallup poll showed that the great majority of adults have "enough time" for work, chores, and sleep but not enough time for friends, self, spouse, and children. When time is at a premium, the factors most likely to be negatively affected are personal health, relationships with children, and marriage or romantic relationships.

Recreation and leisure are important contributors to wellness (quality of life). **Leisure** is generally considered to be the opposite of work and includes "doing things we just want to do," as well as "doing nothing." In contrast, **recreation** involves the organized use of free time and typically includes social interaction. Leisure and recreation can contribute to stress reduction and wellness, though leisure activities are not done specifically to achieve these benefits.

The value of recreation and leisure in the busy lives of people in Western culture is evidenced by the emphasis public health officials place on the availability and accessibility of recreational facilities in communities.

There are many meaningful types of recreation. If fitness is the goal, choose recreational activities involving moderate to vigorous physical activity. Involvement in nonphysical activities also constitutes recreation. For example, reading is an activity that can contribute significantly to other wellness dimensions, such as emotional/mental and spiritual. Passive involvement (spectating) is a third type of participation.

Play is critical to development and a sense of play in adult recreation contributes to wellness. **Play** is distinct from recreation in that it is typically intrinsically motivated and has an imaginative component.

Leisure Time that is free from the demands of work. Leisure is more than free time; it is also an attitude. Leisure activities need not be means to ends (purposeful) but are ends in themselves.

Recreation *Recreation* means creating something anew. In this book, it refers to something that you do for amusement or for fun to help you divert your attention and to refresh yourself (re-create yourself).

Play Activity done of one's own free will. The play experience is fun and intrinsically rewarding, and it is a self-absorbing means of self-expression. It is characterized by a sense of freedom or escape from life's normal rules.

Play has been shown to be important to healthy brain development in humans, and there is considerable evidence for physical, social, and cognitive benefits of play. In children, "free play," or unstructured time for play, seems to be particularly important. This type of play has been linked to a number of positive outcomes, including increased attention in the classroom, better self-regulation, and improved social skills and problem solving. Although much less attention has been given to the value of play in adults, a recent literature review identified benefits of play in adults, including mood enhancement, skill development, and enhanced relationships. Clearly, benefits associated with play have the potential both to prevent stress and to facilitate effective coping with stress.

Time Management

Effective time management helps you adapt to the stresses of modern living. Lack of time is cited by both the general public and experts as a source of stress and a reason for failing to implement healthy lifestyle changes. For college students, managing time is critical to academic success as well as overall well-being. Managing time effectively has become even more of a challenge for college students in recent years, as more and more students are working part- or full-time jobs to support their education (see Figure 1). The following strategies may help you learn to manage your time more effectively.

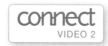

- *Prioritize.* Many people feel that there are not enough hours in the day to do everything that needs to be done. The truth is, they are probably right. If you think about all the things that have to get done, it can seem unmanageable. That is why it is important to prioritize. Many time-management experts advocate the ABC approach as a way to prioritize tasks effectively. Create three lists of things you need to do, with list A including the most urgent tasks and list C containing the least urgent. To help you remember the ABC approach, remember that A tasks must *A*bsolutely get done, B tasks had *B*etter get done, and C tasks *C*ould get done. See Table 2 for a brief description of the ABC approach.

- *Know how you spend your time.* Where does your time go? The answer to this question is the first step toward better time management. Most of us are not fully aware of how we spend our time. If you carry a notebook and write down what you are doing and how long it takes, you can find out exactly where the time goes. You probably need to do this for at least a week. After you complete this exercise, you will know where you need to spend more time. Just as important, monitoring your time will help you identify where you could spend less time. Some common areas where people spend too much time are socializing (in person, by phone, or via email), watching television, playing video games, surfing the Internet, and doing busywork. Lab 17A will give you a chance to evaluate your current use of time.

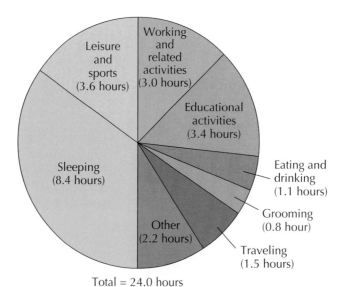

Total = 24.0 hours

Note: Data include individuals, ages 15 to 49, who were enrolled full time at a university or college. Data include averages for non-holiday weekdays.

Figure 1 ▶ Time use on an average weekday for full-time university and college students

Source: Bureau of Labor Statistics, American Time Use Survey.

Table 2 ▶ The ABC System for Time Management

Level of Importance	Description
A	*A tasks* are those that *must* be done, and soon. When accomplished, A tasks may yield extraordinary results. Left undone, they may generate serious, unpleasant, or disastrous consequences. Immediacy is what an A priority task is all about.
B	*B tasks* are those that *should* be done soon. While not as pressing as A tasks, they're still important. They can be postponed, but not for too long. Within a brief time, though, they can easily rise to A status.
C	*C tasks* are those that *could* be done. These tasks could be put off without creating dire consequences. Some can linger in this category almost indefinitely. Others—especially those tied to distant completion dates—will eventually rise to A or B levels as the deadline approaches.

Source: Mancini, M.

- *Write it down.* When things are not too busy, it may be possible to remember what you need to do and when you need to do it without writing it down. During busy times, though, trying to remember everything can lead to big problems. One of the most important steps in effective time management is to write things down. This includes keeping a daily planner to remember your schedule, calendars (weekly and/or monthly) to remember important events and deadlines, and a to-do list (or several, using the ABC approach) to help you remember your goals and priorities. Computers and other digital organizers allow you to keep all of this information in one place.

- *Set goals and deadlines.* In addition to knowing how you spend your time, it is important to know what things need to get done. This includes everything from small tasks that need to get done today to important long-term goals. When setting goals, make sure they are attainable and that the time frame for completing them is reasonable. Some tasks may be more easily accomplished if they are broken down into a series of smaller tasks, each with its own deadline. Setting deadlines for the completion of goals increases the likelihood that you will follow through.

- *Include recreational activities in your schedule in addition to your responsibilities.* Although it may seem that scheduling fun takes away from the enjoyment, you may not find this to be the case. By scheduling your free time,

you can fully enjoy it rather than worrying about other things you "should" be doing.

- *Make the most of the time you have.* To get the most out of your time, know when you do your best work and under what conditions. If you are sharpest in the morning, schedule the most important work to be done during this time. If you study most effectively when you are alone in a quiet place, schedule your studying at a time when you can create that environment. It is also important not to let time that could be productive go to waste. Keep materials with you that will allow you to take advantage of small periods of time (e.g., between classes).

- *Self-assessment of time management can help you improve your ability to manage your time effectively.* Monitoring your progress in time management is helpful in two ways. First, it allows you to see the progress you have made. Success is rewarding in and of itself, but you might also consider rewarding yourself with something tangible when you start out. For example, you might treat yourself to a nice dinner if you finish an important project on time. Monitoring also helps you identify areas in need of further improvement, so that you can adapt your plan to improve your chances of success.

- *Avoid procrastination.* Virtually all of us procrastinate at one time or another, but for many, procrastination can significantly decrease performance and increase stress. A number of causes of procrastination have been identified, including both internal and external influences. Understanding the causes of procrastination can help

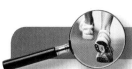

A CLOSER LOOK

Leisure Time

Although Americans find roughly 5 hours each day to engage in leisure activities, the vast majority of time is spent in sedentary activities. For example, the average American spends an average of 2.7 hours each day watching television and only 18 minutes participating in sports, exercise, and recreation. On the positive side, Americans report active efforts to engage in relaxation (average of 17 minutes) and social communication (average of 38 minutes). Search "American Time Use Survey" on the Internet to take a closer look at how time use patterns vary for different segments of the population.

What strategies can you use to decrease sedentary time and increase active recreation?

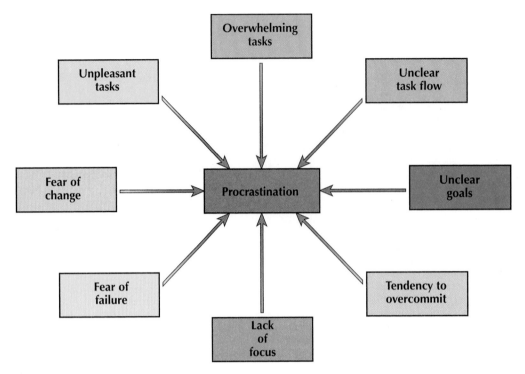

Figure 2 ▶ Causes of procrastination.

Source: Mancini, M.

you find ways to prevent it in the future (see Figure 2). Strategies such as the ABC approach should also help you limit procrastination by getting you to work on the things that are most important first. One of the simplest solutions to procrastination is simply to "get started." The first step toward completing a project is often the most difficult. Once people take the first step, they often find that the task becomes easier, so get started on projects as soon as possible, even if you spend only a short time working.

Stress Management

Stress-management skills can be learned. There is considerable evidence that stress-management training yields both physical and mental health benefits. Positive effects have been noted in a variety of populations.

For example, a recent study found that stress-management training for patients with heart disease resulted in improved cardiovascular function, decreased depression, and lower levels of general distress. Similar results were found following a stress-management intervention provided to women following treatment for breast cancer. Interestingly, and perhaps of more relevance to college students, stress-management training has also been shown to improve academic performance.

One of the most common settings for stress-management training is the workplace. Relaxation training is the most commonly used approach, although cognitive behavioral programs produce the largest benefits. An advantage of cognitive behavioral interventions is that they typically address each of the three types of coping that have been shown to be adaptive. These different coping styles are described in detail in the following section.

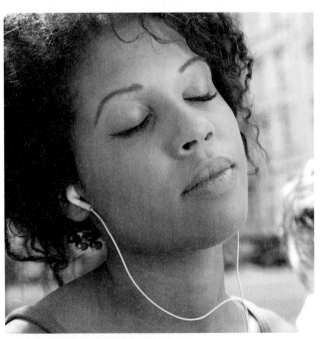

Taking time to relax can help you manage stress.

Table 3 ▶ Strategies for Stress Management

Category	Description
Appraisal-Focused Strategies	**Strategies That Alter Perceptions of the Problem or Your Ability to Cope Effectively with the Problem**
• Cognitive restructuring	• Changing negative or automatic thoughts leading to unnecessary distress
• Seeking knowledge or practicing skills	• Finding ways to increase your confidence in your ability to cope
Emotion-Focused Strategies	**Strategies That Minimize the Emotional and Physical Effects of the Situation**
• Relaxing	• Using relaxation techniques to reduce the symptoms of stress
• Exercising	• Using physical activity to reduce the symptoms of stress
• Expressing your feelings	• Talking with someone about what you are feeling or writing about your emotional experiences
• Spirituality	• Looking for spiritual guidance to provide comfort
Problem-Focused Strategies	**Strategies That Directly Seek to Solve or Minimize the Stressful Situation**
• Systematic problem solving	• Making a plan of action to solve the problem and following through to make the situation better
• Being assertive	• Standing up for your own rights and values while respecting the opinions of others
• Seeking active social support	• Getting help or advice from others who can provide specific assistance for your situation
Avoidant Coping Strategies	**Strategies That Attempt to Distract the Individual from the Problem**
• Ignoring	• Refusing to think about the situation or pretending no problem exists
• Escaping	• Looking for ways to feel better or to stop thinking about the problem, including eating or using nicotine, alcohol, or other drugs
• Suppressing	• Actively trying to suppress emotional experiences or emotional expression
• Ruminating	• Focusing on your negative emotions and what they mean without taking efforts to address the problem

Stress-management training focuses on teaching active coping strategies. Active **coping** strategies are those that attempt to directly affect the source of the stress or to effectively manage the individuals' reactions

HELP **Health is available to Everyone for a Lifetime, and it's Personal**

Many college campuses have resources available to help students address the various causes of stress. Those resources include academic offices to help with time management and scholastic difficulties as well as counseling centers for anxiety, depression, relationships, and other problems. Additionally, offices such as housing, the medical clinic, health promotion, and financial aid can be a resource for a variety of other stressors that often come up.

Do you take advantage of the resources that your college provides to aid in your stress management? Why or why not? What stress management tactics do you use and how important are they in your lifestyle?

connect ACTIVITY

to stress. In contrast, passive coping strategies attempt to direct attention away from the stressor. Active coping strategies can be classified into three basic categories: **appraisal-focused coping, emotion-focused coping,** and **problem-focused coping.** These coping strategies target the emotional and physiological, behavioral, and cognitive aspects of stress, respectively (see Table 3).

Appraisal-focused coping strategies are based on changing the way one perceives the stressor or changing one's perceptions of resources for effectively managing stress. Emotion-focused coping strategies attempt to regulate the emotions resulting from stressful events. In contrast, problem-focused strategies are aimed at changing the source of the stress. While each of these strategies is effective in various circumstances, **avoidant coping** strategies, such as ignoring or escaping the problem or suppressing negative emotions, are likely to be ineffective for almost everyone.

connect VIDEO 3

Coping A person's constantly changing cognitive and psychological efforts to manage stressful situations.

Appraisal-Focused Coping Adapting to stress by changing your perceptions of stress and your resources for coping.

Emotion-Focused Coping Adapting to stress by regulating the emotions that cause or result from stress.

Problem-Focused Coping Adapting to stress by changing the source or cause of stress.

Avoidant Coping Seeking immediate, temporary relief from stress through distraction or self-indulgence (e.g., use of alcohol, tobacco, or other drugs).

Concept 16 described the characteristics associated with positive health outcomes, including optimism, an internal locus of control, self-efficacy, and conscientiousness. Not surprisingly, individuals with these characteristics tend to engage more effectively in adaptive coping strategies.

Coping with most stress requires a variety of thoughts and actions. Stress forces the body to work under less than optimal conditions, yet this is the time when we need to function at our best. Effective coping may require some efforts to regulate the emotional aspects of the stress and other efforts to solve the problem. For example, if you receive a bad grade on an exam, how you view the situation and interpret its meaning will have a major impact on how you feel. You will have to eventually accept your current grade and manage the emotions that accompany this reality. Then, you will need to take active steps to improve your performance on the next exam. It does no good to worry about past events so it is more important to look ahead for ways to address the problem. Coping with this situation may, therefore, require the use of all three coping strategies.

Emotion regulation is a primary goal of both appraisal- and emotion-focused coping. Emotion regulation refers to efforts to manage initial emotional reactions to stress or the resulting emotions and how they are expressed. Thus, both appraisal- and emotion-focused coping are considered emotion regulation strategies. The difference between the two approaches is in the timing: appraisal-focused coping attempts to change the initial emotional experience, whereas emotion-focused coping attempts to manage the emotional experiences that follow appraisal. Efforts to positively reappraise stressful experiences can reduce initial emotional reactions to a stressor but additional efforts may be needed to manage these emotions. Such efforts can be both adaptive and maladaptive. Adaptive approaches include relaxation and meditation, appropriate emotional expression, and efforts to seek social support. Often the latter two approaches go hand-in-hand, as members of one's social support network provide an outlet for expression of emotional distress.

Effective Coping Strategies

Appraisal-focused coping strategies can be effective for certain situations. The way you think about stressful situations (see Table 4) can dramatically impact your emotional experiences. Research has demonstrated that cognitive reappraisal leads to down-regulation of the autonomic and endocrine systems, leading to physical and mental health benefits. Fortunately, even those of us who do not typically engage in reappraisal can learn to use this approach. Research on

Table 4 ▶ Types of Distorted Thinking

Type	Description
1. All-or-none thinking	You look at things in absolute, black-and-white categories.
2. Overgeneralization	You view a negative event as a never-ending pattern of defeat.
3. Mental filter	You dwell on the negatives and ignore the positives.
4. Discounting the positives	You insist that your accomplishments and positive qualities don't count.
5. Jumping to conclusions	(a) Mind reading—you assume that others are reacting negatively to you when there is no definite evidence of this. (b) Fortune telling—you arbitrarily predict that things will turn out badly.
6. Magnification or minimization	You blow things out of proportion or shrink their importance inappropriately.
7. Emotional reasoning	You reason from how you feel: "I feel like an idiot, so I must be one." "I don't feel like doing this, so I'll put it off."
8. Should statements	You criticize yourself or other people with "shoulds" or "shouldn'ts." "Musts," "oughts," and "have tos" are similar offenders.
9. Labeling	You identify with your shortcomings. Instead of saying, "I made a mistake," you tell yourself, "I am a jerk," "a fool," or "a loser."
10. Personalization and blame	You blame yourself for something that you weren't entirely responsible for, or you blame other people and overlook ways that your own attitudes and behaviors might have contributed to the problem.

Source: Burns, D. D.

cognitive therapy approaches for treating anxiety and mood disorders has shown that people can readily learn this skill, and learning to change the way you think can reduce emotional distress. Fortunately, the effectiveness of cognitive reappraisal is not limited to people experiencing anxiety or mood disorders. In a study of workplace stress and health, a cognitive-behavioral intervention that targeted appraisal of stress was more effective than a behavioral coping skills intervention that combined emotion- and problem-focused coping strategies. Thus, the way you think about stressful situations can be as important as how you respond to them.

At one time or another, virtually all people have distorted thinking, which can create unnecessary stress. Distorted thinking is also referred to as negative or automatic thinking. To alleviate stress, it can be useful to recognize some common types of distorted thinking (see Table 4). If you can learn to recognize distorted thinking, you can change the way you think and often reduce your stress levels.

If you have ever used any of the 10 types of distorted thinking described in Table 4, you may find it useful to consider different methods of "untwisting" your thinking and change negative thinking to positive thinking (see Table 5). To try this, think of a recent situation that caused stress. Describe the situation on paper, and see if you used distorted thinking in the situation (see Table 4). If so, write down which types of distorted thinking you used. Finally, determine if any of the guidelines in Table 5 would have been useful. If so, write down the strategy you could have used. When a similar situation arises, you will be prepared to deal with the stressful situation. Repeat this technique, using several situations that have recently caused stress.

Emotion-focused coping strategies are helpful for issues or problems that are not within your control. Relaxation techniques and/or coping strategies can help reduce the negative impact of both physical and

Table 5 ▶ Ten Ways to Untwist Your Thinking

Way	Description
1. Identify the distortion.	Write down your negative thoughts, so you can see which of the 10 types of distorted thinking you are involved in. This will make it easier to think about the problem in a more positive and realistic way.
2. Examine the evidence.	Instead of assuming that your negative thought is true, or if you feel you never do anything right, you can list several things that you have done successfully.
3. Use the double standard method.	Instead of putting yourself down in a harsh, condemning way, talk to yourself in the same compassionate way you would talk to a friend with a similar problem.
4. Use the experimental technique.	Do an experiment to test the validity of your negative thought. For example, if, during an episode of panic you become terrified that you are about to die of a heart attack, you can jog or run up and down several flights of stairs. This will prove that your heart is healthy and strong.
5. Think in shades of gray.	Although this method might sound drab, the effects can be illuminating. Instead of thinking about your problems in all-or-none extremes, evaluate things on a range from 0 to 100. When things do not work out as well as you had hoped, think about the experience as a partial success, rather than a complete failure. See what you can learn from the situation.
6. Use the survey method.	Ask people questions to find out if your thoughts and attitudes are realistic. For example, if you believe that public speaking anxiety is abnormal and shameful, ask several friends if they have ever felt nervous before giving a talk.
7. Define terms.	When you label yourself "inferior," "a fool," or "a loser," ask, "What is the definition of 'a fool'?" You will feel better when you see that there is no such thing as a fool or a loser.
8. Use the semantic method.	Simply substitute language that is less colorful or emotionally loaded. This method is helpful for "should" statements. Instead of telling yourself, "I *shouldn't* have made that mistake," you can say, "It would be better if I hadn't made that mistake."
9. Use reattribution.	Instead of automatically assuming you are "bad" and blaming yourself entirely for a problem, think about the many factors that may have contributed to it. Focus on solving the problem instead of using up all your energy blaming yourself and feeling guilty.
10. Do a cost-benefit analysis.	List the advantages and disadvantages of a feeling (such as getting angry when your plane is late), a negative thought (such as "No matter how hard I try, I always screw up"), or a behavior pattern (such as overeating and lying around in bed when you are depressed). You can also use the cost-benefit analysis to modify a self-defeating belief, such as "I must always be perfect."

Source: Burns, D. D.

emotional consequences of stress. These approaches can slow your heart and respiration rate, relax tense muscles, clear your mind, and help you relax mentally and emotionally. Perhaps most important, these techniques can improve your outlook and help you cope better with the stressful situation. In Lab 17C, you will try several relaxation techniques. However, performing the exercises only once will not prepare you to use relaxation techniques effectively. You must practice learning to relax.

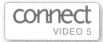

Conscious relaxation techniques reduce stress and tension by directly altering the physical symptoms. When you are stressed, heart rate, blood pressure, and muscle tension all increase to help your body deal with the challenge. Conscious relaxation techniques reduce these normal effects and bring the body back to a more relaxed state. These approaches can also help you manage the negative emotions that result from stressors and your appraisal of those stressors. Most techniques use the "three Rs" of relaxation to help the body and mind relax: (1) reduce mental activity, (2) recognize tension, and (3) reduce respiration. Some relaxation techniques include:

- *Deep breathing and mental imagery.* One of the quickest ways to experience relaxation is through deep breathing. There are many versions of deep breathing exercises. For example, first inhale deeply through your nose for about 4 seconds, making sure that your abdomen rises when you are inhaling. Next, let the air out slowly through your mouth (for about 8 seconds, or twice as long as the inhalation). Repeating these steps for several minutes can help control the body's reaction to stress. See Lab 17C, Figure 3, for detailed instructions on diaphragmatic breathing. Many relaxation approaches combine deep breathing with mental imagery to maximize the relaxation response. This approach involves imagining a pleasant image or scene that you associate with relaxation, such as a peaceful lake or stream. The goal is to imagine the scene as completely as possible using all of your senses. The main advantage of these approaches is that they can be used in any setting, and they take very little time to induce a relaxation response.

- *Jacobson's progressive relaxation method.* You must be able to recognize how a tense muscle feels before you can voluntarily release the tension. In this technique, contract the muscles strongly and then relax. Relax each of the large muscles first and later the small ones. Gradually reduce the contractions in intensity until no movement is visible. The emphasis is always placed on detecting the feeling of tension as the first step in "letting go," or "going negative." Jacobson, a pioneer

in muscle relaxation research, emphasized the importance of relaxing eye and speech muscles, because he believed these muscles trigger the reactions of the total organism more than other muscles.

- *Biofeedback.* Biofeedback training uses machines that monitor certain physiological processes of the body and that provide visual or auditory evidence of what is happening to normally unconscious bodily functions. The evidence, or feedback, is then used to help you decrease these functions. When combined with autogenic training, subjects have learned to relax and reduce the electrical activity in their muscles, lower blood pressure, decrease heart rate, change their brainwaves, and decrease headaches, asthma attacks, and stomach acid secretion.

- *Stretching and rhythmical exercises.* After working long hours at a desk, release tension by getting up frequently to stretch, taking a brisk walk, or by performing "office exercises." Exercising to music or a rhythmic beat can be relaxing and even hypnotic. One popular activity that uses 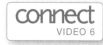 stretching and rhythmic exercise (as well as breathing techniques) is yoga. Many find it to be beneficial in reducing stress, and research has found both physical and mental health benefits associated with yoga.

TECHNOLOGY UPDATE

Instant Biofeedback

Although biofeedback has been used by physicians for decades, it has typically involved patient visits to the doctor to use expensive biofeedback equipment. Fortunately, new technology has increased the portability of biofeedback. There are now several commercially available biofeedback devices that are relatively compact and affordable, and some can simply be connected to your own computer. Examples include StressEraser and MyCalmBeat. More recently, biofeedback programs have been developed as applications for mobile devices. For example, Stress Check is a free application that uses the camera on your smartphone to measure heart rate variability, providing you with feedback about your stress level. You can try using it before and after one of the relaxation techniques described in Lab 17C to find out if you are effectively managing your stress response.

Would you consider using this type of biofeedback application for stress management if it was available on your smartphone?

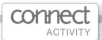

Spirituality and mindfulness can help you cope with stress and daily problems. Besides managing the body's physical response to stress, one must deal with the impact of stress on thoughts and emotions. Although relaxation strategies can impact these dimensions, additional approaches may be necessary to adequately manage these aspects of the stress response.

- *Spirituality.* Studies have shown that spirituality can decrease blood pressure, be a source of internal comfort, and have other calming effects associated with reduced distress. It can also provide confidence to function more effectively, thereby reducing the stresses associated with ineffectiveness at work or in other situations. The health benefits of spirituality do not appear to be restricted to prayer, however. Using a more global measure of spirituality, one study of college students found that spirituality moderated the relationship between stress and health outcomes. For those low in spirituality, stress was associated with higher levels of negative emotion and physical symptoms of illness. Among those higher in spirituality, the link between stress and health outcomes was much weaker.

- *Mindfulness meditation.* While most relaxation techniques seek to distract attention away from distressing emotions, mindfulness meditation encourages the individual to experience fully his or her emotions in a nonjudgmental way. The individual brings full attention to the internal and external experiences that are occurring "in the moment." Although research on mindfulness is just emerging, results look promising. For example, in a study of medical students, a mindfulness-based stress-reduction program led to significant decreases in mood disturbances. In another study, mindfulness meditation reduced the impact of daily stressors, psychological distress, and medical symptoms. Mindfulness may have particular value for individuals with chronic medical conditions. Benefits have been demonstrated with medical conditions such as fibromyalgia, cancer, and coronary artery disease. The nonjudgmental aspect of awareness in mindfulness is critical to the success of this approach. Increased attention to negative emotion that involves an evaluative component (e.g., this emotion is terrible) is often referred to as rumination. There is considerable evidence that rumination leads to negative psychological adjustment, including increased risk for depression.

Appropriately expressing emotion can help you reduce distress. The ability to control emotional outbursts is an adaptive skill that develops with age. As a society, we socialize our children to develop these skills, as they are critical to adaptive functioning in adulthood. At the same time, complete suppression of emotion has long been recognized as potentially harmful to our health. For example, Freud believed that inhibition of emotion contributed to psychological problems. Although it has taken roughly 100 years since Freud's early writing, recent studies have demonstrated that suppression of emotion leads to negative outcomes. In the laboratory, emotional suppression leads to increased physiological stress. Among college students, emotional suppression is related to increased anxiety, sensitivity, depression, and poor social adjustment. Thus, if we want to minimize the potential negative impact of our emotions, we need to find appropriate ways to express them.

We often turn to others to provide an outlet for us to "vent" or "get it off our chest." Although this is a perfectly good way to express emotion, we can also benefit from writing about our stressful experiences. Expressive writing has shown benefits for a wide range of outcomes, from faster wound healing to better adaptation following traumatic events. Writing also seems to help mitigate the effects of stress related to discrimination. For example, a recent study of gay male college students found that writing about stresses related to sexual orientation led to better adjustment 3 months later. Interestingly, the writing experience seemed to provide the most benefit to students who had lower levels of social support. Thus, writing about stressful experiences may provide an important outlet when social support is not readily available. In addition, there is some evidence that sharing one's expressive writing with others has further benefits. In fact, a recent study of college students found that, although both private and shared writing improved psychological outcomes, only shared emotional writing showed benefits on physical symptoms.

Problem-focused coping is most effective in dealing with controllable stressors. While appraisal- and emotion-focused coping may be the most effective means for coping with situations beyond one's control, a problem under personal control may best be addressed by taking action to solve the problem.

Problem solving and assertiveness can help you cope. Each stressful situation has unique circumstances and meaning to the individual. Thus, it is impossible to offer specific information about the best stress management strategy without knowing the source of the stress and how it is affecting a specific person. However, it is possible to offer a framework for consistently responding to difficult situations. A technique called "systematic problem solving" has been shown to improve the likelihood of problem resolution.

The first step is brainstorming, generating every possible solution to the problem. During this stage, do not limit the solutions you generate in any way. Even silly and impractical solutions should be included. After generating a comprehensive list, narrow your focus by eliminating any solutions that do not seem reasonable. Reduce the number of solutions to a reasonable number (four or five), and then carefully evaluate each option. Consider the potential costs and benefits of each approach to aid in making a decision. Once you decide on an approach, carefully plan the implementation of the strategy, anticipating anything that might go wrong and being prepared to alter your plan as necessary.

In some cases, directly addressing the source of stress involves responding assertively. For example, if the source of stress is an employer placing unreasonable demands on your time, the best solution to the problem may involve talking to your boss about the situation. This type of confrontation is difficult for many people concerned about being overly aggressive. However, you can stand up for yourself without infringing on the rights of others.

Many people confuse assertiveness with aggression, leading to passive responses in difficult situations. An aggressive response intimidates others and fulfills one's own needs at the expense of others. In contrast, an assertive response protects your own rights and values while respecting the opinions of others.

Once you are comfortable with the idea of responding assertively, practice or role-play assertive responses with a trusted friend before trying them in the real world. Your friend may provide valuable feedback about your approach, and the practice may increase your self-efficacy for responding and your expectancies for a positive outcome.

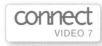

Social Support and Stress Management

Social support is important for effective stress management. **Social support** can play a role in coping with stress, and it has been linked to better physical and mental health outcomes among individuals with chronic stress-related illnesses. For example, in a large group of patients with coronary artery disease, participation in a social support group was associated with lower systolic blood pressure, better social functioning, and better mental health. The improvements in social functioning and mental health were due, at least in part, to improved health behaviors. Social support may also be critical to managing stress in academic settings. A recent study found that a lack of social support from family, teachers, and peers was associated with a lack of academic motivation and subsequent academic failure.

Social support may be particularly important for women. Women may be particularly likely to seek and provide social support when stressed. A paradigm called

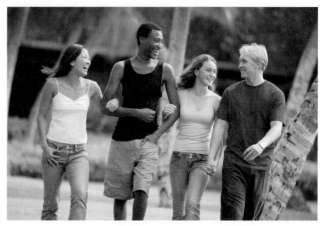

Social support is important for stress management.

the "tend or befriend" model suggests that women have a unique stress response. Women respond to stress by tending to others (nurturing) and affiliating with a social group (befriending). This response is helpful in protecting offspring and reducing the risk for the negative health consequences of stress.

Social support has various sources. Everyone needs someone to turn to for support when feeling overwhelmed. Support can come from friends, family members, clergy, a teacher, a coach, or a professional counselor. Different sources provide different forms of support. Even pets have been shown to be a good source of social support, with consequent health and quality of life benefits. The goal is to identify and nurture relationships that can provide this type of support. In turn, it is important to look for ways to support and assist others.

There are many types of social support. Social support has three main components: informational, material, and emotional. Informational (technical) support includes tips, strategies, and advice that can help a person get through a specific stressful situation. For example, a parent, friend, or co-worker may offer insight into how he or she once resolved similar problems. Material support is direct assistance to get a person through a stressful situation—for example, providing a loan to help pay off a short-term debt. Emotional support is encouragement or sympathy that a person provides to help another cope with a particular challenge.

Regardless of the type of support, it is important that it fosters autonomy. Social support that helps you to become more self-reliant because of increased feelings

Social Support The behavior of others that assists a person in addressing a specific need.

In the News

Social Networking for Social Support

Some have expressed concern that social networking sites (SNS) like Facebook may lead to a deterioration in "real world" social support; however, recent studies suggest that these websites are associated with higher rather than lower levels of social support. A recent study by Pew Internet (www.pewinternet.org) found no differences between SNS and non-SNS users with respect to the number of people in their social networks. However, SNS users were significantly less likely to be socially isolated and reported a larger number of close social ties. The latter difference remained when controlling for demographic variables including gender, age, and education. These results suggest that the use of SNS strengthens rather than weakens social support. A recent study of college students published in *Developmental Psychology* also found support for the social benefits of social network sites though not all outcomes were positive (e.g., possible increases in narcissistic displays).

Do you think your use of social networking sites has improved or worsened the quality of your social network?

of competence is best for developing autonomy. Social support that is controlling or leads to dependence may increase rather than decrease stress over time.

Obtaining good social support requires close relationships. Although we live in a social environment, it is often difficult to ask people for help. Sometimes the nature and severity of our problems may not be apparent to others. Other times, friends may not want to offer suggestions or insight because they do not want to appear too pushy. To obtain good support, one must develop quality personal relationships. Although having a large social support network is helpful, quality seems to be at least as important as quantity. Many individuals report feeling lonely despite having large social networks, and loneliness is associated with negative health behaviors, including smoking and lack of exercise.

Sometimes professional help is necessary to deal with problems related to stress. Although members of your social support network may be able to help you manage many of the stressors you experience, sometimes stress creates problems that require professional help. If you think you might be suffering from posttraumatic stress disorder or depression, there are well-established treatments that can help you function more effectively. Sometimes, professionals can also be helpful in efforts to change negative health behaviors such as alcohol and drug use, or problematic patterns of eating. Thankfully, stigmas associated with these problems have decreased in the past 25 years, leading many more people to seek professional services. In addition, new approaches to treatment are now being developed, including online therapy and mail-based interventions. These approaches have the potential to reach even more people in need of professional help.

Strategies for Action

Some practical steps can help you identify and manage your stress. This concept described strategies and skills for preventing, managing, and coping with stress. For strategies to be effective, they must be used regularly. Several practical steps you can take are described in the following list.

- *Self-assess your stress levels.* Making self-assessments such as those in Labs 16A and 16B can help you identify the sources and the magnitude of stress in your life.

- *Adopt effective coping strategies.* Consistent with the information presented in this concept, learning about and using a variety of appraisal-focused, emotion-focused, and problem-focused strategies will help you manage stress in your daily life.

- *Manage time effectively.* Lab 17A can help you understand your current time use patterns and help you develop a schedule that will allow you to focus on your priorities.

- *Evaluate strategy effectiveness.* Lab 17B will help you assess the effectiveness of various coping strategies. It also provides a basis for altering strategies to manage your stress levels more effectively. Lab 17C will help you to relax tense muscles, an emotion-focused coping strategy. Lab 17D will help you evaluate your current social support system.

connect
ACTIVITY

Web Resources

ABC's of Internet Therapy **www.metanoia.org/imhs**

American Institute of Stress **www.stress.org**

American Psychological Association **www.apa.org**

American Time Use Survey from the Bureau of Labor Statistics **www.bls.gov/tus/**

International Stress Management Association **www.isma.org.uk**

Mental Health Resources **www.mentalhealth.about.com**

National Mental Health Information Center **www.mentalhealth.samhsa.gov**

Time Management for College Students **www.time-management-for-students.com**

Suggested Readings

Girdano, D., G. S. Everly, and D. E. Duseck. 2012. *Controlling Stress and Tension.* 9th ed. Needham Heights, MA: Benjamin Cummings.

Goldin, P. R., and J. J. Gross. 2010. Effects of mindfulness-based stress reduction (MBSR) on emotion regulation in social anxiety disorder. *Emotion* 10:83–91.

Greenberg, J. S. 2011. *Comprehensive Stress Management.* 11th ed. New York: McGraw-Hill.

Hampton, K. N., et al. 2011. Social networking sites and our lives. Pew Research Center's Internet & American Life Project. Available at **http://pewinternet.org/ Reports/2011/Technology-and-social-networks.aspx**

Jacobson, E. 1978. *You Must Relax.* New York: McGraw-Hill.

Keogh, E., F. W. Bond, and P. E. Flaxman. 2006. Improving academic performance and mental health through a stress management intervention: Outcomes and mediators of change. *Behaviour Research and Therapy* 44:339–357.

Low, C. A., A. L. Stanton, and J. E. Bower. 2008. Effects of acceptance-oriented versus evaluative emotional processing on heart rate recovery and habituation. *Emotion* 8:419–424.

Manago, A. M., Taylor, T., and P. M. Greenfield. 2012. Me and my 400 friends: The anatomy of college students' Facebook networks, their communication patterns, and well-being. *Developmental Psychology* 48:369–380.

O'Keefe, E. J., and D. S. Berger. 2007. *Self-Management for College Students: The ABC Approach.* 3rd ed. Hyde Park, NY: Partridge Hill.

Pachankis, J. E., and M. R. Goldfried. 2010. Expressive writing for gay-related stress: Psychosocial benefits and mechanisms underlying improvement. *Journal of Consulting and Clinical Psychology* 78:98–110.

Penedo, F. J., and J. R. Dahn. 2005. Exercise and well-being: A review of mental and physical health benefits associated with physical activity. *Current Opinion in Psychiatry* 18:189–193.

Puterman, E., et al. 2010. The power of exercise: Buffering the effect of chronic stress on telomere length. PLoS ONE 5(5):e10837. doi:10.1371/journal.pone.0010837

Richardson, K. M., and H. R. Rothstein. 2008. Effects of occupational stress management intervention programs: A meta-analysis. *Journal of Occupational Health Psychology* 13:69–93.

Roemmich, J. N., et al. 2009. Protective effect of interval exercise on psychophysiological stress reactivity in children. *Psychophysiology* 46:852–861.

Romas, J. A., and M. Sharma. 2007. *Practical Stress Management: A Comprehensive Workbook for Managing Change and Promoting Health.* 4th ed. San Francisco: Benjamin Cummings.

Seligman, M. E. 1998. *Learned Optimism: How to Change Your Mind and Your Life.* New York: Pocket Books.

Srivastava, S., et al. 2009. The social costs of emotional suppression: A prospective study of the transition to college. *Journal of Personality and Social Psychology* 96:883–897.

Healthy People 2020

The objectives listed below are societal goals designed to help all Americans improve their health between now and the year 2020. They were selected because they relate to the content of this concept.

- Promote quality of life, healthy development, and healthy behaviors across all stages of life.

- Increase screening and treatment of mental health problems.

- Increase levels of social support among adults.

- Increase screening for and reduce rates of depression.

- Increase availability of work-site stress-reduction programs.

- Increase the proportion of primary care facilities that provide mental health treatment.

A national goal is to improve mental health through prevention and by ensuring access to appropriate, quality mental health services. A specific goal is to improve screening and treatment of depression. The increased acceptance of depression as a medical problem has helped many people to seek help. Would you know the signs of depression well enough to recommend that a friend or family member seek help from a doctor?

connect
ACTIVITY

Lab 17A Time Management

Name Jason Herrin   **Section**   **Date**

Purpose: To learn to manage time to meet personal priorities

Procedures

1. Follow the four steps outlined below.
2. Complete the Conclusions and Implications section.

Results

Step 1: Establishing Priorities

1. Check the circles that reflect your priorities in the list below. Add priorities as necessary.
2. Rate each of the priorities you checked. Use a 1 for highest priority, 2 for moderate priority, and 3 for low priority.

Check Priorities	Rating	Check Priorities	Rating	Check Priorities	Rating
✓ More time with family	1	○ More time with boy/girlfriend		✓ More time with spouse	1
✓ More time for leisure	2	✓ More time to relax	3	○ More time to study	
✓ More time for work success	2	✓ More time for physical activity	3	✓ More time to improve myself	2
✓ More time for other recreation	3	○ Other _____		○ Other _____	

Step 2: Monitor Current Time Use

1. On the following daily calendar, keep track of daily time expenditure.
2. Write in exactly what you did for each time block.

7–9 A.M.	9–11 A.M.	11 A.M.–1 P.M.	1–3 P.M.
get dressed / shower Exercise. Check emails	Head to work respond to emails. work	work lunch	work call family

3–5 P.M.	5–7 P.M.	7–9 P.M.	9–11 P.M.
work return home	dinner homework	spend time w/ kids	get kids ready for bed sleep

Step 3: Analyze Your Current Time Use by Using the ABC Method (See Table 2 on page 387)

A Tasks That Must *Absolutely* Get Done	B Tasks That *Better* Get Done	C Tasks That *Could* Be Done
work shower sleep get dressed	Spend time w/ family Eat Emails homework call family	Exercise get kids ready for bed leisure/relax

Step 4: Make a Schedule: Write in Your Planned Activities for the Day

Time	Activities	Time	Activities
6:00 A.M.		3:00 P.M.	work / call family
7:00 A.M.	wake up	4:00 P.M.	work
8:00 A.M.	Exercise / get ready	5:00 P.M.	work / return home
9:00 A.M.	travel to work / emails	6:00 P.M.	dinner
10:00 A.M.	emails / work	7:00 P.M.	homework
11:00 A.M.	work	8:00 P.M.	homework / kids
12:00 P.M.	work	9:00 P.M.	kids
1:00 P.M.	lunch	10:00 P.M.	relax
2:00 P.M.	work	11:00 P.M.	sleep

Conclusions and Implications: In several sentences, discuss how you might modify your schedule to find more time for important priorities.

My problem is I am so busy that I have little time for myself. I get little time with my wife alone and even less time by myself. This makes it difficult when a time conflict occurs and causes more stress. I need to just balance what little time I do have and perhaps take a vacation.

Lab 17B Evaluating Coping Strategies

Name	Section	Date

Purpose: To learn how to use appropriate coping strategies that work best for you

Procedures

1. Think of five recent stressful experiences that caused you some concern, anxiety, or distress. Describe these situations in Chart 1. Then use Chart 2 to make a rating for changeability, severity, and duration. Assign one number for each category for each situation.
2. In Chart 3, place a check for each coping strategy that you used in coping with each of the five situations you described.
3. Answer the questions in the Conclusions and Implications section.

Results

Chart 1 Stressful Situations

Think of five different stressful situations. Appraise each situation and assign a score (changeability, severity, duration) using the scale in Chart 2.

Briefly describe the situation.	Changeability	Severity	Duration
1. Fights w/ wife	3	4	2
2. stress from boss	2	3	1
3. kids acting out	2	2	1
4. money being tight	3	4	3
5. renters being difficult	3	3	1

Chart 2 Appraisal of the Stressful Situations

Use this chart to rate the five situations you described in Chart 1. Assign a number for changeability, severity, and duration for each situation in Chart 1.

	1	2	3	4	5
Was the situation changeable?	Completely within my control	Mostly within my control	Both in and out of my control	Mostly out of my control	Completely outside of my control
What was the severity of the stress?	Very minor	Fairly minor	Moderate	Fairly major	Very major
What was the duration of the stress?	Short-term (weeks)	Moderately short	Moderate (months)	Moderately long	Long (months to year)

Chart 3 Coping Strategies

Directions: Think about your response to the five stressful situations you recently experienced and check the strategies that you used in each situation. List use of other strategies as appropriate.

Coping Strategy	Situation 1	Situation 2	Situation 3	Situation 4	Situation 5
1. I apologized or corrected the problem as best I could.	✓	✓	✓		
2. I ignored the problem and hoped that it would go away.	✓	✓	✓		
3. I told myself to forget about it and grew as a person from the experience.	✓	✓	✓		
4. I tried to make myself feel better by eating, drinking, or smoking.					
5. I prayed or sought spiritual meaning from the situation.	✓			✓	
6. I expressed anger to try to change the situation.	✓	✓	✓		
7. I took active steps to make things work out better.	✓	✓	✓	✓	
8. I used music, images, or deep breathing to help me relax.	✓				
9. I tried to keep my feelings to myself and kept moving forward.	✓	✓		✓	
10. I pursued leisure or recreational activity to help me feel better.	✓	✓	✓	✓	
11. I talked to someone who could provide advice or help me with the problem.	✓	✓	✓		
12. I talked to someone about what I was feeling or experiencing.	✓	✓	✓	✓	
13. Other _____					
14. Other _____					
15. Other _____					

Conclusions and Implications: In several sentences, discuss the coping strategies you used. What were the ones you used the most? Are these the ones you typically use? Were they effective? Would you consider other strategies in the future?

In very stressful situations I sought relief through prayer or through leisure activities. I am seeing a therapist and he helps me deal with my stress. Meeting with him has helped me handle future situations more effectively. I will continue to use these.

Lab 17C Relaxation Exercises

Name	Section	Date

Purpose: To gain experience with specific relaxation exercises and to evaluate their effectiveness

Procedures

1. Choose two of the relaxation exercises included in Chart 1 of this lab (see page 402) and read through the written instructions until you have a basic understanding of the exercises. Think through the specific aspects of the exercise until you have the process figured out.
2. Find a quiet place to try one of the exercises and follow the procedures as best you can. It is not possible to provide detailed instructions, but the information should be sufficient to give you a basic understanding of the exercises.
3. On another day try a different exercise.
4. Answer the questions in the Results section. Then complete the Conclusions and Implications section.

Results

1. Which of the two exercises did you try? (List them below.)

> 1. Jaws
> 2. Lower Back

2. Have you done either of the exercises before? ⊗ Yes   ◯ No

3. Was one relaxation exercise more effective or better suited to you than the others? Which one?

> Lower back exercise was more effective

Conclusions and Implications

In several sentences, discuss whether or not you feel that relaxation exercises will be a part of your wellness program. In what ways might you benefit from relaxation training? If you do not think you have a problem with relaxation, explain why.

> I think I will try these relaxation exercises.
> I believe I am good at relaxation. I still
> need to practice more methods though

Chart 1 Descriptions of Relaxation Exercises

A. Progressive Relaxation

Progressive relaxation uses active (conscious) mechanisms to achieve a state of relaxation. The technique involves alternating phases of muscle contraction (tension) and muscle relaxation (tension release). Muscle groups are activated one body segment at a time, incorporating all regions of the body by the end of the routine. Begin by lying on your back in a quiet place with eyes closed. Alternately contract and relax each of the muscles below—following the procedures described below. Begin with the dominant side of the body first; repeat on the nondominant side.

1. Hand and forearm—Make a fist.
2. Biceps—Flex elbows.
3. Triceps—Straighten arm.
4. Forehead—Raise your eyebrows and wrinkle forehead.
5. Cheeks and nose—Wrinkle nose and squint.
6. Jaws—Clench teeth.
7. Lips and tongue—Press lips together and tongue to roof of mouth, teeth apart.
8. Neck and throat—Tuck chin and push head backward against floor (if lying) or chair (if sitting).
9. Shoulder and upper back—Hunch shoulders to ears.
10. Abdomen—Suck abdomen inward.
11. Lower back—Arch back.
12. Thighs and buttocks—Squeeze buttocks together, push heels into floor (if lying) or chair rung (if sitting).
13. Calves—Pull instep and toes toward shins.
14. Toes—curl toes.

Muscle contraction phase: Inhale as you contract the designated muscle for 3–5 seconds. Use only a moderate level of tension.

Muscle relaxation phase: Exhale, relaxing the muscle and releasing tension for 6–10 seconds. Think of relaxation words such as warm, calm, peaceful, and serene.

Relax every muscle in your body at the end of the exercise.

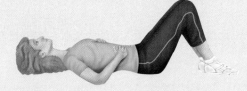

Figure 3 ▶ Diaphragmatic breathing.

B. Diapraghmatic Breathing

This exercise will help improve awareness of using deep abdominal breathing over shallower chest-type breathing. To begin, lie on your back with knees bent and feet on the floor. Place your right hand over your abdomen and left hand over your chest. Your hands will be used to monitor breathing technique. Slowly inhale through the nose by allowing the abdomen to rise under your right hand. Concentrate on expanding the abdomen for 4 seconds. Continue inhaling another 2 seconds allowing the chest to rise under your left hand. Exhale through your mouth in reverse order (for about 8 seconds, or twice as long as inhalation). Relax the chest first, feeling it sink beneath the left hand and then the abdomen, allowing it to sink beneath the right hand. Repeat 4–5 times. Discontinue if you become light-headed.

C. Show Gun

This is a form of Qigong, a Chinese meditation technique. The basic principles of tai chi are to maintain balance, use the entire body to achieve movement, unite movement with awareness (mind) and breathing (chi), and to keep the body upright. Tai chi involves holding the body in specific positions, or "forms." To execute the basic form, stand straight, feet shoulder-width apart and parallel with one another. Your knees should be bent and turned outward slightly with knees over the foot. Your hands are on belly button with palms facing body (men place hands right on left and women left on right), fingers are straight, spread slightly and relaxed.

1. Bring arms in front of body at a 30-degree angle to the plane of the back, palms face downward. Reach up to shoulder height with arms moving up and to the sides. (Breathe in, allowing belly to move out as you raise arms upward.)
2. When hands reach shoulder height, turn palms up and move hands to head, allowing wrists to drop down. Imagine energy (chi) flowing from palms to top of head. (Continue breathing in.)
3. Imagine energy flowing down through a central line of the body. Follow the energy with hands, point fingers toward one another, palms down, move arms downward in front of the midline of face and chest. (Breathe out as arms lower.)
4. Two inches bellow belly button stop, cross palms, and move hands together.
5. Lower hands toward sides. (Complete breathing out.)
6. Repeat.

Lab 17D Evaluating Levels of Social Support

Name	Section	Date

Purpose: To evaluate your level of social support and to identify ways that you can find additional support

Procedures

1. Answer each question in Chart 1 by placing a check in the box below Not True, Somewhat True, or Very True. Place the number value of each answer in the score box to the right.
2. Sum the scores (in the smaller boxes) for each question to get subscale scores for the three social support areas.
3. Record your three subscores in the Results section on the next page. Total your subscores to get a total social support score.
4. Determine your ratings for each of the three social support subscores and for your total social support score using Chart 2 on the next page.
5. Answer the questions in the Conclusions and Implications section.

Chart 1 Social Support Questionnaire

These questions assess various aspects of social support. Base your answer on your actual degree of support, not on the type of support that you would like to have. Place a check in the space that best represents what is true for you.

Social Support Questions	Not True 1	Somewhat True 2	Very True 3	Score
1. I have close personal ties with my relatives.				
2. I have close relationships with a number of friends.				
3. I have a deep and meaningful relationship with a spouse or close friend.				
			Access to social support score:	
4. I have parents and relatives who take the time to listen and understand me.				
5. I have friends or co-workers whom I can confide in and trust when problems come up.				
6. I have a nonjudgmental spouse or close friend who supports me when I need help.				
			Degree of social support score:	
7. I feel comfortable asking others for advice or assistance.				
8. I have confidence in my social skills and enjoy opportunities for new social contacts.				
9. I am willing to open up and discuss my personal life with others.				
			Getting social support score:	

Results

Scores and Ratings

(Use Chart 2 to obtain ratings.)

Access to social support score [ ]   Rating [ ]

Degree of social support score [ ]   Rating [ ]

Getting social support score [ ]   Rating [ ]

Total social support score [ ]   Rating [ ]
(sum of three scores)

Chart 2 Rating Scale for Social Support

Rating	Item Scores	Total Score
High	8–9	24–27
Moderate	6–7	18–23
Low	Below 6	Below 18

Conclusions and Implications

1. In several sentences, discuss your overall social support. Do you think your scores and ratings are a true representation of your social support?

2. In several sentences, describe any changes you think you should make to improve your social support system. If you do not think change is necessary, explain why.

Evaluating Fitness and Wellness Products: Becoming an Informed Consumer

LEARNING OBJECTIVES

After completing the study of this concept, you will be able to:

▶ Define quackery and fraud and outline steps that can be taken to avoid being susceptible to them.

▶ Evaluate the effectiveness of different physical activity programs and products.

▶ Select exercise equipment based on effectiveness, safety, and utility, and by avoiding quackery or fraud.

▶ Assess health clubs and exercise leaders (and their qualifications).

▶ Evaluate body composition and weight loss products for effectiveness and safety.

▶ Evaluate nutrition products for effectiveness and safety.

▶ Evaluate other consumer products (e.g., Internet, books, magazines) for various factors.

"Let the buyer beware" is a good motto for the consumer seeking advice or planning a program for developing or maintaining fitness, health, or wellness.

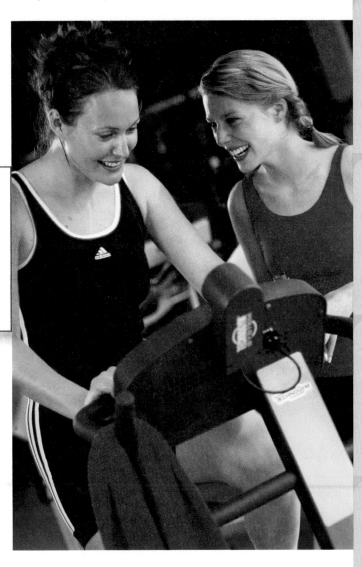

People have always searched for the fountain of youth and an easy, quick, and miraculous route to health and happiness. In current society, this search often focuses on fitness, nutrition, weight loss, or appearance. A variety of products are available that promise weight loss, better health, or improved fitness with little or no effort. The sale of these products can typically be classified as either quackery or fraud, since most do not work.

The dictionary definition of *quack* is "a pretender of medical skill" or "one who talks pretentiously without sound knowledge of the subject discussed." This implies that the promotion of quackery involves deliberate deception, but quacks often believe in what they promote. The consumer watchdog group Quackwatch defines quackery more broadly as "anything involving overpromotion in the field of health." This definition encompasses questionable ideas as well as questionable products and services. The word *fraud* is reserved for situations in which deliberate deception is involved. This concept discusses common myths and provides guidelines to help you be a more informed consumer of fitness, health, and wellness products.

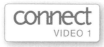

Quacks and Quackery

Quacks can be identified by their unscientific practices. Look for these clues to identify quacks, frauds, and rip-off artists:

- To a large extent, they use testimonials and anecdotes to support their claims rather than the scientific method (controlled experimentation that can be verified by other scientists). There is no such thing as a valid testimonial. Anecdotal evidence is no evidence at all.
- They have something to sell, and they advise you to buy something you would not otherwise have bought.
- They claim everyone can benefit from the product or service they are selling. There is no such thing as a simple, quick, easy, painless remedy for conditions for which medical science has not yet found a remedy.
- They promise quick, miraculous results. A perfect, no-risk treatment does not exist.
- Their claims cover a wide variety of conditions.
- They may offer a money-back guarantee. A guarantee is only as good as the company.
- They claim the treatment or product is approved by the Food and Drug Administration (FDA), but federal law does not permit mentioning the FDA to suggest marketing approval.
- They may claim the support of experts, but the experts are not identified.
- The ingredients in the product are not identified.

- They claim there is a conspiracy against them by "bureaucrats," "organized medicine," the FDA, the American Medical Association (AMA), and other groups. Never believe a doctor who claims the medical community is persecuting him or her or that the government is suppressing a wonderful discovery.
- Their credentials may be irrelevant to the area in which they claim expertise.
- They use scare tactics, such as "If you don't do this, you will die of a heart attack."
- They may appear to be a sympathetic friend who wants to share a new discovery with you.
- They misquote scientific research (or quote out of context) to mislead you; they also mix a little bit of truth with a lot of fiction.
- They cite research or quote from individuals or institutions with questionable reputations.
- They claim it is a new discovery (often originated in Europe). There is never a great medical breakthrough that debuts in an obscure magazine or tabloid.
- The person or organization named is similar to a famous person or credible institution (e.g., the Mayo diet had no connection with the Mayo Clinic).
- They often sell products through the mail or the Internet, which does not allow you to examine the product personally.

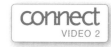

Experts have an educated, scientific base and meet other professional criteria. Unlike quacks, experts base their work on the scientific method. Some characteristics of professional experts are an extended education, an established code of ethics, membership in well-known associations, involvement in the profession as an intern before obtaining credentials, and a commitment to perform an important social service. Some experts require a license. Examples of experts in the fitness, health, and wellness area are medical doctors, nurses, certified fitness leaders, physical educators, registered dietitians, physical therapists, and clinical psychologists. In most cases, you can check if a person has the credentials to be considered an expert before obtaining services. The following list includes some things that can be done to determine a person's expertise.

- Determine the source of the person's education and the nature of the degree and/or certification.
- Check with the person's professional association, a government board, licensing agency, or certifying agency to see if there are any complaints against the person; for example, you can contact your state's medical board to check complaints against physicians.
- Check if the person has credentials to provide the service you are seeking (e.g., a registered dietitian is qualified to give nutrition advice but not medical advice).

Reduce your susceptibility to quackery by being an informed consumer. The three key characteristics that predispose people to health-related quackery are a concern about appearance, health, or performance; a lack of adequate knowledge; and a desire for immediate results. Understanding the principles of exercise and nutrition presented in this book will help you know when something sounds "too good to be true."

When evaluating health-related products or information, carefully consider the quality of your source. Common sources of misinformation are magazines, health food stores, and TV infomercials. These entities all have an economic incentive in promoting the purchase and use of exercise, diet, and weight loss products. Because of freedom of speech laws, it is legal to state opinion through these media. Note, however, that few companies make claims on product labels, since this is false advertising. Follow these additional guidelines to avoid being a victim of quackery:

- Read the ad carefully, especially the small print.
- Do not send cash; use a check, money order, or credit card so you will have a receipt.
- Do not order from a company with only a post office box, unless you know the company.
- Do not let high-pressure sales tactics make you rush into a decision.
- When in doubt, check out the company through your Better Business Bureau (BBB).

Scientific research is a systematic search for truth. Occasionally, companies will mention that their product or program has been scientifically tested, but this does not necessarily mean that the results were positive. Even if a study did show positive results, the study may have been flawed. An article in a prominent scientific journal documented that results of studies, especially small studies that are not well controlled, are often found to be wrong or the effects are not as large as originally thought. The media often highlight the results of novel or unusual findings, and this leads some people to conclude that experts simply "can't make up their minds." In actuality, scientists typically take a cautious approach with any new finding and wait for other studies to confirm the results. Beware of news reports that denounce established evidence based on a single study or "preliminary research." These findings may or may not be confirmed by future studies.

Physical Activity Quackery

There is no "effortless" way to get the benefits from physical activity. Advertisements for exercise that claim to "get you totally fit in 10 minutes" or that their program "will get you fit with little effort" are false. The only way to get fit is to follow the FIT formula for the type of exercise that you

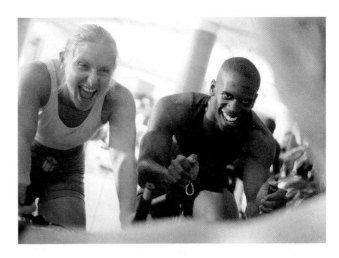

Changing your lifestyle, rather than quick solutions, is the key to health, fitness, and wellness.

choose for meeting specific fitness goals. Claims for exercise that will effortlessly reduce weight or produce significant health benefits are equally false. As noted in previous concepts, there are specific guidelines for physical activity designed for weight loss or maintenance and for achieving health benefits. Beware of those who claim otherwise.

Claims for many forms of exercise are overstated or unsubstantiated. New exercise programs or routines are often promoted as the complete answer for total fitness or a **panacea** for health. Claims for hatha yoga suggest it will help you lose weight, trim inches, strengthen glands and organs, or cure health problems, such as the common cold or arthritis. Hatha yoga can be useful in reducing stress, promoting relaxation, and improving flexibility, but the other claims are overstated.

Similar hype may be used for promoting new pieces of exercise equipment. Each piece of equipment claims to be fun, easy to use, and more effective than other forms of exercise. The benefits from exercise depend on the relative intensity and duration of the activity—and whether it is done regularly over time. The best form of exercise is clearly the one that you are willing and able to do.

Contrary to claims, passive exercises do not provide any benefits for fitness or weight loss. For exercise to be beneficial, the work must be done by contracting skeletal muscles. A variety of **passive exercise** forms have been promoted to try to reduce the effort required to perform regular exercise. Some passive

Panacea A cure-all; a remedy for all ills.

Passive Exercise Exercise in which no voluntary muscle contraction occurs; an outside force moves the body part with no effort by the person.

In the News

Exaggerated Health Claims on Shoes

Shoe companies release new technologies and innovations to attract customers to their products. Some new features include the integration of activity monitoring sensors and links with GPS sensors and music players. These technologies have focused on enhancing the exercise experience, but companies also try to develop new shock absorption technologies or training features aimed at enhancing performance. Some new innovations in shoes include curved heels and soles and shoes that have five pockets for your toes. The new innovations may be attractive to buyers because they are unique, but are they better than other shoes? The jury is still out on the benefits and potential dangers of shoes with special features, but if companies make claims for shoes, they must be able to back the claims. The Federal Trade Commission recently settled a claim against Reebok International. Reebok agreed to pay $25 million in customer refunds because of deceptive advertising of Easy-Tone and RunTone shoes. Under the settlement, Reebok is barred from making claims that toning shoes and apparel are effective in strengthening muscles, or that using the footwear will result in a specific percentage or amount of muscle toning or strengthening, unless the claims are true and backed by scientific evidence. Consumers cannot assume that the FTC or any other agency will protect them against other false claims. Therefore, you should carefully consider the basis for any fitness and health claims on products.

Are you influenced by ads and promotions for new sports and fitness technology? What can you do to make yourself less susceptible to false advertising or over-stated claims?

connect
ACTIVITY

---

devices have value for people with special needs, when used by a qualified person, such as a physical therapist. However, passive devices sold for use by the general public are ineffective. The goal of sellers is to convince people that there is an effortless way to exercise—there is not. The fallacies associated with many past forms of passive exercise, such as fat rolling machines (purported to break up and redistribute fat), seem obvious today, but new approaches come out all the time with different marketing and promotions. The list that follows highlights some of the common forms of passive exercise.

- *Vibrating belts.* These wide canvas or leather belts are driven by an electric motor, causing loose tissue of the body part to shake. They have no beneficial effect on fitness, fat, or figure. They are potentially harmful to the back and if used on the abdomen (especially if used by women during pregnancy, during menstruation, or while an IUD is in place).

- *Vibrating tables and pillows.* Contrary to advertisements, these passive devices (also called toning tables) will not improve posture, trim the body, reduce weight, or develop muscle **tonus.**

- *Continuous passive motion (CPM) tables.* The motor-driven CPM table, unlike the vibrating table, moves body parts repeatedly through a range of motion. Tables are designed to do such things as passively extend the leg at the hip joint and raise the upper trunk in a sit-up-like motion. Advocates claim that the tables remove cellulite, increase circulation and oxygen flow, and eliminate excess water retention. All of these claims are false. Hospitals and rehabilitation centers use a similar machine to maintain range of motion in the legs of knee surgery patients, maintain

integrity of the cartilage, and decrease the incidence of blood clots. Certainly, a healthy person has nothing to gain from using such a device.

- *Motor-driven cycles and rowing machines.* Like all mechanical devices that do the work for the individual, motor-driven machines are not effective in a fitness program. They may help increase circulation and maintain flexibility, but they are not as effective as active exercise. Nonmotorized cycles and rowing machines are good equipment for use in a fitness program.

- *Massage.* Whether done by a certified or licensed massage therapist or a mechanical device, massage is passive, requiring no effort on the part of the individual. It can help increase circulation, induce relaxation, prevent or loosen adhesions, retard muscle atrophy, and serve other therapeutic uses when administered in the clinical setting for medical reasons. However, massage has no useful role in a physical fitness program and will not alter your shape. There is no scientific evidence that it can hasten nerve growth, remove subcutaneous fat, or increase athletic performance. Some athletes (e.g., cyclists) find it aids in recovery from exercise.

- *Magnets.* The law requires magnets marketed with medical claims to obtain clearance from the FDA. To date, the FDA has not approved the marketing of any magnets for medical use, and sellers making medical claims for magnets are in violation of the law.

- *Electrical muscle stimulators.* Neuromuscular electrical stimulators cause the muscle to contract involuntarily. In the hands of qualified medical personnel, muscle stimulators are valuable therapeutic devices. They can increase muscle strength and endurance selectively and aid in the treatment of edema. They can also help prevent atrophy in a patient who is unable to move and may decrease muscle spasms, but in a healthy person they do not have the same value as exercise. The Federal Trade Commission (FTC) has filed false advertising claims against several firms that market exercise stimulators that promise to build *"six-pack abs"* and tone muscles without exercise. These devices, worn over the abdomen, are heavily advertised in infomercials and have been shown to be ineffective and potentially hazardous to health. Electrical stimulators placed on the chest, back, or abdomen can interfere with the normal rhythm of the heart, even for normally healthy people. For those with heart, gastrointestinal, orthopedic, kidney, and other health problems, such as epilepsy, hernia, and varicose veins, they can be especially dangerous. Beware of spas and clinics that use these devices and make claims of fitness enhancement for healthy people.

- *Weighted belts.* Claims have been made that these belts reduce waists, thighs, and hips when worn under the clothing. In reality, they do none of these things and have been reported to cause physical harm. However, when used in a progressive resistance program, wristlet, anklet, or laced-on weights can help produce an overload and, therefore, develop strength or endurance.

- *Inflated, constricting, or nonporous garments.* These garments include rubberized inflated devices (sauna belts and sauna shorts) and paraphernalia that are airtight plastic or rubberized. Evidence indicates that their girth-reducing claims are unwarranted. If exercise is performed while wearing such garments, the exercise, not the garment, may be beneficial. You cannot squeeze fat out of the pores, nor can you melt it.

- *Body wrapping.* Some reducing salons, gyms, and clubs advertise that wrapping the body in bandages soaked in a magic solution will cause a permanent reduction in body girth. This so-called treatment is pure quackery. Tight, constricting bands can temporarily indent the skin and squeeze body fluids into other parts of the body, but the skin or body will regain its original size within minutes or hours. The solution is usually similar to Epsom salts, which can cause fluid to be drawn from tissue. The fluid is water, not fat, and is quickly replaced. Body wrapping may be dangerous to your health; at least one fatality has been documented.

Considerations with Exercise Equipment

Exercise machines are very useful, but take care when determining the type of machine to use. When deciding which machines are best for you, ask yourself these questions.

- *What is your current state of fitness and your current level of physical activity?* Beginners and people with low fitness will want to choose a different piece of equipment than a more advanced exerciser. For example, exercise on a spinning bike would be appropriate for an advanced exerciser. The beginner might choose a regular exercise bicycle instead.

- *What are your goals?* Make sure the machine will help you meet your goals. For example, a resistance machine would be a good choice for building muscle fitness, and a treadmill or an elliptical machine would be a good choice for building cardiovascular fitness.

- *Will you enjoy it?* One limitation of exercise machines is that they are not as fun as doing sports and some other activities. But some machines may be more fun

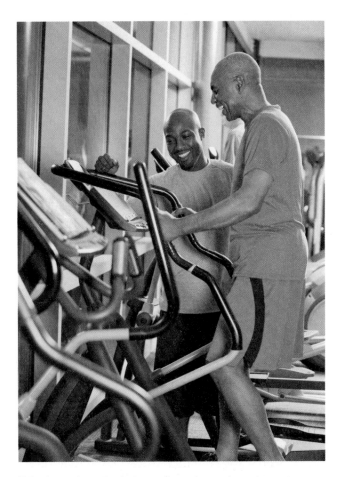

Take time to learn the features of exercise equipment.

Tonus The most frequently misused and abused term in fitness vocabularies. Tonus is the tension developed in a muscle as a result of passive muscle stretch. Tonus cannot be determined by feeling or inspecting a muscle. It has little or nothing to do with the strength of a muscle.

for you than others. Try several machines and consider one that you enjoy the most.

- *Will you stick with it?* Choose a machine you think you can use consistently. Enjoyment is a factor, but so is difficulty. Find a machine that allows you to easily adjust the intensity so you can find a comfortable intensity and gradually increase it over time.

- *Is it safe?* Exercise machines are the source of more than a few injuries. People with limitations (e.g., knee problems) may choose a bicycle rather than a treadmill. Get proper instruction on how to use a machine before trying it.

- *Can it be adjusted to fit your body?* Before you begin exercising, adjust the machine to fit your body. For example, adjust the seat on an exercise bicycle. If you are short or tall, some equipment may not fit you.

Home exercise machines can be very useful, but research your options before making a purchase. Research by the Consumer's Union (Consumer Reports) has shown that well-designed and manufactured exercise machines can be used as an effective means to achieving good health-related physical fitness. When using a piece of equipment at a health club, you can change machines if you don't like the one you are using. If you buy the equipment, you are stuck with it even if you don't like it. Before purchasing, consider the questions provided in the previous section as well as the following:

- *Is this the best piece of equipment for you?* Should you buy a resistance machine, a treadmill, an exercise bicycle, or some other equipment? Consider your goals and fitness needs to help you decide what equipment to buy.

- *Do you have space for it?* If you do not have a space where you can put the equipment and leave it, you will probably not use it regularly. Some equipment is "portable" so that it can be stored when not in use, but it is less likely to be used regularly than equipment that is readily available. The more difficult it is to move equipment, the less likely it is to be used. Consider ceiling height, room width, other uses for the space. Also, do you have space for a TV to watch?

- *Is the space appropriate?* More than a few people have bought equipment thinking they will put it in the TV room or the garage. Be sure all members of the family approve of the location of the equipment before purchasing it. Garages may be appropriate for some machines in some locales, but may be unusable in some very hot or cold climates. Also, some equipment such as free weights may take up extra space.

- *Will you use it?* The best time to buy used exercise equipment is in February or March. This is because many people buy equipment in January to fulfill a New Year's resolution to be more active. They don't carefully consider the reasons for their purchase and find that they don't use what they have bought. Try out the equipment before you buy, especially when considering expensive machines.

- *Do you need it?* Are there cheaper alternatives? Can you do the same thing less expensively?

- *Have you considered information from a reliable source such as Consumer Reports?* Consumer Reports does regular evaluations of exercise equipment. Consider their ratings and ratings of fitness experts to determine the quality, reliability, and repair records of various machines. Price is also a consideration. In some cases, if you cannot afford a quality machine, it might be wise to wait rather than to buy something that may not last. Finally, consider the product warranty and the cost of repairs if you do not get a warranty.

- *Is the dealer reputable?* Select a company or store that has been in business for a while and is a member of the Better Business Bureau. Compare prices for similar equipment. Beware of dealers who try to sell you extra attachments or accessories you won't use.

Be aware of the limitations of exercise machines and devices. Although exercise machines can be useful in carrying out your personal exercise plan, they are not without limitations. Some of these limitations are described here.

- *Many pieces of equipment are for a single purpose.* A machine that builds cardiovascular fitness may do little for muscle fitness or flexibility.

- *Monitors on machines are often inaccurate.* Studies have shown that machines that provide feedback often overestimate energy expenditure (calories expended).

- *Claims for the benefits of some machines are exaggerated.* Claims that machines can get you in the "fat burning zone" or that promise high-calorie expenditure with "low effort" are examples of quackery and should be discounted.

- *Some home equipment is not cost effective.* Will you get significant benefits from high-cost items? Consider low-cost equipment, such as exercise bands, exercise balls, and low-cost weights.

The use of hand weights and wrist weights while walking, running, dancing, or bench-stepping can increase the energy expended but require caution. Various devices, such as wrist, arm, or ankle weights and small, handheld weights, have been marketed as aids for increasing the energy expenditure in activities such as walking, running, and other forms of aerobic exercise. Step benches are another device that can be used to increase energy expenditure for aerobic exercise.

The practice of carrying weights is controversial. Carrying weights (not more than 1 to 3 pounds) while doing aerobic dance, walking, and other aerobic activities can increase energy expenditure, but the effect is negligible unless the arms are pumped (bending the elbow and raising the weight to shoulder height and then extending the elbow as the arm swings down). This energy output is comparable to a slow jog. Some experts caution that pumping the arms using weights can increase the risk for injury and suggest that the benefit of added energy expenditure is not worth the added risk for injury. Also, gripping weights while exercising can cause an increase in blood pressure.

Those who choose to use weights while doing aerobic activity are at less risk for injury if they use wrist weights rather than handheld weights. Arm movements should be limited to a range of motion below the shoulder level. Coronary patients and people with shoulder or elbow joint problems are advised not to use hand or wrist weights. Ankle weights are not recommended because they may alter your gait and stress the knees.

Consideration with Health Clubs and Leaders

Consider the credentials of a fitness leader or personal trainer before making a selection. Individuals with a college degree in physical education, physical therapy, exercise science, or kinesiology are recommended, as well as certifications from reputable organizations, such as the American College of Sports Medicine (ACSM). The ACSM offers several certifications with differing levels of expertise and education ranging from certified personal trainer to registered clinical exercise physiologist. Not all certifications are equal. Some unreputable and unethical organizations require little more than an application and a fee payment.

Consider a number of factors before making decisions about a health or fitness club. Consider the following factors when making your decisions.

- Is access to the facility really essential for you to begin or maintain a program?
- Is the facility convenient? The distance of a facility from home or work will greatly influence whether you use it regularly.
- Determine the qualifications of the personnel, especially of the individual responsible for your program. Is he or she an expert, as defined previously?
- Observe staff conduct to determine if they are available and efficient in day-to-day operations.
- Check to see if your membership can be sold, transferred, or canceled if you move.

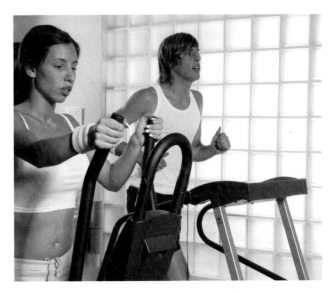

Visit a health club before you join.

- Choose a no-contract or monthly payment option if it is available so you can change your mind. Be prepared to resist options for long-term contracts.
- Check for hidden costs associated with membership (e.g., costs for testing, use of personal training).
- Do not be swayed by promises of quick results.
- Check if the equipment is up to date and maintained.
- Check for cleanliness. Is the facility clean?
- Are quack products sold and pushed? If so, it does not speak well of the professionalism of the staff.
- Are unproven products, such as supplements, sold or pushed to gain income?
- Check to see that towels are provided to wipe machines after use and that weights are replaced after use. If not, it is a good indication that supervision is not adequate.
- Are rules posted? For example, is there a time limit for using machines and is there a dress code?
- Speak with other members to get an insider's perspective on how they have been treated.
- Make a trial visit during the hours when you would expect to use the facility to determine if it is overcrowded, and if you would enjoy the atmosphere.
- Make certain the club is a well-established facility that will not disappear overnight.
- Check its reputation with the Better Business Bureau. Know that the BBB can only tell you if complaints have been made. It does not endorse companies and may lack information on new companies.
- Investigate programs offered by the YMCA/YWCA, local colleges and universities, and municipal park and recreation departments. These agencies often have excellent fitness classes, lower prices, and qualified personnel.

Saunas, steam baths, whirlpools, and hot tubs provide no significant health benefits, and guidelines must be followed to ensure safety. Baths do not melt off fat; fat must be metabolized. The heat and humidity from baths may make you perspire, but it is water, not fat, oozing from the pores.

The effect of such baths is largely psychological, although some temporary relief from aches and pains may result from the heat. The same relief can be had by sitting in a tub of hot water in your bathroom. The following guidelines and precautions should be considered when using a sauna, steam bath, whirlpool, or hot tub:

- Take a soap shower before and after entering.
- Do not wear makeup or skin lotion or oil.
- Wait at least an hour after eating before bathing.
- Cool down after exercise before entering the bath.
- Drink plenty of water before or during the bath.
- Do not wear jewelry.
- Do not sit on a metal stool; do sit on a towel.
- Do not drink alcohol before bathing.
- Get out immediately if you become dizzy; feel hot, chilled, or nauseous; or get a headache.
- Get approval from your physician if you have heart disease, low or high blood pressure, a fever, kidney disease, or diabetes; are obese; are pregnant or think you might be pregnant; or are on medications (especially anticoagulants, stimulants, or tranquilizers).
- Limit use for the elderly and for children.
- Do not exercise in a sauna or steam bath.
- Skin infections can be spread in a bath; make certain it is cleaned regularly and that the hot tub or whirlpool has proper pH and chlorination.
- Follow appropriate guidelines:

  Sauna: should not exceed 190°F (88°C) and duration should not exceed 10 to 15 minutes

  Steam bath: should not exceed 120°F (49°C) and duration should not exceed 6 to 12 minutes

  Whirlpool/hot tub: should not exceed 100°F (37°C) and duration should not exceed 5 to 10 minutes

Having a good tan is often associated with being fit and looking good, but getting tanned can be risky. Tanning salons may claim their lamps are safe because they emit only UVA rays, but these rays can age the skin prematurely, making it look wrinkled and leathery. They may also increase the cancer-producing potential of UVB rays and cause eye damage. Since there is no warning sign of redness, overdosing can occur. Thirty minutes of exposure to UVA can suppress the immune system. Tanning devices can also aggravate certain skin diseases. The Food and Drug Administration advises against the use of any suntan lamp. It is dangerous to use tanning accelerator lotions with the lamps because they can promote burning of the skin. Tanning pills are an even worse choice. They can cause itching, welts, hives, stomach cramps, and diarrhea and can decrease night vision. Tanning in the sun is also hazardous because it damages the skin, making it age prematurely, and it is a cause of skin cancer. Wearing sunscreen with at least a 15 SPF (sun protection factor), sunglasses, and protective clothing (including a hat) are good ideas when exposed to the sun.

Myths and Issues with Body Composition

Getting rid of cellulite does not require a special exercise, diet, cream, or device, as some books and advertisements insist. Cellulite is ordinary fat with a fancy name. You do not need a special treatment or device to get rid of it. In fact, it has no special remedy. To decrease fat, reduce calories and do more physical activity.

Spot-reducing, or losing fat from a specific location on the body, is not possible. When you do physical activity, calories are burned and fat is recruited from all over the body in a genetically determined pattern. You cannot selectively exercise, bump, vibrate, or squeeze the fat from a particular spot. If you are flabby to begin with, local exercise can strengthen the local muscles, causing a change in the contour and the girth of that body part, but exercise affects the muscles, not the fat on that body part. General aerobic exercises are the most effective for burning fat, but you cannot control where the fat comes off.

Surgically sculpting the body with implants and liposuction to acquire physical beauty will not give you physical fitness and may be harmful. Rather than doing it the hard way, an increasing number of people are resorting to surgery and muscle implants to improve their physique. Liposuction is not a weight loss technique but, rather, a contouring procedure. Like any surgery, it has risks, including risks for infection, hematoma, skin slough, other conditions, and death. As noted in Concept 15, a widely advertised product that claims to dissolve fat (Lipodissolve) has not been approved as safe by the FDA, and the FDA has issued a letter to sellers warning them to stop making unsubstantiated claims. Muscle implants give a muscular appearance, but they do not make you stronger or more fit. The implants are not really muscle tissue but, rather, silicon gel or saline, such as that used in breast implants or a hard substitute. Some complications can occur, such as infection and bleeding, and some physicians believe that calf implants may put pressure on the calf muscles and cause them to atrophy. A better way to improve physique and fitness is to engage in proper exercise.

Weight loss quackery is the most common form of consumer fraud. A one-year FTC study found that nearly one quarter of reported fraud cases involved weight loss products or resources. A recent example of fraud in the weight loss industry is the promotion of products containing human chorionic gonadotropin (HCG), a hormone produced by the human placenta and found in the urine of pregnant women. While HCG is FDA-approved as an injectable prescription drug for the treatment of some cases of female infertility and other medical conditions, there are no HCG drug products approved for weight loss. Companies marketed a number of over-the-counter HCG-based products by referring to them as a "homeopathic" therapy for weight loss. The products (sold as oral drops, pellets, and sprays) were actively marketed online and in retail stores such as GNC. The labeling states that the HCG should be taken in conjunction with a very-low-calorie diet; however, there is no scientific evidence HCG increases weight loss beyond that resulting from the caloric restriction. The FDA recently took action against companies selling HCG products. They specifically objected to the labeling of the products as homeopathic since there is no evidence that the use provides health benefits. The warning letters alert the companies that they are violating federal law by selling drugs that have not been approved and by making unsupported claims for the products. Although companies will be forced to stop selling this product, some just repackage products with new names or create new companies with a new line of products. As will be described later, it is difficult for the FDA to keep up with the continual release of new health and weight loss supplements on the market.

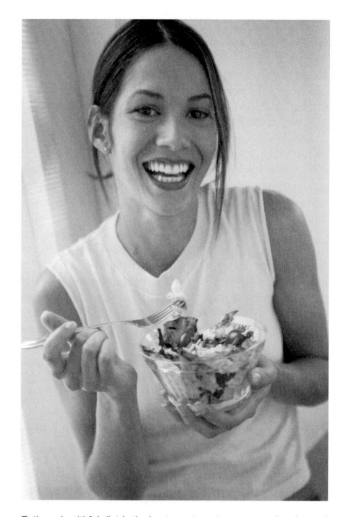

Eating a healthful diet is the best way to get necessary vitamins and minerals and other essential nutrients.

Nutrition Quackery

Diets are a major source of quackery. Basic guidelines for sound eating were described in Concepts 14 and 15. Beware of diets that do not follow these guidelines. Avoid diets that emphasize one nutrient at the expense of others (unbalanced diets), require the purchase of special products, and are proposed by people lacking sound credentials.

It is not true that if a little of something is "good," more is "better." The marketing of nutrition products often relies on convincing people that additional vitamins, minerals, or enzymes are beneficial. It is true that deficiencies of certain compounds may be harmful, but extra amounts don't always provide added protection or improved health. The myth that vitamin C can cure the common cold is based on the fact that deficiencies of vitamin C can lead to scurvy. The same hype is used to sell consumers many other unnecessary supplements. For example, protein supplements are marketed with convincing (and honest) claims that the body needs amino acids to form muscle. The hidden truth is that the body cannot store or use more than it needs.

Beware of energy drinks with "boosts" sold at smoothie shops and fitness clubs. Many restaurants and shops now promote drinks containing "boosts" (a tablespoon or two of a food supplement). Health clubs that sell drinks with supplements are susceptible to the claim that they are selling products for financial gain rather than the best interests of clients. Even if some supplements are effective, which most are not, taking one dose in a drink would be ineffective and a waste of money.

The designations of "herbal" or "natural" on supplements do not ensure safety or efficacy. Many health and nutrition supplements emphasize the word *herbal* because it relates to plants and people assume plants are natural and therefore healthy. There are literally thousands of herbal products and most medicines are derived from plants. However, the fact that herbs are natural does not mean they are safe. The most prominent example is with the herbal stimulant ephedra, which was used in many weight loss supplements. Over 150 deaths and thousands of adverse reactions were attributed to ephedra use before it was banned in 2004. Several other prominent herbal products include Saw Palmetto, an herbal supplement touted as a preventive for prostate cancer, and echinacea, an herb widely used to reduce symptoms of the common cold. While early studies showed some promise for these products, subsequent studies have not supported claims for these supplements. Consumers are encouraged to be careful about claims made for herbal products.

Some popular supplements from animal sources are also highly touted as having unique benefits. Glucosamine, for example, is made from shellfish, and chondroitin is made from the cartilage of sharks and/or cattle. Glucosamine and chondroitin are two of the most widely used supplements other than vitamins and minerals. They are often used to relieve symptoms and pain from osteoarthritis. Results of one large clinical trial suggested that the two supplements, taken together or separately, were no more effective than a placebo; however, a small group of people who had moderate to severe pain did experience some relief after using the supplements. These products probably do no harm but they may also do little for clinical relief of joint problems.

Consumer Protections against Fraud and Quackery

Current legislation does not protect food supplement customers. According to the FDA, a dietary supplement is a product taken by mouth that contains a "dietary ingredient" intended to supplement the diet. These ingredients include vitamins, minerals, herbs and other botanicals, amino acids, and other substances, such as enzymes, organ tissues, glandulars, and metabolites. Supplements come in many forms, including powders, tablets, softgels, capsules, gelcaps, and liquids. The passage of the Dietary Supplements Health and Education Act (DSHEA) in the 1990s shifted the burden of providing assurances of product effectiveness from the FDA to the food supplement industry, which really means it shifted to the consumer. Food supplements are typically not considered to be drugs, so they are not regulated. Unlike drugs and medicines, food supplements need not be proven effective or even safe to be sold in stores. To be removed from stores, they must be proven ineffective or unsafe. Unfortunately, it takes time and often extended court battles for the FBA and other agencies to get some products off the market.

When the DSHEA was passed in 1994, there were also no provisions for assuring that dietary supplements contained the ingredients they claimed to contain. However, the FDA has since instituted a rule requiring supplement manufacturers to provide labels to "insure a consistent product free of contamination, with accurate labeling." This is important because more than a few cases of product contamination have been reported. Under the new regulations, the manufacturer, not the FDA, has to test products to be sure that they are pure and accurately labeled. The FDA monitors the safety of supplements through "adverse events monitoring." This means that the FDA relies on consumers to report problems, or adverse events, rather than performing tests on the contents of products. When reports of problems are filed, the FDA investigates. For this reason, the only way that dangerous products and unscrupulous manufacturers can be identified is if consumers report problems to the FDA. Reports can be made at **www.fda .gov/medwatch/how.htm**. As noted in Table 1, there are other steps that can be taken to help determine if specific supplements contain what they say they do.

Most Americans favor more regulation of the supplement industry. When informed that the FDA does not regulate supplements, more than 80 percent of adults indicate that the FDA should review supplements before they are offered for sale. More than half of adults want more regulation on advertising of supplements and better rules to ensure purity and accurate dosage. Despite the lack of regulation of supplements, nearly half of Americans routinely take supplements and slightly more than half believe in the value of supplements. Interestingly, 44 percent believe that physicians know little or nothing about supplements. More than a few critics point out that self-regulation within the industry has not worked well. They suggest that the public would have more confidence in supplements if the FDA were watching out for their best interests. Table 1 presents some questions that should be asked about food supplements.

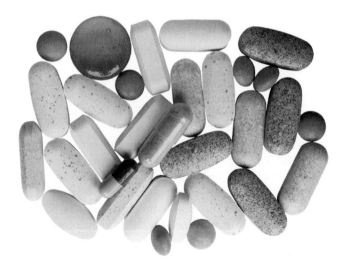

Good consumer skills are important for evaluating health products and for interpreting health claims.

Table 1 ▶ Summary of Important Facts about Food Supplements

The government does not test food supplements to ensure effectiveness or safety. This means that dietary supplements do not need approval of the FDA before they are marketed, and products are not prevented from reaching the market even if no evidence exists as to effectiveness.

Beginning in 2007, the FDA began requiring manufacturers to accurately label the content of supplements and to assure that products are what the manufacturer claims they are. However, the FDA does not test these products and, as noted in the text, relies on consumers to report problems with supplements.

Supplements can have side effects and interact with medicines (see Table 2 for examples).

U.S. Pharmacopia (USP) is a private, nonprofit organization that tests supplements to assure the quality, purity, and strength of a standard unit (dose size and strength). The USP label ensures that a product is what it says it is and that a dose is in the amount advertised. USP periodically tests products and removes its label from those who fail to meet its standards.

Informed-Choice is another nonprofit organization that provides information about dietary supplements. Information on supplements tested by the organization can be found at **www.informed-choice.org.**

Little is known about the long-term effects of most supplement use. For example, melatonin is a hormone that is used for insomnia. Hormones can have strong side effects, and little is known about melatonin's long-term effects. Consider alternative solutions to long-term use of unstudied supplements.

People who sell supplements are not required to have special training. Beware of people who use tactics such as those described in this concept to sell supplements. Avoid verbal information about products, especially information from sellers. Be wary of "third-party" information that cites research out of context or inaccurately.

Consumers should review the evidence carefully before using supplements. Federal guidelines and reports provide the best source of health information. Public confusion about the role of vitamins and minerals led to a formal review by a panel of experts with the National Institutes of Health (NIH). The report noted the value of some vitamin and mineral supplements while not recommending others. It endorsed folic acid supplements for women of childbearing age, calcium and vitamin D to protect against osteoporosis for postmenopausal women, and several other supplements for those with an eye condition called macular degeneration. The board found that there was not enough evidence to support taking a daily multivitamin. The board did not suggest, however, that those already taking a multivitamin stop doing it and did not find evidence that daily multivitamins are harmful. The review board did take a position against

beta-carotene (a form of vitamin A), saying there was no evidence that it is effective. Also, board members warned against taking very high levels of vitamins and minerals (megadoses), noting that they are not beneficial and can be dangerous. The board's cautious recommendations about vitamins were well founded as a recent study reported some negative consequences of long-term use of supplements and vitamins in people who do not have nutritional deficiencies. The study reported increased risk for cardiovascular disease and cancer among older women who took a daily vitamin supplement, even just a multivitamin. Previous studies have questioned the value of some supplements and vitamins, but this study raises questions about whether vitamin supplementation may do more harm than good in generally healthy people. More research is clearly needed.

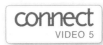

Some additional problems that you should be aware of when considering the use of supplements are described in Table 2. Some other incidents that illustrate that supplements are not always what they appear to be are listed below:

• The founder and former president of Metabolife pled guilty to federal charges that he gave false statements to the FDA. He claimed he had received no complaints about a diet pill containing ephedra (prior to the FDA

Table 2 ▶ Problems Associated with Supplements

Postsurgical problems, including bleeding, irregular heartbeat, and stroke—examples: echinacea, ephedra, ginkgo, kava, St. John's wort, ginseng

Dangerous interactions with medicines—examples: ephedra, St. John's wort (interact with birth control pills and HIV pills)

FDA warnings concerning unsubstantiated claims about herbs added to foods, such as energy bars and water—examples: ginkgo, ginseng, echinacea

Allergic and other physiological reactions; negative effect on decision making—example: GHB

Known ill effects to health—examples: comfrey (kidneys), kava (liver), ephedra (multiple deaths)

Recall because of dangerous effects associated with contamination—examples: PC SPES, Lipokinetix

Action by the FTC because of deceptive advertisements—examples: Exercise in a Bottle, Fat Trapper

Banned by several sporting groups, including the International Olympic Committee, NCAA, and NFL—examples: steroids, androstendione, ephedra (illegal in doses above 10 mg), THC

Contents may not be what they appear to be and dosage information is unknown—example: the International Olympic Committee studied 240 different supplements and found that 18.8 percent of the products contained steroids.

ban of ephedra). In his plea, he admitted the company received thousands of complaints about adverse effects.

- Hi Health, a major supplier of supplements, was fined by the FTC ($450,000) for false and misleading claims for one of its products (Ocular Nutrition).

- Producers of Airborne, a supplement purporting to help the body fight germs in public places, agreed to pay $23.3 million when a lawsuit exposed the fact that no scientists participated in studies cited by the company.

- A one-year FTC study found that 30.2 million adults bought fraudulent products; nearly 7 million people bought fraudulent weight loss products.

- A major supplement company was found guilty of selling bogus pills (e.g., to increase height, breast size, and penis size) that do not work. The company took in more than $77 million, but will pay only $4 million in refunds to customers.

The cost of supplements is substantial. Since the Dietary Supplements Health and Education Act was passed in 1994, the annual sales of food supplements nearly tripled, totaling more than $20 million each year. The cost of food supplements in a bottle (e.g., pills, capsules, powders) is typically very high. For example, a protein supplement can cost as much as $1 per gram. The cost per gram in good food, such as in a chicken breast, is typically a few cents per gram. Also, "protein bars" have a high cost per gram of protein and are sometimes high in empty calories (simple sugars) and/or fat.

In addition to the dollars spent on supplements and the high relative cost of supplements as opposed to food, there are costs to people who experience health problems associated with the use of some supplements. An editorial in a leading national newspaper suggests that "troubling side effects mount" and that "putting customers' health at risk is a high price to pay for a free market in diet supplements."

Be wary of claims made for supplements. The DSHEA has had at least one positive effect. Food supplement labeling must now be truthful. Claims concerning disease prevention, treatment, or diagnosis must be substantiated in order to appear on the product. Unfortunately, the act did not limit false claims if they are not on the product label. The result has been the removal of claims from labels in favor of claims on separate literature, often called third-party literature, because the label makes no claims and the seller (the second party) makes no written claims. Rather, the seller provides claims in literature by other people (a third party). The literature is distributed separately from the product, thus allowing sellers to make unsubstantiated claims for products. Also, the law does not prohibit unproven verbal claims by salespeople. Many medical experts feel that "alternative treatments" should

be subjected to the same type of rigorous scientific testing used to evaluate other medicines. However, as things currently stand, it is up to the consumer to make decisions about the safety and effectiveness of food supplements, so it is especially important to be well informed.

connect
VIDEO 6

Health Literacy and the Internet

Not all books provide information that is sound, reliable, and scientifically accurate. Some material is published on the basis of how popular, famous, or attractive the author is or how sensational or unusual his or her ideas are. Very few movie stars, models, TV personalities, and Olympic athletes are experts in biomechanics, anatomy and physiology, exercise, and other foundations of physical fitness. Having a good figure or physique, being fit, or having gone through a training program does not, in itself, qualify a person to advise others.

After reading the facts presented in this book, you should be able to evaluate whether or not a book, a magazine, or an article on exercise and fitness is valid, reliable, and scientifically sound. To assist you further, Lab 18A lists 10 guidelines.

Not all websites provide information that is sound, reliable, and scientifically accurate. Currently, approximately three-fourths of all teen and young adult computer users seek health information on the Web. But many health websites contain misinformation. Studies show that Wikipedia is the most common source of health information for the general public. One report showed that as many as one half of doctors surveyed used Wikipedia for health information. Many consumers, and some physicians, do not realize that Wikipedia can be edited by anyone and for this reason can contain erroneous information.

A recent study compared prescription drug information from Wikipedia and Medscape Drug Reference and found that Wikipedia had incomplete answers, incorrect information about dosage, and errors of omission about side effects. The authors of the study noted that Wikipedia should be used only as a supplemental source for drug information.

Improving health literacy is a key public health goal for 2020. The Internet has made an almost unlimited amount of health information accessible, but it has proven difficult to ensure that the information is used wisely. The public health service has established key goals to improve public health literacy and the quality of health information on the Internet. The two goals are designed to work together: consumers need access to accurate information, but they also need to know how to

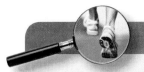

A CLOSER LOOK

Health Information on the Internet

The topic "health" has been the most actively searched topic on the Internet over the past 5 years. Unfortunately, consumers cannot always trust all the information they find on the Web. The best way to ensure good information is to start with good sources. There are a number of credible health websites that provide comprehensive health information on a variety of topics. Some examples include WebMD, Medline Plus, and Medwatch. While these sites provide accurate health information, there are countless others that provide flawed, biased, and even fraudulent information. To combat this, federal agencies and organizations have developed educational resources to help consumers detect quackery and fraud in health-related products and supplements. For example, the Food and Drug Administration's (FDA) Office of Regulatory Affairs recently launched a website designed to educate the public about health-fraud scams (**www.fda.gov/healthfraud**). The site includes educational and video resources, information about recent compliance actions, press releases, and links to the Medwatch site to report a problem with an FDA-regulated product.

Is this type of resource sufficient for educating consumers about health-care fraud and quackery?

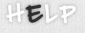

interpret and use the information (health literacy). The content presented in this concept provides a foundation for interpreting health information, but some additional guidelines are provided for effectively using the Internet.

One general rule is to consult at least two or more sources to confirm information. Getting confirmation of information from non-Web sources is also a good idea. Perhaps the most important recommendation is to consider the source of information. In general, government sites are valid sources that contain sound information prepared by experts and based on scientific research. Government sites typically include ".gov" as part of the address. Professional organizations and universities can also be good sources of information. Organizations typically have ".org" and universities typically have ".edu" as part of the address. However, caution should still be used with organizations because starting an organization and obtaining an ".org" address is easy. Your greatest trust can be placed in the sites of stable, credible organizations (see Web Resources in this book). The great majority of websites promoting health products have ".com" in the address because these are commercial sites, which are in business to make a profit. Thus, although some contain good information, they may focus on selling products or services. Therefore, it is important to view content from these sites more critically. The websites listed at the end of each concept fit the general guidelines given here, but you are encouraged to consider the quality of the individual sources when evaluating information from the various sites. The planned expansion of Internet domain names will complicate life on the Internet (see Technology Update).

TECHNOLOGY UPDATE

What about Titanium Necklaces?

Many fitness and sports stores have been selling titanium bracelets as a sports performance aid. The bracelets are fashionable and are promoted by high-profile athletes that are shown wearing the bracelets during training or competition. The website from the leading manufacturer suggests that muscles fatigue because of disruptions in the flow of bio-electric current and the unstated implication is that the bracelets address this in some way. The website mentions a "proprietary process" that allows the titanium to release current into your body but there is no scientific evidence supporting any potential benefits of titanium bracelets on performance or on pain relief (another common claim).

Would you try a product like this based on advertisements and testimonials?

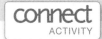

HELP   **Health is available to Everyone for a Lifetime, and it's Personal**
The Internet has become the leading source of health information for Americans. Unfortunately many health websites contain false or misleading information. We all have health problems from time to time and need good information.

If you or a family member has a health problem, what steps will you take to get information that you know to be accurate?

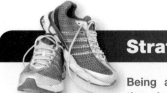

Strategies for Action

Being a good consumer requires time, information, and effort. Taking the time to investigate a product will help you save money and avoid making poor decisions that affect your health, fitness, and wellness. In Lab 18A, you will evaluate an exercise device, a food supplement, a magazine article, or a website. In Lab 18B, you will evaluate a health/wellness or fitness club.

When making decisions about products or services, begin your investigation well in advance of the day when a decision is to be made. Salespeople often suggest that "this offer is only good today," knowing that people often make poor decisions when under pressure.

Web Resources

Center for Science in the Public Interest **www.cspinet.org**
FDA's Health Fraud Scams website **www.fda.gov/healthfraud**
Federal Trade Commission **www.ftc.gov**
Food and Drug Administration **www.fda.gov**
Healthfinder **www.healthfinder.gov**
Health on the Net **www.hon.ch**
Medline Plus **http://medlineplus.gov/**
Medwatch **www.fda.gov/Safety/MedWatch/default.htm**
National Council against Health Fraud **www.ncahf.org**
National Institutes of Health, Health Information **http://health.nih.gov/**
Office of Dietary Supplements **http://ods.od.nih.gov**
Quackwatch **www.quackwatch.org**
U.S. Consumer Information Center **http://publications.usa.gov/USAPubs.php**

Suggested Readings

Anderson, G. M., D. Juurlink, and A. S. Detsky. 2008. Newly approved does not always mean new and improved. *Journal of the American Medical Association* 299(13):1598–1600.

Barrett, S., et al. 2013. *Consumer Health: A Guide to Intelligent Decisions.* 9th ed. New York: McGraw-Hill Higher Education.

Brokowski, L. 2009. Evaluation of pharmacist use and perception of Wikipedia as a drug information resource. *Annals of Pharmacotherapy* 43(11):1912–1913.

Consumer Reports. 2010. Dangerous Supplements. *Consumer Reports* 75(9):16.

Corbin, C. B. 2007. Dietary supplements: Making informed decisions. *ACSM's Health & Fitness Journal* 11(5):1–6.

Fox, S., and S. Jones. 2009. *The Social Life of Health Information: America's Pursuit of Health Takes Place on a Widening Network of Both Online and Offline Sources.* Washington, DC: Pew Internet & American Life Project.

Mursu, J. et al. 2011. Dietary supplements and mortality rate in older women: The Iowa Women's Health Study. *Archives of Internal Medicine* 171(18):1625–1633.

Seifert, S. M., et al. 2011. Health effects of energy drinks on children, adolescents, and young adults. *Pediatrics* 127(3):511–528.

Should you buy this now? Usually not, based on our tests of 15 infomercial products. 2010. *Consumer Reports* 75(2):16–20.

Swaim, D. P. 2009. Exercise equipment: Assessing the advertised claims. *ACSM's Health and Fitness Journal* 13(5):8–11.

Healthy People 2020

The objectives listed below are societal goals designed to help all Americans improve their health between now and the year 2020. They were selected because they relate to the content of this concept.

- Improve the health literacy of the population.

- Increase percentage of high-quality health-related websites.

- Increase percentage of college students receiving information on priority risk behavior areas.

- Create social and physical environments that promote good health for all.

- Increase food safety (variety of areas).

- Reduce adverse events from medical products.

- Reduce medical emergencies that occur from adverse events associated with medicines.

An important national health goal is to improve the health literacy of the population. Yet many people have misconceptions about health and fall prey to people who exploit their lack of information. What are two or three things that you think can be done to improve health literacy?

connect
ACTIVITY

Lab 18A Practicing Consumer Skills: Evaluating Products

Name	Section	Date

Purpose: To evaluate an exercise device, a book, a magazine article, an advertisement, a food supplement, or a website

Procedures

1. Evaluate an exercise device, a book, an article, a newspaper or magazine advertisement, a food supplement, or a website. Place an X in the circle by the item you choose to evaluate. Attach a copy if you evaluate an advertisement.
2. Read each of the 10 evaluation factors for the item you selected. Place an X in the circle by the factors that describe the item you are evaluating.
3. Total the number of X marks to determine a score for the item being evaluated. The higher the score, the more likely it is to be safe and/or effective.
4. Answer the questions in the Conclusions and Implications section.

Results

Directions: Place an X in the circle by the product you evaluated. Place an X over the circle by each true statement. Provide information about the product in the space provided.

Exercise Device

1. The exercise device requires effort consistent with the FIT formula.
2. The exercise device is safe and the exercise done using the device is safe.
3. There are no claims that the device uses exercise that is effortless.
4. Exercise using the device is fun or is a type that you might do regularly.
5. There are no claims using gimmick words, such as *tone, cellulite, quick,* or *spot fat reduction.*
6. The seller's credentials are sound.
7. The product does something for you that cannot be done without it.
8. You can return the device if you do not like it (the seller has been in business for a long time).
9. The cost of the product is justified by the potential benefits.
10. The device is easy to store or you have a place to permanently use the equipment without storing it.

Exercise Device

Name of device: _____
_____
_____

Description and manufacturer:
_____
_____
_____

Book or Article

Author(s): _____
_____
_____

Journal article or book title: _____
_____
_____

Journal name or name of publisher:
_____
_____
_____

Date of publication: _____
_____
_____

Advertisement

Source: _____
_____
_____

Book/Article/Advertisement

1. The credentials of the author are sound. He or she has a degree in an area related to the content of the book or magazine.*
2. The facts in the article are consistent with the facts described in this book.
3. The author does not claim "quick" or "miraculous" results.
4. There are no claims about the spot reduction of fat or other unfounded claims.
5. The author/advertisement is not selling a product.
6. Reputable experts are cited.
7. The article does not promote unsafe exercises or products.
8. New discoveries from exotic places are not cited.
9. The article/advertisement does not rely on testimonials by nonexpert, famous people.
10. The author/advertisement does not make claims that the AMA, the FDA, or another legitimate organization is trying to suppress information.

*Not applicable for advertisement.

Food Supplement

1. The seller is not the prime source of product information.

2. The seller has been in business for a long time and has a good reputation.

3. There is scientific evidence of product effectiveness.

4. There is clear evidence about the side effects of the active ingredients.

5. The long-term effectiveness and safety of the product are cited.

6. You are sure of the content of the product.

7. You have information that the manufacturer is reputable.

8. The known benefits are worth the cost.

9. There is evidence that you can get benefits from this product that cannot be obtained from good food.

10. There are no claims that use quack words or claims about conspiracies against the product by reputable organizations.

Food Supplement

Name: _____
_____
_____

Purported benefit: _____
_____
_____

Manufacturer/seller: _____
_____
_____

Dose and active ingredient: _____
_____
_____

Website

Web address: _____
_____
_____

Type of information provided: ____
_____
_____

Organization or person responsible for information: _____
_____
_____

Website

1. The site does not sell products associated with information provided.

2. The provider is a person, an organization (org), or a governmental agency (gov) with a sound reputation.

3. The site does not use quack words.

4. The site does not try to discredit well-established organizations or governmental agencies.

5. The site does not rely on testimonials, celebrities, or people with unknown credentials.

6. The site is well regarded by experts (e.g., check ratings on sites such as at http://navigator.tufts.edu).

7. The site has a history of providing good information.

8. The site provides complete information that is documented by research.

9. No claims of quick cures or miracle results are made.

10. The site provides information consistent with information provided in this text.

Conclusions and Implications

Total the number of Xs for the device, book/magazine, advertisement, food supplement, or website:

In several sentences, give your assessment of the product. Did it score well? Would you use/buy the product? Explain.

Lab 18B Evaluating a Health/Wellness or Fitness Club

Name	Section	Date

Purpose: To practice evaluating a health club (various combinations of the words *health, wellness,* and *fitness* are often used for these clubs)

Procedures

1. Choose a club and make a visit.
2. Listen carefully to all that is said and ask lots of questions.
3. Look carefully all around as you are given the tour of the facilities; ask what the exercises or the equipment does for you, or ask leading questions, such as, "Will this take inches off my hips?"
4. As soon as you leave the club, rate it, using Chart 1. Space is provided for notes in Chart 1.

Chart 1 Health Club Evaluation Questionnaire

Directions: Place an X over a "yes" or "no" answer. Make notes as necessary.

	Yes	No	Notes
1. Were claims for improvement in weight, figure/physique, or fitness realistic?	○	○	
2. Was a long-term contract (1 to 3 years) encouraged?	○	○	
3. Was the sales pitch high-pressure to make an immediate decision?	○	○	
4. Were you given a copy of the contract to read at home?	○	○	
5. Did the fine print include objectionable clauses?	○	○	
6. Did they ask you about medical readiness?	○	○	
7. Did they sell diet supplements as a sideline?	○	○	
8. Did they have passive equipment?	○	○	
9. Did they have cardiovascular training equipment or facilities (cycles, track, pool, aerobic dance)?	○	○	
10. Did they make unscientific claims for the equipment, exercise, baths, or diet supplements?	○	○	
11. Were the facilities clean?	○	○	
12. Were the facilities crowded?	○	○	
13. Were there days and hours when the facilities were open but would not be available to you?	○	○	
14. Were there limits on the number of minutes you could use a piece of equipment?	○	○	
15. Did the floor personnel closely supervise and assist clients?	○	○	
16. Were the floor personnel qualified experts?	○	○	
17. Were the managers/owners qualified experts?	○	○	
18. Has the club been in business at this location for a year or more?	○	○	

Results

1. Score the chart as follows:

   A. Give 1 point for each "no" answer for items 2, 3, 5, 7, 8, 10, 12, 13, and 14 and place the score in the box.

   Total A ☐

   B. Give 1 point for each "yes" answer for items 1, 4, 6, 9, 11, and 18 and place the score in the box.

   Total B ☐

   Total A and B above and place the score in the box.

   Total A and B ☐

   C. Give 1 point for each "yes" answer for items 15, 16, and 17 and place the score in the box.

   Total C ☐

2. A total score of 12–15 points on items A and B suggests the club rates at least fair, compared with other clubs.

3. A score of 3 on item C indicates that the personnel are qualified and suggests that you could expect to get accurate technical advice from the staff.

4. Regardless of the total scores, you would have to decide the importance of each item to you personally, as well as evaluate other considerations, such as cost, location, and personalities of the clients and the personnel, to decide if this would be a good place for you or your friends to join.

Conclusions and Implications: In several sentences, discuss your conclusion about the quality of this club and whether you think it would fit your needs if you wanted to belong.

Toward Optimal Health and Wellness: Planning for Healthy Lifestyle Change

LEARNING OBJECTIVES

After completing the study of this concept, you will be able to:

▶ Assess inherited health risks.

▶ Describe how to access and use the health-care system effectively.

▶ Explain the importance of environmental influences on lifestyle (as well as the impact of our lifestyles on our environment).

▶ List the key healthy lifestyles that influence health and wellness.

▶ Explain how personal actions and interactions influence the adoption of healthy lifestyles.

▶ Apply behavioral skills to plan and follow personal health and fitness programs.

In addition to healthy lifestyles, other factors such as heredity, health care, the environment, cognitions and emotions, and personal actions and interactions contribute to good health, wellness, and fitness.

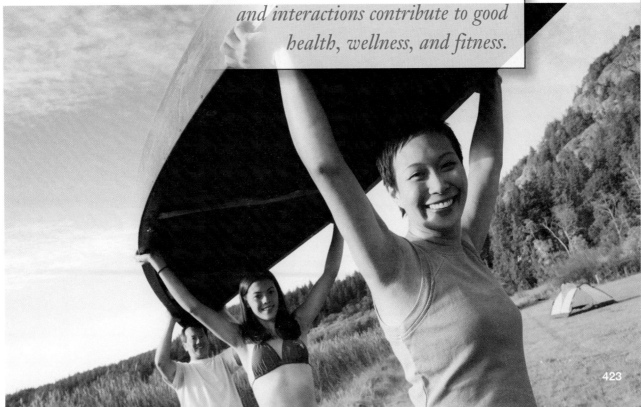

The broad vision of Healthy People 2020 is to create "a society in which all people live long, healthy lives." Two major missions of the 2020 objectives are "to identify nationwide health improvement priorities and increase public awareness and understanding of the determinants of health, disease, and disability and the opportunity for progress." The first concept in this book introduced you to a model that explained the many factors influencing health, wellness, and fitness (see Figure 1). The focus of this book has been on changing factors over which you have control. For this reason, much of the discussion has centered on changing lifestyles, because lifestyles impact health, wellness, and fitness more than any of the other factors. As shown in the figure, you have the most control over the lifestyles you lead, reasonable control over your cognitions/emotions, some control over your environment and use of health care, but relatively little control over heredity factors. This final concept provides information about these other factors and overall strategies for optimizing your health.

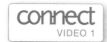

Understand Inherited Risks and Strengths

Learn about your family health history and take stock of inherited risk. Many health conditions and risks are linked to or influenced by your genetics. If members of your immediate or extended family have had specific diseases or health problems, you may have a greater risk or likelihood of the same condition. Your DNA contains the instructions for building the proteins that control the structure and function of all the cells in your body. Abnormalities in DNA can provide the wrong set of instructions and lead to faulty cell growth or function. There are clear genetic influences on risks for obesity, cardiovascular disease risk factors, diabetes, and many forms of cancer. At present it is not possible for people to truly know their genetic risk profile, but it may be possible in the future with more comprehensive genetic testing.

Take action to diminish risk factors for which you have a predisposition. As mentioned, research shows strong familial aggregation of certain chronic

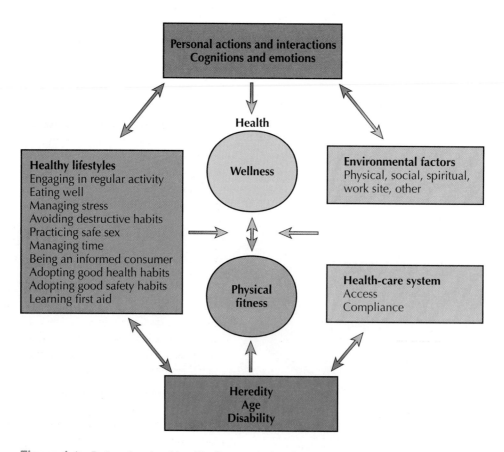

Figure 1 ▶ Determinants of health, fitness, and wellness.

disease risk factors (e.g., obesity, diabetes, cholesterol, blood pressure) as well as some cancers. While you cannot change your heredity risks, you can take steps to reduce your risks for certain inherited conditions. Specifically, adopting healthy lifestyles may significantly reduce inherited risks for certain diseases. A recent study computed obesity risk scores based on the presence or absence of 32 genes known to increase weight status. The genetic risk score was associated with an individual's inherited risk for being overweight but risk was influenced by lifestyle behaviors. An active lifestyle (marked by the presence of a brisk daily walk) reduced the genetic influence by 50 percent while a sedentary lifestyle (marked by watching television four hours a day) increased the genetic influence by 50 percent. Eating a healthy diet, managing stress, and not smoking are other key lifestyles that would likely contribute to lowering inherited risks for disease.

Use the Health-Care System Effectively

Follow sound medical advice and recommendations. The medical system can provide individuals with supportive, personalized health care, but people have to seek consultation and follow advice for it to be effective (see Table 1). Some basic strategies for accessing the medical system effectively are summarized below:

- *Get medical insurance.* People who think they save money by avoiding the payment of insurance premiums place themselves (and their families) at risk and may not really save money.

Table 1 ▶ Facts about Personal Physicians and Health Insurance

- More women than men have a regular physician.
- More than half of young men have no personal doctor.
- Three times more women than men have visited a doctor in the past year.
- Women are more aware of health issues than men.
- Nearly half of men wait a week or more to see a doctor when ill.
- Many men see sickness as "unmanly."
- Married men see doctors more frequently than single men because their wives prompt them.
- Lack of health insurance results in fewer doctor's visits, less frequent health screening, and less access to prescribed medicine.

- *Investigate and then identify a hospital and regular doctor.* Check with other physicians you know and trust for referrals. Check with your state medical board and national directories (e.g., Directory of Board Certified Medical Specialists, www.abms.org) for specialist certifications or fellowships. Choose an accredited emergency center near your home and a hospital that is accredited and grants privileges to your personal doctors.

- *Get periodic medical exams.* Do not wait until something is wrong before you seek medical advice. A yearly preventive physical exam is recommended for adults over the age of 40. Younger people should have an exam at least every 2 years.

- *Follow appropriate screening recommendations.* Many illnesses and chronic conditions can be effectively treated if they are identified early in the disease process. Following cancer screening guidelines is particularly important (e.g., mammograms for women and prostate tests for men). Breast and testicular self-exams are also important for detection.

- *Ask questions.* Do not be afraid to speak up. Prepare questions for doctors and other medical personnel. The American College of Surgeons suggests several questions before surgeries: What are the reasons for the surgery? Are there alternatives? What will happen if I don't have the procedure? What are the risks? What are the long-term effects and problems? How will the procedure impact my quality of life and future health?

- *Understand effects of medications.* Seek out information about medicines and supplements so you understand their intended effect. Read the inserts that come with the medicine and ask your doctor and pharmacist about correct dosage and information concerning when to take the medication. The FDA recently simplified drug inserts to help you understand the information that comes with medicine. Track your medicine and supplement use and share it with your physician.

- *Consider potential side effects of medicines you take.* Most medications are tested for use with certain populations and they may not be safe or effective for all people. Consider the safety and potential risks. Side effects from preventable adverse reactions to medicines account for more than 1.5 million deaths each year. When medicine is prescribed, ask for details. Ask why the medicine was prescribed and the nature of side effects. Ask if the medicine interacts with other medicines or supplements.

- *If you have doubts about medical advice, get a second opinion.* As many as 30 percent of original diagnoses are incorrect or differ from second opinions. Don't worry about offending your doctor by getting another opinion. Good doctors encourage this.

In the News

Does Zinc Help with Treatment of the Common Cold?

The common cold is one of the top causes of visits to the doctor and absenteeism from school and work. It is typically caused by the rhinovirus and there are no proven treatments. While colds may not be preventable, evidence has been accumulating on the benefits of taking supplemental zinc to shorten the length and severity of colds. A variety of products are available to provide supplemental zinc (e.g., Zicam), which is thought to work by slowing the replication of the virus. A respected Cochrane Review examined 25 years of research and concluded that zinc treatments are beneficial in reducing the duration and severity of the common cold in healthy people when taken within 24 hours of onset of symptoms. A meta-analysis in the *Canadian Medical Association Journal* reviewed 17 controlled trials and reported that zinc shortened the duration of cold symptoms in adults by 2 to 3 days. Higher doses of zinc were also associated with better outcomes but surprisingly no effect was observed in children. The results are promising but additional trials are needed.

Would you consider using zinc supplements or do you need more evidence? Explain your answer and describe how you approach new health products or supplements that are being promoted.

connect
ACTIVITY

- *Make your wishes for health care known.* Have a medical power of attorney. This document spells out the treatments you desire in the case of severe illness. Without such a document, your loved ones may not be able to make decisions consistent with your wishes. Be sure your loved ones have a similar document so that you can help them carry out their wishes.

Become a wise health- and medical-care consumer. Medical illiteracy and lack of health-care information are linked to higher than normal death rates. This is why improving medical literacy is such a high priority for public health officials. Some strategies for becoming a better health- and medical-care consumer are below:

- *Become familiar with the symptoms of common medical problems.* If symptoms persist, seek medical help. Many deaths can be prevented if early warning signs of medical problems are heeded.

- *Practice good hygiene.* The recent fears about dangerous versions of flu (e.g., H1N1) led to increased awareness about good hygiene. There was debate over whether regular hand washing impacts the spread of H1N1, but it is clearly the best defense against the common cold and other respiratory diseases. Always wash hands before preparing food or eating and after using the toilet, touching animals, handling garbage, coughing, or blowing your nose. Avoid sharing cups and utensils and use hand sanitizers when you don't have access to water.

- *Stay home when you are sick.* Most companies urge sick employees to stay home to prevent spreading illness to others. According to one survey, 40 percent of employees say they have gotten the flu at work. This is possibly because most workers feel guilty staying home or pressure to go to work even when sick. Sick workers are less productive, and working when sick lengthens recovery time.

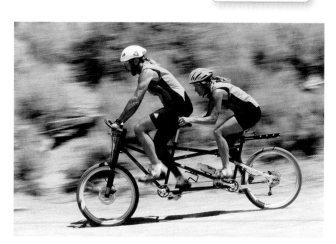

Physical activity contributes to fitness, wellness, and quality of life.

- *Carefully review the credibility and accuracy of new health information.* As described in Concept 23, there are many examples of misleading claims and fraud in the health and fitness industry. Even news reports from credible scientific studies can exert too much influence on consumer decisions. It takes years for scientific consensus to emerge, so carefully review new health claims. (See In the News.)

Consider Environmental Influences on Your Health

Understand how environmental factors shape your behaviors. As described throughout the book, environmental factors influence your health and well-being. Experts in obesity research have coined the term *obesogenic environments* to specifically describe how aspects of our environment contribute to overeating and lack of physical activity. To live healthy, it is important to understand how environmental

A positive _physical_ environment helps make the healthy choice the easy choice.

- **Access to physical activity and healthy foods:** A healthy environment supports efforts to adopt healthy lifestyles by making it easier to be active and to eat healthy. Parks, trails, green spaces provide opportunities to be active. Farmers' markets, health sections of grocery stores, and food co-ops make it easier to select healthy food.

- **Safe and clean communities:** A pleasant, clean, and safe environment encourages healthy living and the adoption of healthy lifestyles. Clean water and clean air are critical for good health.

A positive _spiritual_ environment helps to support spiritual fulfillment.

- **Opportunities for spiritual development:** Reading spiritual materials, prayer, meditation, and discussions with others provide opportunities to clarify and solidify spiritual beliefs.

- **Access to spiritual community and leadership:** Finding a community for worship provides comfort and a path to fulfillment for many. Consider consultation with those with experience and expertise.

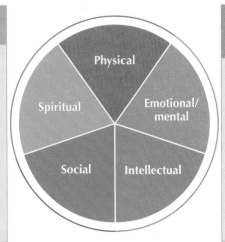

A positive _emotional_ environment can help with adopting healthy lifestyles and managing stress.

- **Supportive personal relationships:** Support by others, especially family members, can help in managing stress and in adopting healthy lifestyles. Unhealthy relationships have the opposite effect.

- **Stress management skills:** Friends, families, and co-workers can provide emotional support to assist in coping and stress management.

A healthy _social_ environment enhances quality of life and supports wellness.

- **Creating a sense of community:** Being a part of the greater community is important to social and mental health. Community-based groups are also important for planning and promoting healthy lifestyles for residents.

- **Using social support:** A strong support network can help in times of need and provide advice, assistance, or support when needed.

A stimulating _intellectual_ environment fosters learning and critical thinking.

- **Access to accurate information:** Whether the source is formal education or self-learning, access to accurate information is essential. Of course, good information is beneficial only if used.

- **Build and maintain cognitions:** A stimulating intellectual environment can promote self-discovery, build cognitive skills, and promote critical thinking.

Figure 2 ▶ The influence of environmental factors on dimensions of wellness.

settings and factors influence our lifestyles. Figure 2 summarizes the broad impact of physical, spiritual, social, intellectual, and emotional environments on personal health and wellness. Specific environmental strategies that you can use for each dimension of wellness are listed below:

- _Strategies for the physical environment._ Living healthy in our modern society can be challenging, but this can

be overcome with good planning. Think ahead about ways to be sitting less during the day and how to add daily physical activity (e.g., commuting and walk breaks). Plan your meals and dining choices to ensure you can make healthier food choices. Avoid smoke-filled establishments, highly polluted environments, and use of toxic products.

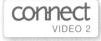

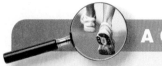

A CLOSER LOOK

City, County, and State Health Ratings

Numerous organizations conduct surveys to determine which cities and states are the healthiest. All use indicators such as access to health care, percentage of people insured, health-care costs, resources (e.g., parks, work-site wellness programs), environmental quality, and personal fitness and health (e.g., percent of population that is overweight, access to fitness centers). Results vary depending on the organization doing the polling, the methods used to compile the data, and the indicators used. The rankings vary considerably but some consistent patterns emerge. In general, health status and wellness appear to be worst in the South. In contrast, health rankings tend to be higher in the West (i.e., mountain states), Midwest, and Northeast. A comprehensive review by the Robert Wood Johnson Foundation ranks the health of individual counties across the country based on objective health indicators. The Well-Being Index by Gallup-Healthways uses a detailed polling system to compare health status and well-being in states across the country. The American Fitness Index of the American College of Sports ranks cities based on availability and usability of physical activity resources.

Do you see any potential public health value by posting this type of information online?

ACTIVITY

- *Strategies for the social and emotional environment.* Find a social community that accommodates your personal and family needs; get involved in community affairs, including those that affect the environment; build relationships with family and friends; provide support for others so that their support will be there for you when you need it; use time-management strategies to help you allocate time for social interactions.

- *Strategies for the spiritual environment.* Pray, meditate, read spiritual materials, participate in spiritual discussions, find a place to worship, provide spiritual support for others, seek spiritual guidance from those with experience and expertise, keep a journal, experience nature, honor relationships, help others.

- *Strategies for the intellectual environment.* Make decisions based on sound information, question simple solutions to complex problems, seek environments that stimulate critical thinking.

Choose to live and work in places that support healthy living. Environmental factors are often out of a person's control. However, you do have some autonomy regarding where you choose to live and work. If physical activity is important to you, find a community with parks and playgrounds and accessible sidewalks, bike paths, jogging trails, swimming facilities, a gym, or health club. Avoid environments that only have fast-food restaurants. Find a social environment that reinforces healthy lifestyles. If possible, work in businesses or settings that support healthy lifestyles. Ideally, the work environment should have adequate space, lighting, and freedom from pollution (tobacco smoke), as well as a healthy physical, social, spiritual, and intellectual environment. Considerable attention has been given recently to characteristics that define healthy work sites, communities, cities, and states (see A Closer Look). This is encouraging because the increased demand for healthy resources could lead to increased supply.

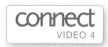
VIDEO 3

Adopt and Maintain Healthy Lifestyles

Consider strategies for adopting healthy lifestyles. Statistics show that more than half of early deaths are caused by unhealthy lifestyles. For this reason, changing lifestyles is the focus of this book. We emphasize priority healthy lifestyles such as being regularly active, eating well, managing stress, avoiding destructive behaviors, and practicing safe sex because they are factors over which we have some control, and if adopted, they have considerable impact on health, wellness, and fitness. (see Figure 1). Being an informed consumer is another healthy lifestyle emphasized in the book since it enables you to understand health information and take appropriate action. Other healthy lifestyles not emphasized in the book include adopting good health and safety habits and learning first aid. Examples of healthy lifestyles in these domains are highlighted in Table 2.

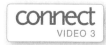
VIDEO 4

Consider the impact of your lifestyle on the health of the environment. The environment clearly influences your lifestyle, but your lifestyle can also have a damaging effect on the environment. Consider our use of fossil fuels. Burning fossil fuels has contributed to depletion of the ozone layer and the associated pattern of global warming. The changes in weather along with the pollution of our air and water compromise our agricultural systems, which in turn threatens our food and water supply. These are just a few examples of the complex

Table 2 ▶ Other Healthy Lifestyles

Lifestyle	Examples
Adopting good personal health habits. Many of these habits, important to optimal health, are considered to be elementary because they are often taught in school or in the home at an early age. In spite of their importance, many adults regularly fail to adopt these behaviors.	• Brushing and flossing teeth • Regular bathing and hand washing • Adequate sleep • Care of ears, eyes, and skin • Limit exposure to loud sounds, including live and recorded music. • Limit sun exposure (e.g., wear protective clothing, hats, and sunglasses) and use sunscreen with high SPF to reduce exposure to ultraviolet rays from the sun.
Adopting good safety habits. Thousands of people die each year and thousands more suffer disabilities or problems that detract from good health and wellness. Not all accidents can be prevented, but we can adopt habits to reduce risk.	• *Automobile accidents.* Wear seat belts, avoid using the phone while driving, do not drink and drive, and do not drive aggressively. • *Water accidents.* Learn to swim, learn CPR, wear life jackets while boating, do not drink while boating. • *Others.* Store guns safely, use smoke alarms, use ladders and electrical equipment safely, and maintain cars, bikes, and motorcycles properly.
Learning first aid. Many deaths could be prevented and the severity of injury could be reduced if those at the sites of emergencies were able to administer first aid.	• Learn cardiopulmonary resuscitation (CPR). New research shows that chest compression alone saves lives even without mouth-to-mouth breathing. • Learn the Heimlich maneuver to assist people who are choking. • Learn basic first aid.

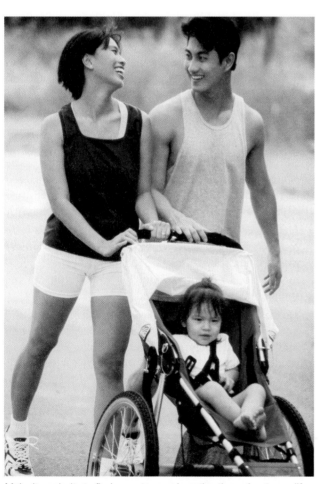

Make it a priority to find ways to remain active throughout your life.

ecological systems going on in the world. There are a number of promising strategies being implemented to address these problems, including the use of alternative energy sources to reduce our consumption of fossil fuels. While technology can solve some of the problem, we cannot completely heal the environment without major efforts from large segments of the population. Individually we can't change the world, but if each person makes small changes, we can together have a big impact. For example, individual efforts to use your car less, recycle, and use less paper can add up to larger changes in society. See Technology Update for an example of a novel, fitness-related technology that may help to change awareness about lifestyles and the environment.

Importance of Personal Actions and Interactions

Consider strategies for taking action and benefiting from personal interactions. The diagram in Figure 1 includes a box labeled "Personal actions and interactions" at the very top of the image. It is at the top for a reason—ultimately, it is what you do that counts. You can learn everything there is to know about fitness, health, and wellness, but if you do not take action and take advantage of your interactions with people and your environments, you will not benefit. As described in this concept (and throughout the book), your actions and interactions have a major influence on all aspects of wellness.

Sustainable Exercise Machines

Interest in energy conservation has led to the development of exercise equipment that harnesses the energy you expend. One leading company (Plug Out Fitness) sells lines of exercise equipment that track energy savings in addition to energy consumption—rather than expending calories you are producing watts! According to estimates from the company, an average exerciser can produce 50 watts of electricity per hour when exercising at a moderate pace. The company believes it may be possible to use that energy by transferring it into the electrical grid. The movement is still in its infancy but there are already sustainable gyms and sustainable dance clubs that are powered by the exercisers in the facility.

Can you envision a future in which human energy is captured and used as part of a more sustainable environment?

Table 3 ▶ Actions and Interactions That Influence Wellness

Dimension of Wellness	Influential Factors
Physical wellness	Pursuing behaviors that are conducive to good physical health (being physically active and maintaining a healthy diet)
Social wellness	Being supportive of family, friends, and co-workers and practicing good communication skills
Emotional wellness	Balancing work and leisure and responding proactively to challenging or stressful situations
Intellectual wellness	Challenging yourself to continually learn and improve in your work and personal life
Spiritual wellness	Praying, meditating, or reflecting on life
Total wellness	Taking responsibility for your own health

Commit to using this information to help plan your approaches for healthy living. (See Table 3.) People who plan are not only more likely to act; they are also more likely to act effectively and more proactively. Many people put off health and wellness, believing they will eventually be able to get control over their lives and their lifestyles. Delaying action will only make it harder to change in the future. As noted in Concept 15, it is much easier to maintain a healthy weight than it is to lose weight after it is gained. This applies to all aspects of healthy living. Do not put off until tomorrow what you can do today. The information in the book can help you create plans for healthy living, but the decision to follow them is up to you.

Consider your cognitions and emotions when planning strategies for action. Much of the information in this book is designed to help you make good decisions about health, wellness, and fitness. Using the guidelines presented throughout this book and using self-management skills can help you make good decisions. As noted in Concept 1, it is also important to consider your emotions when making decisions. Consider these guidelines:

- *Collect and evaluate information before you act.* Become informed before you make important decisions. Get information from reliable sources and consult with others you trust.

- *Emotions will influence certain decisions but should not detract from sound decision-making processes.* Fear and anger are two emotions that can affect your judgment and influence your ability to make decisions. Even love for another person can influence your actions. Get control of your emotions, or seek guidance from others you trust, before making important decisions in emotionally charged situations.

- *Resist pressure to make quick decisions when there is no need to decide quickly.* Salespeople often press for a quick decision to get a sale. Take some time to think before making a quick decision that may be based on emotion rather than critical thinking. Of course, some decisions must be made when emotions are charged (e.g., medical care in an emergency), but, when possible, delaying a decision can be to your advantage.

- *Use stress-management techniques to help you gain control when you must make decisions in emotionally charged situations.* Practice stress-management techniques (see Concepts 16 and 17) so that you can use them effectively when needed.

- *Honor your beliefs and relationships.* Actions and interactions that are inconsistent with basic beliefs and that fail to honor important relationships can result in reduced quality of life.

- *Seek the help of others and provide support for others who need your help.* As already noted, support from friends, family, and significant others can be critical in helping you achieve health, wellness, and fitness. Get help. Do what you can to be there for others who need your help.

- *Consider using professional help.* Most colleges have health center programs that provide free, confidential assistance or referral. Many businesses have employee

Health is available to Everyone for a Lifetime, and it's Personal

Some people rely on personal trainers to help motivate them to stay active. Health coaches and life planners are increasingly common for helping people learn how to live healthy and balanced lifestyles. These support systems can be useful, but the hope is that you now have the background and insights to do these things on your own. Motivation and confidence are important for adopting and maintaining a healthy lifestyle but there are no shortcuts or ways to store up good health in the bank. Healthy lifestyles must be maintained over time to provide continued benefits.

Do you have the skills to take responsibility for your health, fitness, and wellness?

connect
ACTIVITY

assistance programs (EAP), providing counselors who will help you or your family members find ways to solve a particular problem. Other programs and support groups help with lifestyle changes. For example, most hospitals and many health organizations have hotlines that provide referral services for establishing healthy lifestyles.

Consider your personal beliefs and philosophy when making decisions. Though science can help you make good decisions and solve problems, most experts tell you that there is more to it than that. Your personal philosophy and beliefs play a role. The following are factors to consider:

- *Clarify your personal philosophy and consider a new way of thinking.* Health, wellness, and fitness are often subjective. Making comparisons to other people can result in setting personal standards impossible to achieve. For example, achieving the body fat of a model seen on TV or performing like a professional athlete is not realistic for most of us. For this reason, the standards for health, wellness, and fitness in this book are based on health criteria rather than comparative criteria. Adhering to the HELP philosophy can help you adopt a new way of thinking. This philosophy suggests that each person should use health (H) as the basis for making decisions rather than comparisons with others. This is something that everyone (E) can do for a lifetime (L). It allows each of us to set personal (P) goals that are realistic and possible to attain.

- *Allow for spontaneity.* The reliance on science emphasized in this book can help you make good choices. But if you are to live life fully, you sometimes must allow yourself to be spontaneous. In doing so, the key is to be consistent with your personal philosophy so that your spontaneous actions will be enriching rather than a source of future regret.

- *Believe that you can make a difference.* As noted previously, you make your own choices. Though heredity and several other factors are out of your control, the choices that you make are yours. Believing that your actions make a difference is critical to taking action and making changes when necessary, allowing you to be healthy, well, and fit for a lifetime.

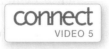

Strategies for Action

Develop and follow a plan for healthy living. You do not have full control over health and wellness factors, but it is important to take control over those you can. In Concept 2, you learned about the six steps involved in planning for a healthy lifestyle change. The labs at the end of this concept help you to use these six steps. Lab 19A helps you identify areas in which you especially need to prepare for lifestyle changes. Lab 19B helps you prepare for making lifestyle change from the list presented in Figure 1. Lab 19C is designed to help you plan a personal physical activity program. This lab utilizes results compiled from the fitness-related concepts in the book and provides a culminating personal fitness plan.

connect
VIDEO 5

Formal steps can become less formal with experience. The labs in this concept use a structured approach to self-assessment and planning. It is important to learn this process but it is likely that you will eventually adopt less formalized procedures on your own. Few of us will go through life doing formal fitness assessments every month, writing down goals weekly, or self-monitoring activity daily. However, the more a person does self-assessments, the more he or she is aware of personal fitness status. This awareness reduces the need for frequent testing. For example, a person who does regular heart-rate monitoring knows when he or she is in the target zone without counting heart rate every minute. The same is true of other self-management skills.

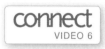
connect
VIDEO 6

With experience, you can use the techniques less formally to manage your lifestyle in the future.

connect
ACTIVITY

Web Resources

Academy of Nutrition and Dietetics **www.eatright.org**

ACSMs American Fitness Index **www.americanfitnessindex.org**

American College Health Association **www.acha.org**

American Heart Association (search CPR)
www.americanheart.org

CDC Healthy Places Network **www.cdc.gov/healthyplaces/**

County Health Rankings-Robert Wood Johnson Foundation
www.countyhealthrankings.org

Gallup-Healthyways Well-Being Index **www.well-beingindex**
.com

Healthfinder **www.healthfinder.gov**

Healthy People 2020 **www.healthypeople.gov/hp2020**

Mayo Clinic **www.mayoclinic.com**

National Health Interview Survey **www.cdc.gov/nchs/nhis.htm**

Prevention Institute **www.preventioninstitute.org/**

Research America **www.researchamerica.org**

U.S. Consumer Information Center **http://publications.usa**
.gov/USAPubs.php

World Health Organization **www.who.int**

Suggested Readings

Boehm, J. K., and L. D. Kubzansky. 2012. The heart's content: The association between positive psychological well-being and cardiovascular health. *Psychological Bulletin.* Published online April 12.

Bray, S. R. 2007. Self-efficacy for coping with barriers helps students stay physically active during transition to their first year at a university. *Research Quarterly for Exercise and Sport* 78(1):61–70.

Central Intelligence Agency. 2012. *The World Fact Book.* Washington, DC: CIA.

Duhigg, C. 2012. *The Power of Habit.* New York: Random House.

Eime, R. M. 2010. Does sports club participation contribute to health-related quality of life? *Medicine and Science in Sports and Exercise* 42(5):1022–1028.

Nagao, K., et al. 2007. Cardiopulmonary resuscitation by bystanders with chest compression only (SOS-KANTO): An observational study. *Lancet* 369(9565):920–926.

Qi, Q., et al. 2012. Genetic predisposition to dyslipidemia and type 2 diabetes risk in two prospective cohorts. *Diabetes* 61(3):745–752.

Qi, Q., et al. 2012. Weight-loss diets modify glucose-dependent insulinotropic polypeptide receptor rs2287019 genotype effects on changes in body weight, fasting glucose, and insulin resistance: The Preventing Overweight Using Novel Dietary Strategies trial. *American Journal of Clinical Nutrition* 95(2):506–513.

Steptoe, A., and J. Wardle. 2011. Positive affect measured using ecological momentary assessment and survival in older men and women. *Proceedings of the National Academy of Sciences* 108(45):18244–18248.

Taylor, S. 2011. *Health Psychology.* 8th ed. New York: McGraw-Hill.

Trust for America's Health. 2008. Blueprint for a Healthier America. Washington, DC: Trust for America's Health. Available at **http://healthyamericans.org/report/55/**
blueprint-for-healthier-america

World Health Organization. 2009. Global Health Risks. Geneva: WHO. Available at **www.who.int/publications/en**

Xu, J., and R. E. Roberts. 2010. The power of positive emotions: It's a matter of life or death—Subjective well-being and longevity over 28 years in a general population. *Health Psychology* 29(1):9–19.

Healthy People 2020

The objectives listed below are societal goals designed to help all Americans improve their health between now and the year 2020. They were selected because they relate to the content of this concept.

- Attain high-quality, longer lives free of preventable disease, injury, and premature death.
- Achieve health equity and eliminate disparities.
- Create healthy social and physical environments.
- Promote quality of life across all stages of life.
- Increase public awareness and understanding of the determinants of health, disease, and disability.
- Improve the health literacy of the population.

- Increase percentage of college students receiving information on priority risk-behavior areas.
- Increase percentage of people with health-care providers who involve them in decisions about health care.
- Increase recycling and environmental health efforts.
- Increase proportion of adults who have social support.

Two of the primary national health goals are "attaining high-quality life (wellness)" and "attaining longer lives free of preventable disease, injury, and premature death." In Concept 1, you reflected on these two goals. Reflect again on these goals. What can you do to achieve these two goals for you personally and what can people do in general to accomplish them?

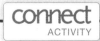

Lab 19A Assessing Factors That Influence Health, Wellness, and Fitness

Name Jason Herrin

Section

Date 4/21/16

Purpose: To assess the factors that relate to health, wellness, and fitness

Chart 1 Assessment Questionnaire: Factors That Influence Health, Wellness, and Fitness

Factor	Very True	Somewhat True	Not True At All	Score
Heredity				
1. I have checked my family history for medical problems.	③	②	①	3
2. I have taken steps to overcome hereditary predispositions.	③	②	①	3
			Heredity Score =	6
Health Care				
3. I have health insurance.	③	②	①	3
4. I get regular medical exams and have my own doctor.	③	②	①	2
5. I get treatment early, rather than waiting until problems get serious	③	②	①	3
6. I carefully investigate my health problems before making decisions.	③	②	①	3
			Health-Care Score =	11
Environment				
7. My physical environment is healthy.	③	②	①	2
8. My social environment is healthy.	③	②	①	2
9. My spiritual environment is healthy.	③	②	①	3
10. My intellectual environment is healthy.	③	②	①	2
11. My work environment is healthy.	③	②	①	2
12. My environment fosters healthy lifestyles.	③	②	①	2
			Environment Score =	13
Lifestyles				
13. I am physically active on a regular basis.	③	②	①	3
14. I eat well.	③	②	①	2
15. I use effective techniques for managing stress.	③	②	①	2
16. I avoid destructive behaviors.	③	②	①	2
17. I practice safe sex.	③	②	①	3
18. I manage my time effectively.	③	②	①	2
19. I evaluate information carefully and am an informed consumer.	③	②	①	3
20. My personal health habits are good.	③	②	①	2
21. My safety habits are good.	③	②	①	2
22. I know first aid and can use it if needed.	③	②	①	2
			Lifestyles Score =	23
Personal Actions and Interactions				
23. I collect and evaluate information before I act.	③	②	①	2
0. I plan before I take action.	③	②	①	2
25. I am good about taking action when I know it is good for me.	③	②	①	2
26. I honor my beliefs and relationships.	③	②	①	3
27. I seek help when I need it.	③	②	①	3
			Personal Actions/Interactions Score =	12

Procedures

1. Answer each of the questions in Chart 1 on page 433. Consider the information in this concept as you answer each question. The five factors assessed in the questionnaire are from Figure 1, page 424.
2. Calculate the scores for heredity (sum items 1 and 2), health care (sum items 3–6), environment (sum items 7–12), lifestyles (sum items 13–22), and actions/interactions (sum items 23–27).
3. Determine ratings for each of the scores using the Rating Chart.
4. Record your scores and ratings in the Results chart. Record your comments in the Conclusions and Implications section.

Results

Factor	Score	Rating
Heredity	6	healthy
Health care	11	healthy
Environment	13	marginal
Lifestyles	23	marginal
Actions/interactions	12	marginal

Rating Chart

Factor	Healthy	Marginal	Needs Attention
Heredity	6	4–5	Below 4
Health care	11–12	9–10	Below 9
Environment	16–18	13–15	Below 13
Lifestyles	26–30	20–25	Below 20
Actions/ interactions	13–15	10–12	Below 10

Conclusions and Implications

1. In the space below, discuss your scores for the five factors (sums of several questions) identified in Chart 1. Use several sentences to identify specific areas that need attention and changes that you could make to improve.

> Overall my scores are marginal to healthy. I direct more attention to health care, environment, lifestyles, and actions. There are a lot of areas to improve so I need to just pick a few at a time and focus on them.

2. For any individual item on Chart 1, a score of 1 is considered low. You might have a high score on a set of questions and still have a low score in one area that indicates a need for attention. In several sentences, discuss actions you could take to make changes related to individual questions.

> I did not score a 1 on any of the questions but I did have areas where I can improve. I am going to choose a few areas of focus and work on those.

Lab 19B Planning for Improved Health, Wellness, and Fitness

Name	Section	Date

Purpose: To plan to make changes in areas that can most contribute to improved health, wellness, and fitness

Procedures

1. Experts agree that it is best not to make too many changes all at once. Focusing attention on one or two things at a time will produce better results. Based on your assessments made in Lab 19A, select two areas in which you would like to make changes. Choose one from the list related to health care and environment and one related to lifestyle change. Place a check by those areas in Chart 1 in the Results section. Because Lab 19C is devoted to physical activity, it is not included in the list. You may want to make additional copies of this lab for use in making other changes in the future.

2. Use Chart 2 to determine your Stage of Change for the changes you have identified. Since you have identified these as an area of need, it is unlikely that you would identify the stage of maintenance. If you are at maintenance, you can select a different area of change that would be more useful.

3. In the appropriate locations, record the change you want to make related to your environment or health care. State your reasons, your specific goal(s), your written statement of the plan for change, and a statement about how you will self-monitor and evaluate the effectiveness of the changes made. In Chart 3, record similar information for the lifestyle change you identified.

Results

Chart 1

Check one in each column.

Area of Change	✔	Area of Change	✔
Health insurance		Eating well	
Medical checkups		Managing stress	
Selecting a doctor		Avoiding destructive habits	
Physical environment		Practicing safe sex	
Social environment	✓	Managing time	✓
Spiritual environment		Becoming a better consumer	
Intellectual environment		Improving health habits	✓
Work environment		Improving safety habits	✓
Environment for lifestyles	✓	Learning first aid	

Chart 2

List the two areas of change identified in Chart 1. Make a rating using the diagram at the right.

Identified Area of Change	Stage of Change Rating
1. Social env. ~~safety habits~~	preparation
2. safety	contemplation

Maintenance	The change has lasted at least 6 months.
Action	"I have made some short-term changes."
Preparation	"I am getting ready to change."
Contemplation	"I am thinking about a change."
Precontemplation	"I don't want to change."

Note: Some of the areas identified in this lab relate to personal information. It is appropriate not to divulge personal information to others (including your instructor) if you choose not to. For this reason, you may choose not to address certain problems in this lab. You are encouraged to take steps to make changes independent of this assignment and to consult privately with your instructor to get assistance.

Chart 3 Making Changes for Improved Health, Wellness, and Fitness

Describe First Area of Change (from Chart 1)	**Describe Second Area of Change (from Chart 1)**

Step 1: State Reasons for Making Change

I need people to support my health

Step 1: State Reasons for Making Change

Safety. - I want to be more safe.

Step 2: Self-Assessment of Need for Change
List your stage from Chart 2.

preparation

Step 2: Self-Assessment of Need for Change
List your stage from Chart 2.

contemplation

Step 3: State Your Specific Goals for Change
State several specific and realistic goals.

- go to the gym
- involve wife in my health
- involve family in health

Step 3: State Your Specific Goals for Change
State several specific and realistic goals.

- Follow driving laws (don't speed)
- stretch every morning

Step 4: Identify Activities or Actions for Change
List specific activities you will do or actions you will take to meet your goals.

- set alarm for gym
- plan gymtime
- bring wife

Step 4: Identify Activities or Actions for Change
List specific activities you will do or actions you will take to meet your goals.

- stretch
- practice safe driving

Step 5: Write a Plan; Include a Timetable
Expected start date:

April 17

Expected finish date:

April 23

Days of week and times: list times below days.

Mon.	Tue.	Wed.	Th.	Fri.	Sat.	Sun.
7:00 AM	7:00 AM		7:00 AM			7:00 AM

Location: Where will you do the plan?

Gym / home

Step 5: Write a Plan; Include a Timetable
Expected start date:

April 17

Expected finish date:

April 23

Days of week and times: list times below days.

Mon.	Tue.	Wed.	Th.	Fri.	Sat.	Sun.
7:00 AM	7:00 AM		7:00 AM			7:00 AM

Location: Where will you do the plan?

Home

Step 6: Evaluate Your Plan
How will you self-monitor and evaluate to determine if the plan is working?

Much better

Step 6: Evaluate Your Plan
How will you self-monitor and evaluate to determine if the plan is working?

Much better

Lab 19C Planning Your Personal Physical Activity Program

Name	Section	Date

Purpose: To establish a comprehensive plan of lifestyle physical activity and to self-monitor progress in your plan (note: you may want to reread the concept on planning for physical activity before completing this lab)

Procedures

Step 1. Establishing Your Reasons

In the spaces provided below, list several of your principal reasons for doing a comprehensive activity plan.

1. Health
2. consistency
3. stress management
4. self esteem
5.
6.

Step 2. Identify Your Needs Using Fitness Self-Assessments and Ratings of Stage of Change for Various Activities

In Chart 1, rate your fitness by placing an X over the circle by the appropriate rating for each part of fitness. Use your results obtained from previous labs or perform the self-assessments again to determine your ratings. If you took more than one self-assessment for one component of physical fitness, select the rating that you think best describes your true fitness for that fitness component. If you were unable to do a self-assessment for some reason, check the "No Results" circle.

Chart 1 Rating for Self-Assessments

	Rating				
Health-Related Fitness Tests	High-Performance Zone	Good Fitness Zone	Marginal Zone	Low Zone	No Results
1. Cardiovascular: 12-minute run (Chart 6, page 133)	○	⊗	○	○	○
2. Cardiovascular: step test (Chart 2, page 131)	○	⊗	○	○	○
3. Cardiovascular: bicycle test (Chart 5, page 133)	○	⊗	○	○	○
4. Cardiovascular: walking test (Chart 1, page 131)	⊗	○	○	○	○
5. Cardiovascular: swim test (Chart 7, page 134)	○	⊗	○	○	○
6. Flexibility: sit-and-reach test (Chart 1, page 220)	○	⊗	○	○	○
7. Flexibility: shoulder flexibility (Chart 1, page 220)	⊗	○	○	○	○
8. Flexibility: hamstring/hip flexibility (Chart 1, page 220)	○	⊗	○	○	○
9. Flexibility: trunk rotation (Chart 1, page 220)	○	⊗	○	○	○
10. Strength: isometric grip (Chart 3, page 190)	○	⊗	○	○	○
11. Strength: 1 RM upper body (Chart 2, page 188)	○	⊗	○	○	○

Chart 1 Rating for Self-Assessments, *continued*

Health-Related Fitness Tests	Rating				
	High-Performance	Good Fitness	Marginal	Low	No Results
12. Strength: 1 RM lower body (Chart 2, page 188)	⊗	○	○	○	○
13. Muscular endurance: curl-up (Chart 4, page 190)	○	⊗	○	○	○
14. Muscular endurance: 90-degree push-up (Chart 4, page 190)	○	○	⊗	○	○
15. Muscular endurance: flexed arm support (Chart 5, page 190)	○	○	⊗	○	○
16. Fitness rating: skinfold (Chart 1, page 306)	○	⊗	○	○	○
17. Body mass index (Chart 7, page 311)	○	○	⊗	○	○

Skill-Related Fitness and Other Self-Assessments	Rating				
	Excellent	Very Good or Good	Fair	Poor	No Results
1. Agility (Chart 1, page 281)	○	⊗	○	○	○
2. Balance (Chart 2, page 282)	⊗	○	○	○	○
3. Coordination (Chart 3, page 282)	⊗	○	○	○	○
4. Power (Chart 4, page 283)	○	⊗	○	○	○
5. Reaction time (Chart 5, page 283)	○	⊗	○	○	○
6. Speed (Chart 6, page 284)	○	⊗	○	○	○
7. Fitness of the back (Chart 2, page 258)	○	⊗	○	○	○
8. Posture (Chart 2, page 261)	○	○	⊗	○	○

Summarize Your Fitness Ratings Using the Results Above	Rating				
	High-Performance	Good Fitness	Marginal	Low	No Results
Cardiovascular	○	⊗	○	○	○
Flexibility	⊗	○	○	○	○
Strength	○	⊗	○	○	○
Muscular Endurance	○	○	⊗	○	○
Body fatness	○	○	⊗	○	○

	Excellent	Very Good or Good	Fair	Poor	No Results
Skill-related fitness	○	⊗	○	○	○
Posture and fitness of the back	○	○	⊗	○	○

Rate your stage of change for each of the different types of activities from the physical activity pyramid. Make an X over the circle beside the stage that best represents your behavior for each of the five types of activity in the lower three levels of the pyramid. A description of the various stages is provided below to help you make your ratings.

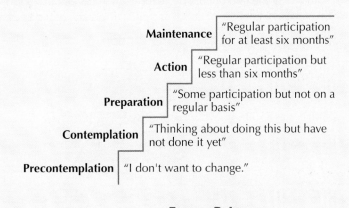

Maintenance | "Regular participation for at least six months"

Action | "Regular participation but less than six months"

Preparation | "Some participation but not on a regular basis"

Contemplation | "Thinking about doing this but have not done it yet"

Precontemplation | "I don't want to change."

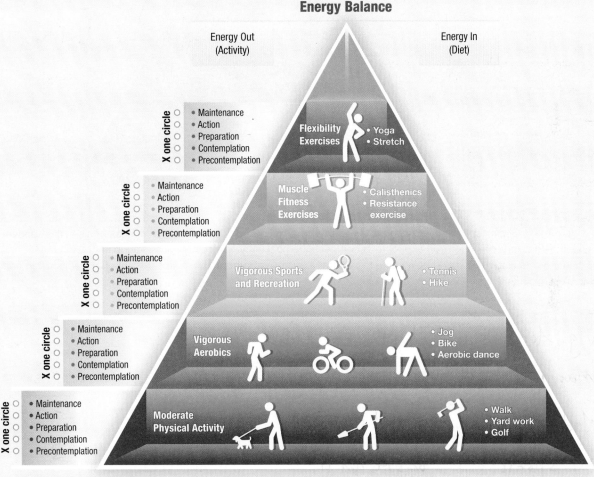

Energy Balance

Energy Out (Activity)　　　　　Energy In (Diet)

X one circle
- Maintenance
- Action
- Preparation
- Contemplation
- Precontemplation

Flexibility Exercises · Yoga · Stretch

X one circle
- Maintenance
- Action
- Preparation
- Contemplation
- Precontemplation

Muscle Fitness Exercises · Calisthenics · Resistance exercise

X one circle
- Maintenance
- Action
- Preparation
- Contemplation
- Precontemplation

Vigorous Sports and Recreation · Tennis · Hike

X one circle
- Maintenance
- Action
- Preparation
- Contemplation
- Precontemplation

Vigorous Aerobics · Jog · Bike · Aerobic dance

X one circle
- Maintenance
- Action
- Preparation
- Contemplation
- Precontemplation

Moderate Physical Activity · Walk · Yard work · Golf

*150 minutes of moderate or 75 minutes of vigorous activity per week is recommended; moderate and vigorous activity can be combined to meet guidelines.

Avoid Inactivity

Source: C. B. Corbin

In Step 1, you wrote down some general reasons for developing your physical activity plan. Setting goals requires more specific statements of goals that are realistic and achievable. For people who are at the contemplation or preparation stage for a specific type of activity, it is recommended that you write only short-term physical activity goals (no more than 4 weeks). Those at the action or maintenance level may choose short-term goals to start with, or if you have a good history of adherence, choose long-term goals (longer than 4 weeks). Precontemplators are not considered because they would not be doing this activity.

Step 3. Set Specific Goals

Chart 2 Setting Goals

Physical Activity Goals. Place an X over the appropriate circle for the number of days and weeks for each type of activity. Write the number of exercises or minutes of activities you plan in each of the five areas.

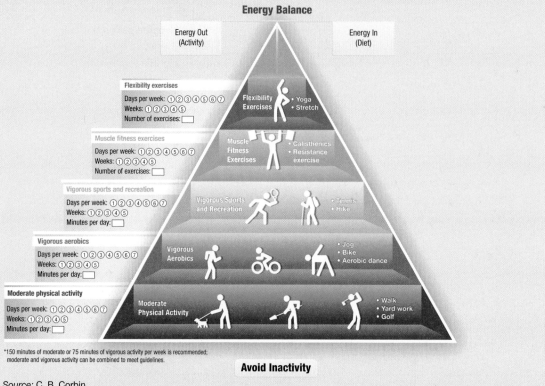

Source: C. B. Corbin

Physical Fitness Goals (for People at Action or Maintenance Only). Write specific physical fitness goals in the spaces provided below. Indicate when you expect to accomplish the goal (in weeks). Examples include improving the 12-minute run to a specific score, being able to perform a specific number of push-ups, attaining a specific BMI, and being able to achieve a specific score on a flexibility test.

Part of Fitness	Description of Specific Performance	Weeks to Goal
Vig. Acrobics	Tobata exccises	3
Muscle fitness	Upper body weights	3
Mod. Phys. Act.	Walk / stairs	3
Vig Sports.	Basketball	3

Step 4. Selecting Activities

In Chart 3, indicate the specific activities you plan to perform from each area of the physical activity pyramid. If the activity you expect to perform is listed, note the number of minutes or reps/sets you plan to perform. If the activity you want to perform is not listed, write the name of the activity or exercise in the space designated as "Other." For lifestyle activities, active aerobics, and active sports and recreation, indicate the length of time the activity will be performed each day. For flexibility, muscle fitness exercises, and exercises for back and neck, indicate the number of repetitions for each exercise.

Chart 3 Lifetime Physical Activity Selections

✔	Lifestyle Activities	Min./Day	✔	Active Aerobics	Min./Day	✔	Active Sports and Recreation	Min./Day
	Walking	40		Aerobic exercise machines			Basketball	30
	Yard work	15		Bicycling			Bowling	
	Active housework	15		Circuit training or calisthenics			Golf	
	Gardening			Dance or step aerobics			Karate/judo	
	Social dancing			Hiking or backpacking			Mountain climbing	
	Occupational activity	120		Jogging or running (or walking)	30		Racquetball	
	Wheeling in wheelchair			Skating/cross-country skiing			Skating	
	Bicycling to work or store			Swimming			Softball	
	Other:			Water activity			Skiing	
	Other:			Other:			Soccer	
	Other:			Other:			Volleyball	
	Other:			Other:			Other:	
	Other:			Other:			Other:	
	Other:			Other:			Other:	
	Other:			Other:			Other:	

✔	Flexibility Exercises	Reps/Sets	✔	Muscle Fitness Exercises	Reps/Sets	✔	Exercises for Back and Neck	Reps/Sets
	Calf stretch	10/5		Bench or seated press	10/3		Back saver stretch	10/3
	Hip and thigh stretch	10/3		Biceps curl	10/3		Single knee to chest	10/3
	Sitting stretch	10/3		Triceps curl	10/3		Low back stretch	12/3
	Hamstring stretch	10/3		Lat pull down	10/3		Hip/thigh stretch	10/3
	Back stretch (leg hug)	10/3		Seated rowing	10/3		Pelvic tilt	10/3
	Trunk twist	10/3		Wrist curl	10/3		Bridging	
	Pectoral stretch	10/3		Knee extension			Wall slide	
	Arm stretch	10/3		Heel raise			Pelvic stabilizer	
	Other:			Half-squat skiing			Neck rotation	
	Other:			Lunge			Isometric neck exercise	10/5
	Other:			Toe press			Chin tuck	
	Other:			Crunch or reverse curl			Trapezius stretch	
	Other:			Other:			Other:	
	Other:			Other:			Other:	
	Other:			Other:			Other:	

Step 5. Preparing a Written Plan

In Chart 4, place a check in the shaded boxes for each activity you will perform for each day you will do it. Indicate the time of day you expect to perform the activity or exercise (Example: 7:30 to 8 A.M. or 6 to 6:30 P.M.). In the spaces labeled "Warm-Up Exercises" and "Cool-Down Exercises," check the warm-up and cool-down exercises you expect to perform. Indicate the number of reps you will use for each exercise.

Chart 4 My Physical Activity Plan

✔	Monday	Time	✔	Tuesday	Time	✔	Wednesday	Time
	Lifestyle activity	120		Lifestyle activity	90		Lifestyle activity	90
	Active aerobics			Active aerobics	30		Active aerobics	30
	Active sports/rec.	30		Active sports/rec.			Active sports/rec.	30
	Flexibility exercises*	15		Flexibility exercises*	15		Flexibility exercises*	15
	Muscle fitness exercises*			Muscle fitness exercises*			Muscle fitness exercises*	30
	Back/neck exercises*			Back/neck exercises*	15		Back/neck exercises*	
	Warm-up exercises	30		Warm-up exercises	15		Warm-up exercises	30
	Other:			Other:			Other:	

✔	Thursday	Time	✔	Friday	Time	✔	Saturday	Time
	Lifestyle activity	90		Lifestyle activity	120		Lifestyle activity	90
	Active aerobics			Active aerobics	30		Active aerobics	
	Active sports/rec.	30		Active sports/rec.			Active sports/rec.	60
	Flexibility exercises*	15		Flexibility exercises*	30		Flexibility exercises*	15
	Muscle fitness exercises*	30		Muscle fitness exercises*			Muscle fitness exercises*	
	Back/neck exercises*	15		Back/neck exercises*			Back/neck exercises*	15
	Warm-up exercises	15		Warm-up exercises	15		Warm-up exercises	
	Other:			Other:			Other:	

✔	Sunday	Time	✔	Warm-Up Exercises	Reps	✔	Cool-Down Exercises	Reps
	Lifestyle activity	20		Walk or jog 1–2 min.	3		Walk or jog 1–2 min.	3
	Active aerobics			Calf stretch	4		Calf stretch	5
	Active sports/rec.			Hamstring stretch	2		Hamstring stretch	
	Flexibility exercises*	30		Leg hug			Leg hug	
	Muscle fitness exercises*	30		Sitting side stretch	2		Sitting side stretch	
	Back/neck exercises*			Zipper			Zipper	
	Warm-up exercises	30		Other:			Other:	
	Other:			Other:			Other:	

*Perform the specific exercises you checked in Chart 3.

442

Step 6. Keeping Records of Progress and Evaluating Your Plan

Make copies of Chart 4 (one for each week that you plan to keep records). Each day, make a check by the activities you actually performed. Include the times when you actually did the activities in your plan. Periodically check your goals to see if they have been accomplished. At some point, it will be necessary to reestablish your goals and create a revised activity plan.

Results

After performing your plan for a specific period of time, answer the question in the space provided.

How long have you been performing the plan?

Conclusions and Implications

1. In several sentences, discuss your adherence to the plan. Have you been able to stick with the plan? If so, do you think it is a plan you can do for a lifetime? If not, why do you think you are unable to do your plan?

2. In several sentences, discuss how you might modify your plan in the future.

3. In several sentences, discuss your goals for your program. Do you think you will meet your goals? Why or why not?

Appendix A
Metric Conversion Charts

Chart 1 Traditional/Metric Measurement Conversions

	Metrics to Traditional	Traditional to Metrics
Length	centimeters to inches: cm $\times$ .39 = 1 in.	inches to centimeters: in. $\times$ 2.54 = cm
	meters to feet: m $\times$ 3.3 = ft.	feet to meters: ft. $\times$ .3048 = m
	meters to yards: m $\times$ 1.09 = yd.	yards to meters: yd. $\times$ 0.92 = m
	kilometers to miles: km $\times$ 0.6 = mi.	miles to kilometers: mi. $\times$ 1.6 = km
Weight (Mass)	grams to ounces: g $\times$ 0.0352 = oz.	ounces to grams: oz. $\times$ 28.41 = g
	kilograms to pounds: kg $\times$ 2.2 = lb.	pounds to kilograms: lb. $\times$ 0.45 = kg
Volume	milliliters to fluid ounces: ml $\times$ 0.03 = fl. oz.	fluid ounces to milliliters: fl. oz. $\times$ 29.573 = ml
	liters to quarts: l $\times$ 1.06 = qt.	quarts to liters: qt. $\times$ 0.95 = l
	liters to gallons: l $\times$ 0.264 = gal.	gallons to liters: gal. $\times$ 3.8 = l

Chart 2 Isometric Strength Rating Scale (kg)—page 190

Classification	Men			Women		
	Left Grip	Right Grip	Total Score	Left Grip	Right Grip	Total Score
High-performance zone	57+	61+	118+	34+	39+	73+
Good fitness zone	45–56	50–60	95–117	27–33	32–38	59–72
Marginal zone	41–44	43–49	84–94	20–26	23–31	43–58
Low zone	<41	<43	<84	<20	<23	<43

Suitable for use by young adults between 18 and 30 years of age. After 30, an adjustment of 0.5 of 1 percent per year is appropriate because some loss of muscle tissue typically occurs as you grow older.

Chart 3 Power Rating Scale—page 283

Classification	Men	Women
Excellent	68 cm+	60 cm+
Very good	53–67 cm	48–59 cm
Good	42–52 cm	37–47 cm
Fair	31–41 cm	27–36 cm
Poor	<32 cm	<27 cm

Chart 4 Reaction Time Rating Scale—page 283

Classification	Score in Inches	Score in Centimeters
Excellent	>21	>52
Very good	19″–21	48–52
Good	16″–18 ¾	41–47
Fair	13″–15 ¾	33–40
Poor	<13	<33

Chart 5 Speed Rating Scale—page 284

Classification	Men		Women	
	Yards	Meters	Yards	Meters
Excellent	24+	22+	22+	20+
Very good	22–23	20–21.9	20–21	18–19.9
Good	18–21	16.5–19.9	16–19	14.5–17.9
Fair	16–17	14.5–16.4	14–15	13–14.4
Poor	<16	<14.5	<14	<13

Canada's Food Guide to Healthy Eating

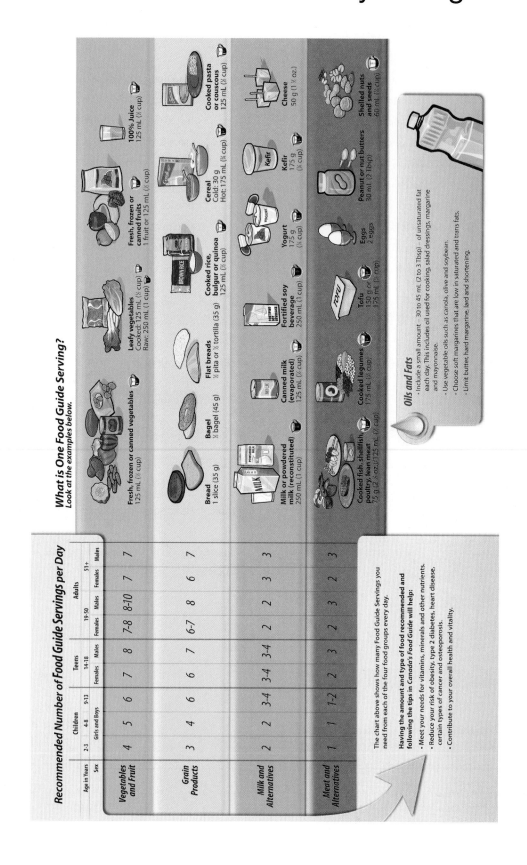

Recommended Number of Food Guide Servings per Day

Age in Years	Children			Teens		Adults				
	2-3	4-8	9-13	14-18		19-50		51+		
Sex	Girls and Boys			Females	Males	Females	Males	Females	Males	
Vegetables and Fruit	4	5	6	7	8	7-8	8-10	7	7	
Grain Products	3	4	6	6	7	6-7	8	6	7	
Milk and Alternatives	2	2	3-4	3-4	3-4	2	2	3	3	
Meat and Alternatives	1	1	1-2	2	3	2	3	2	3	

The chart above shows how many Food Guide Servings you need from each of the four food groups every day.

Having the amount and type of food recommended and following the tips in *Canada's Food Guide* will help:

• Meet your needs for vitamins, minerals and other nutrients.
• Reduce your risk of obesity, type 2 diabetes, heart disease, certain types of cancer and osteoporosis.
• Contribute to your overall health and vitality.

What is One Food Guide Serving?
Look at the examples below.

Vegetables and Fruit

Fresh, frozen or canned vegetables
125 mL (½ cup)

Leafy vegetables
Cooked: 125 mL (½ cup)
Raw: 250 mL (1 cup)

Fresh, frozen or canned fruits
1 fruit or 125 mL (½ cup)

100% Juice
125 mL (½ cup)

Grain Products

Bread
1 slice (35 g)

Bagel
½ bagel (45 g)

Flat breads
½ pita or ½ tortilla (35 g)

Cooked rice, bulgur or quinoa
125 mL (½ cup)

Cereal
Cold: 30 g
Hot: 175 mL (¾ cup)

Cooked pasta or couscous
125 mL (½ cup)

Milk and Alternatives

Milk or powdered milk (reconstituted)
250 mL (1 cup)

Canned milk (evaporated)
125 mL (½ cup)

Fortified soy beverage
250 mL (1 cup)

Yogurt
175 g
(¾ cup)

Kefir
175 g
(¾ cup)

Cheese
50 g (1 ½ oz.)

Meat and Alternatives

Cooked fish, shellfish, poultry, lean meat
75 g (2 ½ oz.)/125 mL (½ cup)

Cooked legumes
175 mL (¾ cup)

Tofu
150 g or
175 mL (¾ cup)

Eggs
2 eggs

Peanut or nut butters
30 mL (2 Tbsp)

Shelled nuts and seeds
60 mL (¼ cup)

Oils and Fats

• Include a small amount – 30 to 45 mL (2 to 3 Tbsp) – of unsaturated fat each day. This includes oil used for cooking, salad dressings, margarine and mayonnaise.
• Use vegetable oils such as canola, olive and soybean.
• Choose soft margarines that are low in saturated and trans fats.
• Limit butter, hard margarine, lard and shortening.

Make each Food Guide Serving count...
wherever you are – at home, at school, at work or when eating out!

▸ **Eat at least one dark green and one orange vegetable each day.**
- Go for dark green vegetables such as broccoli, romaine lettuce and spinach.
- Go for orange vegetables such as carrots, sweet potatoes and winter squash.

▸ **Choose vegetables and fruit prepared with little or no added fat, sugar or salt.**
- Enjoy vegetables steamed, baked or stir-fried instead of deep-fried.

▸ **Have vegetables and fruit more often than juice.**

▸ **Make at least half of your grain products whole grain each day.**
- Eat a variety of whole grains such as barley, brown rice, oats, quinoa and wild rice.
- Enjoy whole grain breads, oatmeal or whole wheat pasta.

▸ **Choose grain products that are lower in fat, sugar or salt.**
- Compare the Nutrition Facts table on labels to make wise choices.
- Enjoy the true taste of grain products. When adding sauces or spreads, use small amounts.

▸ **Drink skim, 1%, or 2% milk each day.**
- Have 500 mL (2 cups) of milk every day for adequate vitamin D.
- Drink fortified soy beverages if you do not drink milk.

▸ **Select lower fat milk alternatives.**
- Compare the Nutrition Facts table on yogurts or cheeses to make wise choices.

▸ **Have meat alternatives such as beans, lentils and tofu often.**

▸ **Eat at least two Food Guide Servings of fish each week.***
- Choose fish such as char, herring, mackerel, salmon, sardines and trout.

▸ **Select lean meat and alternatives prepared with little or no added fat or salt.**
- Trim the visible fat from meats. Remove the skin on poultry.
- Use cooking methods such as roasting, baking or poaching that require little or no added fat.
- If you eat luncheon meats, sausages or prepackaged meats, choose those lower in salt (sodium) and fat.

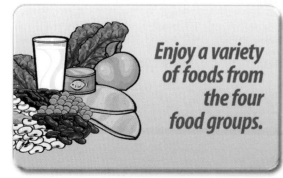

Enjoy a variety of foods from the four food groups.

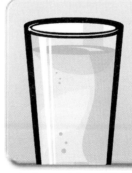

Satisfy your thirst with water!

Drink water regularly. It's a calorie-free way to quench your thirst. Drink more water in hot weather or when you are very active.

* Health Canada provides advice for limiting exposure to mercury from certain types of fish. Refer to www.healthcanada.gc.ca for the latest information.

Appendix C
Calories of Protein, Carbohydrates, and Fats in Foods

Food Choice	Total Calories	Protein Calories	Carbohydrate Calories	Fat Calories
Breakfast				
Scrambled egg (1 lg.)	111	29	7	75
Fried egg (1 lg.)	99	26	1	72
Pancake (1-6)	146	19	67	58
Syrup (1 T[4])	60	0	60	0
French toast (1 slice)	180	23	49	108
Waffle (7-inch)	245	28	100	117
Biscuit (medium)	104	8	52	44
Bran muffin (medium)	104	11	63	31
White toast (slice)	68	9	52	7
Wheat toast (slice)	67	14	52	6
Peanut butter (1 T)	94	15	11	68
Yogurt (8 oz. plain)	227	39	161	27
Orange juice (8 oz.)	114	8	100	6
Apple juice (8 oz.)	117	1	116	0
Soft drink (12 oz.)	144	0	144	0
Bacon (2 slices)	86	15	2	70
Sausage (1 link)	141	11	0	130
Sausage (1 patty)	284	23	0	261
Grits (8 oz.)	125	11	110	4
Hash browns (8 oz.)	355	18	178	159
French fries (reg.)	239	12	115	112
Donut, cake	125	4	61	60
Donut, glazed	164	8	87	69
Sweet roll	317	22	136	159
Cake (medium slice)	274	14	175	85
Ice cream (8 oz.)	257	15	108	134
Cream cheese (T)	52	4	1	47
Jelly (T)	49	0	49	0
Jam (T)	54	0	54	0
Coffee (cup)	0	0	0	0
Tea (cup)	0	0	0	0
Cream (T)	32	2	2	28
Sugar (t)	15	0	15	0
Corn flakes (8 oz.)	97	8	87	2
Wheat flakes (8 oz.)	106	12	90	4
Oatmeal (8 oz.)	132	19	92	21
Strawberries (8 oz.)	55	4	46	5
Orange (medium)	64	6	57	1
Apple (medium)	96	1	86	9
Banana (medium)	101	4	95	2
Cantaloupe (half)	82	7	73	2
Grapefruit (half)	40	2	37	1
Custard pie (slice)	285	20	188	77
Fruit pie (slice)	350	14	259	77
Fritter (medium)	132	11	54	67
Skim milk (8 oz.)	88	36	52	0

Food Choice	Total Calories	Protein Calories	Carbohydrate Calories	Fat Calories
Whole milk (8 oz.)	159	33	48	78
Butter (pat)	36	0	0	36
Margarine (pat)	36	0	0	36
Lunch				
Hamburger (reg. FF[1])	255	48	120	89
Cheeseburger (reg. FF)	307	61	120	126
Doubleburger (FF)	563	101	163	299
¼ lb. burger (FF)	427	73	137	217
Doublecheese burger (FF)	670	174	134	362
Doublecheese baconburger (FF)	724	138	174	340
Hot dog (FF)	214	36	54	124
Chili dog (FF)	320	51	90	179
Pizza, cheese (slice FF)	290	116	116	58
Pizza, meat (slice FF)	360	126	126	108
Pizza, everything (slice FF)	510	179	173	158
Sandwich, roast beef (FF)	350	88	126	137
Sandwich, bologna	313	44	106	163
Sandwich, bologna-cheese	428	69	158	201
Sandwich, ham-cheese (FF)	380	91	133	156
Sandwich, peanut butter	281	39	118	124
Sandwich, PB and jelly	330	40	168	122
Sandwich, egg salad	330	40	109	181
Sandwich, tuna salad	390	101	109	180
Sandwich, fish (FF)	432	56	147	229
French fries (reg. FF)	239	12	115	112
French fries (lg. FF)	406	20	195	191
Onion rings (reg. FF)	274	14	112	148
Chili (8 oz.)	260	49	62	148
Bean soup (8 oz.)	355	67	181	107
Beef noodle soup (8 oz.)	140	32	59	49
Tomato soup (8 oz.)	180	14	121	45
Vegetable soup (8 oz.)	160	21	107	32
Small salad, plain	37	6	27	4
Small salad, French dressing	152	8	50	94
Small salad, Italian dressing	162	8	28	126
Small salad, bleu cheese	184	13	28	143
Potato salad (8 oz.)	248	27	159	62
Cole slaw (8 oz.)	180	0	25	155
Macaroni and cheese (8 oz.)	230	37	103	90
Beef taco (FF)	186	59	56	71
Bean burrito (FF)	343	45	192	106
Meat burrito (FF)	466	158	196	112
Mexican rice (FF)	213	17	160	36
Mexican beans (FF)	168	42	82	44
Fried chicken breast (FF)	436	262	13	161
Broiled chicken breast	284	224	0	60

The principal reference for the calculation of values used in this appendix was the *Nutritive Value of Foods*, published by the United States Department of Agriculture, Washington, DC, Home and Gardens Bulletin, No. 72, although other published sources were consulted, including Jacobson, M., and S. Fritschner. *The Fast-Food Guide* (an excellent source of information about fast foods). New York: Workman.

Notes:
1. FF by a food indicates that it is typical of a food served in a fast food restaurant.
2. Your portions of foods may be larger or smaller than those listed here. For this reason, you may wish to select a food more than once (e.g., two hamburgers) or select only a portion of a serving (i.e., divide the calories in half for a half portion).
3. An oz. equals 28.35 grams.
4. T = tablespoon and t = teaspoon.

Food Choice	Total Calories	Protein Calories	Carbohydrate Calories	Fat Calories
Broiled fish	228	82	32	114
Fish stick (1 stick FF)	50	18	8	24
Fried egg	99	26	1	72
Donut	125	4	61	60
Potato chips (small bag)	115	3	39	73
Soft drink (12 oz.)	144	0	144	0
Apple juice (8 oz.)	117	1	116	0
Skim milk (8 oz.)	88	36	52	0
Whole milk (8 oz.)	159	33	48	78
Diet drink (12 oz.)	0	0	0	0
Mustard (t)	4	0	4	0
Catsup (t)	6	0	6	0
Mayonnaise (T)	100	0	0	100
Fruit pie	350	14	259	77
Cheesecake (slice)	400	56	132	212
Ice cream (8 oz.)	257	15	108	134
Coffee (8 oz.)	0	0	0	0
Tea (8 oz.)	0	0	0	0
Dinner				
Hamburger (reg. FF)	255	48	120	89
Cheeseburger (reg. FF)	307	61	120	126
Doubleburger (FF)	563	101	163	299
¼ lb. burger (FF)	427	73	137	217
Doublecheese burger (FF)	670	174	134	362
Doublecheese baconburger (FF)	724	138	174	412
Hot dog (FF)	214	36	54	124
Chili dog (FF)	320	51	90	179
Pizza, cheese (slice FF)	290	116	116	58
Pizza, meat (slice FF)	360	126	126	108
Pizza, everything (slice FF)	510	179	173	158
Steak (8 oz.)	880	290	0	590
French fried shrimp (6 oz.)	360	133	68	158
Roast beef (8 oz.)	440	268	0	172
Liver (8 oz.)	520	250	52	218
Corned beef (8 oz.)	493	242	0	251
Meat loaf (8 oz.)	711	228	35	448
Ham (8 oz.)	540	178	0	362
Spaghetti, no meat (13 oz.)	400	56	220	124
Spaghetti, meat (13 oz.)	500	115	230	155
Baked potato (medium)	90	12	78	0
Cooked carrots (8 oz.)	71	12	59	0
Cooked spinach (8 oz.)	50	18	18	14
Corn (1 ear)	70	10	52	8
Cooked green beans (8 oz.)	54	11	43	0
Cooked broccoli (8 oz.)	60	19	26	15
Cooked cabbage	47	12	35	0
French fries (reg. FF)	239	12	115	112
French fries (lg. FF)	406	20	195	191
Onion rings (reg. FF)	274	14	112	148
Chili (8 oz.)	260	49	62	148
Small salad, plain	37	6	27	4
Small salad, French dressing	152	8	50	94
Small salad, Italian dressing	162	8	28	126
Small salad, bleu cheese	184	13	28	143
Potato salad (8 oz.)	248	27	159	62
Cole slaw (8 oz.)	180	0	25	155
Macaroni and cheese (8 oz.)	230	37	103	90
Beef Taco (FF)	186	59	56	71
Bean burrito (FF)	343	45	192	106
Meat burrito (FF)	466	158	196	112

Food Choice	Total Calories	Protein Calories	Carbohydrate Calories	Fat Calories
Mexican rice (FF)	213	17	160	36
Mexican beans (FF)	168	42	82	44
Fried chicken breast (FF)	436	262	13	161
Broiled chicken breast	284	224	0	60
Broiled fish	228	82	32	114
Fish stick (1 stick FF)	50	18	8	24
Soft drink (12 oz.)	144	0	144	0
Apple juice (8 oz.)	117	1	116	0
Skim milk (8 oz.)	88	36	52	0
Whole milk (8 oz.)	159	33	48	78
Diet drink (12 oz.)	0	0	0	0
Mustard (t)	4	0	4	0
Catsup (t)	6	0	6	0
Mayonnaise (T)	100	0	0	100
Fruit pie (slice)	350	14	259	77
Cheesecake (slice)	400	56	132	212
Ice cream (8 oz.)	257	15	108	134
Custard pie (slice)	285	20	188	77
Cake (slice)	274	14	175	85
Snacks				
Peanut butter (1 T)	94	15	11	68
Yogurt (8 oz. plain)	227	39	161	27
Orange juice (8 oz.)	114	8	100	6
Apple juice (8 oz.)	117	1	116	0
Soft drink (12 oz.)	144	0	144	0
Donut, cake	125	4	61	60
Donut, glazed	164	8	87	69
Sweet roll	317	22	136	159
Cake (medium slice)	274	14	175	85
Ice cream (8 oz.)	257	15	108	134
Softserve cone (reg.)	240	10	89	134
Ice cream sandwich bar	210	40	82	88
Strawberries (8 oz.)	55	4	46	5
Orange (medium)	64	6	57	1
Apple (medium)	96	1	86	9
Banana (medium)	101	4	95	2
Cantaloupe (half)	82	7	73	2
Grapefruit (half)	40	2	37	1
Celery stick	5	2	3	0
Carrot (medium)	20	3	17	0
Raisins (4 oz.)	210	6	204	0
Watermelon (4" × 6" slice)	115	8	99	8
Chocolate chip cookie	60	3	9	48
Brownie	145	6	26	113
Oatmeal cookie	65	3	13	49
Sandwich cookie	200	8	112	80
Custard pie (slice)	285	20	188	77
Fruit pie (slice)	350	14	259	77
Gelatin (4 oz.)	70	4	32	34
Fritter (medium)	132	11	54	67
Skim milk (8 oz.)	88	36	52	0
Diet drink	0	0	0	0
Potato chips (small bag)	115	3	39	73
Roasted peanuts (1.3 oz.)	210	34	25	151
Chocolate candy bar (1 oz.)	145	7	61	77
Choc. almond candy bar (1 oz.)	265	38	74	164
Saltine cracker	18	1	1	16
Popped corn	40	7	33	0
Cheese nachos	471	63	194	214

Credits

Text Credits

2: *Healthy People 2020.* www.healthypeople.gov/ HP2020. **4:** Trust for America's Health. 2008. *Blueprint for a Healthier America.* Washington, DC: Trust for America's Health. http://healthyamericans .org/report/55/blueprint-for-healthier-america. **12:** Institute of Medicine. 2004. *Insuring America's Health: Principles and Recommendations.* Washington, DC: The National Academies Press. **15:** Mokdad, A. H. et al. 2004. Actual causes of death in the United States, 2000. *Journal of the American Medical Association* 291(10):1238–1245. **25:** Buettner, D. 2008. *The Blue Zones: Lessons for Living Longer from People Who've Lived the Longest.* Washington, DC: The National Geographic Society. **26:** Christakis, N. A., and J. H. Fowler. 2007. The spread of obesity in a large social network over 32 years. *New England Journal of Medicine* 375(4):370–379. **44:** ACSM. 2010. *ACSM's Guidelines for Exercise Testing and Prescription.* 8th ed. Philadelphia: Lippincott, Williams & Wilkins. **44:** United States Department of Health and Human Services. 1996. *Physical Activity and Health: A Report of the Surgeon General.* Washington, DC: USDHHS. http://www.cdc.gov/nccdphp/sgr/index .htm. **65:** Health Canada. 1986. *Achieving Health for All: A Framework for Health.* **65:** USDHHS. 2008. *Physical Activity Guidelines for Americans.* Atlanta, GA: Author. http://www.health.gov/ paguidelines. **69:** National Cholesterol Education Program. 2001. *Third Report of the National Cholesterol Education Program.* Atlanta, GA: National Institutes of Health. Publication No. 02-5215. www.nhlbi.nih.gov/guidelines/cholesterol/atp-3full.pdf. **71:** National Heart Lung and Blood Institute. 2012. *What Is High Blood Pressure?* http://www.nhlbi.nih.gov/health/health-topics/ topics/hbp. **73:** National Cholesterol Education Program. 2012. *Framingham Risk Assessment Tool.* http://hp2010.nhlbihin.net/atpiii/calculator.asp. **75:** National Center for Health Statistics. 2012. *Obesity and Overweight.* www.cdc.gov/nchs/fastats/ overwt.htm. **78:** Kennedy, J. F. 1960. The soft American. *Sports Illustrated* 13(26):14–23. **90:** Blair, S. N. 2009. Physical inactivity: The biggest public health problem of the 21st century. *British Journal of Sports Medicine* 43(1):1–2. **90:** Corbin, C. B. 2012. *The Physical Activity Pyramid.* Used by permission. The source is the same for all subsequent uses of the pyramid.

93: Centers for Disease Control and Prevention. 2007. Prevalence of regular physical activity among adults—United States. *Morbidity and Mortality Weekly Reports* 56(46):1209–1212. **93:** Barnes, P. M., et al. 2009. Early release of selected estimates based on data from the January– June 2009 National Health Interview Survey. National Center for Health Statistics. www.cdc .gov/nchs/nhis/released200912.htm. **105:** Levine, J. A. 2007. Nonexercise activity thermogenesis— Liberating the life-force. *Journal of Internal Medicine* 263(3):273–287. **108:** Ainsworth, B. E. 2000. Compendium of physical activities: An update of activity codes and MET intensities. *Medicine and Science in Sports and Exercise* 32 (Suppl):S498–S516. **110:** National Association of Realtor. 2011. *The 2011 Community Preference Survey.* http://www.stablecommunities.org/sites/all/files/ library/1608/smartgrowthcommsurveyresults2011 .pdf. **121:** Blair, S. N., et al. 1989. Physical fitness and all-cause mortality. A prospective study of healthy men and women. *Journal of the American Medical Association* 363(17):2395– 2401. **125:** Timmons, J. A., et al. 2010. Using molecular classification to predict gains in maximal aerobic capacity following endurance exercise training in humans. *Journal of Applied Physiology* 108(6):1487–1496. **127, 135:** Borg, G. 1982. Psychophysical bases of perceived exertion. *Medicine and Science in Sports and Exercise* 14 (5):377–381. **147:** Knab, A. M., et al. 2011. 45-minute vigorous exercise bout increases metabolic rate for 14 hours. *Medicine and Science in Sports and Exercise* 43(9):1643–1648. **149:** Sporting Goods Manufacturers Association. www.sgma .com. **150:** Sporting Goods Manufacturers Association. www.sgma.com. **158:** Compendium of Physical Activities. http://prevention.sph .sc.edu/tools/docs/documents_compendium.pdf. **162:** Williams, M. A., et al. 2007. Resistance exercise in individuals with and without cardiovascular disease. 2007 update: A scientific statement from the American Heart Association Council on Clinical Cardiology and Council on Nutrition, Physical Activity, and Metabolism. *Circulation* 116(5):572– 584. **163:** Growing Stronger: Strength Training for Older Adults. www.cdc.gov/physicalactivity/ growingstronger/index.html. **165:** Technogym, www.technogym.com. **167:** CrossFit Games, http://games.crossfit.com. **175:** P90X, www .beachbody.com/P90X. **203:** Pereles, D., A. Roth,

and D. J. S. Thompson. 2010. A large, randomized, prospective study of the impact of a pre-run stretch on the risk of injury in teenage and older runners. *USA Track and Field.* http://www.usatf .org/stretchStudy/StretchStudyReport.pdf. **210:** Thompson, W. R. 2011. Worldwide survey of fitness trends for 2012. *ACSM's Health and Fitness Journal* 15(6):9–18. **210:** FICSIT. www.ncbi.nlm .nih.gov/pubmed/8617895. **270:** Gibala, M. 2012. Active voice: Is high-intensity interval training a time-efficient exercise strategy to promote health? *Sports Medicine Bulletin,* February 28. **273:** Brittenham, G. 1992. Plyometric exercise. A word of caution. *Journal of Physical Education, Recreation and Dance* 63(1):20–23. **281:** Adams, W., et al. 1965. *Foundations of Physical Activity.* Champaign, IL: Stipes and Co. **291:** World Health Organization. BMI Classification. http://apps.who.int/bmi/ index.jsp?introPage=intro_3.html. **295:** Wang, Y., et al. 2008. Will all Americans become overweight or obese? Estimating the progression and cost of the U.S. obesity epidemic. *Obesity* 16(10):2323– 2330. **295:** Lee, C. D., A. S. Jackson, and S. N. Blair. 1998. US Weight Guidelines: It is also important to consider cardiorespiratory fitness. *International Journal of Obesity* 22(supplement 2):S2. **305:** Welk, G. J., and S. N. Blair. 2008. Health benefits of physical activity and fitness in children. In G. J. Welk and M. D. Meredith (Eds.), *Fitnessgram/Activitygram Reference Guide.* Dallas, TX: The Cooper Institute. http://www.cooper institute.org/reference-guide. **308:** Baumgartner, T. A., and A. S. Jackson. 1999. *Measurement for Evaluation in Physical Education and Exercise Science.* Dubuque, IA: W. C. Brown Publishers. **310:** Metropolitan Life Insurance Company. www.metlife .com. **310:** U. S. Department of Agriculture, www .usda.gov, and Department of Health and Human Services. www.hhs.gov. **324:** USDA 2010. www .choosemyplate.gov. **328:** American Heart Association 2009. *AHA Scientific Statement: Dietary Sugars Intake and Cardiovascular Health.* http:// circ.ahajournals.org/content/120/11/1011 .abstract. **328:** American Dietetics Association. 2008. www.eatright.org/About/Content.aspx? id=8355&terms=fiber. **328:** International Agency of Research on Cancer. www.iarc.fr. **331:** Williams, M. H. 2001. *Nutrition for Health, Fitness, and Sports.* 6th ed. St. Louis: McGraw-Hill. **334:** Manore, M. M. 2001. Vitamins and minerals: Part II. Who needs supplements? *ACSM's Health* *and Fitness Journal* 5(3):30–34. **336:** U.S. Food and Drug Administration. www.fda.gov. **339:** Harris Interactive. 2011. Healthy eating habits differ the most between the old and the young. www.harrisinteractive.com/NewsRoom/HarrisPolls/tabid/447/mid/1508/articleId/762/ctl/ReadCustom%20Default/Default.aspx. **351:** International Food Information Council. 2012. *2012 Food & Health Survey: Consumer Attitudes toward Food Safety, Nutrition and Health.* www.foodinsight.org. **354:** Wansink, B. 2007. *Mindless Eating: Why We Eat More Than We Think.* New York: Bantam Books. **355:** American College of Sports Medicine. www.acsm.org/about-acsm/media-room/acsm-in-the-news/2011/08/01/acsm-position-stand-on-physical-activity-and-weight-loss-now-available. **356:** BodyMedia Fit. www.bodymedia.com. **358:** Northern Manhattan Study. 2011. Diet soda may raise odds of vascular events; salt linked to stroke risk. http://newsroom.heart.org/pr/aha/1249.aspx. **368:** Kanner, A. D., et al. 1981. Comparison of two modes of stress measurement: Daily hassles and uplifts versus major life events. *Journal of Behavioral Medicine* 4:1–39. **369:** American Psychological Association, 2012. *Stress In America,* www.apa.org/news/press/releases/stress/index.aspx. **370:** Gallagher, R. P. 2011. National Survey of Counseling Center Directors 2011. The International Association of Counseling Services, Inc. Monograph Series Number 8T. www.iacsinc.org/2011%20NSCCD.pdf. **370:** Gallup-Wellbeing Poll. www.gallup.com/poll/wellbeing.aspx. **371:** Selye, H. 1956. *The Stress of Life.* New York: McGraw-Hill. **373:** Thomas, J. L., et al. 2010. Prevalence of mental health problems and functional impairment among active component National Guard soldiers 3 and 12 months following combat in Iraq. *Archives of General Psychiatry* 67:614–623. **380:** Sarason, I. G., J. H. Johnson, and J. M. Siegel. 1978. Assessing the impact of life changes: Development of the life experiences survey. *Journal of Consulting and Clinical Psychology* 46(5):932–946. **386–387:** American Time Use Survey from the Bureau of Labor Statistics. www.bls.gov/tus. **387:** Mancini, M. 2003. *Time Management.* McGraw-Hill: Blacklick, OH. **390:** Burns, D. D. 1999. *The Feeling Good Handbook.* Plume: New York. **395:** Pew Internet. www.pewinternet.org. **395:** Manago, A. M., T. Taylor, and P. M. Greenfield. 2012. Me and my 400 friends: The anatomy of college students' Facebook networks, their communication patterns, and well-being. *Developmental Psychology* 48:369–380. **408:** Federal Trade Commission. http://www.ftc.gov/opa/2011/09/reebok.shtm. **409:** Federal Trade Commission. http://www.ftc.gov/bcp/edu/microsites/redflag. **415:** National Institutes of Health. http://health.nih.gov/topic/VitaminandMineralSupplements. **426:** Science, M., et al. 2012. Zinc or the treatment of the common cold: A systematic review and meta-analysis of randomized controlled trials. *Canadian Medical Association Journal* 184(10):E551–561.

Photo Credits

1: Rubberball/Getty Images. **2:** © BananaStock/PunchStock. **4:** (left) MichaelSvoboda/Getty Images, (right) © JLP/Jose L. Paleez/Corbis. **8:** (clockwise, from top left) © Royalty-Free/Jupiterimages, © Thinkstock Images/Jupiterimages, Stockbyte/Getty Images, © Royalty-Free/Corbis, © Tom & Dee Ann McCarthy/Corbis. **10:** (clockwise, from top left) © PhotoDisc/Getty Images, © Ryan McVay/Getty Images, © Brand X Pictures/Punchstock, Dorgie Productions/Getty Images, © Royalty-Free/Getty Images, © Karl Weatherly/Getty Images. **21:** Ingram Publishing. **23:** © LWA-Stephen Welstead/Corbis. **28:** Getty Images/Photodisc. **31:** (left) © BananaStock/PunchStock, (right) © Royalty-Free/PunchStock. **33:** © Jose Luis Pelaez, Inc./Corbis. **43:** Getty Images. **44:** © Digital Vision/PunchStock. **47:** Courtesy of Vibram USA. **49:** © Liquidlibrary/PictureQuest. **51:** © Dennis Welsh/PunchStock. **65:** Aurora Open/Whit Richardson/Getty Images. **78:** Blend Images/Getty Images. **85:** Eyewire/Getty Images. **91:** © Bob Winsett/Corbis. **92:** Signature Treadmill Desks. **101:** © Jim Cummins/Corbis. **104:** PureStock/Getty Images. **107:** The McGraw-Hill Companies, Inc./Christopher Kerrigan, photographer. **110:** Photo provided by NYCewheels.com. **111:** Image Source/Corbis. **117:** Comstock Images. **124:** Photodisc/Getty Images. **127:** (left) © Creatas Images/PunchStock, (right) © PhotoDisc/Getty Images. **139:** Ingram Publishing. **143:** © Thinkstock Images/JupiterImages.

145: Ryan McVay/Getty Images. **146:** Courtesy of Professional Disc Golf Association. **147:** JupiterImages/Creatas/Alamy. **159:** Royalty-Free/Corbis. **160:** © Corbis—All Rights Reserved. **164:** Image provided courtesy of Technogym, Inc. **166:** Mark Ahn Creative Services (with appreciation to Orangetheory Fitness®, Chandler, AZ). **166:** (bottom) Blend Images/Getty Images. **170:** © Royalty-Free/Corbis. **189:** © Charles B. Corbin. **199:** © Royalty-Free/Corbis. **204:** © Royalty-Free/Corbis. **206:** RubberBall/Alamy. **210:** © PhotoDisc/Getty Images. **212:** © Royalty-Free/JupiterImages. **225:** Ryan McVay/Getty Images. **231:** ©Thinkstock Images/Jupiterimages. **232:** ©Thinkstock Images/Jupiterimages. **236:** (top) Jonathon Ross/Cutcaster. **236:** (photo of woman standing, two photos of women lying down) Mark Ahn Creative Services (with appreciation to Orangetheory Fitness®, Chandler, AZ). **237:** (top left, 3 photos of woman lifting boxes) Ken Karp for MMH, (bottom right) © Creatas Images/Jupiter Images, (bottom left) © Stockdisc/PunchStock, (top right) Ingram Publishing/SuperStock. **265:** U.S. Air Force photo by Staff Sgt. Desiree N. Palacios. **267:** © David Pu'u/Corbis. **268:** Ingram Publishing. **271:** © Brand X Pictures/Superstock. **272:** © Corbis—All Rights Reserved. **274:** (all images) Rubberball/Getty Images. **289:** © Royalty-Free/Jupiter Images. **292:** ©JGI/Blend Images LLC. **302:** (left) © Jose Luis Pelaez Inc/Blend Images LLC, (right) © Peter Ciresa/Index Stock Imagery. **328:** © Image Shop/Corbis. **329:** Blend Images/Getty Images. **332:** © BananaStock/PunchStock. **340:** © PhotoDisc/Getty Images. **349:** Jack Hollingsworth/Blend Images LLC. **355:** Teo Lannie/GettyImages. **356:** © Photo courtesy of BodyMedia, Inc. **358:** © Jose Luis Palaez, Inc./Corbis. **367:** © McGraw-Hill Companies, Inc./Gary He, photographer. **369:** © James Russell/Corbis. **372:** © Corbis. **383:** © Royalty-Free/Corbis. **388:** © Fancy Photography/Veer. **394:** Design Pics/Don Hammond. **405:** © Imageshop/Punchstock. **407:** © Royalty-Free/Corbis. **409:** © Ariel Skelley/Getty Images. **411:** © Ingram Publishing/SuperStock. **413:** © Jose Luis Pelaez, Inc./Corbis. **414:** © Stockbyte. **423:** © Jeremy Woodhouse/Blend Images LLC. **426:** © Pixtal/SuperStock. **429:** © Getty Images/Purestock.

Index